WORKBOOK TO ACCOMPANY

ADMINISTRATIVE MEDICAL ASSISTING

Seventh Edition

Linda L. French, CMA-C (AAMA), NCICS, CPC
Formerly, Instructor and Business Consultant, Administrative Medical Assisting, Medical Terminology, and Medical Insurance Billing and Coding
Simi Valley Adult School and Career Institute, Simi Valley, California
Ventura College, Ventura, California
Oxnard College, Oxnard, California
Santa Barbara Business College, Ventura, California

Marilyn T. Fordney, CMA-AC (AAMA)
Formerly, Instructor of Medical Insurance, Medical Terminology, Medical Machine Transcription, and Medical Office Procedures
Ventura College, Ventura, California

DELMAR
CENGAGE Learning

Australia • Brazil • Japan • Korea • Mexico • Singapore • Spain • United Kingdom • United States

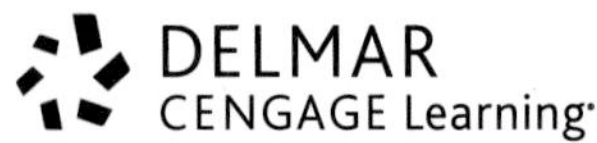

Workbook to Accompany Administrative Medical Assisting, Seventh Edition
Linda L. French, Marilyn T. Fordney

Vice President, Editorial: Dave Garza
Director of Learning Solutions: Matthew Kane
Executive Editor: Rhonda Dearborn
Managing Editor: Marah Bellegarde
Senior Product Manager: Sarah Prime
Product Manager: Lauren Whalen
Vice President, Marketing: Jennifer Baker
Marketing Director: Wendy E. Mapstone
Senior Marketing Manager: Nancy Bradshaw
Marketing Coordinator: Piper Huntington
Production Director: Wendy Troeger
Production Manager: Andrew Crouth
Content Project Manager: Brooke Greenhouse
Senior Art Director: Jack Pendleton
Technology Project Manager: Ben Knapp

Library of Congress Control Number: 2012932314

ISBN-13: 978-1-133-27857-3

ISBN-10: 1-133-27857-4

Delmar
5 Maxwell Drive
Clifton Park, NY 12065-2919
USA

Cengage Learning is a leading provider of customized learning solutions with office locations around the globe, including Singapore, the United Kingdom, Australia, Mexico, Brazil, and Japan. Locate your local office at: **international.cengage.com/region**

Cengage Learning products are represented in Canada by Nelson Education, Ltd.

To learn more about Delmar, visit **www.cengage.com/delmar**

Purchase any of our products at your local college store or at our preferred online store **www.cengagebrain.com**

Notice to the Reader

Publisher does not warrant or guarantee any of the products described herein or perform any independent analysis in connection with any of the product information contained herein. Publisher does not assume, and expressly disclaims, any obligation to obtain and include information other than that provided to it by the manufacturer. The reader is expressly warned to consider and adopt all safety precautions that might be indicated by the activities described herein and to avoid all potential hazards. By following the instructions contained herein, the reader willingly assumes all risks in connection with such instructions. The publisher makes no representations or warranties of any kind, including but not limited to, the warranties of fitness for particular purpose or merchantability, nor are any such representations implied with respect to the material set forth herein, and the publisher takes no responsibility with respect to such material. The publisher shall not be liable for any special, consequential, or exemplary damages resulting, in whole or part, from the readers' use of, or reliance upon, this material.

Printed in the United States of America
6 7 8 9 10 18 17 16

CONTENTS

ACKNOWLEDGMENTS

This *Workbook* has grown to include hundreds of chapter review questions, expanded critical thinking exercises, and more than 150 Job Skills. With this edition, computerized exercises have been developed to incorporate the use of Medical Office Simulated Software (MOSS) 2.0 so students can be trained in both hands-on and computerized skills. I gratefully acknowledge the work of Cindy Correa, who shared her expertise of MOSS and diligently developed exercises to incorporate the computerized medical office as part of this edition's learning package. These practice exercises will increase students' knowledge of how the computer is used in a medical office, familiarize them with common tasks in commercial medical software, and train them in various job skills—thank you, Cindy, for your invaluable contribution.

I wish to express my gratitude for the help and encouragement provided by friends, colleagues, and family, and the staff of Delmar Cengage Learning. And to the people and organizations who so willingly and enthusiastically contributed to the contents of this book, I am ever grateful. Without their expertise, comments, and suggestions, the work would not be as complete as it is.

I extend my sincere thanks to the following people who acted as consultants and assisted in reviewing parts of the manuscript and to the companies that granted permission to use the various forms that are an integral part of this *Workbook*. The realistic forms allow students to complete and master Job Skills so they are ready to enter the workforce. This is our ultimate goal!

Monica Cristorean, NRCMA, CPC
Medical Billing Instructor
Career Colleges of America
South Gate, California

Delux Corporation
500 Main Street
Groton, Massachusetts

Karen Levein, CPC, CPC-I
Medical Office Procedures Instructor
Burbank Adult School
Duarte, California

Medical Arts Press
100 Scheltern Road
Lincolnshire, Illinois

Holly Scheaffer, CPC
Business Manager
Ventura, California

Carolyn Talesfore
Advertising and Promotion Manager
Bibbero Systems, Inc.
Petaluma, California

INTRODUCTION TO THE *WORKBOOK*

PERFORMANCE OBJECTIVES

Performance objectives for the *Workbook* are listed at the beginning of each chapter. For this edition, Job Skills that satisfy each objective are also listed. Although review questions and critical thinking exercises are included for each chapter, objectives for these are too numerous to list.

INSTRUCTIONS TO THE STUDENT

This *Workbook* has been prepared for those who use *Administrative Medical Assisting* as a text. The *Workbook* Job Skills combined with the theory learned in the *textbook* meet the educational entry-level competencies outlined by the Commission on Accreditation of Allied Health Education Programs (CAAHEP) and the Accrediting Bureau of Health Education Schools (ABHES) as well as the educational components of the American Association of Medical Assistants Occupational Analysis of the CMA (AAMA) from 2007/2008 and the American Medical Technologists (AMT) Medical Assisting Task List of 2007.

The following components have been developed to make the *Workbook* a complete learning tool, which allows practical application of job skills that will be performed in a physician's office. An asterisk (*) indicates features new to or enhanced for this edition.

Part I: Chapter Exercises*

- **Objectives** are clearly stated with Job Skills listed.*
- **Focus on Certification*** summarizes content listed by the (1) American Association of Medical Assistants for the 2010* Certified Medical Assistant Certification /Recertification Examination, (2) the 2007* Registered Medical Assistant Certification Examination Competencies and Construction Parameters, and (3) Certified Medical Administrative Specialist Competencies and Examination Specifications listed by the American Medical Technologists.
- **Abbreviation and Spelling Review** incorporates medical terminology into a short chart note for each chapter, giving students an opportunity to write definitions for abbreviations and spell medical terms. Answers are found in the *Instructor's Manual.**
- **Review Questions** cover key points in chapters and address areas not covered by the exam-style review questions in the textbook. Review questions help students prepare for a multiple-choice theory test on each chapter studied. Answers are found in the *Instructor's Manual.*
- **Critical Thinking Exercises*** offer students an opportunity to address situations and solve problems realistic to an office setting.
- **MOSS Computer Competency*** exercises are included in Chapters 5, 7, 11, 15, and 16. These exercises provide hands-on practice performing front-office procedures with computerized practice management software. Procedures include patient registration, appointment scheduling, transcription, written correspondence, procedure and payment posting, insurance billing, and patient statements.
- **Job Skills** have been enhanced to include up-to-date forms and technical information and have been expanded to cover and cross-reference the 2008 CAAHEP* and the 2009/2010 ABHES* competencies. They are designed to include a Performance Evaluation Checklist with the directions, thus eliminating the need for a separate form to grade each job skill.

Read through each Job Skill entirely before attempting to begin the assignment. Follow the directions in the *Workbook* where noted and refer to the Procedure in the textbook for step-by-step directions. These directions are comprehensive and written to assist students with the office task, not just the job skill in the *Workbook.* Where noted, refer to the textbook figures for visual examples.

Performance objectives are stated for each exercise. Your instructor will indicate which standards are expected, the time frame for the completion of each exercise, and the accuracy required for individual exercises.

Points are assigned for each job skill for the first, second, and third attempt according to the steps required and difficulty of the task. These may be adjusted by your instructor.

To access the Premium Website, please visit www.CengageBrain.com and use the access code on the Printed Access Card. At the CengageBrain.com home page, search for the ISBN of the text (from the back cover) using the search box at the top of the page. This will take you to the product page where these resources can be found.

Part II: Forms

Blank forms are realistic and similar to those found in medical offices. New ones have been added,* some have been enhanced,* and they are easily removed and require completion for a variety of Job Skills. The forms are also accessible on the premium Website, in order to be completed electronically and saved, or printed and completed manually.

Part III: Appendix for Practon Medical Group, Inc.

Important information is listed in the Practon Medical Group, Inc., reference file, which includes detailed office protocols. Before beginning the Job Skills, tear out the appendix, place it in a three-ring binder, and add section indexes so you can access information quickly to help you complete the *Workbook* Job Skills. The appendix includes (1) medical practice reference material; (2) office policies, including information about the daily routine in the office, office hours, appointment protocols, information regarding telephone calls, and filing routines; (3) payment policies and health insurance guidelines; and (4) directions for using the office fee schedule. A mock fee schedule is provided that lists procedure codes (by sections) in the same order in which they are listed in the *CPT* codebook, descriptions of services, and fees you will need when answering questions that patients might ask and for posting to ledgers and completing insurance forms. Also included are (5) a listing of *CPT* code modifiers with brief descriptions and (6) a sample listing of Medicare *HCPCS Level II* codes with fees.

Part IV: Abbreviation Tables

Abbreviation tables that appear in the *textbook* are conveniently listed to easily locate medical definitions and help decode abbreviations when completing the Abbreviation and Spelling Review lessons, answering questions, and performing Job Skills.

Part V: Medical Office Simulation Software* (MOSS) 2.0

The MOSS 2.0 Computer Competency activities in Chapters 5, 7, 11, 15, and 16 in this *Workbook* are designed to be used with Medical Office Simulation Software (MOSS) 2.0 (single-user version). Instructions for installing, signing on, and navigating within MOSS 2.0 are included in this section. Refer to this section prior to starting the exercises in Chapter 5 of this *Workbook*. For additional MOSS 2.0 support, log on to the MOSS Information, Training, and Support Site at www.cengage.com/community/moss.

Additional Items Needed

If you do not have a background in medical terminology, you need to obtain and use a good medical dictionary. In addition to the blank forms included in this *Workbook*, you will need the following items. Check them off as you obtain them for your coursework.

_______ 1 three-ring binder with index tabs

_______ 1 folder with pockets to hand in assignments

_______ 3 manila file folders

_______ 3 name labels for manila folders

_______ 50 sheets of 8½″ by 11″ white typing or computer paper

_______ 60 3″ by 5″ white file cards

_______ 2 white number 10 envelopes (9½″ by 4″)

_______ rubber bands, paper clips, pens, highlighter pen set (5 colors), pencils, transparent tape

Optional items:

_______ 7 white number 10 envelopes (large)

_______ 7 white number 6 envelopes (small)

Notebook Content Suggestions

It is a good idea to remove the reference appendix (Part III) and the Abbreviation Tables (Part IV) from the *Workbook* and place them in a notebook. You may want to remove the blank forms (Part II), which may be photocopied prior to use. The forms may also be accessed on the Premium Website at www.CengageBrain.com and completed online and printed, or printed and completed by hand. Following are several items from the textbook that you may also want to include:

Insurance Form Template for Medicare	Figure 16-10
Insurance Form Template for Medicare/Medigap	Figure 16-12
Insurance Form Template for TRICARE	Figure 16-13
List of Evaluation and Management *CPT* Codes	Tables 17-2 and 17-3
Comprehensive List of *CPT* Modifiers	Table 17-4
CMS-1500 Claim Form Field-by-Field Instructions	Appendix A
Commercial Insurance Template	Figure A-1
Glossary Pages	G1-G14

Portfolio

Saving your completed work in a portfolio is strongly suggested. You may wish to take it to a job interview in order to present the type of job skills you have acquired and the level of work you have performed during your course of study. You will need a three-ring binder with indexes to organize the material and develop a table of contents. You should add items to this folder as you progress through the course. There are several ways to accomplish this, but a simple way would be according to job duties (e.g., appointment scheduling, telephone techniques, insurance coding and claim forms, letter composition, bookkeeping, payroll, and so forth). Your instructor may suggest additional items to include or a specific arrangement of all items.

The content of this portfolio is evidence of your administrative skills and is a good indication of your organizational abilities as well as the neatness and completeness of your work.

WORKBOOK JOB SKILL EXERCISES

PART I

Chapter Exercises

- Objectives
- Focus on Certification
- Abbreviation and Spelling Review
- Review Questions
- Critical Thinking Exercises
- MOSS Computer Competency
- Job Skills with Performance Evaluation Checklists

CHAPTER 1

A Career as an Administrative Medical Assistant

OBJECTIVES

After completing the exercises, the student will be able to:

1. Enhance knowledge of medical terminology, interpret abbreviations, and accurately spell medical words.
2. List the duties of an administrative medical assistant.
3. Name specialty areas that utilize administrative skills.
4. State important interpersonal skills for medical assistants.
5. List attributes for good team interaction.
6. Name the stages of dying.
7. Complete a self-assessment of interpersonal skills and professional attributes to identify strengths and weaknesses.
8. Participate in a self-assessment on stress to evaluate the risk.
9. Role-play two scenarios to demonstrate empathy.
10. Research organizations and support groups in the local community for the terminally ill.
11. Interpret and accurately spell medical terms and abbreviations (Job Skill 1-1).
12. Use the Internet to look up key terms and hear pronunciations (Job Skill 1-2).
13. Prioritize a task list to practice time management skills (Job Skill 1-3).
14. Use the Internet to obtain information about certification or registration (Job Skill 1-4).

15. Use the Internet to perform a self-test of anatomy and physiology or medical terminology (Job Skill 1-5).
16. Develop a medical practice survey (Job Skill 1-6).

FOCUS ON CERTIFICATION*

CMA Content Summary

- Medical terminology
- Death and dying
- Defense mechanisms
- Professionalism
- Empathy/sympathy
- Understanding emotional behavior
- Internet services
- Time management

RMA Content Summary

- Medical terminology
- Abbreviations and symbols
- Licensure, certification, registration
- Credentialing requirements
- Professional development and conduct
- Interpersonal skills and relations
- Instructing patients

CMAS Content Summary

- Medical terminology
- Professionalism
- Continuing education

STOP AND THINK CASE SCENARIOS AND EXAM-STYLE REVIEW QUESTIONS

Refer to the end of Chapter 1 in the *textbook*.

Review Questions

Review the objectives, glossary, and chapter information before completing the following review questions.

1. In a customer service–oriented practice, the elements of customer service are demonstrated by the ______________________, ______________________, and ______________________.
2. True or False. Each employee and patient has the same idea about what "good" service means.
   ____
3. Define "flextime." ____
4. Name some specialty areas in which administrative skills may be used in a health care career.
   a. ____
   b. ____

*This *Workbook* and the accompanying *textbook* meet the entry-level administrative and general competencies for the CMA outlined by the AAMA Examination Content Outline and Occupational Analysis and for the RMA and CMAS outlined by the AMT Competencies, Construction Parameters, and Examination Specifications (see Competency Grid in Appendix B of the *textbook*).

c. ____________________

d. ____________________

e. ____________________

5. A medical transcriptionist is now also known as a ____________________ or ____________________.

6. Of the duties an administrative medical assistant might perform,

   a. List two that require interpersonal skills.

   ____

   ____

   b. List five that require keyboard input skills (assume you work in a computerized office).

   ____

   ____

   ____

   ____

   ____

   c. List five that require basic math skills.

   ____

   ____

   ____

   ____

   ____

   d. List five that require other clerical skills.

   ____

   ____

   ____

   ____

   ____

7. In addition to the many duties that an administrative medical assistant performs, there are various interpersonal skills required. Name five that you would like to be known for.

   a. ____________________

   b. ____________________

   c. ____________________

   d. ____________________

   e. ____________________

8. When trying to understand a viewpoint or evaluating a patient's behavior, it is important to ____________________ and ____________________.

9. An emergency has occurred in Dr. Practon's office. Name the behavior the medical assistant must exhibit to patients.

   a. ______

   b. ______

   c. ______

   d. ______

   e. ______

10. List some attributes an employee needs for good team interaction.

    a. ______

    b. ______

    c. ______

    d. ______

    e. ______

    f. ______

11. What must a health care worker be aware of and understand in order to avoid work-related emotional and psychological problems? ______

12. When patients receive unfortunate news about themselves or loved ones, how should medical assistants act, and what are some things that can be done to help? ______

    ______

    ______

13. List the stages of dying.

    a. ______

    b. ______

    c. ______

    d. ______

    e. ______

14. What is the name of the national foundation that offers medical care and support to patients and family members dealing with a terminal illness or the loss of a loved one?

    ______

15. Define "stress," and name one thing that has caused stress in your life.

    ______

    ______

16. How does a medical assistant's excellent grooming reflect the image and management of the medical office?

    ______

    ______

17. Give the names of two national organizations that certify or register medical assistants trained in both clinical and administrative areas.

   a. ______________________________

   b. ______________________________

18. Name five ways a medical assistant can keep knowledge of research and new techniques current.

   a. ______________________________

   b. ______________________________

   c. ______________________________

   d. ______________________________

   e. ______________________________

Critical Thinking Exercises

1. Another medical assistant in the office criticizes a patient behind his or her back for wearing bizarre clothes. What would your response be? ______________________________

   ____

2. Following are some questions that will help you do an interpersonal skill and professional attribute self-assessment. Read each of them carefully and try to answer them honestly. After you have completed them, identify and mark your strengths with an ***S*** and your weaknesses with a ***W***. This will not only help you to know what areas you need to work on but also help you determine which type of job you may be best suited for.

   ________ a. Are you considerate of others?

   ________ b. Do you treat people with respect?

   ________ c. Do you have a kind, friendly, and good-natured manner?

   ________ d. Do you have the ability to be discreet and keep information confidential?

   ________ e. Do you have a positive attitude?

   ________ f. Can you smile easily?

   ________ g. Can you listen instead of talking all the time?

   ________ h. Are you polite?

   ________ i. Can you be sympathetic and empathetic and discern the difference?

   ________ j. Are you reliable and dependable?

   ________ k. Are you honest and trustworthy?

   ________ l. Can you accept responsibility?

   ________ m. Can you remain calm during an emergency?

   ________ n. Are you well groomed, with a neat appearance?

   ________ o. Are you a team player?

   ________ p. Are you patient?

   ________ q. Do you reserve judgment of others?

   ________ r. Do you have good judgment?

________ s. Are you willing to learn?

________ t. Do you accept criticism?

________ u. Are you sensitive to the feelings of others?

________ v. Can you remain free from bias?

3. Answer "yes" or "no" to complete this self-assessment to gain a better understanding of how to handle stress:
   a. Do you prefer to work alone rather than with coworkers? ________
   b. Do you give more than you receive in work relationships? ________
   c. Is it hard for you to establish warm relationships with your coworkers and peers? ________
   d. Do you have someone whom you can trust to discuss personal problems and keep the information confidential? ________
   e. Do you have a difficult time saying "no" and often overload yourself as a result? ________
   f. Do you guard yourself against talking, trusting, and feeling? ________
   g. Do you often get irritated, frustrated, or even angry when performing your regular work tasks? ________
   h. Do you often do things yourself rather than take the time to show someone else how to do them? ________
   i. Do you easily accept help from others? ________
   j. Do you place the needs of others before your own? ________
   k. Do you obtain your personal identity from your profession? ________
   l. Are most of your needs met by helping others? ________
   m. Do you feel guilty when you take a vacation or time to "play" or rest? ________
4. Role-play the following scenarios demonstrating empathy:
   a. A patient has been diagnosed with cancer and the prognosis looks very poor. You are left alone with the patient and his spouse. Demonstrate empathy as you interact with the patient and his family.
   b. Your coworker has just been told that she has had her hours cut and she is very angry. Respond with empathy.
5. Research organizations and support groups in the local community for the terminally ill. Make a list of available resources. ________

JOB SKILL 1-1
Interpret and Accurately Spell Medical Terms and Abbreviations

Name ______________________________ Date ______________ Score ________

Performance Objective

Task: Decode abbreviations.

Conditions: Use pen or pencil. Refer to Procedure 1-1 in the textbook for step-by-step directions.

Standards: Complete all steps listed in this skill in ________ minutes with a minimum score of ________. (Time element and accuracy criteria may be given by instructor.)

Time: **Start:** ____________ **Completed:** ____________ **Total:** ____________ minutes

Scoring: One point for each step performed satisfactorily unless otherwise listed or weighted by instructor.

Directions with Performance Evaluation Checklist

Read the following patient's chart note and write the meanings for the abbreviations listed following the note. To decode any abbreviations you do not understand or that appear unfamiliar to you, refer to the list of abbreviations in Part IV of this *Workbook*. Medical terms in the chart note are *italicized*; study them for spelling. Use your medical dictionary to look up their definitions. Your instructor may give a test for the spelling and definition of the words and abbreviations. Note: Although abbreviations are not presented in Chapter 1 of the textbook, they appear throughout the text, and a chart note with medical terms and abbreviations is presented at the beginning of each chapter of the *Workbook* entitled "Abbreviation and Spelling Review" to offer students the opportunity to learn these terms. Refer back to Procedure 1-1 in the textbook while doing these.

Bart J. Stephens

September 15, 20XX Routine PE. Ht 6 ft. Wt 163 lb. P 70. BP 130/70. Pt $\bar{s}$ complaints. *Systemic* Ex neg. except for Grade I *pulmonic murmur*. EKG, CBC, UA, & chest x-ray films neg. IMP: No disease. Rx: *Tetanus toxoid* booster, 0.5 ml. Ret p.r.n.

Fran Practon, MD

Fran Practon, MD

1st Attempt	2nd Attempt	3rd Attempt		
______	______	______	Gather materials (equipment and supplies) listed under "Conditions."	
______	______	______	1. PE	______________________
______	______	______	2. Ht	______________________
______	______	______	3. ft	______________________
______	______	______	4. wt	______________________
______	______	______	5. lb	______________________
______	______	______	6. P	______________________
______	______	______	7. BP	______________________
______	______	______	8. pt	______________________
______	______	______	9. $\bar{s}$	______________________

JOB SKILL 1-1 *(continued)*

______	______	______	10. Ex ______
______	______	______	11. neg. ______
______	______	______	12. EKG ______
______	______	______	13. CBC ______
______	______	______	14. UA ______
______	______	______	15. IMP ______
______	______	______	16. Rx ______
______	______	______	17. ml ______
______	______	______	18. ret ______
______	______	______	19. p.r.n. ______
______	______	______	Complete within specified time.
____/21	____/21	____/21	**Total points earned** (To obtain a percentage score, divide the total points earned by the number of points possible.)

Comments:

Evaluator's Signature: ______________________ **Need to Repeat:** ______________

National Curriculum Competency: CAAHEP: Cognitive: IV.C.11; Psychomotor: IV. P.3 ABHES: 3.d

JOB SKILL 1-2
Use the Internet to Look Up Key Terms and Hear Pronunciation

Name ______________________________ Date ____________ Score ______

Performance Objective

Task: Use an Internet online dictionary to look up key terms and hear the words pronounced.

Conditions: Computer with Internet hookup. *Textbook* key terms or abbreviations.

Standards: Complete all steps listed in this job skill in _______ minutes with a minimum score of _______. (Time element and accuracy criteria may be given by instructor.)

Time: **Start:** __________ **Completed:** __________ **Total:** __________ minutes

Scoring: One point for each step performed satisfactorily unless otherwise listed or weighted by instructor.

Directions with Performance Evaluation Checklist

The Merriam-Webster Online Dictionary (http://www.merriam-webster.com) can be used to hear pronunciations for key terms in the *textbook*. Select "Dictionary" for most of the key terms or "Medical" for medical terms. A "Thesaurus" can be selected for antonyms and synonyms. "English/Spanish" may be selected to help translate from one language to the other. You may refer back to this Job Skill any time you need a pronunciation. Key terms are defined within each chapter as well as in the glossary at the end of the *textbook*. Abbreviations are listed in various tables throughout the *textbook* and in Part IV of this *Workbook*.

1st Attempt	2nd Attempt	3rd Attempt	
______	______	______	Gather materials (equipment and supplies) listed under "Conditions."
______	______	______	1. Use a computer, obtain an Internet connection, and go to: http://www.merriam-webster.com
______	______	______	2. Under "Merriam-Webster Online Search" select "Dictionary" or "Medical" depending on the type of word. For this exercise select "Dictionary."
______	______	______	3. Type the term in the blank box that says, "Enter word or phrase." Type the first key term in Chapter 1, "accreditation."
______	______	______	4. Click "Search." There will be a listing as follows:
____/2	____/2	____/2	5. The "Main Entry" for the word will appear. Write the root for the term "accreditation." ______________________________
______	______	______	6. The phonetic pronunciation guide will appear next. Click on the sound symbol next to the main entry. A pop-up window will appear with the term and another sound symbol. Click on the sound symbol as many times as necessary to learn how to pronounce the word.
____/2	____/2	____/2	7. Next, the "function" or part of speech will be listed (e.g., adjective, noun, verb, or abbreviation). Scan to find the term "accreditation" and list the part of speech. ______________________________
____/2	____/2	____/2	8. The etymology will be listed next. Type in the term "etymology" and write a simple definition. ______________________________

JOB SKILL 1-2 *(continued)*

____/2 ____/2 ____/2 9. Type the term "antonym" and write a simple definition. ____________

____

____/2 ____/2 ____/2 10. Type the term "synonym" and write a simple definition. ____________

____

____/2 ____/2 ____/2 11. The term will then be used in a sentence; a definition and often a synonym will be listed. What is the synonym for "accredit"?

____

______ ______ ______ Complete within specified time.

____/19 ____/19 ____/19 **Total points earned** (To obtain a percentage score, divide the total points earned by the number of points possible.)

Comments:

Evaluator's Signature: ________________________________ **Need to Repeat:** ____________

National Curriculum Competency: CAAHEP: Psychomotor: IV.P.3 (Ch 1–20)	ABHES: 3.a–d (Ch 1–20)

JOB SKILL 1-3
Prioritize a Task List to Practice Time Management Skills

Name ______________________________ Date ______________ Score ________

Performance Objective

Task: Study each task listed and prioritize.

Condition: Task list, paper, and pen or pencil.

Standards: Complete all steps listed in this skill in _______ minutes with a minimum score of _______. (Time element and accuracy criteria may be given by instructor.)

Time: **Start:** ____________ **Completed:** ____________ **Total:** ____________ minutes

Scoring: One point for each step performed satisfactorily unless otherwise listed or weighted by instructor.

Directions with Performance Evaluation Checklist

You are an administrative medical assistant who has arrived at work at 9:00 a.m. The office manager has opened the back door to let you in but only one other staff member has arrived who is a clinical medical assistant. She is running laboratory controls and getting the treatment rooms ready. The office manager says to you, "I received a telephone call from two coworkers. Due to an accident on the freeway they will not be arriving until approximately 9:30 a.m. Will you please cover the front until they arrive? The charts have already been pulled for today's patients and the telephone is still on the answering service. When you are able, please call them to pick up the messages and switch the telephone over to the office." Following are typical tasks that need to be done:

Task List

_____ Call the answering service and record all messages.

_____ Call your husband to let him know what time you will meet him for lunch.

_____ Go make coffee in the lunchroom.

_____ Turn on the lights in the front office and waiting room.

_____ Unlock the waiting room door.

_____ Print financial accounts or pull ledgers for patients who will be seen today.

_____ Straighten your desk in the back office.

_____ Look to see what is on your task list for today.

_____ Invite the patients who are waiting outside into the office.

_____ Open the drapes.

JOB SKILL 1-3 *(continued)*

Directions with Performance Evaluation Checklist

1st Attempt	2nd Attempt	3rd Attempt	
_______	_______	_______	Gather materials (equipment and supplies) listed under "Conditions."
_______	_______	_______	1. Study each task to determine which is the most important, the next most important, and so forth down to the least important.
____/10	____/10	____/10	2. Mark the most important number 1, the next in priority number 2, and so forth, with number 10 being the least important; use common sense.
____/10	____/10	____/10	3. List comments for the rationale you used to help you determine the order of priority.
_______	_______	_______	Complete within specified time.
____/23	____/23	____/23	**Total points earned** (To obtain a percentage score, divide the total points earned by the number of points possible.)

Comments:

Evaluator's Signature: ______________________________ **Need to Repeat:** __________

National Curriculum Competency: CAAHEP: Cognitive: V.C.13; Affective: V.A.2

JOB SKILL 1-4
Use the Internet to Obtain Information on Certification or Registration

Name ______________________________ Date ______________ Score ________

Performance Objective

Task: Research certification or registration via the Internet.

Conditions: Computer with Internet connection and references from Table 1-1 in the textbook.

Standards: Complete all steps listed in this skill in _______ minutes with a minimum score of _______. (Time element and accuracy criteria may be given by instructor.)

Time: **Start:** ____________ **Completed:** ____________ **Total:** ____________ minutes

Scoring: One point for each step performed satisfactorily unless otherwise listed or weighted by instructor.

Directions with Performance Evaluation Checklist

1st Attempt	2nd Attempt	3rd Attempt	
_______	_______	_______	Gather materials (equipment and supplies) listed under "Conditions."
_______	_______	_______	1. Study Table 1-1 to determine what areas of certification or registration interest you.
_______	_______	_______	2. Access the Internet.
_______	_______	_______	3. Type in the Web site address from the column on the right side of the table for the organization(s) you have selected (e.g., Certified Bookkeeper = http://www.aipb.org).
_______	_______	_______	4. Select key terms ("certification," "registration," or "about" the program).
_____/4	_____/4	_____/4	5. Print the information to read and share with your class, and label a file folder to keep it for future reference.
_______	_______	_______	Complete within specified time.
____/10	____/10	____/10	**Total points earned** (To obtain a percentage score, divide the total points earned by the number of points possible.)

Comments:

Evaluator's Signature: ______________________________ **Need to Repeat:** ______________

National Curriculum Competency: CAAHEP: Psychomotor: V.P.7

JOB SKILL 1-5
Use the Internet to Perform a Self-Test of Anatomy and Physiology or Medical Terminology

Name ______________________________ Date ____________ Score ________

Performance Objective

Task: Test your knowledge of anatomy and physiology or medical terminology via the Internet. If you have not completed your course of study in anatomy and physiology or medical terminology, you may use this job skill to test your knowledge at a later time.

Conditions: Computer with Internet connection.

Standards: Complete all steps listed in this job skill in _______ minutes with a minimum score of _______. (Time element and accuracy criteria may be given by instructor.)

Time: **Start:** ____________ **Completed:** ____________ **Total:** ____________ minutes

Scoring: One point for each step performed satisfactorily unless otherwise listed or weighted by instructor.

Directions with Performance Evaluation Checklist

1st Attempt	2nd Attempt	3rd Attempt	
_______	_______	_______	Gather materials (equipment and supplies) listed under "Conditions."
_______	_______	_______	1. Access the Internet.
_______	_______	_______	2. Type in the Web site address for the American Association of Medical Assistants: http://www.aama-ntl.org
_______	_______	_______	3. Highlight "CMA (AAMA) Exam," then select "Prepare for the CMA (AAMA) Exam."
_______	_______	_______	4. Select either "anatomy and physiology" or "medical terminology practice exam."
_______	_______	_______	5. Read the instructions and download, open, and print the answer form.
_______	_______	_______	6. Read each question and mark the answer.
____/50	____/50	____/50	7. Compare your answers with the answer key, which is listed directly after the questions.
_______	_______	_______	8. Make note of the questions you need to study.
_______	_______	_______	Complete within specified time.
____/59	____/59	____/59	**Total points earned** (To obtain a percentage score, divide the total points earned by the number of points possible.)

JOB SKILL 1-5 (*continued*)

Comments:

Evaluator's Signature: ______________________ **Need to Repeat:** __________

National Curriculum Competency: CAAHEP: Cognitive: I.C.1–4	ABHES: 2.b

JOB SKILL 1-6
Develop a Medical Practice Survey

Name ____ Date ______________ Score ________

Performance Objective

Task: Design a patient satisfaction survey form.

Conditions: White 8½″ by 11″ paper, pen or pencil, and computer if available.

Standards: Complete all steps listed in this skill in _______ minutes with a minimum score of ________. (Time element and accuracy criteria may be given by instructor.)

Time: **Start:** ____________ **Completed:** ____________ **Total:** ____________ minutes

Scoring: One point for each step performed satisfactorily unless otherwise listed or weighted by instructor.

Directions with Performance Evaluation Checklist

1st Attempt	2nd Attempt	3rd Attempt	
_____	_____	_____	Gather materials (equipment and supplies) listed under "Conditions."
____/5	____/5	____/5	1. Design your own survey form using the reference material on Practon Medical Group, Inc., found in Part III of this *Workbook*.
____/5	____/5	____/5	2. Formulate at least five questions that address patient satisfaction.
_____	_____	_____	Complete within specified time.
___/12	___/12	___/12	**Total points earned** (To obtain a percentage score, divide the total points earned by the number of points possible.)

Comments:

Evaluator's Signature: ________________________________ **Need to Repeat:** ____________

National Curriculum Competency: ABHES: 8.a, dd

CHAPTER 2

The Health Care Environment: Past, Present, and Future

OBJECTIVES

After completing the exercises, the student will be able to:

1. Identify contributions of historic medical pioneers.
2. List the benefits of using managed care and a traditional health care system.
3. Differentiate the types of health care settings.
4. Use the Internet to research and write an essay about a medical pioneer (Job Skill 2-1).
5. Direct patients to specific hospital departments (Job Skill 2-2).
6. Refer patients to the correct physician specialist (Job Skill 2-3).
7. Define abbreviations for health care professionals (Job Skill 2-4).
8. Determine basic skills needed by the administrative medical assistant (Job Skill 2-5).

FOCUS ON CERTIFICATION*

CMA Content Summary

- Medical terminology
- Working as a team
- Patient advocate
- Patient instruction
- Appropriate referrals
- Prepaid HMO, PPO, POS

*This *Workbook* and the accompanying *textbook* meet the entry-level administrative and general competencies for the CMA outlined by the AAMA Examination Content Outline and Occupational Analysis and for the RMA and CMAS outlined by the AMT Competencies, Construction Parameters, and Examination Specifications (see Competency Grid in Appendix B of the *textbook*).

RMA Content Summary

- Medical terminology
- Patient instruction
- Insurance terminology
- Insurance plans: HMO, PPO, EPO

CMAS Content Summary

- Medical terminology
- Prepare information for referrals
- Private/commercial insurance plans

STOP AND THINK CASE SCENARIOS AND EXAM-STYLE REVIEW QUESTIONS

Refer to the end of Chapter 2 in the *textbook*.

Abbreviation and Spelling Review

Read the following patient's chart note and write the meanings for the abbreviations listed below the note. To decode any abbreviations you do not understand or that appear unfamiliar to you, refer to the list of abbreviations in Part IV of this *Workbook*. Step-by-step directions for this exercise are found in Procedure 1-1 of Chapter 1 in the *textbook*. Medical terms in the chart note are italicized; study them for spelling. Use your medical dictionary to look up their definitions. Your instructor may give a spelling and definition test that includes these words and abbreviations.

> Troy Wenzlau
>
> 36-year-old W male seen as E for Fx L *humerus*. Pt DNS for re-exam last month as scheduled. Pt has been on SD X 3 mo for back pain and was determined P&S from a previous back injury last yr. Given I of *Demerol* 50 mg IM for pain, x-ray L arm ordered. Cast and return to ofc in 2 wks.
>
> Gerald M. Practon, MD
>
> Gerald M. Practon, MD

W ______________________

E ______________________

Fx ______________________

L ______________________

Pt ______________________

DNS ______________________

re-exam ______________________

SD ______________________

X ______________________

mo ______________________

P&S ______________________

yr ______________________

I ______________________

mg ______________________

IM ______________________

ofc ______________________

wks ______________________

Review Questions

Review the objectives, glossary, and chapter information before completing the following review questions.

1. Briefly describe the contribution of each of the following:

   a. Imhotep ____

b. Edward Jenner ____

____

____

c. Frederick Banting ____

____

____

d. Anton van Leeuwenhoek ____

____

____

e. Pierre and Marie Curie ____

____

____

f. Paul Ehrlich ____

____

____

2. Match the pioneer in medicine in the left column with the appropriate item in the right column by writing the letters in the blanks.

________ Ignaz Phillip Semmelweis	a. father of modern anatomy
________ Joseph Lister	b. father of medicine
________ Louis Pasteur	c. founder of nursing
________ Jonas Edward Salk	d. discovered the x-ray
________ Clara Barton	e. developed the first lens strong enough to see bacteria
________ Asclepius	f. discovered how yellow fever is transmitted
________ Ambroise Paré	g. father of bacteriology
________ Walter Reed	h. discovered the vaccine against polio
________ William Harvey	i. Greek god of healing
________ Wilhem C. Roentgen	j. founded the American Red Cross
________ Hippocrates	k. father of sterile surgery
________ Andreas Vesalius	l. father of modern surgery
________ James Marion Sims	m. fought against puerperal fever
________ Florence Nightingale	n. demonstrated circulation of blood
________ Alexander Fleming	o. invented the vaginal speculum
	p. discovered insulin
	q. discovered penicillin

3. Name several factors that contributed to the rise of health care costs as medicine advanced. __________

____

4. List the benefits of using a managed care organization (MCO) and a traditional health care system as you compare and contrast their similarities and differences.

Traditional	Managed Care
a. ______	a. ______
b. ______	b. ______
c. ______	c. ______
d. ______	d. ______
e. ______	e. ______
f. ______	f. ______

5. In a health maintenance organization (HMO), what is a treating physician called? ______

______

6. In a preferred provider organization (PPO), (a) what is the health care provider called and (b) what incentive is there for the patient to use this provider?

a. ______

b. ______

7. In an independent practice association (IPA), how is the physician paid? ______

______

______

8. Why is an exclusive provider organization (EPO) called *exclusive*? ______

______

______

9. What choice of care do patients have when belonging to a point-of-service plan? ______

______

______

10. A variety of specialists practicing medicine together is called: ______

______

______

11. List three services urgent care centers provide that most other practices do not offer.

a. ______

b. ______

c. ______

12. Why should the medical assistant meet the hospital personnel where his or her physician is on staff?

______

13. Name several types of nonprofit hospitals.

a. ______ d. ______

b. ______ e. ______

c. ______

14. Name three important factors to consider when choosing a reliable laboratory.

    a. ____________________

    b. ____________________

    c. ____________________

Critical Thinking Exercises

1. Choose the type of health care *setting* you would like to work in and list the *reasons* for your choice.

   Setting: ____________________

   Reasons: ____________________

2. Debate the right of the physician to practice or not practice "concierge" medicine. ____________________

3. Determine the job duties of an administrative medical assistant working in a patient-centered medical home. ____________________

4. As a member of a multidisciplinary team, name several ways you, as an administrative medical assistant, can act as a patient advocate.

   a. ____________________

   b. ____________________

   c. ____________________

JOB SKILL 2-1
Use the Internet to Research and Write an Essay about a Medical Pioneer

Name ______________________________ Date ______________ Score ________

Performance Objective

Task: Use the Internet to look up information on a historical figure who contributed to medicine. Write a one-page essay describing their contribution. *Note:* If directed by instructor, this job skill may be done using library references.

Conditions: Computer with Internet connection, paper, and printer.

Standards: Complete all steps listed in this job skill in _______ minutes with a minimum score of _______. (Time element and accuracy criteria may be given by instructor.)

Time: **Start:** ____________ **Completed:** ____________ **Total:** ____________ minutes

Scoring: One point for each step performed satisfactorily unless otherwise listed or weighted by instructor.

Directions with Performance Evaluation Checklist

1st Attempt	2nd Attempt	3rd Attempt	
______	______	______	Gather materials (equipment and supplies) listed under "Conditions."
______	______	______	1. Turn on computer and establish an Internet connection. Use a search engine such as Yahoo, Google, GoodSearch, or one of your favorites.
____/3	____/3	____/3	2. Type in the key words "famous medical discoveries" or "inventor," then name a procedure or piece of medical equipment you would like to learn the history of, for example, "wheelchair inventor." Select a pioneer not already mentioned in the *textbook*.
____/2	____/2	____/2	3. After selecting the subject to write about, search for two more references containing information.
____/3	____/3	____/3	4. Print each of the references, read and study the material.
____/5	____/5	____/5	5. Type a one-page essay describing the historical figure or invention. Do not copy the text; use language at the level patients would understand if you were to read it to them.
______	______	______	6. Include a cover page with title.
____/3	____/3	____/3	7. Include a bibliography naming your references. To learn how Internet references are cited, search: "Columbia format for citing web research."
______	______	______	Complete within specified time.
____/20	____/20	____/20	**Total points earned** (To obtain a percentage score, divide the total points earned by the number of points possible.)

JOB SKILL 2-1 *(continued)*

Comments:

Evaluator's Signature: ______________________________ **Need to Repeat:** ____________

National Curriculum Competency: CAAHEP: Cognitive: IV.C.8, IV.C.12; Psychomotor: IV.P.2; Affective I.A.2, IV.A.7	ABHES: 8.a, c, e, jj

JOB SKILL 2-2
Direct Patients to Specific Hospital Departments

Name ______________________________ Date ______________ Score ________

Performance Objective

Task: Make determinations to direct patients to specific hospital departments.

Conditions: Use pen or pencil. Refer to *textbook* Figure 2-5A and Figure 2-5B (hospital departments) and Procedure 2-1 for step-by-step directions.

Standards: Complete all steps listed in this skill in _______ minutes with a minimum score of _______. (Time element and accuracy criteria may be given by instructor.)

Time: **Start:** ___________ **Completed:** ___________ **Total:** ___________ minutes

Scoring: One point for each step performed satisfactorily unless otherwise listed or weighted by instructor.

Directions with Performance Evaluation Checklist

In many situations, the administrative medical assistant will be interacting with the hospital. A knowledge of various hospital departments and the services they offer is helpful in order to expediently schedule tests, arrange surgery, obtain test results, and refer patients. In the following scenario, you are the administrative assistant in Dr. Gerald Practon's office. A patient, Reiko Kimon, was discharged from the hospital last week and has various questions. List the correct hospital department you would direct the patient to.

1st Attempt	2nd Attempt	3rd Attempt	
_____	_____	_____	Gather materials (equipment and supplies) listed under "Conditions."
_____	_____	_____	1. Where does she go to pick up a copy of her operative report?
_____	_____	_____	2. Where can she attend a nutritional education class?
_____	_____	_____	3. Where does she go for a urinalysis?
_____	_____	_____	4. She has a question about the medication that was given to her when she left the hospital.
_____	_____	_____	5. Should she use a bronchodilator before she goes to have a pulmonary function test?
_____	_____	_____	6. She would like to personally tell the hospital president how wonderfully she was cared for during her hospital stay.
_____	_____	_____	7. She would like to speak to the physician who admitted her when she first arrived by ambulance at the hospital.
_____	_____	_____	8. She would like to know whether anyone has found a convalescent hospital for her mother, who is an inpatient and soon to be discharged.
_____	_____	_____	9. She would like to schedule occupational therapy.
_____	_____	_____	10. She does not understand a hospital bill and would like it explained.
_____	_____	_____	11. She would like the name of the new OB-GYN doctor from San Francisco who is performing deliveries at the hospital.
_____	_____	_____	12. She has a question regarding the contrast media that will be given to her before a bone scan.
_____	_____	_____	13. She would like to pick up a preparation kit for a barium enema.

JOB SKILL 2-2 *(continued)*

______ ______ ______ 14. She has a question regarding an old refund that should have been sent to her by now.

______ ______ ______ 15. She would like to speak to the utilization review nurse who was assigned to her case.

______ ______ ______ 16. She would like to know if she can wear her wedding ring in the MRI machine.

______ ______ ______ 17. She would like to know how to dress for the treadmill test.

______ ______ ______ 18. She would like to know the preparation for a sigmoidoscopy that is scheduled.

______ ______ ______ 19. She would like to know what time to arrive for a blood transfusion.

______ ______ ______ 20. You are attentive, courteous and diplomatic while demonstrating sensitivity when communicating with the patient and hospital personnel.

______ ______ ______ Complete within specified time.

____/22 ____/22 ____/22 **Total points earned** (To obtain a percentage score, divide the total points earned by the number of points possible.)

Comments:

Evaluator's Signature: ______________________________ **Need to Repeat:** ____________

National Curriculum Competency: CAAHEP: Affective: IV.A.2, VII.A.2	ABHES: 8.aa, 11.b.8

JOB SKILL 2-3
Refer Patients to the Correct Physician Specialist

Name ______________________________ Date ______________ Score ________

Performance Objective

Task: Match the correct specialist with the patient's complaint.

Conditions: Use pen or pencil. Refer to *textbook* Table 2-3 for a list of medical specialties with descriptions and Procedure 2-2 for step-by-step directions.

Standards: Complete all steps listed in this skill in _______ minutes with a minimum score of _______. (Time element and accuracy criteria may be given by instructor.)

Time: **Start:** ____________ **Completed:** ____________ **Total:** ____________ minutes

Scoring: One point for each step performed satisfactorily unless otherwise listed or weighted by instructor.

Directions with Performance Evaluation Checklist

In many situations, administrative medical assistants deal with the authorization referral process. They may also handle patients being referred by primary care physicians to specialists. To enhance understanding of these processes, consider the patients' problems and match their complaints with the correct specialist.

1st Attempt	2nd Attempt	3rd Attempt	Patient Complaint	Specialist
______	______	______	Gather materials (equipment and supplies) listed under "Conditions."	
______	______	______	1. ______ Pregnant	A. Allergist
______	______	______	2. ______ Operation	B. Dermatologist
______	______	______	3. ______ Microbiology report	C. Neonatologist
______	______	______	4. ______ Bladder and kidney problems	D. Neurologist
______	______	______	5. ______ Chronic runny nose from dust	E. Nuclear medicine
______	______	______	6. ______ Severe depression	F. Obstetrician
______	______	______	7. ______ Face lift	G. Ophthalmologist
______	______	______	8. ______ Premature infant	H. Orthopedic surgeon
______	______	______	9. ______ Infant DPT injection	I. Otolaryngologist
______	______	______	10. ______ Ear discharge	J. Pathologist
______	______	______	11. ______ X-rays	K. Pediatrician
______	______	______	12. ______ Fractured bone	L. Physiatrist
______	______	______	13. ______ Rehabilitation for chronic back pain	M. Plastic surgeon N. Psychiatrist
______	______	______	14. ______ Multiple sclerosis (disease of nervous system)	O. Radiologist
______	______	______	15. ______ Glaucoma (increased pressure in eye)	P. Surgeon Q. Urologist
______	______	______	16. ______ Severe case of skin psoriasis	
______	______	______	17. ______ Bone scan (radionuclear)	

JOB SKILL 2-3 *(continued)*

______ ______ ______ Complete within specified time.

____/19 ____/19 ____/19 **Total points earned** (To obtain a percentage score, divide the total points earned by the number of points possible.)

Comments:

Evaluator's Signature: ____________________________________ **Need to Repeat:** ______________

National Curriculum Competency: CAAHEP: Psychomotor: IV.P.5	ABHES: 8.a, 8.gg

JOB SKILL 2-4
Define Abbreviations for Health Care Professionals

Name ______________________________ Date ______________ Score ________

Performance Objective

Task: Match terms for health care professionals with correct abbreviations.

Conditions: Use pen or pencil. Refer to Table 2-4 in the *textbook* for a list of physician specialists, health care professionals, and abbreviations. See Procedure 1-1 in Chapter 1 of the *textbook* for step-by-step directions.

Standards: Complete all steps listed in this skill in _______ minutes with a minimum score of _______. (Time element and accuracy criteria may be given by instructor.)

Time: **Start:** ____________ **Completed:** ____________ **Total:** ____________ minutes

Scoring: One point for each step performed satisfactorily unless otherwise listed or weighted by instructor.

Directions with Performance Evaluation Checklist

Read the following scenario, decode the abbreviations for the appropriate physician specialists and health care professionals, and write the correct term on the line provided.

Laverne M. Stinowski May 15, 20XX

Mrs. Stinowski was brought by ambulance to the hospital and was cared for by an EMT. In the emergency room she was treated by a DEM. During her hospital stay she was seen daily by the MD, who was also a FACS. After discharge, Mrs. Stinowski visited the physician's private office and was processed in by a CMA (AAMA). An LVN drew her blood and escorted her to the treatment room. The physician was out of the office, so an RNP saw Mrs. Stinowski. An order was given for her to see an RPT. The blood test was read in the laboratory by an MT (ASCP). The patient's record was typed by a CMT, and her insurance claim was processed by a CPC. The patient went home, and the PA-C was in charge of ordering the patient a VN for the following day.

Gerald M. Practon, MD

Gerald M. Practon, MD

1st Attempt	2nd Attempt	3rd Attempt	
_______	_______	_______	Gather materials (equipment and supplies) listed under "Conditions."
_______	_______	_______	1. EMT ______________________________
_______	_______	_______	2. DEM ______________________________
_______	_______	_______	3. MD ______________________________
_______	_______	_______	4. FACS ______________________________
_______	_______	_______	5. CMA (AAMA) ______________________________
_______	_______	_______	6. LVN ______________________________
_______	_______	_______	7. RNP ______________________________
_______	_______	_______	8. RPT ______________________________
_______	_______	_______	9. MT (ASCP) ______________________________

JOB SKILL 2-4 (*continued*)

______	______	______	10. CMT ______________________________
______	______	______	11. CPC ______________________________
______	______	______	12. PA-C______________________________
______	______	______	13. VN ______________________________
______	______	______	Complete within specified time.
___/15	___/15	___/15	**Total points earned** (To obtain a percentage score, divide the total points earned by the number of points possible.)

Comments:

Evaluator's Signature: ______________________________ **Need to Repeat:** ______________

National Curriculum Competency: ABHES: 3.d, 8.gg

JOB SKILL 2-5
Determine Basic Skills Needed by the Administrative Medical Assistant

Name ______________________________ Date ______________ Score ________

Performance Objective

Task: Review job requirements and determine basic skills necessary for the administrative medical assistant.

Conditions: Use pen or pencil. Refer to the list of medical specialties and administrative medical assistant job requirements found in Table 2-3 of the *textbook*.

Standards: Complete all steps listed in this skill in _______ minutes with a minimum score of _______. (Time element and accuracy criteria may be given by instructor.)

Time: **Start:** ____________ **Completed:** ____________ **Total:** ____________ minutes

Scoring: One point for each step performed satisfactorily unless otherwise listed or weighted by instructor.

Directions with Performance Evaluation Checklist

Record some basic skills the administrative medical assistant needs. You will see these skills occurring repetitiously under the different specialties listed in *textbook* Table 2-3.

1st Attempt	2nd Attempt	3rd Attempt	
_____	_____	_____	Gather materials (equipment and supplies) listed under "Conditions."
_____	_____	_____	1. ____________________
_____	_____	_____	2. ____________________
_____	_____	_____	3. ____________________
_____	_____	_____	4. ____________________
_____	_____	_____	5. ____________________
_____	_____	_____	6. ____________________
_____	_____	_____	7. ____________________
_____	_____	_____	8. ____________________
_____	_____	_____	Complete within specified time.
___/10	___/10	___/10	**Total points earned** (To obtain a percentage score, divide the total points earned by the number of points possible.)

Comments:

Evaluator's Signature: ______________________________ **Need to Repeat:** ____________

National Curriculum Competency: Skills listed are part of CAAHEP and ABHES competencies.

CHAPTER 3

Medicolegal and Ethical Responsibilities

OBJECTIVES

After completing the exercises, the student will be able to:

1. Write meanings for chart note abbreviations.
2. Enhance spelling skills by learning new medical words.
3. Use critical thinking skills to answer legal questions.
4. List personal ethics and set professional ethical goals (Job Skill 3-1).
5. Complete an authorization form to release medical records (Job Skill 3-2).
6. Download state-specific scope of practice laws and determine parameters for a medical assistant (Job Skill 3-3).
7. Compose a letter of withdrawal (Job Skill 3-4).
8. View a MedWatch online form and learn submitting requirements (Job Skill 3-5).
9. Print the *Patient Care Partnership* online brochure and apply it to the medical office setting (Job Skill 3-6).
10. Download and compare state-specific advance directives (Job Skill 3-7).

FOCUS ON CERTIFICATION*

CMA Content Summary

- Medical practice acts (physician license)
- Advance directives
- Anatomical gifts
- Reportable incidences

*This *Workbook* and the accompanying *textbook* meet the entry-level administrative and general competencies for the CMA outlined by the AAMA Examination Content Outline and Occupational Analysis and for the RMA and CMAS outlined by the AMT Competencies, Construction Parameters, and Examination Specifications (see Competency Grid in Appendix B of the *textbook*).

- Public health statutes
- HIPAA
- Consent/authorization
- Right to privacy
- Drug and alcohol rehabilitation records
- HIV-related issues
- *Subpoena duces tecum*
- Physician-patient relationship (contract/noncompliance)
- Responsibility and rights (physician/patient/medical assistant)
- Third-party agreements
- Professional liability
- Standard of care
- Arbitration
- Affirmative defenses
- Comparative/contributory negligence
- Termination of care
- Medicolegal terms and doctrines
- Releasing information
- Tort law
- Ethical standards (AAMA/AMA)
- Bioethics
- Liability coverage

RMA Content Summary

- Types of consents
- Federal and state laws
- HIPAA
- Privacy acts
- Scope of practice
- Patient Bill of Rights
- Licensure
- Legal terminology
- Medical ethics (AMA)
- Legal responsibilities
- Good Samaritan Act
- Emergency first aid
- Mandatory reporting guidelines

CMAS Content Summary

- Principles of medical laws and ethics (AMA)
- Scope of practice
- Disclosure laws
- Unethical practices
- Confidentiality
- Protected health information

STOP AND THINK CASE SCENARIOS AND EXAM-STYLE REVIEW QUESTIONS

Refer to the end of Chapter 3 in the *textbook*.

Abbreviation and Spelling Review

Read the following patient's chart note and write the meanings for the abbreviations listed below the note. To decide any abbreviations you do not understand or that appear unfamiliar to you, refer to the list of abbreviations in Part IV of this *Workbook*. Step-by-step directions for this exercise are in Procedure 1-1 of Chapter 1 in the *textbook*. Medical terms in the chart note are italicized; study them for spelling. Use your medical dictionary to look up their definitions. Your instructor may give a spelling and definition test that includes these words and abbreviations.

David K. Chung

September 20, 20XX HX: *Diarrhea* 3 days. T 99°F. No A. Cough producing yellow *sputum*. *Wheezing* in lt base. Moderate PND. Rec *vaporizer* and *amoxicillin* 250 mg p.o. q.8h. Diag URI. Etiol. unknown. Ordered CXR, CBC, & UA. Retn 2 wks.

Gerald Practon, MD

Gerald Practon, MD

HX	______	h.	______
T	______	diag	______
F	______	URI	______
A	______	etiol.	______
lt	______	CXR	______
PND	______	CBC	______
rec	______	UA	______
mg	______	retn	______
p.o.	______	wks	______
q.	______		

Review Questions

Review the objectives, glossary, and chapter information before completing the following review questions.

1. Match the terms in the left column with the definitions in the right column by writing the letters in the blanks.

______ Oath of Hippocrates	a.	information in a medical record
______ medical ethics	b.	code of conduct, courtesy, and manners customary in the medical profession
______ bioethics	c.	moral principles and standards in the medical profession
______ privileged information	d.	modern code of ethics
______ medical etiquette	e.	branch of ethics concerning moral issues, questions, and problems that arise in the practice of medicine and in biomedical research
______ Principles of Medical Ethics	f.	first standards of medical conduct and ethics

2. HIPAA stands for ______.
3. According to Title II of HIPAA law, name several ways in which HIPAA affects a medical practice.
   a. ______
   b. ______
   c. ______
   d. ______
4. Information about a patient's past, present, or future health condition that contains personal identifying data is called ______.
5. What does the privacy rule provide? ______

   ______

   ______
6. State three key things you would tell a new employee about patient confidentiality.
   a. ______
   b. ______
   c. ______

7. What are the three items a voluntary signed consent form covers?

   a. ______________________________

   b. ______________________________

   c. ______________________________

8. What form must be obtained for use and disclosure of protected health information? ______________________________

   ____

9. State the definition of a compliance plan. ______________________________

   ____

   ____

10. What is the common term for litigation? ______________________________

11. Another phrase used for medical malpractice is ______________________________.

12. Name two types of medical professional liability insurance.

    a. ______________________________

    b. ______________________________

13. A physician is legally responsible for any act you perform while in his or her employ. The legal phrase used to describe this responsibility is ______________________________, and it means ______________________________.

14. Name three circumstances in which a minor may become emancipated.

    a. ______________________________

    b. ______________________________

    c. ______________________________

15. Define *tort*. ______________________________

16. Match the words in the left column with the definitions in the right column by writing the letters in the blanks.

________ malfeasance	a. carelessness or negligence by a professional person
________ misfeasance	b. lawful treatment done in the wrong way
________ nonfeasance	c. failure of the physician to do anything
________ malpractice	d. reckless disregard for the safety of another; being indifferent to an injury that could occur
________ criminal negligence	e. wrongful treatment of the patient

17. Name the three principal defenses in a malpractice lawsuit.

    a. ______________________________

    b. ______________________________

    c. ______________________________

18. Name three types of bonding.

    a. ______________________________

    b. ______________________________

    c. ______________________________

19. Name three alternatives to the litigation process.

 a. ______________________________

 b. ______________________________

 c. ______________________________

Critical Thinking Exercises

1. A sales representative from the Hope Surgical Company brings a case of bourbon for your physician. Can your physician ethically accept this gift? Why or why not? ______________________________

2. Betty Harper is given a booklet on the office policies that explains charges for missed appointments, telephone calls, and insurance form completion. She brings two insurance forms, and you bill her for this service. Is this ethical? ______________________________

3. You overhear Linda Mason telling another patient in the reception room that another physician is treating her for her stomach ulcer. You know Dr. Practon is also treating her for this same condition in addition to her high blood pressure. What should you do? ______________________________

4. Margaret Silsbee, a patient of Fran Practon, MD, is seen on October 5, 2010, for a pelvic examination. Although she has insurance, she pays cash for the visit and asks that you not bill the insurance company. The following month, her insurance company requests all of her medical records. State what you would do and why. ______________________________

5. Gary Ryan has an outstanding bill of $200. You receive a signed authorization form for release of information from Dr. Homer's office requesting a copy of his progress notes since surgery. Can you ethically withhold this information until Mr. Ryan pays his bill? ______________________________

6. An insurance company sends Dr. Practon a request for the records of Jerry Osborne. A signed authorization accompanies the request. The medical record indicates that the physician discussed HIV testing, and the patient refused the test. What would you do? ______________________________

7. Martin P. Finley is examined, and the physician discovers a wart recurring on the patient's thumb. Mr. Finley asks the physician to remove it. In this instance, what kind of contract exists? ______________________________

8. A tow truck has a head-on collision on a rural highway 25 miles out of town. Dr. O'Halloran is driving along and notices the accident. He stops, finds a victim of the accident bleeding profusely, and renders first aid. Will he be held liable for any medical complication in aiding this victim? ____________________

   Name the law that governs this situation. ____________________

9. Candice Goodson, a 15-year-old, comes into the office and requests an examination for herself and her baby. Can the physician care for the infant and Candice without Candice's parents' consent? ____________________ Why or why not? ____________________

   ____

   ____

10. Dr. Gerald Practon receives a request from a social worker for medical records on a minor who is a ward of the court. The minor has signed a release. What would you do? ____________________

    ____

    ____

11. Give two examples of tort law as it applies to the medical assistant.

    a. ____________________

    b. ____________________

12. Dr. Rodriguez examines Mr. Garcia and diagnoses a gallstone. He reports this to the patient and recommends surgery. The patient says he agrees to the surgery. Are all conditions of informed consent present in this case? ____________________

    If not, name any that might be missing. ____________________

    ____

13. A subpoena is served on Dr. Bradley in regard to patient Teri Sanchez. In this instance, is a patient release-of-information form necessary? ____________________

14. Mrs. Marinacci states she wishes to donate her kidneys for transplant when she dies. How does she legally record her wishes? ____________________

    ____

    ____

JOB SKILL 3-1
List Personal Ethics and Set Professional Ethical Goals

Name ________________________________ Date ______________ Score ________

Performance Objective

Task: List your personal ethics that may affect professional ethics. Determine weak areas and set goals to become more professionally ethically centered for the future.

Conditions: Quiet area for reflection and an ethical partner to work with. Paper and pen or pencil.

Standards: Complete all steps listed in this job skill in _______ minutes with a minimum score of _______. (Time element and accuracy criteria may be given by instructor.)

Time: **Start:** ____________ **Completed:** ____________ **Total:** ____________ minutes

Scoring: One point for each step performed satisfactorily unless otherwise listed or weighted by instructor.

Directions with Performance Evaluation Checklist

1st Attempt	2nd Attempt	3rd Attempt	
______	______	______	Gather materials (equipment and supplies) listed under "Conditions."
______	______	______	1. Find a quiet area so you can reflect and think about the personal ethics you obtain and how they may influence your professional career as a medical assistant.
____/5	____/5	____/5	2. Write down five personal ethics that might affect your professional ethics as a medical assistant. a. ______________________ b. ______________________ c. ______________________ d. ______________________ e. ______________________
____/2	____/2	____/2	3. State one situation where your personal ethics may interfere or contradict the professional ethics of a medical assistant. ______________________ ______________________ ______________________
____/2	____/2	____/2	4. Determine a situation where you need to separate personal from professional ethics (e.g., this could be how you feel about a bioethical situation). ______________________ ______________________ ______________________
____/3	____/3	____/3	5. Determine three key goals to become more ethically centered for the future (you may determine more). a. ______________________ b. ______________________ c. ______________________

JOB SKILL 3-1 *(continued)*

____/3 ____/3 ____/3 6. Pledge to make more time to achieve the goals by giving less priority or more priority to the following:

a. ____________________

b. ____________________

c. ____________________

______ ______ ______ 7. Select a support person and together determine ways he or she can help you. This person's name is: ____________________

____/2 ____/2 ____/2 8. Select a method to maintain your momentum and record your weekly progress. ____________________

____

______ ______ ______ 9. Determine a reward for achieving your milestone and becoming a more professionally ethical person.

______ ______ ______ Complete within specified time.

____/22 ____/22 ____/22 **Total points earned** (To obtain a percentage score, divide the total points earned by the number of points possible.)

Comments:

Evaluator's Signature: ____________________ **Need to Repeat:** ____________

National Curriculum Competency: CAAHEP: Cognitive: X.C.1, X.C.2, X.C.5; Psychomotor: X.P.2	ABHES: 11.b.1

JOB SKILL 3-2

Complete an Authorization Form to Release Medical Records

Name ______________________ Date ____________ Score ________

Performance Objective

Task: Apply HIPAA rules to protect patient privacy when completing an authorization form to release medical information.

Conditions: Use patient demographic information (found below), Authorization for Release of Information (Form 1) found in Part II of this *Workbook*, and pen. Refer to Figure 3-9 for an illustration and Procedure 3-1 for step-by-step directions in the *textbook*. Refer to Medical Practice Reference Material (Part III of the *Workbook*) for physician and practice data.

Standards: Complete all steps listed in this job skill in _______ minutes with a minimum score of _______. (Time element and accuracy criteria may be given by instructor.)

Time: **Start:** __________ **Completed:** __________ **Total:** __________ minutes

Scoring: One point for each step performed satisfactorily unless otherwise listed or weighted by instructor.

Directions with Performance Evaluation Checklist

Scenario: Patient Michele Ramsey (7796 Bluebird Street, Woodland Hills, XY 12345, telephone [555] 937-7102, DOB 04/08/1950, medical record #2078) comes into the office stating that the company she works for will be closing its local office and she is transferring to another city. She would like her medical records sent to her new physician (Margaret Birgelaitis, MD, 66948 Santa Clara Circle, Anytown, XY 12345-0000, telephone [555] 482-0010). Obtain and complete the correct authorization form to process this request. Ms. Ramsey was first seen on 02/13/1996 and last seen on 09/03/2012. Today's date is 10/10/2012 and the authorization will expire at the end of the calendar year.

1st Attempt	2nd Attempt	3rd Attempt	
_____	_____	_____	Gather materials (equipment and supplies) listed under "Conditions."
____/10	____/10	____/10	1. Complete Section A of the form with the following: Patient identifying information, medical practice information, person receiving information, and the reason for and description of the request.
____/3	____/3	____/3	2. Complete Section B of the form and highlight the areas the patient needs to complete or initial.
____/6	____/6	____/6	3. Complete Section C of the form and highlight the areas the patient needs to complete or initial.
_____	_____	_____	Complete within specified time.
____/21	____/21	____/21	**Total points earned** (To obtain a percentage score, divide the total points earned by the number of points possible.)

Comments:

Evaluator's Signature: ______________________ **Need to Repeat:** __________

National Curriculum Competency: CAAHEP: Cognitive: IX.C.2, IX.C.3; Psychomotor: IX.P.1, IX.P.3, IX.P.8; Affective: X.A.2 ABHES: 4.b, 11.b.3

JOB SKILL 3-3

Download State-Specific Scope of Practice Laws and Determine Parameters for a Medical Assistant

Name ______________________________ Date ____________ Score ________

Performance Objective

Task: Use the Internet to download Medical Assisting Scope of Practice Laws for the state in which you live. Review the laws, identify areas of practice, select a topic, and write a summary of what is included in your state.

Conditions: Computer with Internet connection and printer. Paper and pen or pencil.

Standards: Complete all steps listed in this job skill in _______ minutes with a minimum score of _______. (Time element and accuracy criteria may be given by instructor.)

Time: **Start:** ____________ **Completed:** ____________ **Total:** ____________ minutes

Scoring: One point for each step performed satisfactorily unless otherwise listed or weighted by instructor.

Directions with Performance Evaluation Checklist

Check with your instructor: You may want to do this job skill as a cooperative learning effort with several other students, depending on the state information available and the number of students in your class.

1st Attempt	2nd Attempt	3rd Attempt	
_____	_____	_____	Gather materials (equipment and supplies) listed under "Conditions."
_____	_____	_____	1. Turn on the computer and obtain an Internet connection. Go to the Web site for the American Association of Medical Assistants: http://www.aama-ntl.org
_____	_____	_____	2. Click on "Employers," then "Key State Scope of Practice Laws."
_____	_____	_____	3. Select the state in which you live. If your state is not listed, click on "Questions Regarding Your State." The "Occupational Analysis of the CMA" can also be reviewed for basic medical assisting competencies.
____/5	____/5	____/5	4. Select an area to research or frequently asked questions (FAQ) to report on. Print and read the material. Note: Your instructor may direct you to a specific topic, law, or medical task prohibition.
___/10	___/10	___/10	5. Write a paragraph on your findings.
____/2	____/2	____/2	6. What may be the consequences of not working within the legal scope of practice? ____
_____	_____	_____	Complete within specified time.
___/22	___/22	___/22	**Total points earned** (To obtain a percentage score, divide the total points earned by the number of points possible.)

Comments:

Evaluator's Signature: ______________________________ **Need to Repeat:** ____________

National Curriculum Competency: CAAHEP: Cognitive: IV.C.8, IX.C.1; Psychomotor: IX.P.2; Affective: IX.A.2 ABHES: 1.e, 11.b.9

JOB SKILL 3-4
Compose a Letter of Withdrawal

Name ______________________________ Date ______________ Score ________

Performance Objective

Task: Compose a letter of withdrawal from Dr. Gerald Practon to a patient who has failed to pay his medical bill.

Conditions: White paper (8½" by 11"), computer. Refer to Part III of the *Workbook* for letterhead reference information. Refer to Figure 3-11 in the *textbook* for an illustration of a letter and sample wording.

Standards: Complete all steps listed in this skill in ________ minutes with a minimum score of ________. (Time element and accuracy criteria may be given by instructor.)

Time: **Start:** ____________ **Completed:** ____________ **Total:** ____________ minutes

Scoring: One point for each step performed satisfactorily unless otherwise listed or weighted by instructor.

Directions with Performance Evaluation Checklist

Patrick C. Pieper of 697 Williams Street, Woodland Hills, XY 12345 has received medical services amounting to $525. He provided insurance information at the time services were rendered but he is not eligible for medical coverage or benefits under the plan. He has received four statements and made two promises to pay over the telephone, which he has not kept. Dr. Gerald Practon would now like to send a letter of withdrawal and is allowing Mr. Pieper 30 days to locate another physician. He will be referred to the Ventura County Medical Society, (555) 676-5544, if he is unable to locate a new physician. Compose a personal letter of withdrawal on Dr. Practon's letterhead stating the above information.

1st Attempt	2nd Attempt	3rd Attempt	
______	______	______	Gather materials (equipment and supplies) listed under "Conditions."
____/5	____/5	____/5	1. Using a computer, prepare a letterhead that contains the Practon group name, street address, city, state, zip, and telephone number.
______	______	______	2. Format the letter in block style (everything aligned to the left) or modified block style (as in Figure 3-11).
______	______	______	3. Include the current date.
______	______	______	4. Include the inside address.
______	______	______	5. Include a salutation.
___/20	___/20	___/20	6. Compose a letter including the reason for withdrawing from the patient's care, number of days Dr. Practon will be available to attend to Mr. Pieper, referral source for finding a physician, and release of medical record information.
____/2	____/2	____/2	7. Apply ethical principles (honesty and integrity) in your choice of words as you compose this letter.
____/2	____/2	____/2	8. Include a closing and Dr. Practon's typed and signed signature.

JOB SKILL 3-4 *(continued)*

_______	_______	_______	9. Include initials of the letter composer.
_______	_______	_______	10. Include a list of items that are enclosed with the letter.
_______	_______	_______	Complete within specified time.
____/37	____/37	____/37	**Total points earned** (To obtain a percentage score, divide the total points earned by the number of points possible.)

Comments:

Evaluator's Signature: ______________________________ **Need to Repeat:** ____________

National Curriculum Competency: CAAHEP: Cognitive: IV.C.8; Affective: X.A.1	ABHES: 4.b, c

JOB SKILL 3-5

View a MedWatch Online Form and Learn Submitting Requirements

Name ______________________________ Date ____________ Score ______

Performance Objective

Task: View a MedWatch Online Voluntary Reporting Form (3500) and note uses for, areas for completion, and submission requirements.

Conditions: Computer with Internet connection. Pen or pencil.

Standards: Complete all steps listed in this job skill in ______ minutes with a minimum score of ______. (Time element and accuracy criteria may be given by instructor.)

Time: **Start:** __________ **Completed:** __________ **Total:** __________ minutes

Scoring: One point for each step performed satisfactorily unless otherwise listed or weighted by instructor.

Directions with Performance Evaluation Checklist

The U. S. Food and Drug Administration states "the MedWatch online form is used to report serious adverse events for human medical products, including potential and actual product use errors and product quality problems associated with the use of (1) FDA-regulated drugs, (2) biologics, (3) medical devices [including in-vitro diagnostics], and (4) special nutritional products and cosmetics."

1st Attempt	2nd Attempt	3rd Attempt	
______	______	______	Gather materials (equipment and supplies) listed under "Conditions."
______	______	______	1. Turn on the computer and obtain an Internet connection. Go to the U.S. Food and Drug Administration Web site: http://www.accessdata.fda.gov/scripts/medwatch/
___/15	___/15	___/15	2. Click on and read the "MedWatch HIPAA Compliance page" and answer the following questions:

a. The HIPAA Privacy Rule permits reporting of adverse events "to the ______________________ and directly to the ______."

b. "The Rule permits entities to disclose PHI without authorization for

____________________ ____________________

____________________ ____________________."

c. "The FDA relies on the voluntary reporting of ____________

__________ __________ or __________ __________

that you suspect are associated with a drug or medical device you have

________, ______________, or ____________."

1st Attempt	2nd Attempt	3rd Attempt	
___/3	___/3	___/3	3. Read "What NOT to Report to MedWatch Using Online Form 3500." What are the three areas not to report?

a. ____

b. ____

c. ____

JOB SKILL 3-5 *(continued)*

____/15 ____/15 ____/15 4. Click the "BEGIN" button to view parts of the form and answer the following questions:

a. The first section (A) contains ____

____.

b. The next section (B) asks you to:

(1) ____

(2) ____

(3) ____

(4) ____

(5) ____

(6) ____

(7) ____

______ ______ ______ Complete within specified time.

____/36 ____/36 ____/36 **Total points earned** (To obtain a percentage score, divide the total points earned by the number of points possible.)

Comments:

Evaluator's Signature: ________________________________ **Need to Repeat:** ____________

National Curriculum Competency: CAAHEP: Cognitive: IX.C.14, X.C.4; Psychomotor: IX.P.8, X.P.1	ABHES: 11.b.3

JOB SKILL 3-6

Print the *Patient Care Partnership* Online Brochure and Apply It to the Medical Office Setting

Name ______________________________ Date ____________ Score ________

Performance Objective

Task: View the *Patient Care Partnership* brochure (formerly the Patients' Bill of Rights) online and apply it to the medical office setting.

Conditions: Computer with Internet connection and printer. Paper, pen or pencil.

Standards: Complete all steps listed in this job skill in ________ minutes with a minimum score of ________. (Time element and accuracy criteria may be given by instructor.)

Time: **Start:** ____________ **Completed:** ____________ **Total:** ____________ minutes

Scoring: One point for each step performed satisfactorily unless otherwise listed or weighted by instructor.

Directions with Performance Evaluation Checklist

1st Attempt	2nd Attempt	3rd Attempt	
______	______	______	Gather materials (equipment and supplies) listed under "Conditions."
______	______	______	1. Turn on the computer and obtain an Internet connection. Go to the American Hospital Association Web site: http://www.aha.org
______	______	______	2. Click on "About" then "Patient Care Partnership."
______	______	______	3. Select your language (e.g., English). The file will download and the brochure may be printed. Note: This file may also be viewed online to obtain information.
____/6	____/6	____/6	4. Read the *Patient Care Partnership* and write the six areas this brochure addresses:

a. ____

b. ____

c. ____

d. ____

e. ____

f. ____

1st Attempt	2nd Attempt	3rd Attempt	
____/18	____/18	____/18	5. Relate each of these areas to the medical office and write a brief statement about the basic points:

a. **Example:** When you come to our medical facility, our first priority is to provide you with the care you need, when you need it, with skill, compassion, and respect.

b. ____

____

____

JOB SKILL 3-6 *(continued)*

c. ______________________________

____

____

d. ______________________________

____

____

e. ______________________________

____

____

f. ______________________________

____

____

____/3	____/3	____/3	6. Circle the above items (a–f) that show sensitivity to patients' rights.
______	______	______	Complete within specified time.
____/32	____/32	____/32	**Total points earned** (To obtain a percentage score, divide the total points earned by the number of points possible.)

Comments:

Evaluator's Signature: ______________________________ **Need to Repeat:** ____________

National Curriculum Competency: CAAHEP: Cognitive: IX.C.4; Psychomotor: IX.P.5; Affective: IX.A.1

JOB SKILL 3-7
Download and Compare State-Specific Advance Directives

Name ______________________________ Date ______________ Score ________

Performance Objective

Task: Download your state-specific advance directive. Read and compare it to the example shown in the *textbook.*

Conditions: Computer with Internet connection and printer. Sample advance directive (Figure 3-17) found in the *textbook.* Paper and pen or pencil.

Standards: Complete all steps listed in this job skill in ________ minutes with a minimum score of ________. (Time element and accuracy criteria may be given by instructor.)

Time: **Start:** __________ **Completed:** __________ **Total:** __________ minutes

Scoring: One point for each step performed satisfactorily unless otherwise listed or weighted by instructor.

Directions with Performance Evaluation Checklist

Each state has an advance directive found on the Caring Connections Web site. Some are two pages and others are as long as eight pages. Try to locate the unique features found in your state's directive.

1st Attempt	2nd Attempt	3rd Attempt	
______	______	______	Gather materials (equipment and supplies) listed under "Conditions."
______	______	______	1. Turn on the computer and obtain an Internet connection. Go to the Caring Connections Web site: http://www.caringinfo.org/
______	______	______	2. Click on "Download Your State Specific Advance Directive."
______	______	______	3. Each state is listed. Click on your state.
______	______	______	4. Print and read the advance directive.
______	______	______	5. Now, look at the example in the *textbook* (Figure 3-17).
____/5	____/5	____/5	6. Compare your state's advance directive to the one found in the *textbook* and list some of the differences: ______________________________ ______________________________ ______________________________ ______________________________ ______________________________ ______________________________
______	______	______	Complete within specified time.
____/12	____/12	____/12	**Total points earned** (To obtain a percentage score, divide the total points earned by the number of points possible.)

JOB SKILL 3-7 *(continued)*

Comments:

Evaluator's Signature: ______________________ **Need to Repeat:** ______________

National Curriculum Competency: CAAHEP: Cognitive: IX.C.10.f, g

CHAPTER 4

The Art of Communication

OBJECTIVES

After completing the exercises, the student will be able to:

1. Write the meaning for chart note abbreviations.
2. Enhance spelling skills by learning new medical terms.
3. Answer questions relating to all aspects of the communication cycle.
4. Demonstrate body language (Job Skill 4-1).
5. Use the Internet to research active listening skills and write a report (Job Skill 4-2).
6. Communicate with a child via role-playing (Job Skill 4-3).
7. Communicate with an older adult via role-playing (Job Skill 4-4).
8. Name unique qualities of other cultures (Job Skill 4-5).
9. Communicate with a hearing-impaired patient via role-playing (Job Skill 4-6).
10. Communicate with a visually impaired patient via role-playing (Job Skill 4-7).
11. Communicate with a speech-impaired patient via role-playing (Job Skill 4-8).
12. Communicate with a patient who has an impaired level of understanding via role-playing (Job Skill 4-9).
13. Communicate with an anxious patient via role-playing (Job Skill 4-10).
14. Communicate with an angry patient via role-playing (Job Skill 4-11).
15. Communicate with a patient and his or her family members and friends via role-playing (Job Skill 4-12).
16. Communicate with a coworker on the health care team via role-playing (Job Skill 4-13).

FOCUS ON CERTIFICATION*

CMA Content Summary

- Medical terminology
- Developmental/behavioral theories
- Human growth and development
- Adapting communication
- Verbal and nonverbal communication
- Listening skills
- Communication barriers
- Professional communication
- Patient interviewing techniques
- Evaluating effectiveness of communication

RMA Content Summary

- Medical terminology
- Age-specific responses
- Professional conduct
- Communication methods
- Cultural and ethnic differences
- Prejudice
- Interpersonal relations
- Verbal/oral communication skills
- Active listening skills
- History-taking techniques
- Subjective and objective information

CMAS Content Summary

- Medical terminology
- Human relation skills
- Professionalism
- Interview questions
- Oral communication

STOP AND THINK CASE SCENARIOS AND EXAM-STYLE REVIEW QUESTIONS

Refer to the end of Chapter 4 in the *textbook*.

ABBREVIATION AND SPELLING REVIEW

Read the following patient's chart note and write the meanings for the abbreviations listed below the note. To decode any abbreviations you do not understand or that appear unfamiliar to you, refer to the list of abbreviations in Part IV of this *Workbook*. Step-by-step directions for this exercise are found in Procedure 1-1 of Chapter 1 in the *textbook*. Medical terms in the chart note are italicized; study them for spelling. Use your medical dictionary to look up their definitions. Your instructor may give a spelling and definition test that includes these words and abbreviations.

> Leslee Armstrong
>
> 32-year-old Cauc female came in for init visit CO chr pelvic pain, HA, and slt shortness of breath. No ALL. Performed H & P. PMH revealed FUO, PID and *chronic* UTI. Ordered lab work and M. Patient NYD. Pt to have re ch in approx 3 days. R/O STD.
>
> *Gerald Practon, MD*
>
> Gerald Practon, MD

*This *Workbook* and the accompanying *textbook* meet the entry-level administrative and general competencies for the CMA outlined by the AAMA Examination Content Outline and Occupational Analysis and for the RMA and CMAS outlined by the AMT Competencies, Construction Parameters, and Examination Specifications (see Competency Grid in Appendix B of the *textbook*).

Cauc	______	PID	______
Init	______	UTI	______
CO	______	lab	______
chr	______	M	______
HA	______	NYD	______
slt	______	Pt	______
ALL	______	re ch	______
H & P	______	approx	______
PMH	______	R/O	______
FUO	______	STD	______

Review Questions

Review the objectives, glossary, and chapter information before completing the following review questions.

1. Of all the professionals that make up a health care team, who has the most interaction with the patient? ______
2. Name the basic elements of the communication cycle.
   a. ______
   b. ______
   c. ______
   d. ______
   e. ______
3. List, in order of importance, the top three ways humans communicate messages.
   a. ______
   b. ______
   c. ______
4. Name four forms of communication, including the most productive.
   a. ______
   b. ______
   c. ______
   d. ______
5. When interviewing a patient, what is the key to obtaining accurate information and what should you avoid?
   a. key: ______
   b. avoid: ______
6. What is the number one reason for the failure of relationships? ______
7. When does trust begin to develop between the physician and the patient? ______

8. What is the term used when a patient refuses to follow the doctor's treatment plan? ________________

____

9. Describe defensive behavior. ____

____

____

10. Briefly name and describe the five levels of needs according to Maslow's hierarchy theory.

a. ____

b. ____

c. ____

d. ____

e. ____

11. How can the meaning of spoken words change? ________________________________

____

12. What is a "double message"? ____

____

13. What is a "comfort zone" and why does it vary? ________________________________

____

14. Why do we all need to feel as if we are being listened to? ________________________

____

15. What is the difference between active listening and reflective listening? ____________

____

16. When trying to encourage a patient to open up and talk, what type of feedback is recommended and why? ____

____

17. A silent pause may be used to:

a. ____

b. ____

c. ____

d. ____

e. ____

f. ____

g. ____

18. Why is a professional health care interpreter preferred over a family member when translation is needed?

____

____

____

____

19. Why is it important to keep an open mind when dealing with patients of varied ethnic backgrounds?

____

____

20. The following suggestions are made for patients with special needs. State the type of impairment that would match the recommendation listed.

 a. use verbal descriptions _______________

 b. use simple words and short phrases, allowing plenty of time for the patient to digest what you have said

 ____

 c. eliminate background noises _______________

 d. look directly at the patient when you are speaking _______________

21. Name three of the "outward" signs of anxiety.

 a. _______________

 b. _______________

 c. _______________

Critical Thinking Exercises

1. Name one or more common colloquialisms that may confuse a message. _______________

____

____

2. Think about and describe one circumstance in which a person's body language did not match what he or she was saying. _______________

____

____

3. The physician has asked you to convey the following message to a patient. Translate the message into layman's terms so it can be understood. Note: You may need to look up some terms in a medical dictionary. "The patient's chronic diverticulosis has caused acute gastritis, which is resolving. The patient's cystitis and urethritis are unrelated and the ciprofloxacin will help clear that up."

____

____

____

____

____

4. What are some environmental elements in your classroom that may interfere with active listening and communication? _______________

____

5. Suggestions are listed in the *textbook* for how to deal with an angry patient. Can you think of a time when you were really angry and the person dealing with you:

   a. made the matter worse? Describe how. ____________________

   ____

   b. was able to help you dissipate your anger? Describe how. ____________________

   ____

6. In this chapter you read this powerful statement:

   > *In their research, psychologists have learned that the manner in which the medical staff interacts with a sick person can foster wellness or it can unintentionally aggravate a physical condition . . . that preserving the patient's mental state is often more important than performing expert medical skills.*

   What do you feel your responsibility is as a member of a health care team, and how does communication play a role in this?

   ____

   ____

   ____

   ____

   ____

   ____

7. Respond to the following situations:

   a. A patient, Mrs. Takuchi, stops at your desk on the way out, complaining that the physician wanted to give her an injection but she will not let anybody jab a needle into her and put something into her body. What would you say?

   ____

   ____

   ____

   b. The clinical medical assistant, Susan Owens, complains that you did not order the supplies she had requested in time. What would your response be?

   ____

   ____

   ____

JOB SKILL 4-1
Demonstrate Body Language

Name ______________________________ Date ______________ Score ________

Performance Objective

Task: Demonstrate positive and negative body language.

Conditions: Two or more persons; props may be used. Note: This exercise may be performed as a "role-playing" exercise by dividing the class into teams of two or more. One person or team demonstrates the body language, and the other person or team guesses what feelings the first is trying to display.

Standards: Complete all steps listed in this skill in _______ minutes with a minimum score of _______. (Time element and accuracy criteria may be given by instructor.)

Time: **Start:** ____________ **Completed:** ____________ **Total:** ____________ minutes

Scoring: One point for each step performed satisfactorily unless otherwise listed or weighted by instructor.

Directions with Performance Evaluation Checklist

1st Attempt	2nd Attempt	3rd Attempt	
_______	_______	_______	Gather materials (equipment and supplies) listed under "Conditions."
_______	_______	_______	1. Study the various types of body language described in the *textbook* under *Nonverbal Communication*.
____/10	____/10	____/10	2. Without speaking, use body language to convey the way you are feeling or may feel at times.
_______	_______	_______	Complete within specified time.
____/12	____/12	____/12	**Total points earned** (To obtain a percentage score, divide the total points earned by the number of points possible.)

Comments:

Evaluator's Signature: ______________________________ **Need to Repeat:** ______________

National Curriculum Competency: CAAHEP: Cognitive: IV.C.2; Psychomotor: IV.P.11; Affective: IV.A.3 ABHES: 8.ii

JOB SKILL 4-2
Use the Internet to Research Active Listening Skills and Write a Report

Name ______________________________ Date ______________ Score ________

Performance Objective

Task: Use the Internet to research active listening skills and write a short report.

Conditions: Refer to the section *Active Listening* and Procedure 4-1 in the *textbook*. Computer with Internet connection; printer, paper, and pen or pencil.

Standards: Complete all steps listed in this job skill in _______ minutes with a minimum score of _______. (Time element and accuracy criteria may be given by instructor.)

Time: **Start:** ____________ **Completed:** ____________ **Total:** ____________ minutes

Scoring: One point for each step performed satisfactorily unless otherwise listed or weighted by instructor.

Directions with Performance Evaluation Checklist

You will be writing a one-page essay on listening skills. Optional: This report may be presented orally, depending on instructor directions.

1st Attempt	2nd Attempt	3rd Attempt	
_______	_______	_______	Gather materials (equipment and supplies) listed under "Conditions."
____/5	____/5	____/5	1. Read the *Active Listening* section in the *textbook* and note key points.
_______	_______	_______	2. Turn on the computer and obtain an Internet connection. Go to your favorite search engine (e.g., Google, GoodSearch, Yahoo).
____/5	____/5	____/5	3. Key one of the following to begin your search: "Active Listening," "Effective Listening," "Good Listening Skills," or "Improving Listening Skills," and look for information or articles about listening.
____/5	____/5	____/5	4. Take notes on ways to improve your listening that are not already mentioned in the *textbook*.
___/10	___/10	___/10	5. Write a short one-page essay on listening skills and include five things that you are going to do to improve in this area.
_______	_______	_______	Complete within specified time.
___/28	___/28	___/28	**Total points earned** (To obtain a percentage score, divide the total points earned by the number of points possible.)

Comments:

Evaluator's Signature: ______________________________ **Need to Repeat:** ____________

National Curriculum Competency: CAAHEP: Affective: IV.A.2	ABHES: 8.aa

INSTRUCTOR: Job Skills 4-3, 4-4, and 4-6 through 4-13 involve communication role-playing. Two or three students are needed to complete each job skill and you may want to assign one or more job skills to each group. Job Skill 4-12 (Communicate with a Patient and His or Her Family Members and Friends via Role-Playing) is the most comprehensive and if time is limited it would be the best choice to satisfy all of the CAAHEP or ABHES competencies.

JOB SKILL 4-3
Communicate with a Child via Role-Playing

Name ______________________________ Date ____________ Score ________

Performance Objective

Task: Role-play to learn how to communicate with a child.

Conditions: Three students who will role-play a communication scenario. Refer to Procedure 4-2 in the *textbook*.

Standards: Complete all steps listed in this job skill in _______ minutes with a minimum score of _______. (Time element and accuracy criteria may be given by instructor.)

Time: **Start:** ____________ **Completed:** ____________ **Total:** ____________ minutes

Scoring: One point for each step performed satisfactorily unless otherwise listed or weighted by instructor.

Directions with Performance Evaluation Checklist

Scenario: A father comes into the office with Kara, his 6-year-old daughter. He says she has been pulling her left ear and complaining of pain. She appears bashful, is clinging to her father, and is crying softly. Role-play the communication between the administrative medical assistant, father, and child as you prepare her to be taken to the treatment room for the examination.

1st Attempt	2nd Attempt	3rd Attempt	
_____	_____	_____	Gather materials (equipment and supplies) listed under "Conditions."
____/2	____/2	____/2	1. Position yourself at the child's eye level.
____/2	____/2	____/2	2. Talk at a level the child understands.
____/2	____/2	____/2	3. Speak with a soft, low-pitched voice, consoling the child.
____/2	____/2	____/2	4. Ask simple questions making sure they are understood.
____/2	____/2	____/2	5. Allow the child to be involved.
____/2	____/2	____/2	6. Offer a toy or prop to gain attention and cooperation.
____/2	____/2	____/2	7. Allow the child to express fear and cry.
____/2	____/2	____/2	8. Recognize that the child may be stressed and accept the child's behavior, showing sensitivity and empathy.
____/2	____/2	____/2	9. Encourage feedback making sure the message is understood.
_____	_____	_____	Complete within specified time.
____/20	____/20	____/20	**Total points earned** (To obtain a percentage score, divide the total points earned by the number of points possible.)

JOB SKILL 4-3 *(continued)*

Comments:

Evaluator's Signature: ______________________________ **Need to Repeat:** ____________

National Curriculum Competency: CAAHEP: Cognitive: IV.C.7; Affective: IV.A.5, 7, 8, 10	ABHES: 8.cc

JOB SKILL 4-4
Communicate with an Older Adult via Role-Playing

Name ______________________________ Date ______________ Score ________

Performance Objective

Task: Role-play to learn how to communicate with an older adult.

Conditions: Three students who will role-play a communication scenario. Refer to Procedure 4-3 in the *textbook.*

Standards: Complete all steps listed in this job skill in _______ minutes with a minimum score of _______. (Time element and accuracy criteria may be given by instructor.)

Time: **Start:** ____________ **Completed:** ____________ **Total:** ____________ minutes

Scoring: One point for each step performed satisfactorily unless otherwise listed or weighted by instructor.

Directions with Performance Evaluation Checklist

Scenario: A 93-year-old man comes into the office with his daughter. She says he has urinary frequency. He seems a little confused and the daughter keeps trying to manipulate the conversation when the administrative medical assistant is attempting to talk to him. Role-play the communication between the administrative medical assistant, the older adult, and the daughter.

1st Attempt	2nd Attempt	3rd Attempt	
_______	_______	_______	Gather materials (equipment and supplies) listed under "Conditions."
____/2	____/2	____/2	1. Approach the patient in a friendly manner and look directly at him while speaking; do not prejudge.
____/2	____/2	____/2	2. Speak clearly and slowly; offer simple explanations.
____/2	____/2	____/2	3. Form short sentences and ask brief questions.
____/2	____/2	____/2	4. Analyze communication and encourage responses and feedback.
____/2	____/2	____/2	5. Rephrase statements or questions as necessary.
____/2	____/2	____/2	6. React calmly if or when the patient seemed confused or forgetful.
____/2	____/2	____/2	7. Do not make excuses for the patient.
____/2	____/2	____/2	8. Tell the patient when you did not understand him; ask the patient to repeat what was said.
____/2	____/2	____/2	9. Be gentle but honest and truthful when communicating; do not mislead the patient.
____/2	____/2	____/2	10. Offer written instructions.
_______	_______	_______	Complete within specified time.
____/22	____/22	____/22	**Total points earned** (To obtain a percentage score, divide the total points earned by the number of points possible.)

Comments:

Evaluator's Signature: ______________________________ **Need to Repeat:** ______________

National Curriculum Competency: CAAHEP: Cognitive: IV.C.7; Psychomotor: IV.P.5; Affective: IV.A.7, 8, 10 ABHES: 8.cc, kk

JOB SKILL 4-5
Name Unique Qualities of Other Cultures

Name ______________________________ Date ____________ Score ________

Performance Objective

Task: Research and discover unique qualities of other cultures in order to help you understand and serve patients in your geographical area.

Conditions: This will vary according to region but could include library and Internet research, personal interviews, or personal reports (see *Resources* at the end of Chapter 4 in the *textbook*).

Standards: Complete all steps listed in this skill in _______ minutes with a minimum score of _______. (Time element and accuracy criteria may be given by instructor.)

Time: **Start:** ____________ **Completed:** ____________ **Total:** ____________ minutes

Scoring: One point for each step performed satisfactorily unless otherwise listed or weighted by instructor.

Directions with Performance Evaluation Checklist

1st Attempt	2nd Attempt	3rd Attempt	
______	______	______	Gather materials (equipment and supplies) listed under "Conditions."
______	______	______	1. Determine which culture you will be researching and what method you will use to discover unique qualities. If you live in an area where there is little ethnic diversity, you may want to look at the migration statistics for your state.
______	______	______	2. Determine which unique features would have an impact on communication.
______	______	______	3. Determine which unique features would have an impact on the delivery of health care.
______	______	______	4. Select one quality that you admire from a culture that is different from yours.
____/10	____/10	____/10	5. Write a one-page summary of unique qualities and be prepared to present it orally to your class.
______	______	______	Complete within specified time.
____/16	____/16	____/16	**Total points earned** (To obtain a percentage score, divide the total points earned by the number of points possible.)

Comments:

Evaluator's Signature: ______________________________ **Need to Repeat:** ____________

National Curriculum Competency: CAAHEP: Cognitive: IV.C.7, X.C.3; Affective: IV.A.10	ABHES: 5.g, 8.kk

JOB SKILL 4-6

Communicate with a Hearing-Impaired Patient via Role-Playing

Name ______________________________ Date ______________ Score ________

Performance Objective

Task: Role-play to learn how to communicate with a hearing-impaired patient.

Conditions: Two students who will role-play a communication scenario. Refer to Procedure 4-4 in the *textbook.*

Standards: Complete all steps listed in this job skill in _______ minutes with a minimum score of _______. (Time element and accuracy criteria may be given by instructor.)

Time: **Start:** ___________ **Completed:** ___________ **Total:** ___________ minutes

Scoring: One point for each step performed satisfactorily unless otherwise listed or weighted by instructor.

Directions with Performance Evaluation Checklist

Scenario: Mr. Osborn, a 60-year-old man, comes into the office with a large hearing device on his right ear. He is there for a physical examination and it has been several years since his last appointment. You are responsible for obtaining a new history form and updating his registration information. Role-play the communication between the administrative medical assistant and the patient.

1st Attempt	2nd Attempt	3rd Attempt	
_____	_____	_____	Gather materials (equipment and supplies) listed under "Conditions."
____/2	____/2	____/2	1. Select a quiet place to communicate and give the patient your complete attention.
____/2	____/2	____/2	2. Eliminate distractions or background noises.
____/2	____/2	____/2	3. Choose a good seating arrangement, sitting on the side of the patient's good ear.
____/2	____/2	____/2	4. Face the patient in an area of good light.
____/2	____/2	____/2	5. Touch the patient lightly, as necessary, to gain his attention.
____/2	____/2	____/2	6. Speak in a natural tone, slowly, and distinctly, enunciate clearly and use a low-pitched voice.
____/2	____/2	____/2	7. Use short, simple sentences and repeat or rephrase as necessary.
____/2	____/2	____/2	8. Use gestures as needed.
____/2	____/2	____/2	9. Write down words or phrases that you have difficulty communicating.
____/2	____/2	____/2	10. Practice active listening techniques and get feedback by asking questions to verify understanding.
_____	_____	_____	Complete within specified time.
____/22	____/22	____/22	**Total points earned** (To obtain a percentage score, divide the total points earned by the number of points possible.)

Comments:

Evaluator's Signature: ______________________________ **Need to Repeat:** ____________

National Curriculum Competency: CAAHEP: Cognitive: IV.C.3, 4, 5; Psychomotor: IV.P.5; Affective: IV.A.2, 3, 8 ABHES: 5.b, 8.kk

JOB SKILL 4-7
Communicate with a Visually Impaired Patient via Role-Playing

Name ______________________________ Date ______________ Score ________

Performance Objective

Task: Role-play to learn how to communicate with a visually impaired patient.

Conditions: Two students who will role-play a communication scenario. Refer to Procedure 4-5 in the *textbook*.

Standards: Complete all steps listed in this job skill in _______ minutes with a minimum score of _______. (Time element and accuracy criteria may be given by instructor.)

Time: **Start:** ____________ **Completed:** ____________ **Total:** ____________ minutes

Scoring: One point for each step performed satisfactorily unless otherwise listed or weighted by instructor.

Directions with Performance Evaluation Checklist

Scenario: Mrs. Gretna, a 50-year-old legally blind patient, comes into the office to have her back checked. She is complaining of lumbar pain. The physician has asked you to escort Mrs. Gretna to his office where he would like to obtain information before the clinical medical assistant escorts her into an examination room. Role-play the communication between the administrative medical assistant and the patient.

1st Attempt	2nd Attempt	3rd Attempt	
_______	_______	_______	Gather materials (equipment and supplies) listed under "Conditions."
____/2	____/2	____/2	1. Approach the patient cheerfully and identify yourself by name.
____/2	____/2	____/2	2. Look directly at the patient, greet her by name and speak clearly in a normal tone and speed.
____/2	____/2	____/2	3. Inform the patient of others who are in the same room or area.
____/2	____/2	____/2	4. Let the patient know exactly what you will be doing.
____/2	____/2	____/2	5. Ask the patient if you could take her hand to show her the surroundings.
____/2	____/2	____/2	6. Escort the patient to the physician's office, look for obstacles along the way, and provide verbal cues.
____/2	____/2	____/2	7. Inform the patient of the location and tell her when you leave the room; knock before reentering, even if the door was left open.
____/2	____/2	____/2	8. Explain the sounds of unusual noises and office machines.
____/2	____/2	____/2	9. Use large-print material when available.
_______	_______	_______	Complete within specified time.
___/20	___/20	___/20	**Total points earned** (To obtain a percentage score, divide the total points earned by the number of points possible.)

Comments:

Evaluator's Signature: ______________________________ **Need to Repeat:** ______________

National Curriculum Competency: CAAHEP: Cognitive: IV.C.3, 4, 5; Affective: IV.A.8	ABHES: 5.b, 8.kk

JOB SKILL 4-8
Communicate with a Speech-Impaired Patient via Role-Playing

Name ______________________________ Date ______________ Score ________

Performance Objective

Task: Role-play to learn how to communicate with a speech-impaired patient.

Conditions: Two or three students who will role-play a communication scenario. Refer to Procedure 4-6 in the *textbook*.

Standards: Complete all steps listed in this job skill in _______ minutes with a minimum score of _______. (Time element and accuracy criteria may be given by instructor.)

Time: **Start:** ____________ **Completed:** ____________ **Total:** ____________ minutes

Scoring: One point for each step performed satisfactorily unless otherwise listed or weighted by instructor.

Directions with Performance Evaluation Checklist

Scenario: Michelle Kunup, a 40-year-old woman, comes into the office to see the neurologist for a consultation and is escorted by her husband. She has just had a major stroke and was released from the hospital last week. She is walking fine and has full use of her arms and so forth but her speech has been affected. Role-play the communication between the administrative medical assistant and the patient.

1st Attempt	2nd Attempt	3rd Attempt	
______	______	______	Gather materials (equipment and supplies) listed under "Conditions."
____/2	____/2	____/2	1. Look directly at the patient without making her feel self-conscious.
____/2	____/2	____/2	2. Allow the patient time to think through what she is going to say; give her time to speak.
____/2	____/2	____/2	3. Do not speak for the patient or rush the conversation.
____/2	____/2	____/2	4. Do not pretend to understand; ask her to repeat as necessary.
____/2	____/2	____/2	5. Act in a courteous manner and do not shout; show sensitivity.
____/2	____/2	____/2	6. Offer a notepad as necessary.
______	______	______	Complete within specified time.
____/14	____/14	____/14	**Total points earned** (To obtain a percentage score, divide the total points earned by the number of points possible.)

Comments:

Evaluator's Signature: ______________________________ **Need to Repeat:** ____________

National Curriculum Competency: CAAHEP: Cognitive: IV.C.3, 4; Affective: IV.A.5	ABHES: 5.b, 8.kk

JOB SKILL 4-9

Communicate with a Patient Who Has an Impaired Level of Understanding via Role-Playing

Name ______________________________ Date ____________ Score ________

Performance Objective

Task: Role-play to learn how to communicate with a patient who has an impaired level of understanding.

Conditions: Three students who will role-play a communication scenario. Refer to Procedure 4-7 in the *textbook.*

Standards: Complete all steps listed in this job skill in ________ minutes with a minimum score of ________. (Time element and accuracy criteria may be given by instructor.)

Time: **Start:** ____________ **Completed:** ____________ **Total:** ____________ minutes

Scoring: One point for each step performed satisfactorily unless otherwise listed or weighted by instructor.

Directions with Performance Evaluation Checklist

Scenario: Pricilla Longfellow, a 30-year-old woman, comes into Dr. Fran Practon's office with her mother. She is having an ingrown toenail looked at today to see if surgery is needed. She has experienced traumatic brain injury from an automobile accident that occurred when she was 18 years old. She has difficulty speaking and has a level of understanding somewhere between that of a 5- and a 7-year-old. You will be greeting her at the reception desk and collecting a copayment. The patient is emphatic about wanting to see the physician herself and tells her mother, "I can do it by myself, I don't need you." Role-play the communication between the administrative medical assistant, the patient, and her mother.

1st Attempt	2nd Attempt	3rd Attempt	
_____	_____	_____	Gather materials (equipment and supplies) listed under "Conditions."
_____/2	_____/2	_____/2	1. Greet the patient warmly; address the patient by name.
_____/2	_____/2	_____/2	2. Act professionally and keep the conversation focused.
_____/2	_____/2	_____/2	3. Speak slowly and in a calm manner.
_____/2	_____/2	_____/2	4. Select simple words and short phrases.
_____/2	_____/2	_____/2	5. Use verbal and nonverbal cues.
_____/2	_____/2	_____/2	6. Use tone of voice to express concern; do not raise your voice.
_____/2	_____/2	_____/2	7. Repeat and rephrase the message as necessary.
_____/2	_____/2	_____/2	8. Use demonstration when appropriate to reinforce the message.
_____/2	_____/2	_____/2	9. Allow more time than usual.
_____/2	_____/2	_____/2	10. Reassure the patient and do not overload her with information.
_____/2	_____/2	_____/2	11. Inform the patient of what to expect prior to it happening.
_____/2	_____/2	_____/2	12. Exhibit tolerance and sensitivity; do not force answers.
_____/2	_____/2	_____/2	13. Remind the patient why she is at the physician's office; orient her to reality.

JOB SKILL 4-9 *(continued)*

_______ _______ _______ Complete within specified time.

____/28 ____/28 ____/28 **Total points earned** (To obtain a percentage score, divide the total points earned by the number of points possible.)

Comments:

Evaluator's Signature: ______________________________ **Need to Repeat:** ____________

National Curriculum Competency: CAAHEP: Cognitive: IV.C.3, 4, 7; Psychomotor: IV.P.5; Affective: IV.A.5, 7	ABHES: 5.b, 8.kk

JOB SKILL 4-10
Communicate with an Anxious Patient via Role-Playing

Name ______________________________ Date ______________ Score ________

Performance Objective

Task: Role-play to learn how to communicate with an anxious patient.

Conditions: Two students who will role-play a communication scenario. Refer to Procedure 4-8 in the *textbook*.

Standards: Complete all steps listed in this job skill in _______ minutes with a minimum score of _______. (Time element and accuracy criteria may be given by instructor.)

Time: **Start:** ____________ **Completed:** ____________ **Total:** ____________ minutes

Scoring: One point for each step performed satisfactorily unless otherwise listed or weighted by instructor.

Directions with Performance Evaluation Checklist

Scenario: Jessica McMullin, a 20-year-old woman, presents as a new patient. She looks frightened and is shaking when she fills out the paperwork. You later find out that she has a lump in her breast and her aunt died of breast cancer. Role-play the communication between the administrative medical assistant and the patient.

1st Attempt	2nd Attempt	3rd Attempt	
______	______	______	Gather materials (equipment and supplies) listed under "Conditions."
____/2	____/2	____/2	1. Recognize the signs of anxiety and acknowledge them.
____/2	____/2	____/2	2. Pinpointe possible sources of anxiety.
____/2	____/2	____/2	3. Make the patient feel as comfortable as possible.
____/2	____/2	____/2	4. Give the patient personal space.
____/2	____/2	____/2	5. Demonstrate a warm and caring attitude.
____/2	____/2	____/2	6. Speak with confidence and calmness; ask the patient to describe what is causing her anxiety. Allow her to describe her feelings and thoughts.
____/2	____/2	____/2	7. Listen attentively without interruption.
____/2	____/2	____/2	8. Maintain eye contact and keep an open posture.
____/2	____/2	____/2	9. Accept the patient's thoughts and feelings; demonstrate empathy.
____/2	____/2	____/2	10. Help the patient recognize the anxiety and cope with it by providing information and suggesting relaxation techniques.
______	______	______	Complete within specified time.
____/22	____/22	____/22	**Total points earned** (To obtain a percentage score, divide the total points earned by the number of points possible.)

Comments:

Evaluator's Signature: ______________________________ **Need to Repeat:** ______________

National Curriculum Competency: CAAHEP: Cognitive: IV.C.3, 4, 7; Psychomotor: IV.P.5; Affective: IV.A.4, 5 — ABHES: 5.b, 8.bb, kk

JOB SKILL 4-11
Communicate with an Angry Patient via Role-Playing

Name ______________________ Date ____________ Score ________

Performance Objective

Task: Role-play to learn how to communicate with an angry patient.

Conditions: Two students who will role-play a communication scenario. Refer to Procedure 4-9 in the *textbook*.

Standards: Complete all steps listed in this job skill in ______ minutes with a minimum score of ______. (Time element and accuracy criteria may be given by instructor.)

Time: **Start:** ____________ **Completed:** ____________ **Total:** ____________ minutes

Scoring: One point for each step performed satisfactorily unless otherwise listed or weighted by instructor.

Directions with Performance Evaluation Checklist

Scenario: Mr. Murray VanNelson, a retired male patient, comes into the office and checks in at the window. He seems agitated and sits down in a full waiting room and stares at the receptionist with a nasty look on his face. It is almost as if steam is coming out of his ears. You later find out that he is mad because he feels he always has to wait for the doctor and no one respects the time it takes out of his day each time an appointment is necessary. Role-play the communication between the administrative medical assistant and the patient.

1st Attempt	2nd Attempt	3rd Attempt	
______	______	______	Gather materials (equipment and supplies) listed under "Conditions."
____/2	____/2	____/2	1. Recognize that the patient is angry; do not ignore him.
____/2	____/2	____/2	2. Honor the patient's personal space.
____/2	____/2	____/2	3. Keep an open posture, maintain eye contact, and position yourself at the patient's eye level.
____/2	____/2	____/2	4. Remain calm showing that you care about his feelings; demonstrate positive body language and respect.
____/2	____/2	____/2	5. Focus on why the patient is there.
____/2	____/2	____/2	6. Listen attentively with an open mind and ask the patient to describe the cause of his anger and how it makes him feel. Let him vent openly.
____/2	____/2	____/2	7. Do not take a defensive attitude or try to talk the patient out of being angry.
____/2	____/2	____/2	8. Allow the patient time alone.
____/2	____/2	____/2	9. Determine a time frame to get back to the patient with a solution.
______	______	______	Complete within specified time.
____/20	____/20	____/20	**Total points earned** (To obtain a percentage score, divide the total points earned by the number of points possible.)

Comments:

Evaluator's Signature: ______________________ **Need to Repeat:** ____________

National Curriculum Competency: CAAHEP: Cognitive: IV.C.3, 4, 7; Psychomotor: IV.P.11; Affective: IV.A.4, 5, 10	ABHES: 5.b, 8.aa, ii, kk

JOB SKILL 4-12
Communicate with a Patient and His or Her Family Members and Friends via Role-Playing

Name ______________________________ Date ____________ Score ______

Performance Objective

Task: Role-play to learn how to communicate with a patient and his or her family and friends.

Conditions: Two students who will role-play a communication scenario. Refer to Procedure 4-10 in the *textbook.*

Standards: Complete all steps listed in this job skill in ______ minutes with a minimum score of ______. (Time element and accuracy criteria may be given by instructor.)

Time: **Start:** __________ **Completed:** __________ **Total:** __________ minutes

Scoring: One point for each step performed satisfactorily unless otherwise listed or weighted by instructor.

Directions with Performance Evaluation Checklist

Scenario: You are an administrative medial assistant and the office manager has asked you to speak to Mrs. Madelyn Wilson when she comes in today about charges that were denied by Medicare. She just moved into the area in March 2012 and had a 24-hour Holter monitor put on in your office on April 2, 2012. The results were positive, showing that the patient goes in and out of a bigeminal rhythm. However, she had this same service done in January 2012 by a physician where she used to live; the results were negative. Medicare pays for one Holter monitor every 6 months. When she received these services you had her sign an Advance Beneficiary Notice (ABN) and advised her that Medicare might not pay for the services. You can legally bill her and expect to receive payment; however, you have done so and she has not paid. It is June 10, 2012 (after your conversation, she pays the bill in full). Optional: You may role-play a family member or friend who is accompanying the patient to the office to expand this exercise (*three students will be needed*).

1st Attempt	2nd Attempt	3rd Attempt	
____	____	____	Gather materials (equipment and supplies) listed under "Conditions."
____/2	____/2	____/2	1. Pay attention to your personal appearance, knowing that it will affect the patient's responses.
____/2	____/2	____/2	2. Warmly greet the patient and offer her a seat in a private, comfortable area.
____/2	____/2	____/2	3. Introduce yourself and explain why you would like to have a conversation with her.
____/2	____/2	____/2	4. Use a genuine approach and respect her comfort zone.
____/2	____/2	____/2	5. Display a positive attitude and focus on the patient with your undivided attention.
____/2	____/2	____/2	6. Demonstrate confidence while communicating accurately and succinctly.
____/2	____/2	____/2	7. Display sensitivity and empathy while putting the patient at ease and acknowledging any sources of anxiety.
____/2	____/2	____/2	8. Listen carefully to comments and allow time for questions.
____/2	____/2	____/2	9. Answer questions honestly.
____/2	____/2	____/2	10. Obtain feedback so you are sure that the message has been received correctly.

JOB SKILL 4-12 *(continued)*

____/2	____/2	____/2	11. Offer support and guidance; reward the patient's compliance with praise.
______	______	______	Complete within specified time.
____/24	____/24	____/24	**Total points earned** (To obtain a percentage score, divide the total points earned by the number of points possible.)

Comments:

Evaluator's Signature: ______________________ **Need to Repeat:** __________

National Curriculum Competency: CAAHEP: Cognitive: IV.C.5; Psychomotor: IV.P.5; Affective: IV.A.1, 4, 5, 6, 8, 9	ABHES: 8.bb, ii, kk

JOB SKILL 4-13
Communicate with a Coworker on the Health Care Team via Role-Playing

Name _______________ Date _______________ Score _______________

Performance Objective

Task: Role-play to learn how to communicate with a coworker on the health care team.

Conditions: Two students who will role-play a communication scenario. Refer to Procedure 4-11 in the *textbook.*

Standards: Complete all steps listed in this job skill in _______ minutes with a minimum score of _______. (Time element and accuracy criteria may be given by instructor.)

Time: **Start:** _______ **Completed:** _______ **Total:** _______ minutes

Scoring: One point for each step performed satisfactorily unless otherwise listed or weighted by instructor.

Directions with Performance Evaluation Checklist

Scenario: You are the receptionist and have just opened the office and switched all calls from the answering service. Patients have been waiting at the door and now come into the office wanting to check in. Sheryl, a coworker, is trying to tell you about her weekend, but you do not have time to listen to her. How can you respond without hurting her feelings and be able to give your full attention to your job? Role-play the communication between the administrative medical assistant and the coworker.

1st Attempt	2nd Attempt	3rd Attempt	
_____	_____	_____	Gather materials (equipment and supplies) listed under "Conditions."
____/2	____/2	____/2	1. Be polite and cheerful, use a friendly approach.
____/2	____/2	____/2	2. Use correct names and titles.
____/2	____/2	____/2	3. Use tack and diplomacy when attempting to resolve the problem.
____/2	____/2	____/2	4. Speak calmly and respectfully; do not become angry or defensive.
____/2	____/2	____/2	5. Use proper channels of communication. Try to work out the problem.
____/2	____/2	____/2	6. Do not judge; instead practice empathy.
____/2	____/2	____/2	7. Have a positive attitude.
____/2	____/2	____/2	8. Bring the issue that bothered you to the forefront.
____/2	____/2	____/2	9. Perform all your duties and responsibilities cheerfully.
____/2	____/2	____/2	10. Avoid gossip, arguments, and uncomplimentary statements.
____/2	____/2	____/2	11. Do not complain; instead be a problem solver.
_____	_____	_____	Complete within specified time.
____/24	____/24	____/24	**Total points earned** (To obtain a percentage score, divide the total points earned by the number of points possible.)

Comments:

Evaluator's Signature: _______________ **Need to Repeat:** _______________

National Curriculum Competency: CAAHEP: Cognitive: IV.C.15; Affective: IV.A.5	ABHES: 8.aa, kk

CHAPTER 5

Receptionist and the Medical Office Environment

OBJECTIVES

After completing the exercises, the student will be able to:

1. Write meanings for chart note abbreviations.
2. Enhance spelling skills by learning new medical words.
3. Respond to medical office emergencies.
4. Prepare a patient registration form (Job Skill 5-1).
5. Prepare an application form for a disabled person placard (Job Skill 5-2).
6. Research community resources for patient referrals and patient education (Job Skill 5-3).
7. Assess and use proper body mechanics (Job Skill 5-4).
8. Evaluate the work or school environment and develop a safety plan (Job Skill 5-5).
9. Take steps to prevent and prepare for fires in a health care setting (Job Skill 5-6).
10. Demonstrate proper use of a fire extinguisher (Job Skill 5-7).
11. Determine potential disaster hazards in your local community (Job Skill 5-8).
12. Develop an emergency response template with an evacuation plan (Job Skill 5-9).

FOCUS ON CERTIFICATION*

CMA Content Summary

- Medical terminology pertaining to the receptionist
- Professional communication and behavior
- Maintaining confidentiality
- Physical environment of the medical office
- Office maintenance (facility, furniture, and equipment)
- Patient information booklet

RMA Content Summary

- Medical terminology pertaining to the receptionist
- Patient instruction
- Patient instruction regarding: health and wellness, nutrition, hygiene, treatment and medications, pre- and post-operative care, body mechanics, personal and physical safety
- Patient brochures and informational materials
- Communicating, greeting and receiving patients
- Basic emergency triage in coordinating patient arrivals
- Screen visitors and sales persons
- Patient demographic information
- Confidentiality during check-in procedures
- Preparing patient records
- Assist patients into exam rooms

CMA Content Summary

- Receive and process patients and visitors
- Screen visitors and vendors
- Coordinate patient flow into examination rooms

STOP AND THINK CASE SCENARIOS AND EXAM-STYLE REVIEW QUESTIONS

Refer to the end of Chapter 5 in the *textbook*.

Abbreviation and Spelling Review

Read the following patients' chart notes and write the meanings for the abbreviations listed below the note. To decode any abbreviations you do not understand or that appear unfamiliar to you, refer to the list of abbreviations in Part IV of this *Workbook*. Step-by-step directions for this exercise are found in Procedure 1-1 of Chapter 1 in the *textbook*. Medical terms in the chart note are italicized; study them for spelling. Use your medical dictionary to look up their definitions. Your instructor may give a spelling and definition test that includes these words and abbreviations.

DATE	PROGRESS
10/1/20XX	**Maria D. Gomez**, well-developed Hispanic ♀ fell on sharp object at 9 a.m. Laceration of L lower lip 0.5 cm. Tr.: cleaned, sutured, & drained. DTaP inj. Retn in 5 days. *Fran Practon, MD* Fran Practon, MD

*This *Workbook* and the accompanying *textbook* meet the entry-level administrative and general competencies for the CMA outlined by the AAMA Examination Content Outline and Occupational Analysis and for the RMA and CMAS outlined by the AMT Competencies, Construction Parameters, and Examination Specifications (see Competency Grid in Appendix B of the *textbook*).

♀	________________	Tr.	________________
a.m.	________________	DTaP	________________
L	________________	inj.	________________
cm	________________	retn	________________

DATE	**PROGRESS**
10/1/20XX	**Barry K. Wesson** This white ♂ had severe pain Ⓛ sternoclavicular area. Chest clear to P&A, EKG, ō. AP&L chest XR-N. Demerol 75mg for pain Dx neuralgia.
	Fran Practon, MD Fran Practon, MD

♂	________________	AP&L	________________
Ⓛ	________________	XR	________________
P&A	________________	N	________________
EKG	________________	mg	________________
ō	________________	Dx	________________

Review Questions

Review the objectives, glossary, and chapter information before completing the following review questions.

1. Why are first impressions so important in a medical setting? ________________

____

2. What benefits are attained by patients and the physician when the receptionist is attentive to patients' needs? ________________

____

____

3. Name several things that are necessary for a person to be successful when multitasking.
   a. ________________
   b. ________________
   c. ________________
   d. ________________

4. If you are asked in the evening to pull the records of all patients who will be seen the following day, in what order should they be organized? ________________

____

____

5. What should you check for in each chart after pulling it to be sure the chart is complete and ready for the physician prior to the patient's arrival? ________________

____

____

6. What safeguard can be taken against the mispronunciation of a patient's name? ______________________

____

____

7. When greeting patients, what is the easiest way to customize requests and comments to prevent sounding like a broken record? ____

____

____

8. Is calling out a patient's name who is seated in the reception area a violation of HIPAA? Why or why not? ____

____

____

9. When addressing patients, when should surnames be used? ______________________________

____

____

10. List alternatives to using a standard patient sign-in log so patient names and "reason for visit" are not viewed by others.

    a. ____

    b. ____

    c. ____

    d. ____

    e. ____

11. What is the leading nonviolent crime in America?

    a. burglary

    b. drug violations

    c. car theft

    d. identity theft

    e. embezzlement

12. The "Red Flags Rule" offers:

    a. a disaster preparedness plan mandated by the federal government

    b. guidelines for a written prevention and detection program for identity theft

    c. fire alert symbols

    d. hazard warning labels

    e. rules for medical offices regarding patients with disabilities

13. List typical ways patients can be registered or preregistered in a medical office.

    a. ____

    b. ____

    c. ____

    d. ____

14. Does a primary care physician with a managed care plan need an authorization prior to seeing a new patient? ______________________

15. What steps need to be taken before releasing PHI to a patient's family member? ______________________

____

____

16. You are the receptionist and have just found out the doctor will be an hour late. Name three options that can be given to waiting patients.

a. ______________________

b. ______________________

c. ______________________

17. List six special considerations that the office staff can provide a disabled or geriatric patient.

a. ______________________

b. ______________________

c. ______________________

d. ______________________

e. ______________________

f. ______________________

18. List five community resources that can be of value to patients. Note: These need not be on the list from the *textbook*.

a. ______________________

b. ______________________

c. ______________________

d. ______________________

e. ______________________

19. If your office has an open reception area, what are three things you need to take into consideration on a daily basis to protect patient confidentiality?

a. ______________________

b. ______________________

c. ______________________

20. When you visit a physician's office, what are some things that favorably impress you in the reception area?

____

____

____

____

____

21. Write the "general duty" clause from the Occupational Safety and Health Act, which is the basis of compliance mandated by OSHA. ____________________

____

____

____

____

22. True or False? PPE shall be provided by the employer at no cost to the employee. ____________________

23. Define the term *ergonomics:* ____________________

____

____

24. Medical offices may be the target of theft because of ____________________ ____________; therefore, the medical assistant needs to be aware of how to help keep the office secure.

25. What are three common causes of major injury in the workplace? ____________________

____

____

26. List 10 electrical-related items, areas, or situations to check to prevent an electrical fire and keep from receiving an electrical burn or shock.

a. ____________________

b. ____________________

c. ____________________

d. ____________________

e. ____________________

f. ____________________

g. ____________________

h. ____________________

i. ____________________

j. ____________________

27. Three sources needed to start a fire are ____________, ____________, and ____________.

28. When starting a fire, common sources of ignition are:

a. electrical equipment and machinery

b. hot surfaces

c. matches and open flames

d. smoking

e. all of the above

29. Explain what Material Safety Data Sheets are and their use in the medical office. ____________________

____

____

____

30. State what the acronym RACER stands for.

    R. ______________________________

    A. ______________________________

    C. ______________________________

    E. ______________________________

    R. ______________________________

31. Name the type of fire extinguisher listed below and the type of burning material it is used on.

    a. Class A: ____________________ Used on: ____________________

    b. Class B: ____________________ Used on: ____________________

    c. Class C: ____________________ Used on: ____________________

    d. Class D: ____________________ Used on: ____________________

32. Define *disaster response plan*: ______________________________

    ____

    ____

    ____

33. Name the four colors used on a hazardous material label and state what type of hazard the color represents:

    a. Color: ____________________ Represents: ____________________

    b. Color: ____________________ Represents: ____________________

    c. Color: ____________________ Represents: ____________________

    d. Color: ____________________ Represents: ____________________

34. The medical receptionist needs to maintain a ______________ attitude, react ______________, and follow ______________________________ in a situation that demands immediate attention, such as an office medical emergency.

Critical Thinking Exercises

Study the office situations. Use critical thinking skills, tact, and consideration to determine and record your responses. Indicate the situations you have difficulty handling by circling the corresponding numbers in red and bringing them to class for discussion.

1. An impatient Mr. Griffin complains about being kept waiting. How would you respond? ______________

   ____

   ____

   ____

   ____

   ____

   ____

2. A patient, Mr. Avery, invites you to have lunch with him. What would you do?

3. Despite a "No Smoking" sign, a patient in the waiting room, Mrs. Wilson, lights a cigarette. What would you do or say?

4. An overtalkative patient, Mrs. Crowe, is bothering you while you are trying to complete a number of tasks before the next patient arrives. What would you do?

5. A patient, Mr. Mendez, comes into the reception room, arrives at your desk or window, and asks your advice about some medication he has seen advertised. What would be your response?

6. A patient, Mrs. Jeffers, asks you when she will be through with her treatment. She has just finished seeing the physician and comes to your desk to make her return appointment. What would be your response?

7. Mrs. Jones comes up to your desk and asks you if you think cigarette smoking is harmful. What would you say?

8. A friend of yours stops in to see you at the office and wants to "visit." She remains at your desk for 15 minutes talking. The reception room is full of patients. What would you say?

9. Mr. Carson, a blind patient, comes to your office for medical care. How would you handle this patient during his visit?

10. A patient, Mrs. Jesse Bacon, has just had an appointment and thinks that the physician is withholding information from her. She stops by your desk and inquires, "What do you think the chances are of my returning to work on Monday?" How would you respond?

11. An elderly female patient, accompanied by her husband, has arrived for an emergency appointment. She seems to be in pain and is barely able to walk. What should be your immediate response?

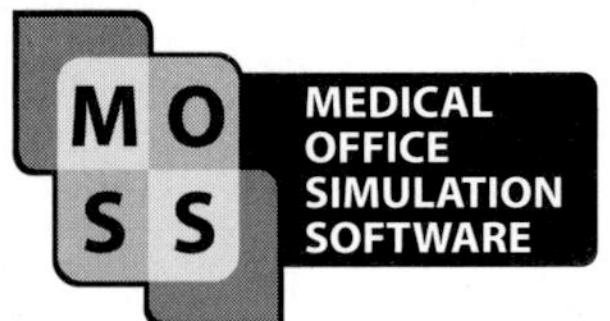

Computer Competency

Getting Started with Medical Office Simulation Software (MOSS) 2.0

Refer to the instructions in Part V of this *Workbook* to install the program. Once installed, double click on the MOSS 2.0 icon on the desktop or select MOSS 2.0 from the Programs list to launch the program. At the logon screen, the username and password is automatically populated for you. Click *OK*. This brings you to the Main Menu, the starting point for all exercises in this *Workbook*. To close MOSS 2.0, click the Exit icon on the top right corner of the Main Menu. Part V of this *Workbook* also contains information on creating backup files, restoring backup databases, and other helpful support information on using the program.

Today's Date Is Monday, 10/21/2013

Simulation: You are the front desk receptionist for Drs. Heath and Schwartz of Douglasville Medicine Associates. Your responsibility this morning is to greet patients as they arrive, check the confidential patient sign-in log, and then review the patient's registration screen in MOSS. Complete the registration information for patients Albertson, Ashby, Ybarra, Merricks, and Cartwright as indicated in each exercise. **You will need to reference the MOSS Source Documents (Insurance Cards and Registration Forms) found at the end of this section to complete the exercises.**

1. Registering Patient Josephine Albertson

Patient Albertson is an existing patient of the practice and Dr. Heath is her physician. Whenever existing patients visit the office, their registration information will need to be reviewed and updated for any changes to address, phone number, or insurance coverage. The office privacy notice will also need to be obtained as required.

A. After greeting Ms. Albertson and checking her in with the sign-in log, review her registration information in MOSS by clicking on *Patient Registration* from the *Main Menu*.

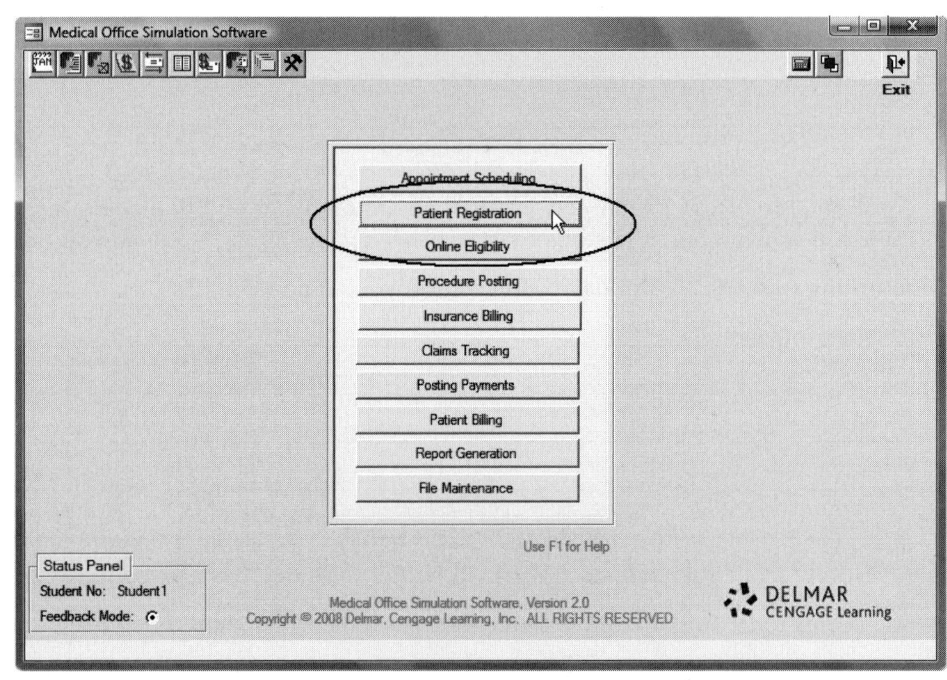

© Cengage Learning 2013

B. The *Patient Registration* search window appears. Highlight her name in the list of existing patients, and click *Select.*

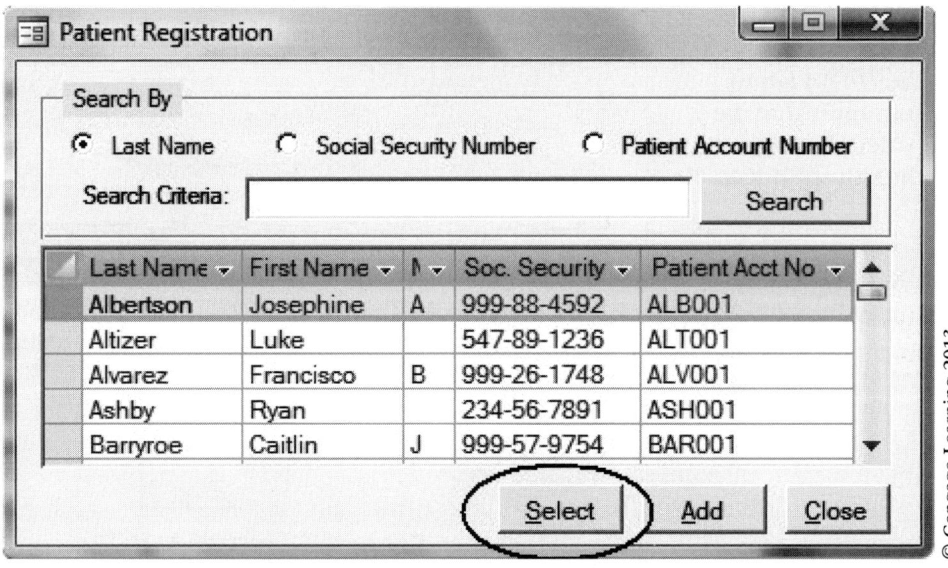

C. Clicking on the tabs along the top of the registration screen allows you to view the information for Ms. Albertson.

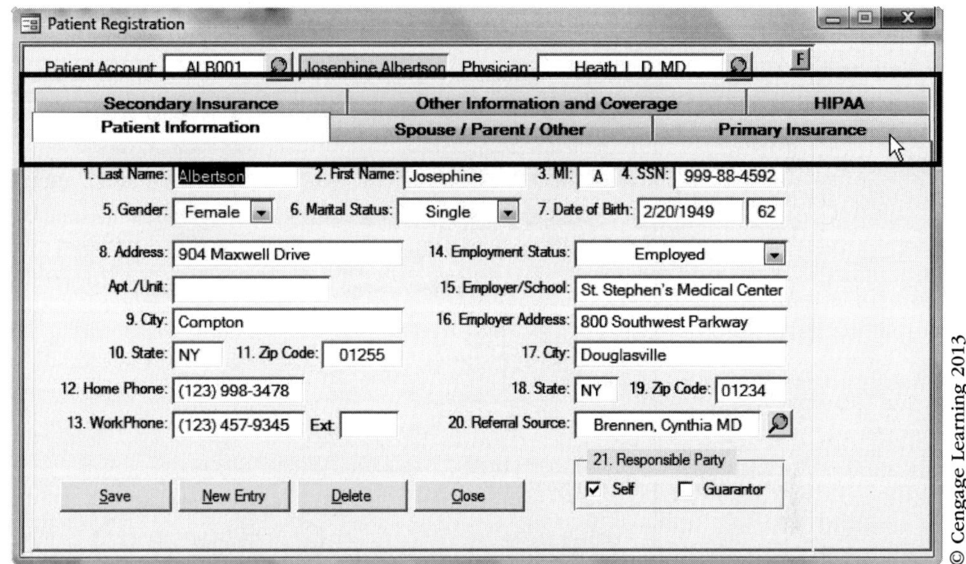

D. The patient advises you that all of her information is current. You will only need to obtain a signed office privacy notice. From the *HIPAA* tab, print a privacy notice for the patient to have, and obtain her signature. Close the privacy notice to return to the *HIPAA* screen.

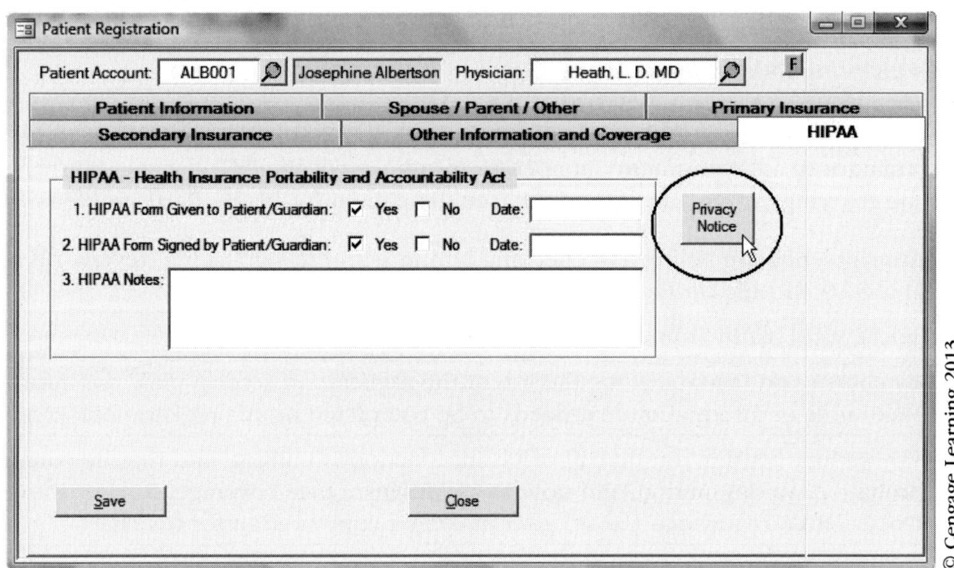

E. Input today's date in Fields 1 and 2 of the *HIPAA* tab to document that the patient has signed the privacy notice.

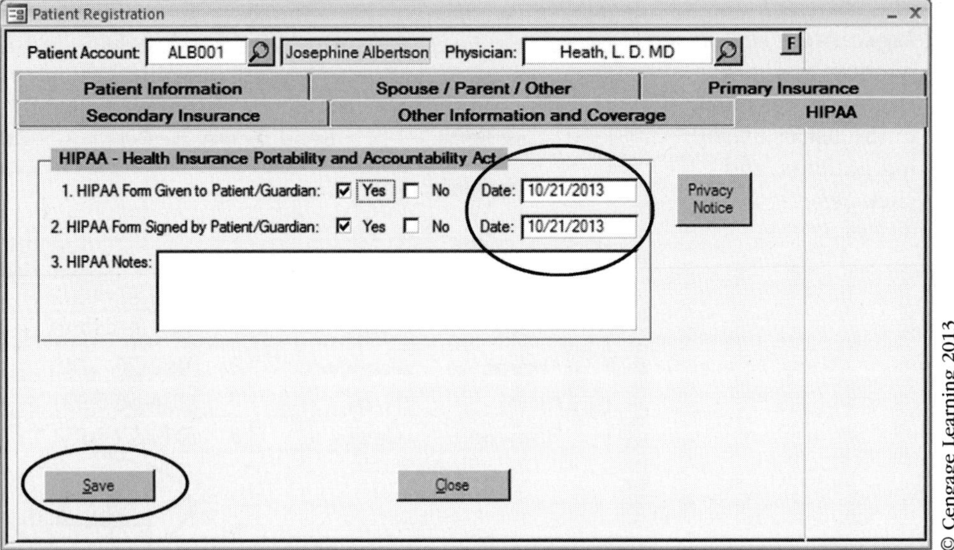

F. Save the record, clicking through all prompts.

G. Click on the *Close* button until you return to the *Main Menu.*

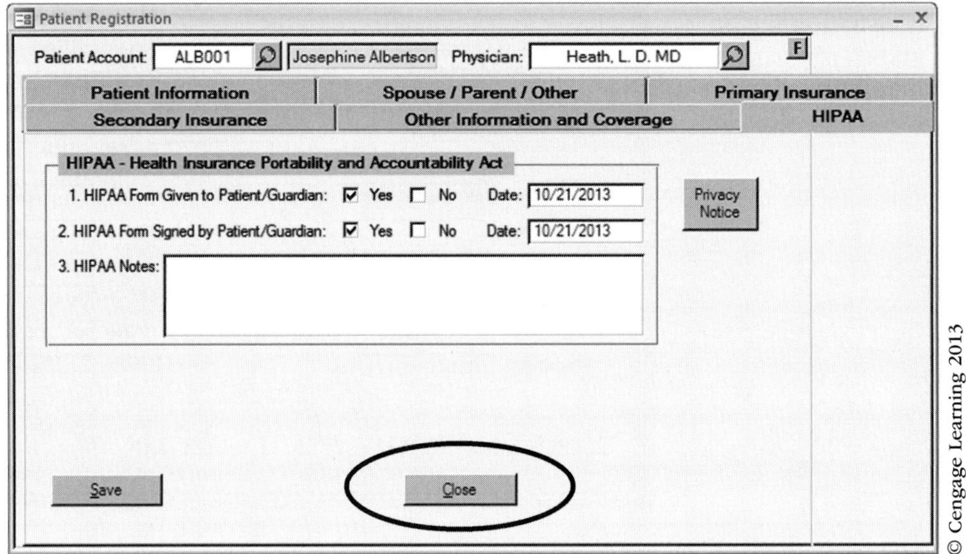

2. Registering Patient Ryan Ashby

Patient Ashby is an existing patient of the practice and Dr. Murray is his primary care physician (PCP). Whenever existing patients visit the office, their registration information will need to be reviewed and updated for any changes to address, phone number, or insurance coverage. Today, Dr. Murray is out of town. Dr. Heath will be covering for Dr. Murray and will see the patient for his medical problem.

A. After greeting Mr. Ashby and checking him in with the sign-in log, review his registration information in MOSS by clicking on *Patient Registration* from the *Main Menu.*

B. Select *Ryan Ashby* from the list of existing patients.

C. By clicking on the tabs along the top of the registration screen, view the information for Mr. Ashby. Make note of information that needs to be completed on his registration screen.

D. The patient advises you that all of his information is current, and that he completed his three-month probation waiting period, and now has HMO insurance coverage. Review the insurance card **(Source Documents: Insurance Cards)** after making a copy or scan for his chart.

E. Enter the information from the insurance card on to the *Primary Insurance* screen in MOSS. Douglasville Medicine Associates participates and takes assignment with Signal HMO Click *Save.*

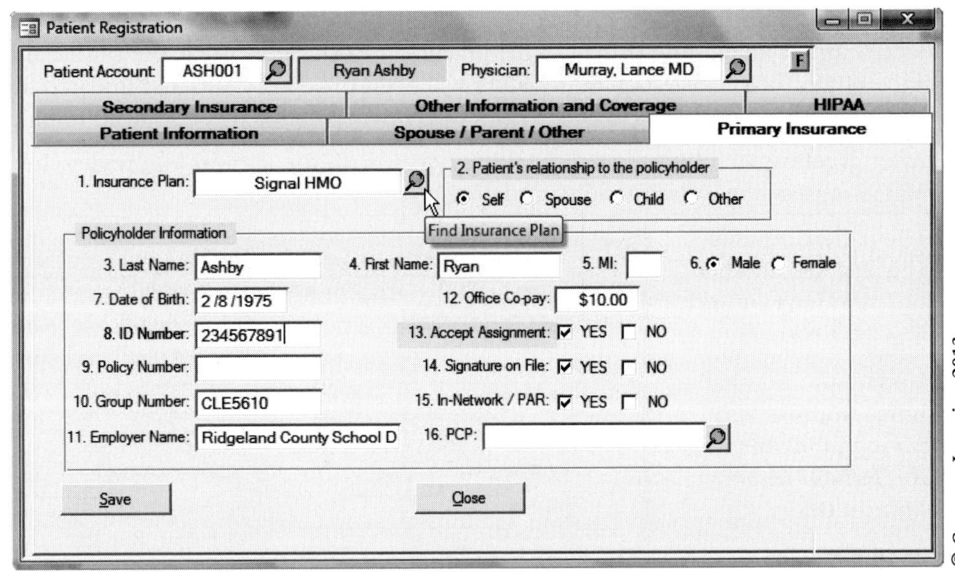

F. Complete the employer address and phone number on the *Patient Information* tab, and *Save.*

Ridgeland County School District

342 N. Industry Way

Douglasville, NY 01236

(123) 521-5561

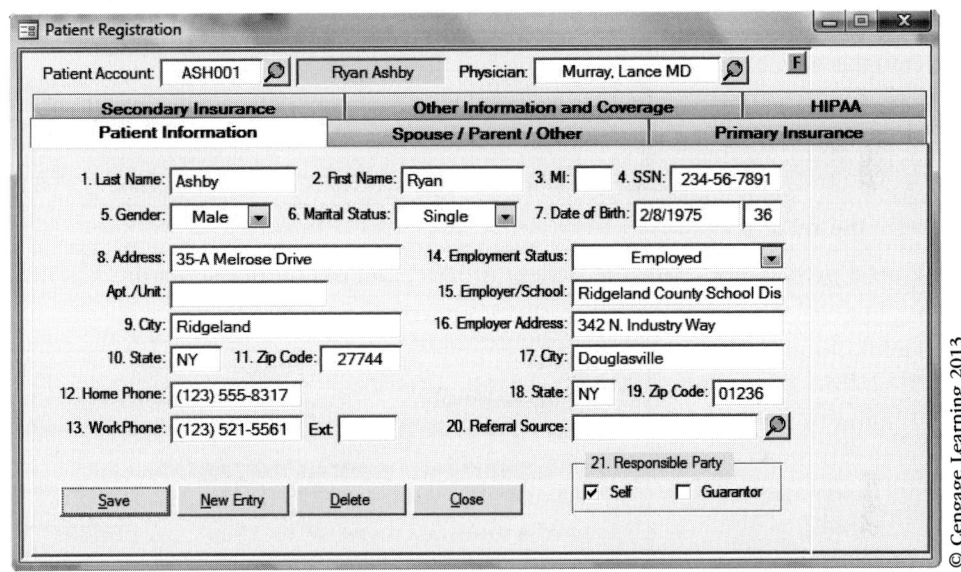

G. Print a copy of the office privacy notice to give to the patient. Provide the date in Fields 1 and 2 of the *HIPAA* tab to indicate that the patient has been given the latest privacy form, and *Save.*

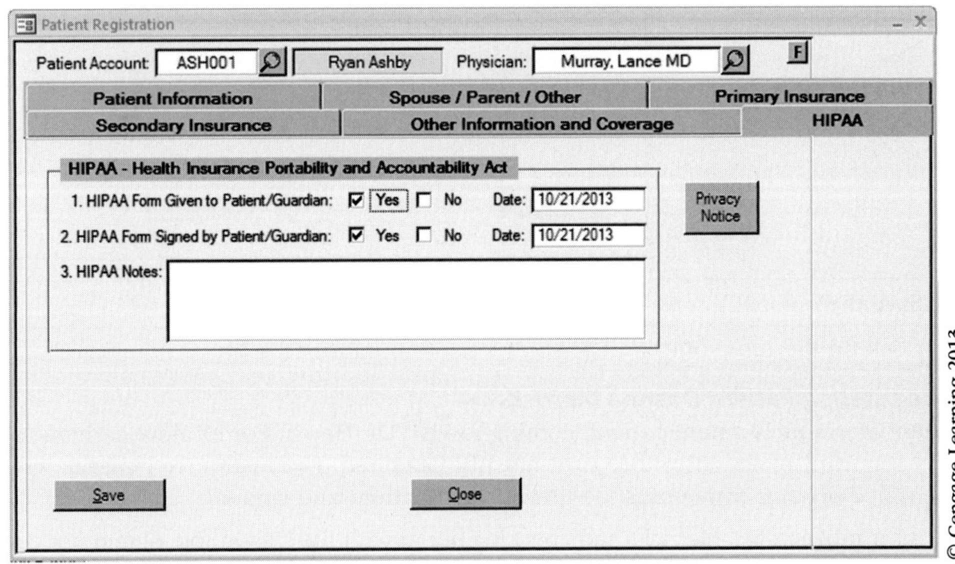

H. Click on the *Close* button until you return to the *Main Menu.*

3. Registering Patient Elane Ybarra

Patient Ybarra is an existing patient of the practice, and Dr. Schwartz is her physician. Whenever existing patients visit the office, their registration information will need to be reviewed and updated for any changes to address, phone number, or insurance coverage. The office privacy notice will also need to be obtained as required.

A. After greeting Mrs. Ybarra and checking her in with the sign-in log, review her registration screen in MOSS for any data that requires updating.

B. The patient advises you that she and her husband have moved to a new address.

Update the new home address and phone number on the *Patient Information* tab.

2518 Slate Drive

Apt. 302

Douglasville, NY 01236

(123) 457-2116

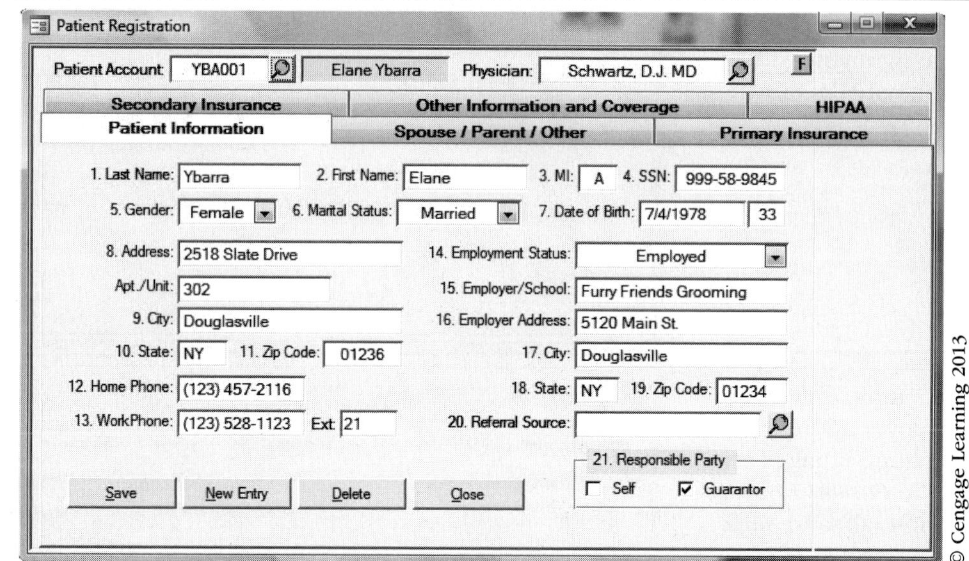

© Cengage Learning 2013

C. Save the record.

D. Print a privacy notice for the patient to have, and obtain her signature.

E. Provide the date in Fields 1 and 2 of the *HIPAA* tab.

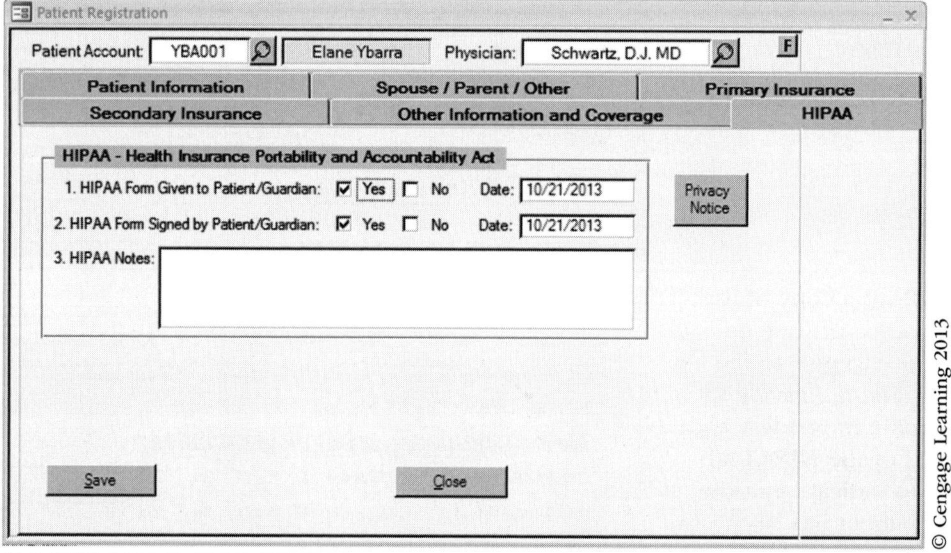

© Cengage Learning 2013

F. Save the record.

G. Click on the *Close* button until you return to the *Main Menu*.

4. Registering Patient Deanna Merricks

Patient Merricks is a new patient, coming to visit Dr. Heath. For all new patients, a registration form and copy (or scan) of the insurance card must be obtained. The insurance benefits will be verified for eligibility. The office privacy notice must be given to the patient and signed.

A. After greeting Ms. Merricks and checking her in with the sign-in log, obtain her completed registration form (**Source Documents: Registration Forms**) and insurance card (**Source Documents: Insurance Cards**).

B. Copy (or scan) the insurance card and return it to the patient.

C. From the patient selection list in *Patient Registration*, click on the *Add* button to add a new patient to MOSS.

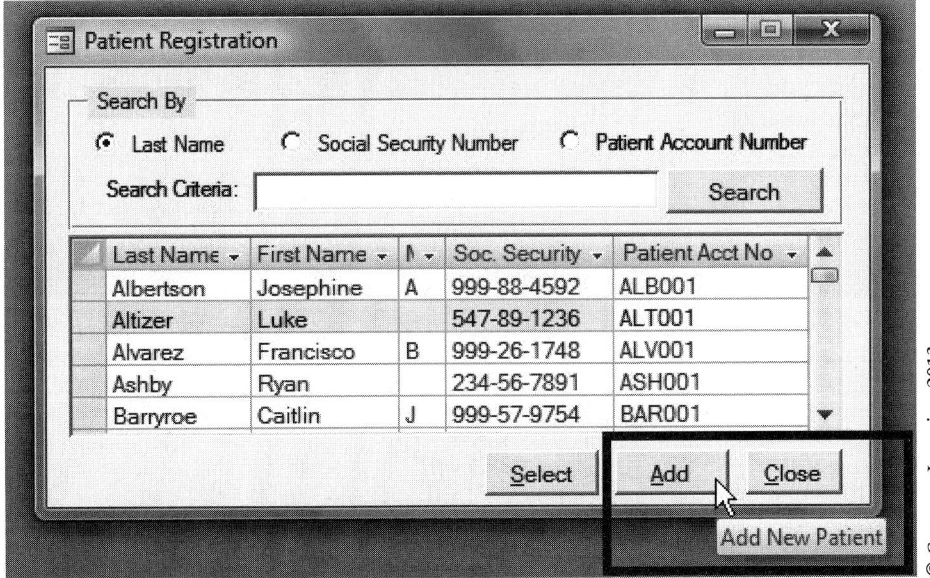

D. Input the demographic information to the *Patient Information* screen, as found on the registration form for *Patient Merricks*.

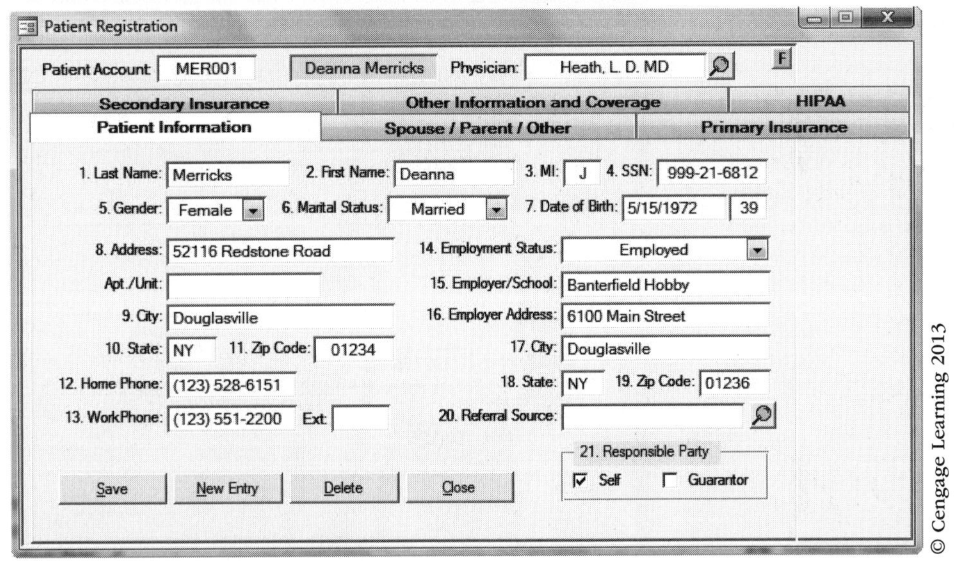

E. Save the record.

F. Input insurance coverage information in the *Primary Insurance* tab. Use the copy of the insurance card to obtain the information. Dr. Heath is a participating physician and takes assignment for this plan.

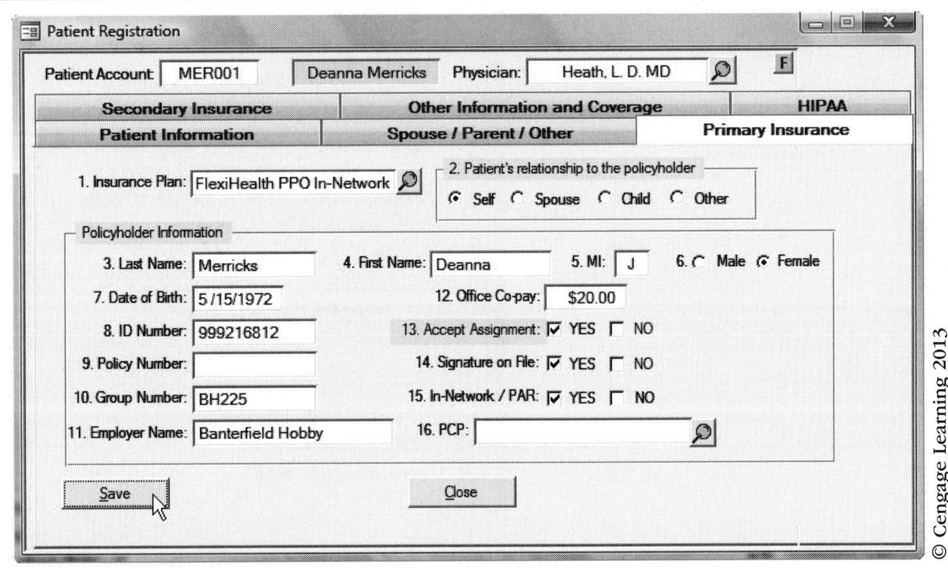

G. Save the record and return to the *Main Menu*.

H. Click on *Online Eligibility* and select *Deanna Merricks*.

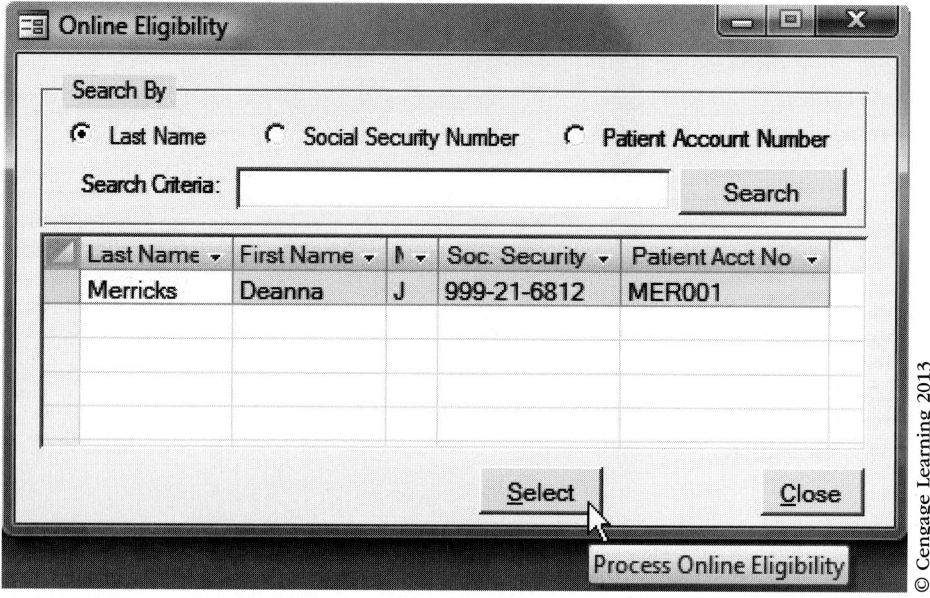

I. To verify benefits, click on *Send to Payer*. MOSS will send the information electronically for eligibility.

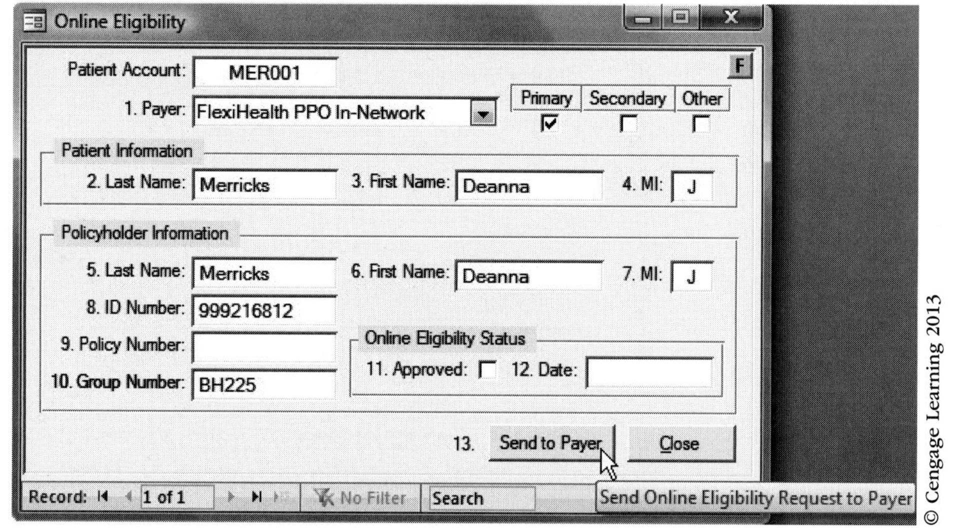

J. View the report, and then print it to include in the patient's file.

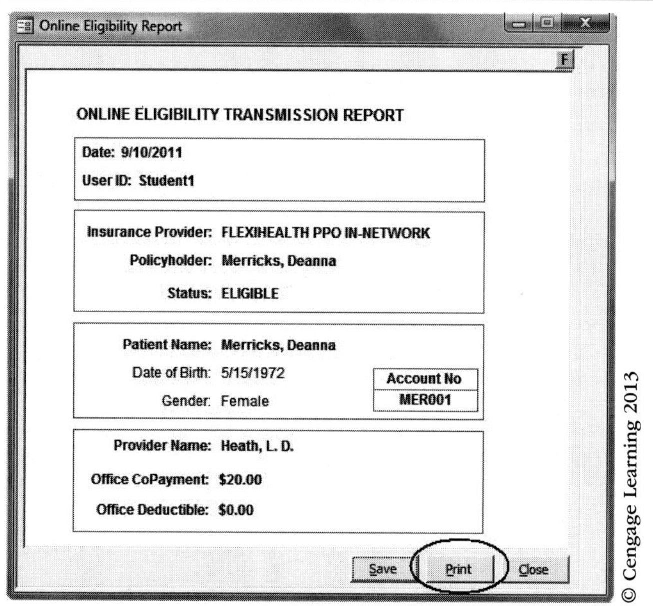

K. Close the *Online Eligibility Report* window, and return to the *Main Menu*. Next, click on *Patient Registration* and select *Patient Merricks*.

L. Print a privacy notice for the patient to have, and obtain her signature.

M. Provide the date in Fields 1 and 2 of the *HIPAA* tab.

N. Save the record.

O. Click on the *Close* button until you return to the *Main Menu*.

5. Registering Patient Tyler Cartwright

Patient Cartwright is a new patient, coming to visit Dr. Heath. For all new patients, a registration form and copy (or scan) of the insurance card must be obtained. The insurance benefits will be verified for eligibility. The office privacy notice must be given to the patient and signed.

A. After greeting Mr. Cartwright and checking him in with the sign-in log, obtain his completed registration form **(Source Documents: Registration Forms)** and insurance card **(Source Documents: Insurance Cards)**.

B. Copy (or scan) the insurance card and return it to the patient.

C. From the patient selection list in *Patient Registration*, click on the *Add* button to add a new patient to MOSS.

D. Input the demographic information to the *Patient Information* screen, as found on the registration form for *Patient Cartwright*.

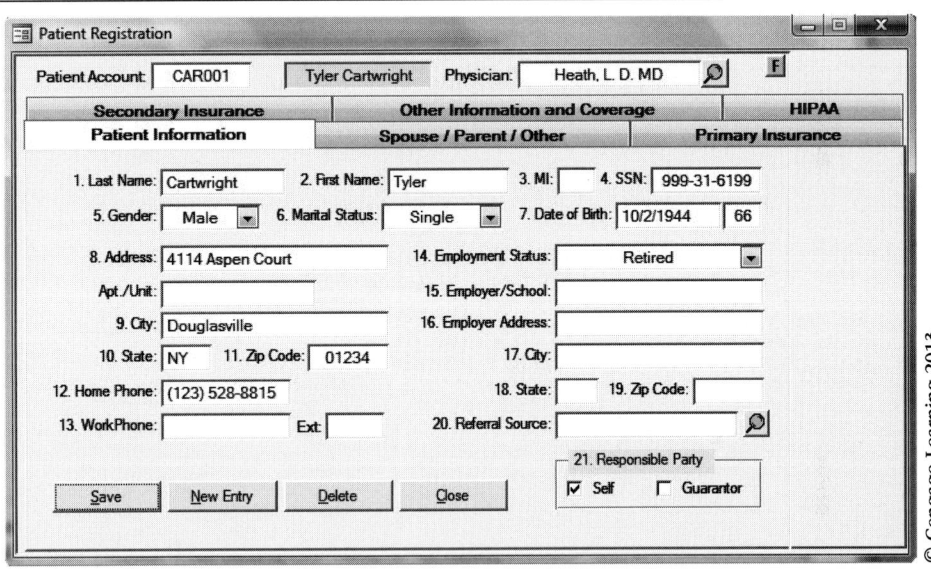

E. Save the record.

F. Input insurance coverage information in the *Primary Insurance* tab. Use the copy of the insurance card to obtain the information. Dr. Heath is a participating physician and takes assignment for this insurance.

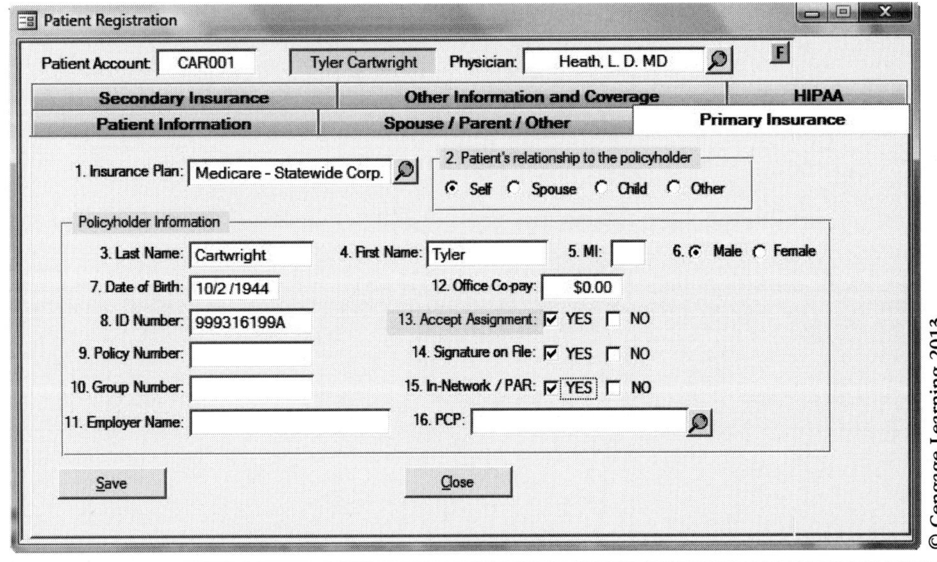

G. Save the record and return to the *Main Menu.*

H. Click on *Online Eligibility* and select *Tyler Cartwright.*

I. To verify benefits, click on *Send to Payer.* MOSS will send the information electronically for eligibility.

J. View the report, and then print it to include in the patient's file.

K. Close the *Online Eligibility Report* window, and return to the *Main Menu.* Next, click on *Patient Registration* and select *Patient Cartwright.*

L. Print a privacy notice for the patient to have, and obtain his signature.

M. Provide the date in Fields 1 and 2 of the *HIPAA* tab.

N. Save the record.

O. Click on the *Close* button until you return to the *Main Menu.*

Computer Competency Source Documents: Insurance Cards

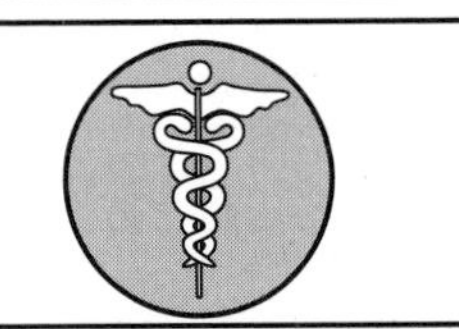

Signal **HMO**

PCP: Douglasville Medicine Associates
L. Murray, M.D.
(123)456-7890

Ryan Ashby 234-56-7891

Copayment Schedule

PCP Office Visits	$ 10.00
Specialists Visits	$ 30.00
Emergency Room	$ 100.00
Hospitalization	Authorization

Preauthorization 800-123-8877

Bank Code
361

Member Group Number: CLE5610

E25/A10
Type of Coverage

Insurer 81564

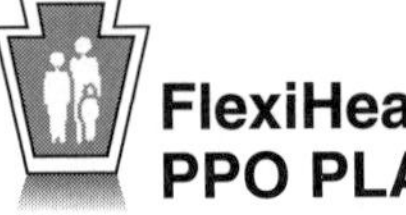

FlexiHealth PPO PLAN

Your Health First SM

Insured: Merricks, Deanna J.
Employer: Banterfield Hobby
Group: BH225

999216812
Network 45A-2

Physician Co-pay: $20.00
Hospital Services: $400.00 Annual deductible.
Surgery & Hospitalization: Requires preauthorization 800-123-3654

MEDICARE 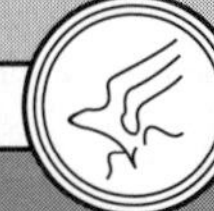 **HEALTH INSURANCE**

HEALTH CARE FINANCING ADMINISTRATION

NAME OF BENEFICIARY
Tyler Cartwright

MEDICARE CLAIM NUMBER
999316199A

SEX
MALE

IS ENTITLED TO

HOSPITAL	(PART A)
MEDICAL	(PART B)

SIGN HERE → *Tyler Cartwright*

Computer Competency Source Documents: Registration Forms

Welcome To Our Office
PLEASE PRINT

NEW PATIENT INFORMATION

Date 10/21/2013

LAST NAME / FIRST NAME / MI	SSN	GENDER	MARITAL STATUS	DATE OF BIRTH
Merricks Deanna J	999216812	Fe	Married	5/15/72

ADDRESS	APT/UNIT	CITY	STATE	ZIP	HOME PH ( )	WORK PH ( ) EXT
52116 Redstone Road		Douglasville	Ny	01234	(123)528-6151	(123)551-2200

EMPLOYER/SCOOL	EMPLOYER ADDRESS	CITY	STATE	ZIP
Banterfield Hobby	6100 Main Street	Douglasville	Ny	01236

REFERRING PHYSICIAN (LAST NAME, FIRST NAME)	ADDRESS	CITY	STATE	ZIP	PHONE

GUARANTOR- Person responsible for payment ☒ self ☐ spouse/other ☐ parent ☐ legal guardian if not "self", please complete the following:

LAST NAME	FIRST NAME	MT	SSN	GENDER	DATE OF BIRTH

ADDRESS (IF DIFFERENT FROM PATIENT)	CITY	STATE	ZIP	HOME PH ( )	ALT. PHONE

EMPLOYER NAME	EMPLOYER ADDRESS	CITY	STATE	ZIP	WORK PHONE EXT

OTHER RESPONSIBLE PARTY:

LAST NAME	FIRST NAME	MI	SSN	GENDER	DATE OF BIRTH	

ADDRESS (IF DIFFERENT FROM PATIENT)	CITY	STATE	ZIP	HOME PH ( )	ALT. PHONE

EMPLOYER NAME	EMPLOYER ADDRESS	CITYSTATE	ZIP	WORK PHONE EXT

INSURANCE - PRIMARY

PLAN NAME	PATIENT RELTIONSHIP TO INSURED:
FlexiHealth PPO	☒ self ☐ spouse ☐ child ☐ other

POLICYHOLDER INFORMATION

LAST NAME / FIRST NAME / MI	DATE OF BIATH	ID #	POLICY #	GROUP #
Merricks Deanna J	5/15/1972	999216812		BH 225
EMPLOYER NAME: Banterfield Hobby	PCP NAME,IF APPLICABLE:			

INSURANCE - SECONDARY

PLAN NAME	PATIENT RELATIONSHIP TO INSURED: ☐ self ☐ spouse ☐ child ☐ other
None	

POLICYHOLDER INFORMATION

LAST NAME / FIRST NAME / MI	DATE OF BIRTH	ID #	POLICY #	GROUP #
EMPLOYER NAME	PCP NAME, IF APPLICABLE:			
ACCIDENT? ☐ YES ☐ NO IF YES, DATE OF INJURY	OCCUR AT WORK? ☐YES ☐ NO	AUTO INVOLVED: ☐YES ☐NO		STATE
NAME OF ATTORNEY	PHONE NUMBER EXT.			

ALL PROFESSIONAL SERVICES RENDERED ARE CHARGED TO THE PATIENT. NECESSARY FORMS WiLL BE COMPLETED TO HELP EXPEDITE INSURANCE CARRIER PAYMENTS. HOWEVER, THE PATIENT IS RESPONSIBLE FDA ALL FEES, REGARDLESS OF INSURANCE COVERAGE. IT IS ALSO CUSTOMARY TO PAY FOR SERVICES WHEN RENDERED UNLESS OTHER ARRANGEMENTS HAVE BEEN MADE IN ADVANCE WITH OUR OFFICE BOOKKEEPER.

INSURANCE AUTHORIZATION AND ASSIGNMENT

Name of Policy holoer Deanna Merricks HIC Number ______

I reuest that payment of authorized medicare/Other Insurance company benefits be made either to me or on my behalf to Dr.Heath for any services furnished me by that party who accepts assignment/physician. Regulations pertaining to Medicare assignment of benefits apply.

I authorize any holder of medical or other information about me to release to the Social Security Administration and CMS or its intermediaries or carriers any information needed for this or a related Medicare claim other Insurance Company claim. I permit a copy of this authorization to be used in place of the original, and request payment of medical insurance benefits either to myself or to the party who accepts assignment. I understand it is mandatory to notify the health care provider of any other party who may be responsible for paying for my treatment. (Section 1128B of the Social Security Act and 31 U.S.C. 3801–3812 provides penalties for withholding this information.) Acknowledgment of Receipt of Privacy Notice - I have been presented with a copy of this provider's Notice of Privacy Policies. detailing how my information may be used and disclosed as permitted under federal and state law. I understand the contents of the notice, and, subject to the following restriction(s) concerning my personal medical Information, I agree to the disclosures named in the Notice;______

Signature Deanna Merricks Date 10/21/2013

Welcome To Our Office **NEW PATIENT INFORMATION** Date 10/21/2013

PLEASE PRINT

LAST NAME	FIRST NAME	MI	SSN	GENDER	MARITAL STATUS	DATE OF BIRTH
Cartwright	Tyler		999-31-6199	Male	Single	10/2/1944

ADDRESS	APT/UNIT	CITY	STATE	ZIP	HOME PH ( )	WORK PH ( ) EXT
4114 Aspen Court		Douglasville	Ny	01234	(123)528-8815	

EMPLOYER/SCOOL	EMPLOYER ADDRESS	CITY	STATE	ZIP
Retired				

REFERRING PHYSICIAN (LAST NAME, FIRST NAME)	ADDRESS	CITY	STATE	ZIP	PHONE

GUARANTOR- Person responsible for payment ☒ self ☐ spouse/other ☐ parent ☐ legal guardian if not "self", please complete the following:

LAST NAME	FIRST NAME	MI	SSN	GENDER	DATE OF BIRTH

ADDRESS (IF DIFFERENT FROM PATIENT)	CITY	STATE	ZIP	HOME PH ( )	ALT. PHONE

EMPLOYER NAME	EMPLOYER ADDRESS	CITY	STATE	ZIP	WORK PHONE EXT

OTHER RESPONSIBLE PARTY:

LAST NAME	FIRST NAME	MI	SSN	GENDER	DATE OF BIRTH	

ADDRESS (IF DIFFERENT FROM PATIENT)	CITY	STATE	ZIP	HOME PH ( )	ALT. PHONE

EMPLOYER NAME	EMPLOYER ADDRESS	CITY	STATE	ZIP	WORK PHONE EXT

INSURANCE - PRIMARY

PLAN NAME	PATIENT RELATIONSHIP TO INSURED:
Medicare- Statewide	☒ self ☐ spouse ☐ chitd ☐ other

POLICYHOLDER INFORMATION

LAST NAME	FIRST NAME	MI	DATE OF BIRTH	ID #	POLICY #	GROUP #
Cartwright	Tyler		10/2/1944	999316199A		
EMPLOYER NAME			PCP NAME,IF APPLICABLE:			
Retired						

INSURANCE - SECONDARY

PLAN NAME	PATIENT RELATIONSHIP TO INSURED ☐ self ☐ spouse ☐ child ☐ other

POLICYHOLDER INFORMATION

LAST NAME	FIRST NAME	MI	DATE OF BIRTH	ID #	POLIY #	GROUP #
EMPLOYER NAME			PCP NAME, IF APPLICBLE:			
ACCIDENT? ☐ YES ☐ NO IF YES, DATE OF INJURY			OCCUR AT WORK? ☐YES ☐ NO	AUTO INVOLED: ☐YES ☐NO		STATE
NAME OF ATTORNEY			PHONE NUMBER EXT.			

ALL PROFESSIONAL SERVICES RENDERED ARE CHARGED TO THE PATIENT. NECESSARY FORMS WiLL BE COMPLETED TO HELP EXPEDITE INSURANCE CARRIER PAYMENTS. HOWEVER, THE PATIENT IS RESPONSIBLE FDA ALL FEES, REGARDLESS OF INSURANCE COVERAGE. IT IS ALSO CUSTOMARY TO PAY FOR SERVICES WHEN RENDERED UNLESS OTHER ARRANGEMENTS HAVE BEEN MADE IN ADVANCE WITH OUR OFFICE BOOKKEEPER.

INSURANCE AUTHORIZATION AND ASSIGNMENT

Name of Policy holoer Tyler Cartwright HIC Number ______

I reuest that payment of authorized medicare/Other Insurance company benefits be made either to me or on my behalf to Dr.Heath for any services furnished me by that party who accepts assignment/physician. Regulations pertaining to Medicare assignment of benefits apply.

I authorize any holder of medical or other information about me to release to the Social Security Administration and CMS or its intermediaries or carriers any information needed for this or a related Medicare claim other Insurance Company claim. I permit a copy of this authorization to be used in place of the original, and request payment of medical insurance benefits either to myself or to the party who accepts assignment. I understand it is mandatory to notify the health care provider of any other party who may be responsible for paying for my treatment. (Section 1128B of the Social Security Act and 31 U.S.C. 3801–3812 provides penalties for withholding this information.) Acknowledgment of Receipt of Privacy Notice - I have been presented with a copy of this provider's Notice of Privacy Policies. detailing how my information may be used and disclosed as permitted under federal and state law. I understand the contents of the notice, and, subject to the following restriction(s) concerning my personal medical Information, I agree to the disclosures named in the Notice;______

Signature Tyler Cartwright Date 10/21/2013

JOB SKILL 5-1
Prepare a Patient Registration Form

Name ______________________________ Date ______________ Score ________

Performance Objective

Task: Become familiar with questions on a patient registration form. Ask a classmate, friend, or family member to write the information requested on the form as one would when visiting a medical office for the first time. Ask for an insurance card and photocopy it if possible. Proofread the form after completion and make corrections or additions to verify that all information is complete.

Conditions: Use Form 2 found in *Workbook* Part II and a pen. Refer to Figure 5-5 and Procedure 5-2 in the *textbook* for an illustration and step-by-step directions.

Standards: Complete all steps listed in this skill in _______ minutes with a minimum score of _______. (Time element and accuracy criteria may be given by instructor.)

Time: **Start:** ____________ **Completed:** ____________ **Total:** ____________ minutes

Scoring: One point for each step performed satisfactorily unless otherwise listed or weighted by instructor.

Directions with Performance Evaluation Checklist

1st Attempt	2nd Attempt	3rd Attempt	
______	______	______	Gather materials (equipment and supplies) listed under "Conditions."
______	______	______	1. Select a classmate, friend, or family member to interview.
______	______	______	2. Direct the person to fill out all areas on the Patient Registration form and put NA in areas that do not apply.
______	______	______	3. Obtain and photocopy insurance card(s) for the file (if possible).
______	______	______	4. Proofread the form for legibility.
____/7	____/7	____/7	5. Verify that the header information (date, account number, insurance number, copayment, work injury, auto accident, date of injury) at the top of the form was completed.
____/20	____/20	____/20	6. Verify that the patient's personal information section is completed and all nonapplicable blanks are marked NA.
____/20	____/20	____/20	7. Verify that the patient's responsible party information section is completed and all nonapplicable blanks are marked NA.
____/20	____/20	____/20	8. Verify that the patient's insurance information section is completed and all nonapplicable blanks are marked NA.
____/3	____/3	____/3	9. Verify that the patient's referral information section is completed and all nonapplicable blanks are marked NA.
____/5	____/5	____/5	10. Verify that the emergency contact section is completed and all nonapplicable blanks are marked NA.
____/4	____/4	____/4	11. Verify that the assignment of benefits name is filled in, the financial agreement is dated and signed, and method of payment is indicated.
______	______	______	Complete within specified time.
____/85	____/85	____/85	**Total points earned** (To obtain a percentage score, divide the total points earned by the number of points possible.)

JOB SKILL 5-1 *(continued)*

Comments:

Evaluator's Signature: ______________________________ **Need to Repeat:** ______________

National Curriculum Competency: CAAHEP: Cognitive: V.C.6	ABHES: 8.a

JOB SKILL 5-2
Prepare an Application Form for a Disabled Person Placard

Name ______________________________ Date ______________ Score ________

Performance Objective

Task: 1. Ask a student, family member, or friend to complete an application form for a disabled person placard, making up a medical condition that is either permanent or temporary; review and verify its completion.

2. Complete the physician portion for physician review and signature.

Conditions: Use Form 3 found in *Workbook* Part II, pen, and the Medical Practice Reference Material found in Part III for physician information. Refer to Figure 5-8 and Procedure 5-3 in the *textbook* for an illustration and step-by-step directions.

Standards: Complete all steps listed in this skill in _______ minutes with a minimum score of _______. (Time element and accuracy criteria may be given by instructor.)

Time: **Start:** ____________ **Completed:** ____________ **Total:** ____________ minutes

Scoring: One point for each step performed satisfactorily unless otherwise listed or weighted by instructor.

Directions with Performance Evaluation Checklist

1st Attempt	2nd Attempt	3rd Attempt	
______	______	______	Gather materials (equipment and supplies) listed under "Conditions."
______	______	______	1. Check to see that the correct box was marked at the top of the form.
____/10	____/10	____/10	2. Complete the applicant's information.
____/2	____/2	____/2	3. Verify that the applicant signed and dated the form.
______	______	______	4. Indicate the reason the patient is applying (1 through 7).
______	______	______	5. Complete the type of disability (temporary, moderate, permanent).
____/7	____/7	____/7	6. Complete the physician's information.
______	______	______	7. Proofread the document before physician review and signature.
______	______	______	Complete within specified time.
____/26	____/26	____/26	**Total points earned** (To obtain a percentage score, divide the total points earned by the number of points possible.)

Comments:

Evaluator's Signature: ______________________________ **Need to Repeat:** ____________

National Curriculum Competency: CAAHEP: Psychomotor: IV.P.13	ABHES: 8.a

JOB SKILL 5-3
Research Community Resources for Patient Referrals and Patient Education

Name ______________________________ Date ______________ Score ________

Performance Objective

Task: Research to determine what materials are available for patient referrals or patient education using the Internet, telephone, or U.S. mail, and order sample items to share with the class.

Conditions: Computer with Internet connection, telephone, or your own stationery and envelope prepared with Practon Medical Group letterhead (Medical Practice Reference Material found in Part III of the *Workbook*). Refer to Procedures 5-4 and 5-5 in the *textbook* for step-by-step directions and the resources listed at the end of the *textbook* chapter.

Standards: Complete all steps listed in this skill in _______ minutes with a minimum score of _______. (Time element and accuracy criteria may be given by instructor.)

Time: **Start:** ____________ **Completed:** ____________ **Total:** ____________ minutes

Scoring: One point for each step performed satisfactorily unless otherwise listed or weighted by instructor.

Directions with Performance Evaluation Checklist

1st Attempt	2nd Attempt	3rd Attempt	
_______	_______	_______	Gather materials (equipment and supplies) listed under "Conditions."
_______	_______	_______	1. Read the resources list at the end of the chapter in the *textbook*.
_______	_______	_______	2. Determine if you would like to research community resources for office referrals or patient education and select a specific topic.
_______	_______	_______	3. Decide whether you will use the Internet, telephone, or write a letter to make a request for resource or patient education material.
____/4	____/4	____/4	4. Contact the appropriate source and determine what resources are available.
_______	_______	_______	5. Request a sample of the item(s) selected.
_______	_______	_______	Complete within specified time.
____/10	____/10	____/10	**Total points earned** (To obtain a percentage score, divide the total points earned by the number of points possible.)

Comments:

Evaluator's Signature: ______________________________ **Need to Repeat:** ____________

National Curriculum Competency: CAAHEP: Psychomotor: XI.P.12	ABHES: 8.e

JOB SKILL 5-4
Assess and Use Proper Body Mechanics

Name ____ Date ______________ Score ________

Performance Objective

Task: List body positions used on the job or in a school setting (i.e., sitting, standing, bending, stooping, lifting) and any repetitive motions used (e.g., computer work). Then assess yourself, naming areas that need changing to comply with ergonomic standards.

Conditions: Refer to the section on ergonomics, Procedure 5-6, and Figure 5-13 through Figure 5-16 in the *textbook*. Work or school environment; computer with printer and paper, pen or pencil.

Standards: Complete all steps listed in this job skill in _______ minutes with a minimum score of _______. (Time element and accuracy criteria may be given by instructor.)

Time: **Start:** _____________ **Completed:** _____________ **Total:** _____________ minutes

Scoring: One point for each step performed satisfactorily unless otherwise listed or weighted by instructor.

Directions with Performance Evaluation Checklist

1st Attempt	2nd Attempt	3rd Attempt	
______	______	______	Gather materials (equipment and supplies) listed under "Conditions."
_____/3	_____/3	_____/3	1. Mentally walk yourself through a work or school day and list all the body positions used. ____ ____
_____/5	_____/5	_____/5	2. Name any repetitive motions you perform. ____
_____/5	_____/5	_____/5	3. Compare the information with the ergonomic standards mentioned or shown in the *textbook*.
_____/5	_____/5	_____/5	4. List areas you need to change to comply with ergonomic standards. ____ ____ ____
_____/3	_____/3	_____/3	5. Determine goals for improving these areas and list ways to remind yourself of ergonomic standards. ____ ____ ____
______	______	______	Complete within specified time.
_____/23	_____/23	_____/23	**Total points earned** (To obtain a percentage score, divide the total points earned by the number of points possible.)

JOB SKILL 5-4 *(continued)*

Comments:

Evaluator's Signature: ______________________ **Need to Repeat:** __________

National Curriculum Competency: CAAHEP: Psychomotor:X1.P.11

JOB SKILL 5-5
Evaluate the Work or School Environment and Develop a Safety Plan

Name ______________________________ Date ______________ Score ________

Performance Objective

Task: Evaluate the work or school environment to identify safe and unsafe working conditions, then develop a plan that provides a safe environment for employees/students and patients.

Conditions: Work or school environment. Refer to "Safe Working Environment" ("Slips, Trips, and Falls" and "Electrical Safety") sections in the *textbook*. Computer with printer and paper; pen or pencil.

Standards: Complete all steps listed in this job skill in ________ minutes with a minimum score of ________. (Time element and accuracy criteria may be given by instructor.)

Time: **Start:** ____________ **Completed:** ____________ **Total:** ____________ minutes

Scoring: One point for each step performed satisfactorily unless otherwise listed or weighted by instructor.

Directions with Performance Evaluation Checklist

1st Attempt	2nd Attempt	3rd Attempt	
______	______	______	Gather materials (equipment and supplies) listed under "Conditions."
____/5	____/5	____/5	1. Perform a walk-through in the office or school setting and look for various areas or objects that could cause an accident.
____/5	____/5	____/5	2. List the dangerous areas or objects that were identified. ________________________________ ________________________________ ________________________________
____/8	____/8	____/8	3. Develop a plan to correct these "risk areas" by naming each area or object and stating what changes need to be made to make the environment safe for workers or students and patients of all ages.
______	______	______	Complete within specified time.
____/20	____/20	____/20	**Total points earned** (To obtain a percentage score, divide the total points earned by the number of points possible.)

Comments:

Evaluator's Signature: ______________________________ **Need to Repeat:** ______________

National Curriculum Competency: CAAHEP: Psychomotor: XI.P.2, 3, 4	ABHES: 8.x

JOB SKILL 5-6
Take Steps to Prevent and Prepare for Fires in a Health Care Setting

Name ______________________________ Date ____________ Score ______

Performance Objective

Task: Follow step-by-step procedures to prevent and prepare for fires in a health care setting.

Conditions: Home, work, or school environment. Refer to *textbook* Procedure 5-7 for step-by-step directions. Computer with printer and paper; pen or pencil.

Standards: Complete all steps listed in this job skill in _______ minutes with a minimum score of _______. (Time element and accuracy criteria may be given by instructor.)

Time: **Start:** ____________ **Completed:** ____________ **Total:** ____________ minutes

Scoring: One point for each step performed satisfactorily unless otherwise listed or weighted by instructor.

Directions with Performance Evaluation Checklist

This job skill may be performed in students' homes rather than in a workplace or school setting. If using a school setting, it may be a collaborative assignment.

1st Attempt	2nd Attempt	3rd Attempt	
_______	_______	_______	Gather materials (equipment and supplies) listed under "Conditions."
_____/2	_____/2	_____/2	1. Conduct a walk-through in your home, workplace, or school setting.
_____/2	_____/2	_____/2	2. Look for and note sources of ignition that contribute to the starting of a fire. ______________________________ ______________________________ ______________________________ ______________________________
_____/2	_____/2	_____/2	3. Look for and note sources of fuel that contribute to the starting of a fire. ______________________________ ______________________________ ______________________________ ______________________________
_____/2	_____/2	_____/2	4. Look for and note sources of oxygen that contribute to the starting of a fire. ______________________________ ______________________________ ______________________________
_____/22	_____/22	_____/22	5. Use the following items listed in Procedure 5-7 as a checklist to prepare for a fire. Indicate a checkmark (✓) when you have completed each of the following (2 points each). Write NA (not applicable) if it does not apply. _____ a. Posted the fire department telephone number. _____ b. Became familiar with the location and operation of fire alarms. _____ c. Learned the location and operation of all fire extinguishers. _____ d. Tested smoke detectors and sprinkler systems.

JOB SKILL 5-6 *(continued)*

_____ e. Developed a floor plan marking the location of fire alarms, fire extinguishers, smoke detectors, stairwells, and routes out of the home, office, or school.

_____ f. Memorized and posted evacuation routes.

_____ g. Determined evacuation procedures for patients with special needs.

_____ h. Ensured good housekeeping practices.

_____ i. Trained or received training and practiced fire drills.

_____ j. Memorized the path between your bed (in a home setting), workstation, or desk and the nearest exit route.

_____ k. Established a meeting place for family members, employees, or students in the event of an evacuation.

_______ _______ _______ Complete within specified time.

____/32 ____/32 ____/32 **Total points earned** (To obtain a percentage score, divide the total points earned by the number of points possible.)

Comments:

Evaluator's Signature: ______________________________ **Need to Repeat:** ______________

National Curriculum Competency: CAAHEP: Psychomotor: XI.P.8

JOB SKILL 5-7
Demonstrate Proper Use of a Fire Extinguisher

Name ______________________________ Date ______________ Score ________

Performance Objective

Task: Demonstrate proper use of a fire extinguisher.

Conditions: Fire extinguisher (can simulate). Refer to *textbook* Procedure 5-8 for step-by-step directions. Computer with printer and paper; pen or pencil.

Standards: Complete all steps listed in this job skill in _______ minutes with a minimum score of _______. (Time element and accuracy criteria may be given by instructor.)

Time: **Start:** ____________ **Completed:** ____________ **Total:** ____________ minutes

Scoring: One point for each step performed satisfactorily unless otherwise listed or weighted by instructor.

Directions with Performance Evaluation Checklist

Scenario: A patient threw a cigarette in a wastebasket in the waiting room of the medical office where you are working. You are the receptionist and saw smoke coming from the basket. You left your desk and by the time you got there a small fire had started. You have several fire extinguishers in the hallway near the waiting room.

1st Attempt	2nd Attempt	3rd Attempt	
_____	_____	_____	Gather materials (equipment and supplies) listed under "Conditions."
____/2	____/2	____/2	1. Select and note the classification of the proper fire extinguisher. ______________________ ______________________
____/6	____/6	____/6	2. Get a ______________________ and successfully demonstrate the steps to put out the fire (you can talk your way through the demonstration indicating what you are doing).
____/2	____/2	____/2	3. Stand ________ feet from the fire.
____/2	____/2	____/2	4. Face the fire with your back to the ______________________.
____/2	____/2	____/2	5. Release the locking mechanism by ______________________.
____/2	____/2	____/2	6. Aim the nozzle at ______________________.
____/2	____/2	____/2	7. Use a ________________ motion until the fire is completely out.
_____	_____	_____	Complete within specified time.
____/20	____/20	____/20	**Total points earned** (To obtain a percentage score, divide the total points earned by the number of points possible.)

Comments:

Evaluator's Signature: ______________________________ **Need to Repeat:** ____________

National Curriculum Competency: CAAHEP: Psychomotor: IX.P.5.b

JOB SKILL 5-8
Determine Potential Disaster Hazards in Your Local Community

Name ______________________________ Date ______________ Score ________

Performance Objective

Task: Evaluate your local community to determine potential hazards and name associated risks.

Conditions: Refer to Procedure 5-9 in the *textbook* for specific guidance. Computer with Internet connection and printer with paper; pen or pencil.

Standards: Complete all steps listed in this job skill in _______ minutes with a minimum score of ________. (Time element and accuracy criteria may be given by instructor.)

Time: **Start:** ____________ **Completed:** ____________ **Total:** ____________ minutes

Scoring: One point for each step performed satisfactorily unless otherwise listed or weighted by instructor.

Directions with Performance Evaluation Checklist

1st Attempt	2nd Attempt	3rd Attempt	
______	______	______	Gather materials (equipment and supplies) listed under "Conditions."
____/3	____/3	____/3	1. Use the list in *textbook* Procedure 5-9 (No. 3) to explore potential hazards in your local community (e.g., earthquakes, tornadoes).
____/5	____/5	____/5	2. Refer to the *Resources* section at the end of Chapter 5 in the *textbook* to locate various Web sites that help determine what risks your region may be exposed to.
____/5	____/5	____/5	3. Use your favorite search engine to look for more information regarding hazards in your area.
____/5	____/5	____/5	4. List all potential hazards found. ________________________________ ________________________________ ________________________________
______	______	______	Complete within specified time.
___/20	___/20	___/20	**Total points earned** (To obtain a percentage score, divide the total points earned by the number of points possible.)

Comments:

Evaluator's Signature: ______________________________ **Need to Repeat:** ______________

National Curriculum Competency: CAAHEP: Psychomotor: XI.P.7

JOB SKILL 5-9
Develop an Emergency Response Template with an Evacuation Plan

Name ______________________________ Date ______________ Score ________

Performance Objective

Task: To develop an emergency response template that can be used with various hazards and determine an evacuation plan, including drawing a diagram of the medical office or school with escape routes.

Conditions: Refer to Procedure 5-9 in the *textbook*. Computer with printer; paper and pen or pencil.

Standards: Complete all steps listed in this job skill in ________ minutes with a minimum score of ________. (Time element and accuracy criteria may be given by instructor.)

Time: **Start:** ____________ **Completed:** ____________ **Total:** ____________ minutes

Scoring: One point for each step performed satisfactorily unless otherwise listed or weighted by instructor.

Directions with Performance Evaluation Checklist

In Steps 1 through 10 you will be developing a generic emergency response template that can be used with various types of emergencies. In Step 11, this job skill can be coupled with Job Skill 5-8 in order to develop actions tailored to the specific risks discovered in your region. This step is optional so completion points have not been assigned.

1st Attempt	2nd Attempt	3rd Attempt	
______	______	______	Gather materials (equipment and supplies) listed under "Conditions."
______	______	______	1. Determine what facility you will use for this exercise (i.e., office or school).
___/18	___/18	___/18	2. Refer to Procedure 5-9 and list the following:

a. Capacity of facility: ______________________________

____

b. Safe places inside and outside facility: ______________________________

____

____

____

c. Alternative site for operation: ______________________________

____

d. Services most likely used during an emergency: ______________________________

____

____

e. Location of quarantine housing: ______________________________

____

____

f. Procedures for closing facility: ______________________________

____

____

JOB SKILL 5-9 *(continued)*

_____/10 _____/10 _____/10 3. State emergencies that may require partial or full evacuation, then draw a diagram of the medical office or school with fire alarms and extinguishers, exits, and escape routes clearly marked (attach).

_____/5 _____/5 _____/5 4. Name emergency supplies needed in the facility. ____________________

____

____

____

_____/5 _____/5 _____/5 5. Identify the role of employees involved in evacuating patients and visitors and define expectations. ____________________

____

____

____

____

_____/2 _____/2 _____/2 6. State where the command post is and who is in command. ____________

____

_____/2 _____/2 _____/2 7. What lines of communication will be used? ____________________

____

_____/5 _____/5 _____/5 8. Write a script for the telephone answering machine. ____________

____

____

____

_____/3 _____/3 _____/3 9. State criteria for calling an end to the emergency and reopening the facility. ____________________

____

_____/2 _____/2 _____/2 10. Identify relevant psychological and emotional issues that may be experienced by responders. ____________________

____

____

Optional: Instructor assigns points 11. Develop an Emergency Operations Plan (EOP) for all potential hazards identified in Job Skill 5-8. Tailor each plan according to specific needs (attach plan).

_______ _______ _______ Complete within specified time.

____/55 ____/55 ____/55 **Total points earned** (To obtain a percentage score, divide the total points earned by the number of points possible.)

Comments:

Evaluator's Signature: ____________________ **Need to Repeat:** ____________

National Curriculum Competency: CAAHEP: Psychomotor: XI.P.7; Affective: XI.A.1, 2

CHAPTER 6

Telephone Procedures

OBJECTIVES

After completing the exercises, the student will be able to:

1. Write meanings for chart note abbreviations.
2. Enhance spelling skills by learning new medical words.
3. Screen incoming telephone calls (Job Skill 6-1).
4. Prepare telephone message forms (Job Skill 6-2).
5. Document telephone messages and physician responses (Job Skill 6-3).
6. Role-play telephone scenario(s) (Job Skill 6-4).

FOCUS ON CERTIFICATION*

CMA Content Summary

- Telephone modalities for incoming and outgoing data
- Prioritizing incoming and outgoing data
- Telephone techniques for incoming calls
- Telephone screening
- Maintaining confidentiality while on the telephone
- Gathering data over the telephone
- Multiple-line competency
- Transferring appropriate calls
- Identifying caller, office, and self
- Taking messages
- Ending telephone calls
- Monitoring special calls (problem calls/emergency calls)

*This *Workbook* and the accompanying *textbook* meet the entry-level administrative and general competencies for the CMA outlined by the AAMA Examination Content Outline and Occupational Analysis and for the RMA and CMAS outlined by the AMT Competencies, Construction Parameters, and Examination Specifications (see Competency Grid in Appendix B of the *textbook*).

RMA Content Summary

- Employ appropriate telephone etiquette
- Perform appropriate telephone techniques
- Instruct patient via telephone
- Inform patients of test results per physician instruction
- Employ active listening skills

CMAS Content Summary

- Address and process incoming telephone calls from outside providers, pharmacies, and vendors
- Employ appropriate telephone etiquette when screening patient calls and addressing office business
- Recognize and employ proper protocols for telephone emergencies

STOP AND THINK CASE SCENARIOS AND EXAM-STYLE REVIEW QUESTIONS

Refer to the end of Chapter 6 in the *textbook*.

Abbreviation and Spelling Review

Read the following patient's chart note and write the meanings for the abbreviations listed below the note. To decode any abbreviations you do not understand or that appear unfamiliar to you, refer to the list of abbreviations in Part IV of this *Workbook*. Step-by-step directions for this exercise are found in Procedure 1-1 of Chapter 1 in the *textbook*. Medical terms in the chart note are italicized; study them for spelling. Use your medical dictionary to look up their definitions. Your instructor may give a spelling and definition test that includes these words and abbreviations.

John F. Mason

October 15, 20XX, Pt comes in PO complaining of *anorexia, nausea, & stomatitis.* CBC reveals RBC 80–90, WBC 60–80, Hgb 17 g/100 ml. Applied $AgNO_3$. Wound healing well. Cont. med. Ordered BUN. Retn 3 days. RO *uremia.*

Gerald Practon, MD

Gerald Practon, MD

Pt	______	ml	______
PO	______	$AgNO_3$	______
CBC	______	Cont.	______
RBC	______	med.	______
WBC	______	BUN	______
Hgb	______	retn	______
g	______	RO	______

Review Questions

Review the objectives, glossary, and chapter information before completing the following review questions.

1. What are three voice components to consider when practicing telephone technique and cultivating a cheerful and calm voice?

 a. ______________ b. ______________ c. ______________

2. What are the two basic things to consider when choosing a telephone system?

 a. ______________

 b. ______________

3. Give four reasons the physician might choose to use a cellular telephone.

 a. ______________

 b. ______________

 c. ______________

 d. ______________

4. All incoming calls should be answered before the ______________ ring.

5. When speaking to an elderly caller, you should be prepared to ______________

 ____

6. When placing outgoing calls, you should always plan your conversation and______________

 ____

7. Name five ways to ensure confidentiality when leaving a message in a voice mail system.

 a. ______________

 b. ______________

 c. ______________

 d. ______________

 e. ______________

8. How does an answering service assist the medical office?______________

 ____

9. Name and define two types of critical situations requiring medical care.

 a. ______________

 ____

 b. ______________

 ____

10. List five telephone procedures that might be discussed in an information booklet presented to a patient on his or her first visit to the office.

  a. ______________________________
  b. ______________________________
  c. ______________________________
  d. ______________________________
  e. ______________________________

11. When telephone lines are busy and calls have to be placed on hold, list several things to consider and actions to take.

  a. ______________________________
  b. ______________________________
  c. ______________________________
  d. ______________________________
  e. ______________________________
  f. ______________________________
  g. ______________________________

12. Name five things that should be included when recording information on a telephone message slip.

  a. ______________________________
  b. ______________________________
  c. ______________________________
  d. ______________________________
  e. ______________________________

13. If no action has been taken on a patient call during the day, what should you do so that the call will not be overlooked in a telephone log? ______________________________

14. Define *conference call* and discuss the procedures for setting up this type of call. ______________________________

Critical Thinking Exercises

1. Dr. Practon reproaches you for having forgotten to make a telephone call he asked you to make. What would you say? ______________________________

2. A patient, Mrs. Braun, wishes to use the physician's telephone. You know she is a talkative person. How would you handle this situation? ____

____

____

____

____

____

3. You are the administrative medical assistant for Drs. Fran and Gerald Practon. Simulate using a telephone to role-play the following scenarios:
   a. Dr. Gerald Practon has asked you to call Marilyn Macy to let her know that her thyroid tests came back normal. She is not home and you reach her answering machine. Leave a message following voice mail guidelines. Later, she calls the office and asks to speak with you. Answer the telephone and tell her the results of her lab work.
   b. You receive a telephone call from Dr. Fran Practon's patient Samantha Delong. She would like to book an appointment for next week; however, before you can schedule her, the telephone rings again and it is Dr. Armstrong, who wants to speak to Dr. Gerald Practon immediately.

JOB SKILL 6-1
Screen Incoming Telephone Calls

Name ______________________________ Date ______________ Score ________

Performance Objective

Task: To screen incoming telephone calls and determine the person or persons the calls should be transferred to.

Conditions: *Textbook* Table 6-1; pen or pencil.

Standards Complete all steps listed in this skill in ________ minutes with a minimum score of ________. (Time element and accuracy criteria may be given by instructor.)

Time: **Start:**____________ **Completed:** ____________ **Total:** ____________ minutes

Scoring: One point for each step performed satisfactorily unless otherwise listed or weighted by instructor.

Directions with Performance Evaluation Checklist

Refer to the *Telephone Decision Grid* (Table 6-1) in the *textbook* to aid in determining how the receptionist would screen and transfer incoming telephone calls. Members of the staff are the physician (MD), office manager (OM), certified medical assistant (CMA [AAMA]), insurance supervisor (INS), and bookkeeper (BK). Write the abbreviations of all those who would be appropriate to receive each telephone call in the space provided. If a message slip would be appropriate, place a check mark on the line (✓).

1st Attempt	2nd Attempt	3rd Attempt	Transfer Call to	Telephone Call Description
			MD OM CMA (AAMA) INS BK	
______	______	______	Gather materials (equipment and supplies) listed under "Conditions."	
______	______	______	1. ______	Daughter wants to talk to her father, the physician, and he is with a patient.
______	______	______	2. ______	Doctor is on another line when a nurse at the hospital telephones regarding a patient. After determining urgency, to whom should the call be directed?
______	______	______	3. ______	New patient, ill, wants to speak to physician about recently prescribed medication.
______	______	______	4. ______	Patient requests laboratory test results.
______	______	______	5. ______	Insurance carrier requests patient information.
______	______	______	6. ______	Doctor's wife calls to inquire about time of medical association dinner, and doctor is involved with an emergency situation.
______	______	______	7. ______	Patient telephones about a recent bill.
______	______	______	8. ______	Pharmacy telephones regarding a new prescription.
______	______	______	9. ______	Attorney telephones physician regarding malpractice matter.
______	______	______	10. ______	Professional society member calls for physician.
______	______	______	11. ______	A mother calls about a child who has sunburn.
______	______	______	12. ______	Pharmacy requests Rx refill for patient.

JOB SKILL 6-1 *(continued)*

______	______	______	13. ______	Family member asks for information about a child who is under the doctor's care.
______	______	______	14. ______	Patient requests telephone consultation with physician, who is out of the office.
______	______	______	15. ______	Pharmaceutical representative asks to make an appointment with physician for sales presentation.
______	______	______	16. ______	Another doctor desires to talk to physician, who is available.
______	______	______	17. ______	OSHA representative calls about making visit to do inspection.
______	______	______	18. ______	Established patient asks to talk to physician, who is unable to take the call.
______	______	______	19. ______	Accountant telephones regarding tax records.
______	______	______	20. ______	Established patient requests Rx refill.
______	______	______	21. ______	Established patient calls to report chest pain.
______	______	______	22. ______	Nurse at convalescent home calls regarding a patient refusing all medications.
______	______	______	23. ______	Telephone referral request is received from another physician, and your doctor is with a patient.
______	______	______	24. ______	Dentist calls to ask if doctor's patient is taking a new drug.
______	______	______	25. ______	Former office employee telephones to request a recommendation for a job.
____/5	____/5	____/5	26. ______	Put check mark by those needing message slips.
______	______	______	Complete within specified time.	
____/32	____/32	____/32	**Total points earned** (To obtain a percentage score, divide the total points earned by the number of points possible.)	

Comments:

Evaluator's Signature: ______________________________ **Need to Repeat:** ______________

National Curriculum Competency: CAAHEP: Psychomotor: I.P.6	ABHES: 9.o.3

JOB SKILL 6-2
Prepare Telephone Message Forms

Name ______________________ Date __________ Score ______

Performance Objective

Task: Evaluate the following incoming telephone calls and determine action to be taken on each call. Complete message forms for all calls that require the transfer of information to message slips.

Conditions: Message slips (Forms 4 through 7 in Part II of the *Workbook*). Refer to Figure 6-5 in the *textbook* for a visual illustration; pen or pencil.

Standards: Complete all steps listed in this skill in _______ minutes with a minimum score of ________. (Time element and accuracy criteria may be given by instructor.)

Time: **Start:** ____________ **Completed:** ____________ **Total:** ____________ minutes

Scoring: One point for each step performed satisfactorily unless otherwise listed or weighted by instructor.

Directions with Performance Evaluation Checklist

It is the morning of Tuesday, November 6, (current year), and both physicians (Fran Practon, MD, and Gerald Practon, MD) are at the hospital and will not be in the office until 1 p.m. Determine which calls may be taken care of immediately (e.g., by making an appointment) and which calls need information transferred to a message slip. Then, indicate what action has been taken on each telephone call and write it on the line following the call (message F.P., made appt., or other action). If a message should be taken, record the necessary information (name of patient and caller, telephone number, if chart is attached, and so forth) on the left portion of the form. Be sure to indicate the date and time of the call and your initials.

On the right portion of the form, record who the message is for (i.e., G.P. or F.P.) and compose the message in a complete but brief statement or question. Refer to call No. 0 for an example:

EXAMPLE

0. (9:15) Marguerite Houston (Mrs. C. F. Houston) calls and sounds upset. She wants to ask Dr. Gerald Practon if she can discontinue the medication he prescribed Friday because she thinks she is allergic to it; she now has a rash on her face. She is due to take her next dose tomorrow morning. You have told her that the doctor is not in the office and that you will ask him to call her (678-7892) as soon as he comes in.

EXAMPLE

	Name of Caller	Tel. #	Reason for Call	Action Taken
Call No. 0	*Marguerite Houston*	*678-7892*	*Can she discontinue medication? Rash on face.*	*Message GP*

PRIORITY ☐

PATIENT Marguerite Houston AGE

CALLER " "

TELEPHONE 678-7892

REFERRED TO

CHART #

CHART ATTACHED ☒ YES ☐ NO

DATE Nov. 6, 20XX TIME 9:15 REC'D BY B.C.

Copyright © 1978 Bibbero Systems, Inc.
Printed in the U.S.A.

TELEPHONE RECORD

MESSAGE G.P.

Rash on face - possibly allergic to newly prescribed medication - call asap.

TEMP ALLERGIES

RESPONSE

PHY/RN INITIALS DATE / / TIME HANDLED BY

FIGURE 6-1

JOB SKILL 6-2 *(continued)*

1st Attempt	2nd Attempt	3rd Attempt	
______	______	______	Gather materials (equipment and supplies) listed under "Conditions."
____/10	____/10	____/10	1. (9:35) Donald Eggert (765-3145) asks to speak to Dr. Fran Practon. He wants to make an appointment for an injection next week. ______________________
____/10	____/10	____/10	2. (9:40) A person calls and refuses to identify himself. He requests information on a patient, Marilyn Turner. ______________________
____/10	____/10	____/10	3. (9:55) A patient, Bruce Jeffers (486-2468), calls to cancel his appointment with Dr. Gerald Practon that is scheduled for this afternoon because he has to leave on a flight to New York tomorrow (N.Y. phone: 542-671-0121). He will make another appointment upon his return late next week. He would like to know what to do about the series of daily injections he has been receiving from Dr. Practon. ______________________
____/10	____/10	____/10	4. (9:58) Phyllis Sperry (678-1162) wants to know the results of the Pap test taken last week by Dr. Fran Practon. (You can find these results in the file and they are normal.) ______________________
____/10	____/10	____/10	5. (10:15) Mr. G. W. Witte (678-5478) represents the General Surgical Supply Company and wants to show the doctors a new instrument. You have suggested he call the next day when you will let him know whether either of the physicians will be able to talk to him or schedule an appointment. ______________________
____/10	____/10	____/10	6. (10:20) Midway Pharmacy (649-3762) calls Dr. Fran Practon and wants to know if a refill is allowed on Philip Stevenson Jr. 's prescription for sleeping pills, No. 8711342. ______________________
____/10	____/10	____/10	7. (10:25) Sylvia Cone (411-8215) calls and asks to speak to Dr. Gerald Practon. She refuses to leave a message and says that it is urgent. ______________________
____/10	____/10	____/10	8. (10:55) Charles Jones (487-6650) calls to ask if the Practons can recommend an eye, ear, and nose specialist. (There is a reference sheet near the telephone.) ______________________
____/10	____/10	____/10	9. (11:00) Mary Lu Practon, the Practons' 14-year-old daughter, calls to report that she is going to Disneyland with the Cone family for the day. She will return home about 9:00 p.m. (Cones' cell phone: 555-678-9000). ______________________
____/10	____/10	____/10	10. (11:05) Betty Knott (678-0076) calls to ask if Dr. Gerald Practon will donate time to give flu injections next Sunday from either 9 to 12 or 1 to 3. She needs to know as soon as possible. She is calling

JOB SKILL 6-2 *(continued)*

from the Reseda Red Cross office on Sepulveda Boulevard, where the injections are to be given.

____

____/10 ____/10 ____/10 11. (11:18) Alan Becker (486-9993) calls and is upset about the bill he received today from Dr. Fran Practon. He thinks the amount is exorbitant, and he asks to speak to Dr. Practon or someone with authority.

____

____/10 ____/10 ____/10 12. (11:20) Patricia Papakostikus (687-4512) calls the office to make an appointment. She is having daily headaches.

____

____/10 ____/10 ____/10 13. (11:30) Dr. Martin Laird (643-1108) calls to ask if Dr. Gerald Practon would like a ride to the AMA meeting tonight. Dr. Practon should let Dr. Laird know before 4:00 p.m.

____

____/10 ____/10 ____/10 14. (11:45) Elizabeth Montague (411-0068) calls to ask if she should continue her medication. She feels fine now. Dr. Gerald Practon is her physician.

____

____/10 ____/10 ____/10 15. (11:50) Alyson Pierce (Mrs. D. M.) (765-9077) calls to ask if Dr. Fran Practon can stop by on her way home tonight at 562 Lynnbrook Avenue, Agoura, to look at her little girl, Courtney, age 3, who has a high fever (103°F). Alyson has no means of transportation. You tell her you will check with the physician as soon as possible and will let her know if this home visit can be worked out.

____

____/10 ____/10 ____/10 Wrote message forms legibly.

_____ _____ _____ Completed within specified time.

____/162 ____/162 ____/162 **Total points earned** (To obtain a percentage score, divide the total points earned by the number of points possible.)

Comments:

Evaluator's Signature: ______________________________ **Need to Repeat:** __________

National Curriculum Competency: CAAHEP: Cognitive: IV.C.12; Psychomotor: IV.P.2, 7, 8	ABHES: 8.hh, jj

JOB SKILL 6-3
Document Telephone Messages and Physician Responses

Name ______________________________________ Date ______________ Score ________

Performance Objective

Task: Document telephone messages and physician responses on telephone message slips. Separate slips and attach to file page for insertion in medical record.

Conditions: One sheet of colored paper, two sheets of telephone message forms (Forms 8 and 9), scissors, cellophane adhesive tape or glue, and pen or pencil. Refer to Figures 6-4 and 6-6 in the *textbook* for visual illustrations.

Standards: Complete all steps listed in this skill in _______ minutes with a minimum score of ________. (Time element and accuracy criteria may be given by instructor.)

Time: **Start:** ____________ **Completed:** ____________ **Total:** ____________ minutes

Scoring: One point for each step performed satisfactorily unless otherwise listed or weighted by instructor.

Directions with Performance Evaluation Checklist

This exercise is for patient Krista Lee Carlisle, Record Number 1181. You will be preparing her chart in Chapter 9 (*Medical Records*). On a sheet of colored paper, key or type "Telephone Messages" in the upper left corner and the patient's name and record number in the upper right corner. Insert the following data on the telephone message slips. When completed, cut apart the message forms and tape or glue them to the sheet of colored paper; retain it for future use.

1st Attempt	2nd Attempt	3rd Attempt	
_______	_______	_______	Gather materials (equipment and supplies) listed under "Conditions."
____/15	____/15	____/15	1. On February 28, 20XX, at 3:00 p.m., Mrs. Robyn Carlisle called Dr. Gerald Practon stating Krista Lee, age 17, is in bed with flu symptoms. She cancelled her appointment for 3/1/XX. Patient's telephone number is 849-7730. Dr. Practon telephoned Mrs. Carlisle at 4:40 p.m. to recommend that Krista Lee drink plenty of fluids; he will prescribe medication if flu symptoms worsen.
____/15	____/15	____/15	2. On March 2, 20XX, at 3:10 p.m., Robyn Carlisle called Dr. Gerald Practon about her daughter, Krista Lee, who has a temperature of 100.2°F. She said Krista is having chest congestion and a persistent dry cough. She asked for a prescription of cough syrup. The family pharmacy is Long's Drug Store (phone: 849-2221). Dr. Practon asks you to fax an order to the pharmacy for Robitussin-PE, 2 teaspoons, every 4 hours. You ordered the medication from the pharmacy and called Mrs. Carlisle at 4:05 p.m. to give her the information.
____/15	____/15	____/15	3. On March 3, 20XX, at 9 a.m., you receive another call from Robyn Carlisle about Krista Lee. She says she thinks Krista has a possible allergy to the medication because she has a rash on her chest; she is continuing to cough and her temperature is 100°F. Dr. Practon returns the call at 11:15 a.m. He tells Robyn to discontinue the Robitussin and suggests an appointment be made for the next day, March 4.
____/15	____/15	____/15	4. Krista Lee sees Dr. Practon on March 4, 20XX, and he prescribes a different cough medication. Dr. Practon asks Mrs. Carlisle to report back in a day or two regarding the rash and cough. Robyn Carlisle calls on March 6, 20XX,

JOB SKILL 6-3 *(continued)*

at 3:30 p.m., saying Krista's rash has disappeared but she still has a cough, which is now producing discolored phlegm; temperature of 100.3°F.

Dr. Practon returns her call at 4:15 p.m. and orders a chest x-ray at College Hospital the following morning and a return appointment the afternoon of March 7. Krista Lee's chart is updated to indicate that she is allergic to codeine.

____/4	____/4	____/4	Wrote message forms legibly.
______	______	______	Complete within specified time.
____/66	____/66	____/66	**Total points earned** (To obtain a percentage score, divide the total points earned by the number of points possible.)

Comments:

Evaluator's Signature: ______________________________ **Need to Repeat:** ____________

National Curriculum Competency: CAAHEP: Cognitive: IV.C.12; Psychomotor: IV.P.2, 7, 8	ABHES: 8.hh, jj

JOB SKILL 6-4
Role-Play Telephone Scenario(s)

Name ______________________________ Date ______________ Score ________

Performance Objective

Task: To role-play a telephone scenario to gain practical experience in telephone technique and critical thinking when determining and managing an emergency call.

Conditions: This scenario is most realistically role-played with two students; one playing the caller and the other playing the medical assistant. Telephone (can simulate as needed) and scenario. Refer to *textbook* Procedure 6-6 for step-by-step directions in identifying and managing emergency calls and Table 6-3 for triage guidance; pen or pencil.

Standards: Complete all steps listed in this job skill in _____ minutes with a minimum score of _____. (Time element and accuracy criteria may be given by instructor.)

Time: **Start:** ____________ **Completed:** ____________ **Total:** ____________ minutes

Scoring: One point for each step performed satisfactorily unless otherwise listed or weighted by instructor.

Directions with Performance Evaluation Checklist

Scenario: Mrs. Ruby Pristine telephones Dr. Practon's office; she is upset and crying. She says that her husband (Mr. Clarence Pristine) fell and she cannot get him up. The student role-playing Mrs. Pristine can "ad lib" Mr. Pristine's condition, thereby making this scenario available to be role-played by different pairs of students who each demonstrate critical thinking skills and telephone technique for a variety of outcomes.

1st Attempt	2nd Attempt	3rd Attempt	
_______	_______	_______	Gather materials (equipment and supplies) listed under "Conditions."
_____/2	_____/2	_____/2	1. Allow the caller to state the problem without interruptions.
_____/5	_____/5	_____/5	2. Ask appropriate questions to determine if the call is an urgent or emergent situation.
_____/2	_____/2	_____/2	3. Maintain a calm, even, low-pitched tone of voice and take deep breaths as necessary to remain composed.
_____/2	_____/2	_____/2	4. Use the caller's and patient's names when asking specific questions.
_____/2	_____/2	_____/2	5. Ask whether the patient has experienced this same problem at a prior time.
_____/2	_____/2	_____/2	6. Ask what is being done, or what the caller had tried to do for the patient.
_____/5	_____/5	_____/5	7. Request that a coworker get the patient's chart while obtaining details about the patient's symptoms, accident description, current status, and any treatment administered.
____/10	____/10	____/10	8. Take action according to the severity of the patient's condition as explained.

JOB SKILL 6-4 *(continued)*

_______ _______ _______ Complete within specified time.

____/32 ____/32 ____/32 **Total points earned** (To obtain a percentage score, divide the total points earned by the number of points possible.)

Comments:

Evaluator's Signature: ______________________________ **Need to Repeat:** ____________

National Curriculum Competency: CAAHEP: Psychomotor: I.P.6, IV.P.7	ABHES: 8.ee, hh; 9.e, o

CHAPTER 7

Appointments

OBJECTIVES

After completing the exercises, the student will be able to:

1. Write meanings for chart note abbreviations.
2. Enhance spelling skills by learning new medical words.
3. Prepare appointment sheets (Job Skill 7-1).
4. Schedule appointments (Job Skill 7-2).
5. Prepare an appointment reference sheet (Job Skill 7-3).
6. Complete appointment cards (Job Skill 7-4).
7. Abstract information and complete a hospital/surgery scheduling form (Job Skill 7-5).
8. Transfer surgery scheduling information to a form letter (Job Skill 7-6).
9. Complete requisition forms for outpatient diagnostic tests (Job Skill 7-7).

FOCUS ON CERTIFICATION*

CMA Content Summary

- Utilizing appointment schedules/types
- Appointment guidelines
- Appointment protocol
- Physician referrals
- Appointment cancellations/no-shows
- Scheduling outside services
- Appointment reminders/recalls

*This *Workbook* and the accompanying *textbook* meet the entry-level administrative and general competencies for the CMA outlined by the AAMA Examination Content Outline and Occupational Analysis and for the RMA and CMAS outlined by the AMT Competencies, Construction Parameters, and Examination Specifications (see Competency Grid in Appendix B of the *textbook*).

RMA Content Summary

- Employ appointment scheduling systems
- Employ proper procedures for cancellations and missed appointments
- Understand referral process
- Understand and manage patient recall system
- Schedule non-office appointments

CMAS Content Summary

- Schedule and monitor patient and visitor appointments
- Address cancellations and missed appointments
- Prepare information for referrals
- Arrange hospital admissions and surgery, and schedule patients for outpatient diagnostic tests

STOP AND THINK CASE SCENARIOS AND EXAM-STYLE REVIEW QUESTIONS

Refer to the end of Chapter 7 in the *textbook*.

Abbreviation and Spelling Review

Read the following patient's chart note and write the meanings for the abbreviations listed below the note. To decode any abbreviations you do not understand or that appear unfamiliar to you, refer to the list of abbreviations in Part IV of this *Workbook*. Step-by-step directions for this exercise are in Procedure 1-1 of Chapter 1 in the *textbook*. Medical terms in the chart note are italicized; study them for spelling. Use your medical dictionary to look up their definitions. Your instructor may give a spelling and definition test that includes these words and abbreviations.

> Dan F. Goodson
>
> September 3, 20XX IV *chemotherapy* started in hospital. Daily hosp PO exams. See op. report giving dx: *superficially infiltrating transitional* cell Ca Class III. Pt DC from hosp 11-1-20XX. Retn for OV 3 p.m. Friday. PT to be started in 1 mo.
>
> Gerald Practon, MD
>
> Gerald Practon, MD

IV	______	DC	______
hosp	______	retn	______
PO	______	OV	______
op.	______	p.m.	______
dx	______	PT	______
Ca	______	mo	______
Pt	______		

Review Questions

Review the objectives, glossary, and chapter information before completing the following review questions.

1. Describe an appointment template. ______________________________

____

2. In a typical office, what time intervals are usually assigned for the following types of patients? Initial visits: ______________________ Follow-up examinations: ______________________

3. What is the name of the sheet used to track the number of patients seen daily for various types of appointments in order to determine a scheduling system? ______________________

____

4. What five factors should be taken into consideration when an appointment book is being selected?

   a. ______________________ d. ______________________

   b. ______________________ e. ______________________

   c. ______________________

5. Why is it advantageous to schedule patient appointments one right after the other? ______________________

____

6. What is the benefit of having a medical assistant make confirmation telephone calls to patients scheduled to be seen within 1 or 2 days? ______________________

7. Which patient flow technique do most physicians' offices use? ______________________

8. Describe true wave scheduling.______________________

____

____

9. What are long wait times equated with? ______________________

10. List four actions the medical assistant might take when an emergency telephone call indicates an immediate response.

    a. ______________________

    b. ______________________

    c. ______________________

    d. ______________________

11. When might an appointment be scheduled for a patient who is habitually late? ______________________

____

12. Besides having a written record of all appointments, why is it important to keep accurate and permanent information? ______________________

13. What systems or devices might a physician use to keep track of out-of-office appointments?

    a. ______________________

    b. ______________________

    c. ______________________

    d. ______________________

    e. ______________________

    f. ______________________

14. Why should postcards not be sent to remind patients of upcoming appointments? ____________________

15. Explain what an appointment reference sheet is and what purpose it serves. ____________________

Critical Thinking Exercises

1. Mrs. Bettle, who has arrived for her appointment 1 hour early, is sure that she has come at the right time. What would you say to her? ____________________

2. After seeing the physician, Mrs. Hall stops at your desk for a new appointment. What do you say to her? ____________________

MOSS MEDICAL OFFICE SIMULATION SOFTWARE

Computer Competency

Today's Date Is Monday, 10/21/2013

Simulation: You are the front desk receptionist for Drs. Heath and Schwartz of Douglasville Medicine Associates. One of your responsibilities is to schedule appointments received by telephone and also to schedule follow-up appointments for patients that have been seen by the physician and are checking out. The physician will indicate when he or she would like to see the patient again on the bottom of the encounter form (superbill). **You will need to reference the MOSS Source Documents (Encounter Forms) found at the end of this section to complete the exercises in this chapter, and later in Chapter 15.**

1. Scheduling Appointments: Patient John Conway

Patient Conway is an existing patient of the practice and Dr. Heath is his physician. The patient has called the office and would like to schedule an appointment for October 29, 2013. Patients who call on the telephone must be screened to distinguish new patients from established patients and to update basic information, such as telephone number and insurance. The reason for the visit is also obtained to determine urgency, physician to be seen, and the time required.

A. After answering the telephone and listening to Mr. Conway's request, click on *Appointment Schedule* from the *Main Menu*.

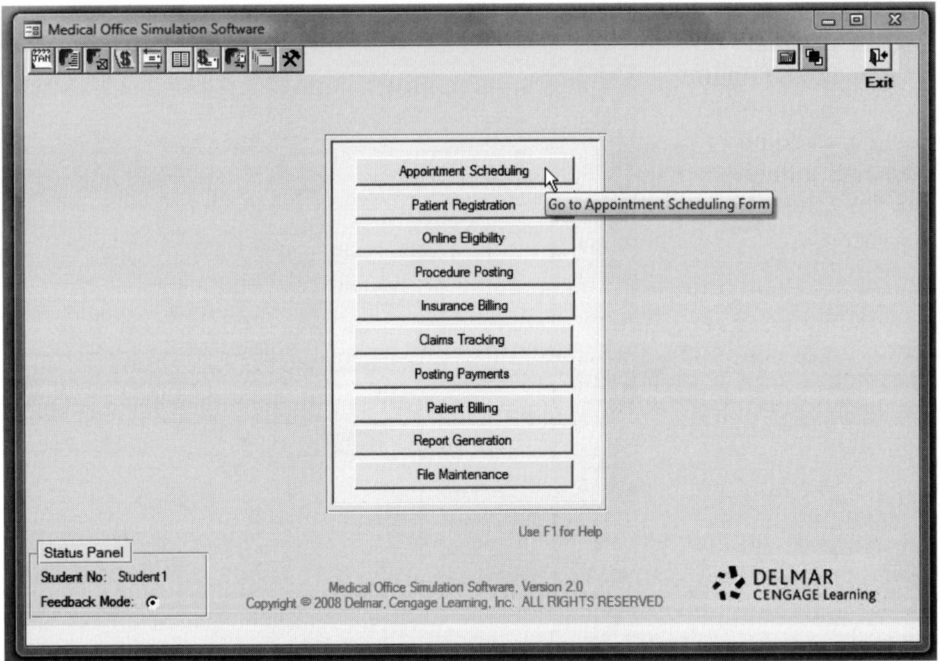

© Cengage Learning 2013

B. When the practice schedule opens, navigate to October 29, 2013, on the calendar. You can either use the Y−/Y+ and M−/M+ keys to navigate to the date, or type 10/29/2013 in the GO TO: field and press *Enter* on the keyboard. Be sure the correct year and month are selected.

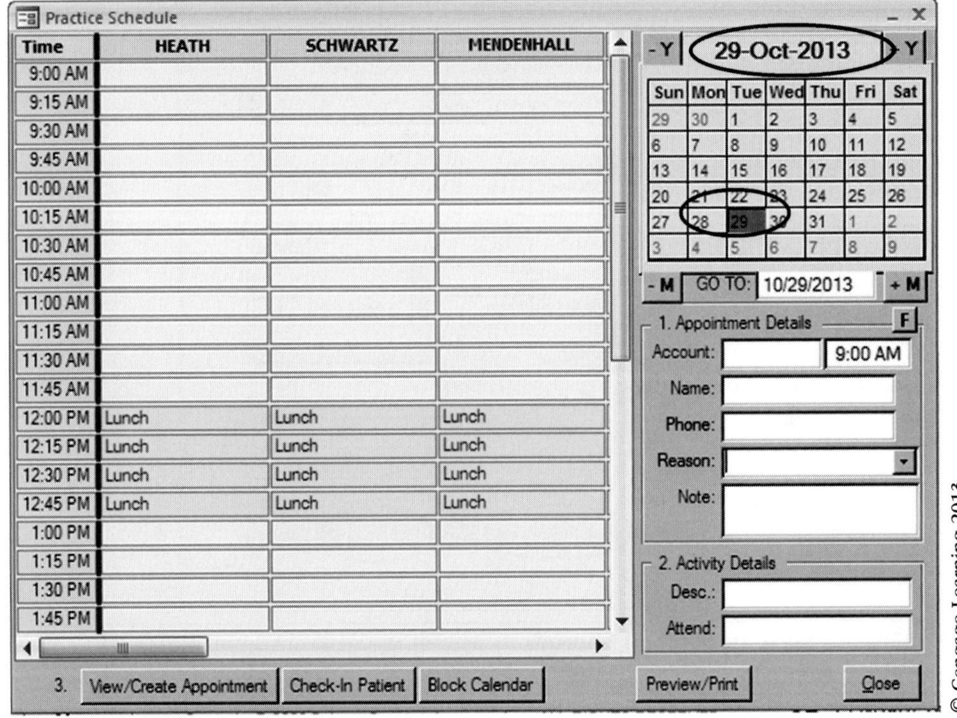

© Cengage Learning 2013

C. Patient Conway indicates he can come to the office October 29, 2013, just before lunch. Double click on the 11:45 slot in the column for Dr. Heath.

D. Search for and select Patient Conway, and then click on *Add* (since you are adding an appointment to the schedule).

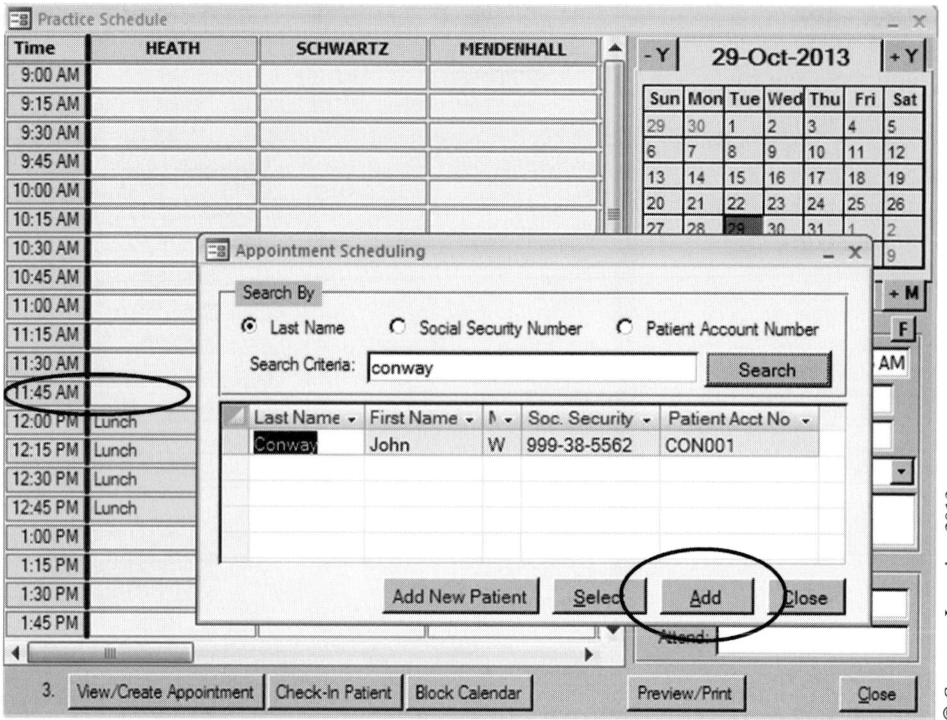

E. In the *Patient Appointment Form* window, select Dr. Heath as the physician. The appointment will be for 15 minutes and the reason is *Office Visit*. In the *Notes* field, enter *Bronchitis* as the patient's reason for seeing the physician.

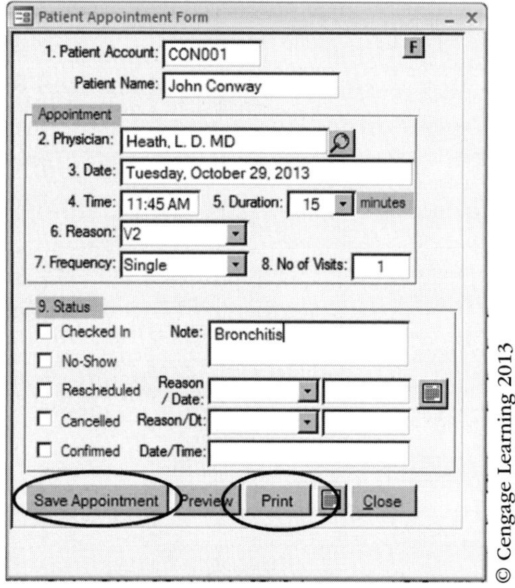

F. Click the *Save Appointment* button to record the appointment. Click *Print* to print out a patient appointment slip.

G. Close the *Patient Appointment Form* window. The appointment now appears in the 11:45 slot in Dr. Heath's column on the practice schedule.

Note to reader: Click on the patient's name on the schedule to view *Appointment Details* on the right side of the screen, below the calendar.

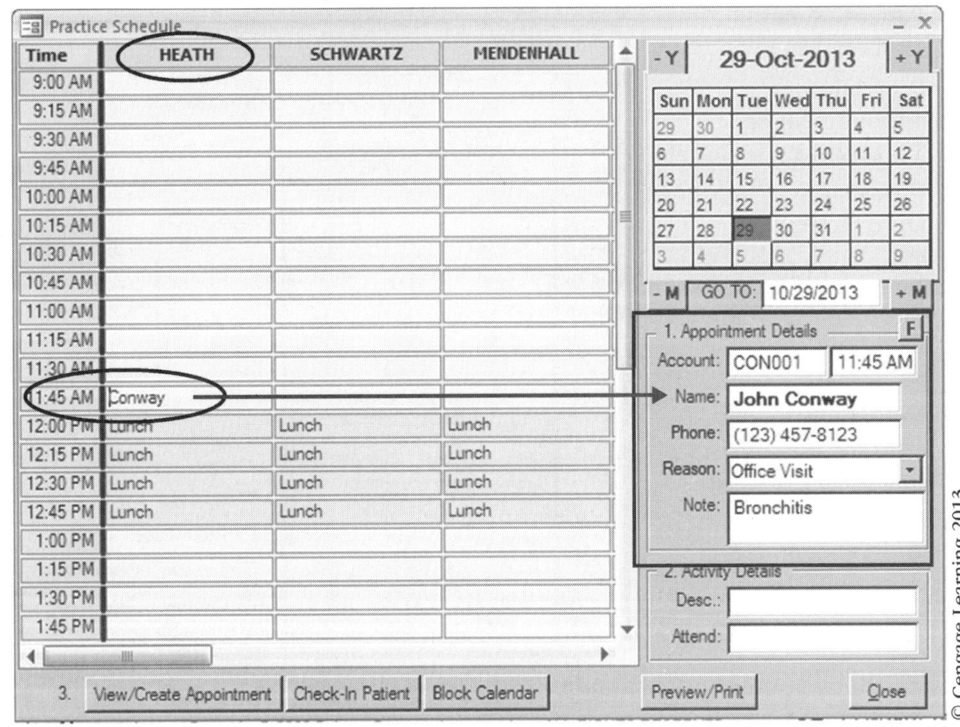

© Cengage Learning 2013

H. Close the practice schedule.

2. Scheduling Appointments: Patients Bradley, Herbert, and Yamagata

Each of the following patients called the office requesting an appointment. Patients who call on the telephone must be screened to distinguish new patients from established patients and to update basic information, such as phone number and insurance. The reason for the visit is also obtained to determine urgency, physician to be seen, and the time required. Schedule each patient using the information given using MOSS.

A. Patient: Aimee Bradley
Schedule appointment on: 10/29/2013

Physician: Dr. D.J. Schwartz

Time: 3:00 p.m.

Reason: Office visit

Duration: 30 minutes

Note: UTI (urinary tract infection)

Print out an appointment slip.

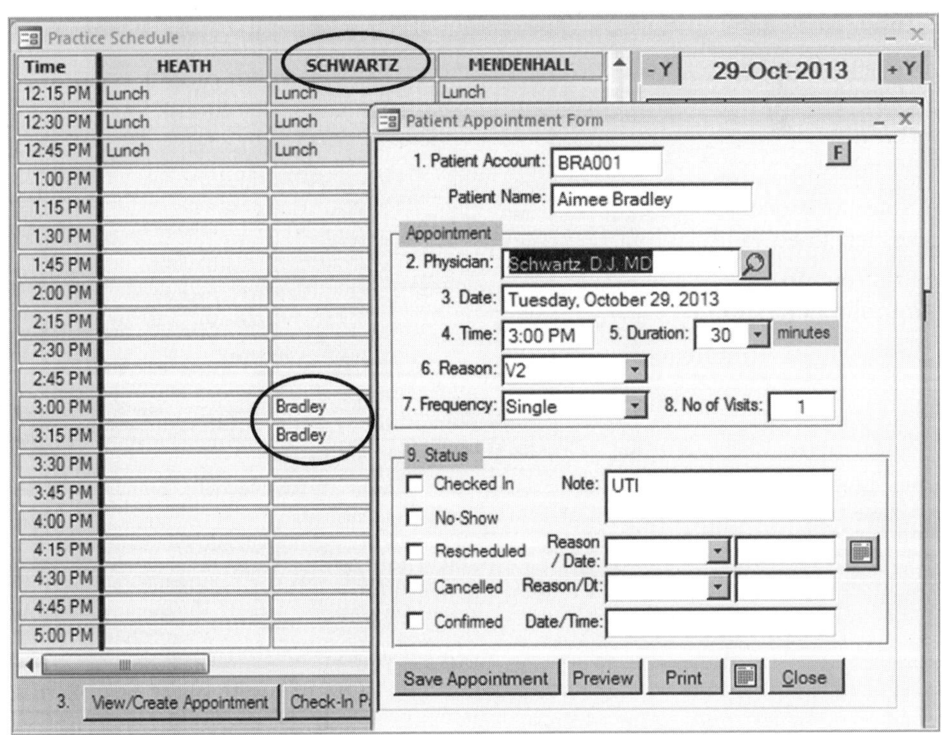

© Cengage Learning 2013

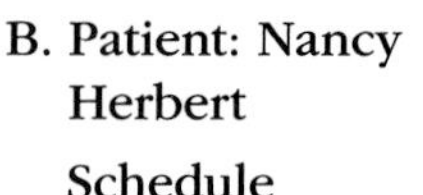

B. Patient: Nancy Herbert
Schedule appointment on: 11/11/2013
Physician: Dr. L.D. Heath
Time: 1:00 p.m.
Reason: Office visit
Duration: 45 minutes
Note: COPD (chronic obstructive pulmonary disease)
Print out an appointment slip.

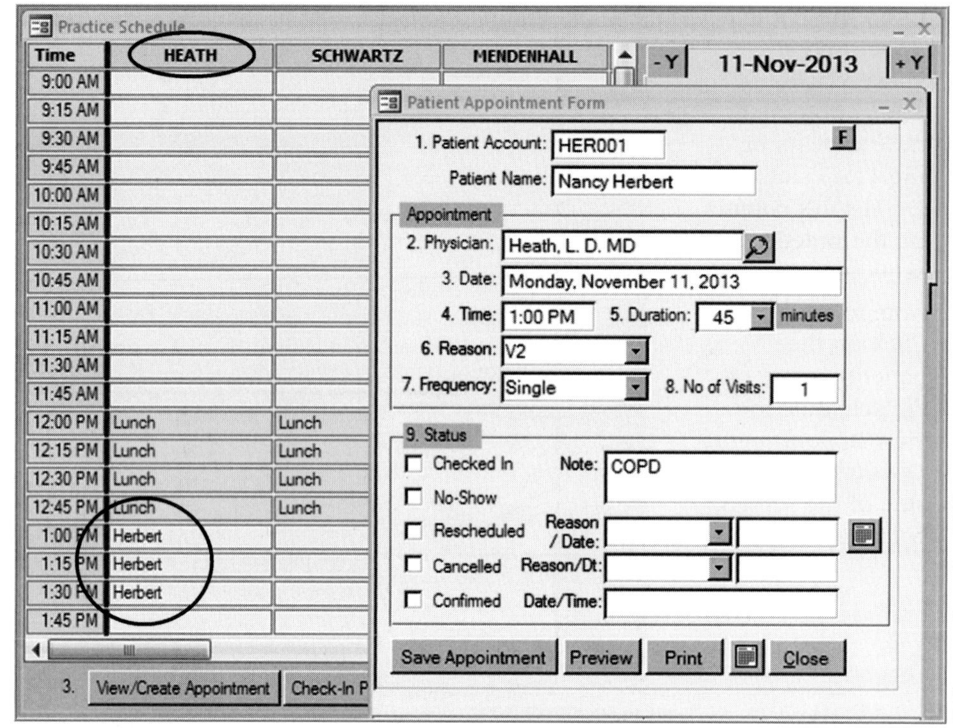

© Cengage Learning 2013

C. Patient: Naomi Yamagata
Schedule appointment on: 11/11/2013
Physician: Dr. D.J. Schwartz
Time: 10:30 a.m.
Reason: Special procedure
Duration: 30 minutes
Note: Arthrocentesis, left knee
Print out an appointment slip.

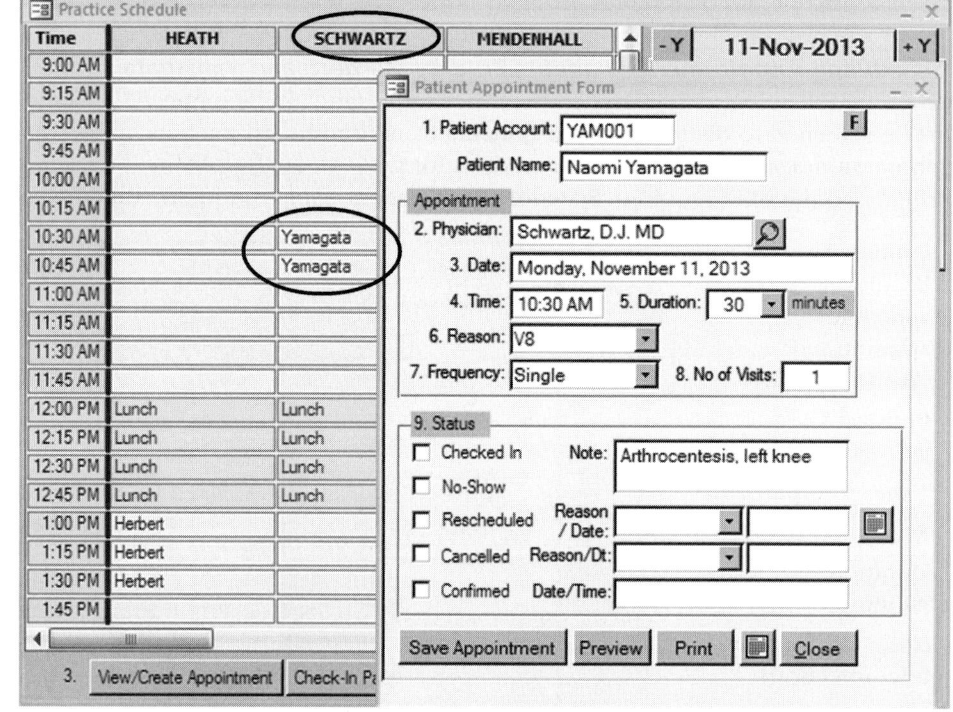

© Cengage Learning 2013

D. Close the practice schedule.

3. Scheduling Follow-up Appointments: Patient Albertson

Patient Albertson has visited the doctor and is at the front desk to check out. The encounter form (superbill) for office patients indicates when the doctor would like to see the patient back in follow-up. Schedule this patient's appointment using MOSS.

A. Patient Albertson stops at the front desk to check out. The medical assistant has returned Encounter Form 2999 to the receptionist, which documents the procedures and diagnoses for today's services. Review the information on the encounter form **(Source Documents: Encounter Forms).**

B. The encounter form indicates that Dr. Heath would like to see the patient in 2 weeks for a follow-up visit. Open the practice schedule by clicking on *Appointment Scheduling* on the MOSS *Main Menu*. Check the schedule to see available time for Dr. Heath 2 weeks from October 21, 2013.

C. The patient indicates that the morning of 11/4/2013 is convenient. Schedule the appointment as follows:

Physician: Dr. Heath

Time: 10:00 a.m.

Reason: Office visit

Duration: 15 minutes

Note: Follow-up viral infection

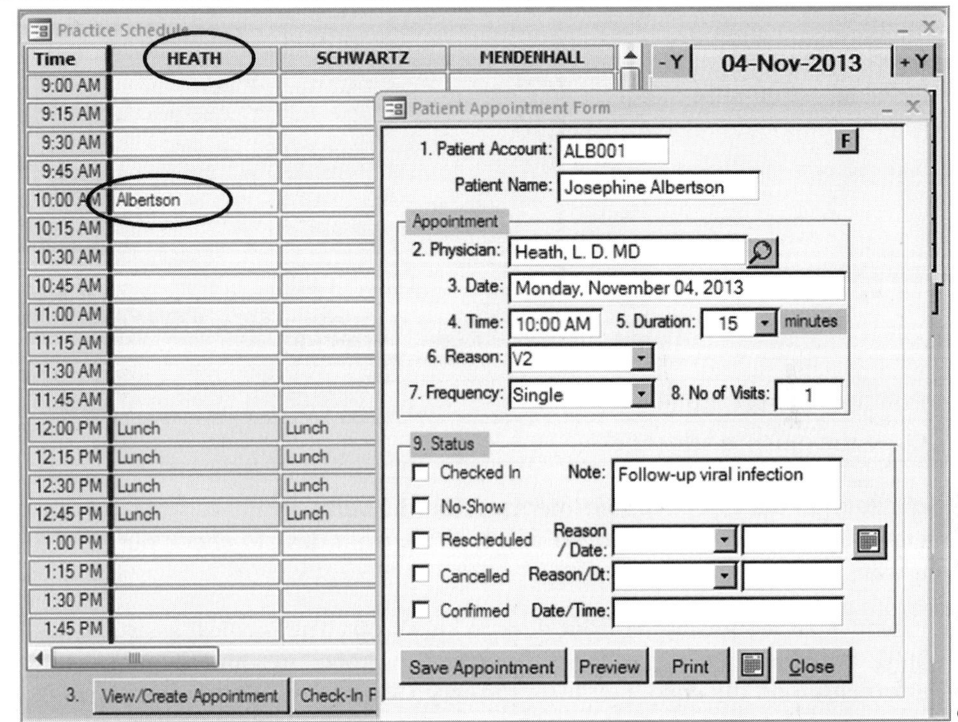

D. Print out an appointment slip.

E. Close the practice schedule.

4. Scheduling Follow-up Appointments: Patient Ashby

Patient Ashby has visited the doctor and is at the front desk to check out. Schedule this patient's appointment using MOSS as indicated.

A. Patient Ashby stops at the front desk to check out. The medical assistant has returned Encounter Form 3000 to the receptionist, which documents the procedures and diagnoses for today's services. Review the information on the encounter form **(Source Documents: Encounter Forms).**

B. The encounter form indicates that Dr. Heath would like to see the patient in 1 month for a follow-up visit. Open the practice schedule by clicking on *Appointment Scheduling* on the MOSS *Main Menu*. Check the schedule to see available time for Dr. Heath 1 month from October 21, 2013.

C. The patient indicates that the morning of 11/18/2013 is convenient. Schedule the appointment as follows:

Physician: Dr. Heath

Time: 11:00 a.m.

Reason: Office visit

Duration: 15 minutes

Note: Follow-up impetigo

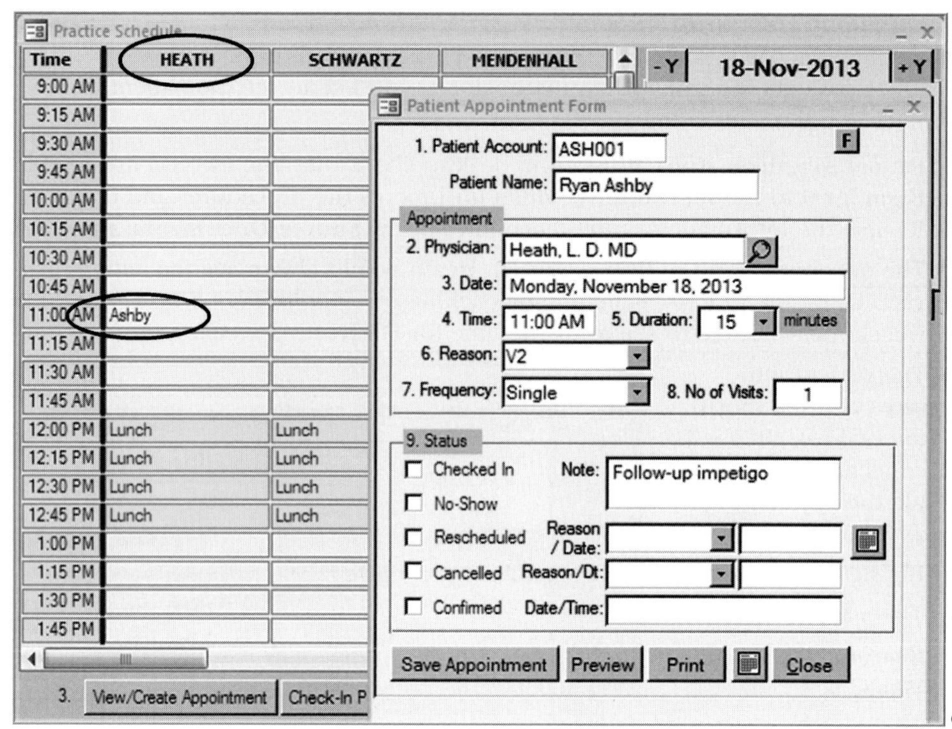

© Cengage Learning 2013

D. Print out an appointment slip.

E. Close the practice schedule.

5. Scheduling Follow-up Appointments: Patient Ybarra

Patient Ybarra has visited the doctor and is at the front desk to check out. Schedule this patient's appointment using MOSS as indicated.

A. Patient Ybarra stops at the front desk to check out. The medical assistant has returned Encounter Form 3001 to the receptionist, which documents the procedures and diagnoses for today's services. Review the information on the encounter form **(Source Documents: Encounter Forms).**

B. The encounter form indicates that Dr. Schwartz would like to see the patient in 3 weeks for a follow-up visit. Open the practice schedule by clicking on *Appointment Scheduling* on the MOSS *Main Menu*. Check the schedule to see available time for Dr. Schwartz 2 weeks from October 21, 2013.

C. The patient indicates that the morning of 11/11/2013 is convenient. Schedule the appointment as follows:

Physician: Dr. Schwartz

Time: 10:00 a.m.

Reason: Office visit

Duration: 30 minutes

Note: Follow-up tonsillitis and GERD (gastroesophageal reflux disease)

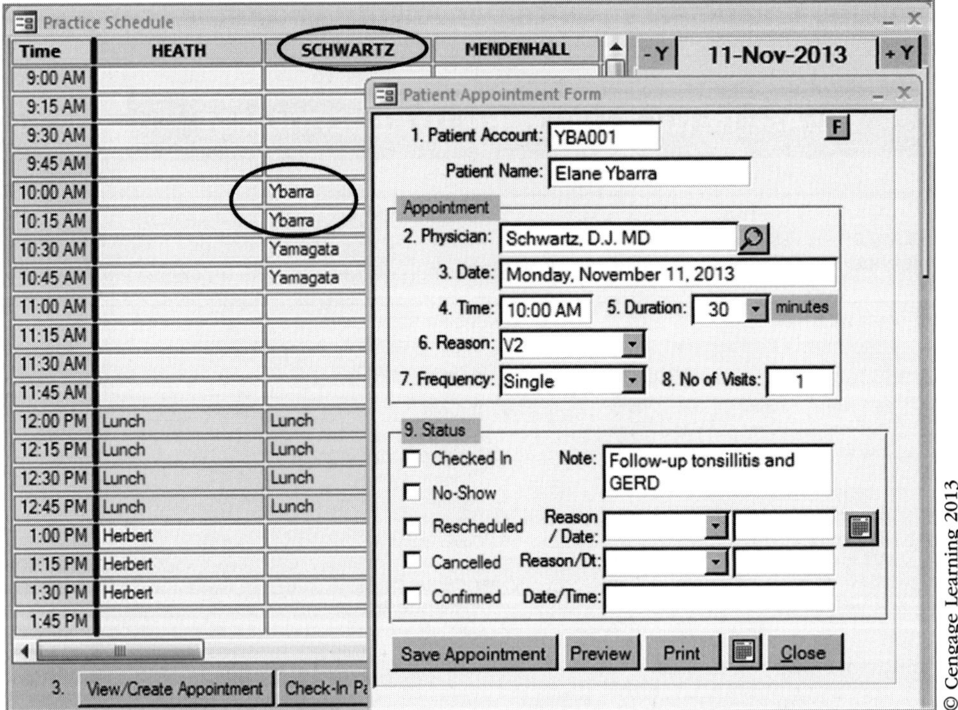

D. Print out an appointment slip.

E. Close the practice schedule.

Computer Competency Source Documents: Encounter Forms

PLEASE RETURN THIS FORM TO RECEPTIONIST

NAME Albertson, Josephine

Receipt No: 2999

PLACE OF SERVICE: (X) OFFICE ( ) NEW YORK COUNTY HOSPITAL ( ) COMMUNITY GENERAL HOSPITAL ( ) RETIREMENT INN NURSING HOME ( ) ____

DATE OF SERVICE 10/21/2013

A. OFFICE VISITS - New Patient

Code	History	Exam	Dec.	Time	
99201	Prob. Foc.	Prob. Foc.	Straight	10 min.	
99202	Ex. Prob. Foc.	Ex. Prob. Foc.	Straight	20 min.	
99203	Detail	Detail	Low	30 min.	
99204	Comp.	Comp.	Mod.	45 min.	
99205	Comp.	Comp.	High	60 min.	

B. OFFICE VISIT - Established Patient

Code	History	Exam	Dec.	Time	
X 99211	(Minimal)	Minimal	Minimal	5 min.	1
99212	Prob. Foc.	Prob. Foc.	Straight	10min.	
99213	Ex. Prob. Foc.	Ex. Prob. Foc.	Low	15 min.	
99214	Detail	Detail	Mod.	25 min.	
99215	Comp.	Comp.	High	40 min.	

C. HOSPITAL CARE

	Dx	Units	Code	
1. Initial Hospital Care (30 min)			99221	
2. Subsequent Care			99231	
3. Critical Care (30-74 min)			99291	
4. each additional 30 min.			99292	
5. Discharge Services			99238	
6. Emergency Room			99282	

D. NURSING HOME CARE

	Dx	Units	Code	
Initial Care - New Pt.				
1. Expanded			99322	
2. Detailed			99323	
Subsequent Care - Estab. Pt.				
3. Problem Focused			99307	
4. Expanded			99308	
5. Detailed			99309	
5. Comprehensive			99310	

E. PROCEDURES

		Code	
1. Arthrocentesis, Small Jt.		20600	
2. Colonoscopy		45378	
3. EKG w/interpretation		93000	
4. X-Ray Chest, PA/LAT		71020	

F. LAB

		Code	
1. Blood Sugar		82947	
2. CBC w/differential		85031	
3. Cholesterol		82465	
4. Comprehensive Metabolic Panel		80053	
5. ESR		85651	
6. Hematocrit		85014	
7. Mono Screen		86308	
8. Pap Smear		88150	
9. Potassium		84132	
10. Preg. Test, Quantitative		84702	
11. Routine Venipuncture		36415	

F. Cont'd

	Dx	Code	Units
12. Strep Screen		87081	
13. UA, Routine w/Micro		81000	
14. UA, Routine w/o Micro		81002	
15. Uric Acid		84550	
16. VDRL		86592	
17. Wet Prep		82710	
18.			

G. INJECTIONS

		Code	
1. Influenza Virus Vaccine		90658	
2. Pneumoccocal Vaccine		90772	
3. Tetanus Toxoids		90703	
4. Therapeutic Subcut/IM		90732	
5. Vaccine Administration		90471	
6. Vaccine - each additional		90472	

H. MISCELLANEOUS

1. ____
2. ____

AMOUNT PAID $ ∅

Mark diagnosis with (1=Primary, 2=Secondary, 3=Tertiary)

DIAGNOSIS NOT LISTED BELOW ____

DIAGNOSIS	ICD-9-CM	1, 2, 3
Abdominal Pain	789.0_	
Allergic Rhinitis, Unspec.	477.9	
Angina Pectoris, Unspec.	413.9	
Anemia, Iron Deficiency, Unspec.	280.9	
Anemia, NOS	285.9	
Anemia, Pernicious	281.0	
Asthma w/ Exacerbation	493.92	
Asthmatic Bronchitis, Unspec.	493.90	
Atrial Fibrillation	427.31	
Atypical Chest Pain, Unspec.	786.59	
Bronchiolitis, due to RSV	466.11	
Bronchitis, Acute	466.0	
Bronchitis, NOS	490	
Cardiac Arrest	427.5	
Cardiopulmonary Disease, Chronic, Unspec.	416.9	
Cellulitis, NOS	682.9	
Congestive Heart Failure, Unspec.	428.0	
Contact Dermatitis NOS	692.9	
COPD NOS	496	
CVA, Acute, NOS	434.91	
CVA, Old or Healed	438.9	
Degenerative Arthritis (Specify Site) ____	715.9	
Dehydration	276.51	
Depression, NOS	311	
Diabetes Mellitus, Type II Controlled	250.00	
Diabetes Mellitus, Type II Controlled	250.02	
Drug Reaction, NOS	995.29	
Dysuria	788.1	
Eczema, NOS	692.2	
Edema	782.3	
Fever, Unknown Origin	780.6	
Gastritis, Acute w/o Hemorrhage	535.00	
Gastroenteritis, NOS	558.9	
Gastroesophageal Reflux	530.81	
Hepatitis A, Infectious	070.1	
Hypercholesterolemia, Pure	272.0	
Hypertension, Unspec.	401.9	
Hypoglycemia NOS	251.2	
Hypokalemia	276.8	
Impetigo	684	
Lymphadenitis, Unspec.	289.3	
Mononucleosis	075	
Myocardial Infarction, Acute, NOS	410.9	
Organic Brain Syndrome	310.9	
Otitis Externa, Acute NOS	380.10	
Otitis Media, Acute NOS	382.9	
Peptic Ulcer Disease	536.9	
Peripheral Vascular Disease NOS	443.9	
Pharyngitis, Acute	462	
Pneumonia, Organism Unspec.	486	
Prostatitis, NOS	601.9	
PVC	427.69	
Rash, Non Specific	782.1	
Seizure Disorder NOS	780.39	
Serous Otitis Media, Chronic, Unspec.	381.10	
Sinusitis, Acute NOS	461.9	
Tonsillitis, Acute	463.	
Upper Respiratory Infection, Acute NOS	465.9	
Urinary Tract Infection, Unspec.	599.0	
Urticaria, Unspec.	708.9	
Vertigo, NOS	780.4	
Viral Infection NOS	079.99	1
Weakness, Generalized	780.79	
Weight Loss, Abnormal	783.21	

ABN: I UNDERSTAND THAT MEDICARE PROBABLY WILL NOT COVER THE SERVICES LISTED BELOW

A.____ B.____ C.____

Date____ Patient Signature____

Doctor's Signature L.D. Heath MD

RETURN:____ Days 2 Weeks ____ Months

DOUGLASVILLE MEDICINE ASSOCIATES
5076 BRAND BLVD., SUITE 401
DOUGLASVILLE, NY 01234
PHONE No. (123) 456-7890
☒ L.D. HEATH, M.D. NPI# 9995010111 ☐ D.J. SCHWARTZ, M.D. NPI# 9995020212
EIN# 00-1234560

REF# 122949 SB (05 07 09) TO REORDER CALL INHEALTH RECORD SYSTEMS 800-477-7374

PLEASE RETURN THIS FORM TO RECEPTIONIST

NAME Ashby, Ryan

Receipt No: 3000

PLACE OF SERVICE: (X) OFFICE ( ) NEW YORK COUNTY HOSPITAL ( ) COMMUNITY GENERAL HOSPITAL ( ) RETIREMENT INN NURSING HOME ( ) ______

DATE OF SERVICE 10/21/2013

A. OFFICE VISITS - New Patient

	Code	History	Exam	Dec.	Time	
___	99201	Prob. Foc.	Prob. Foc.	Straight	10 min.	___
___	99203	Detail	Detail	Low	30 min.	___
___	99204	Comp.	Comp.	Mod.	45 min.	___
___	99205	Comp.	Comp.	High	60 min.	___

B. OFFICE VISIT - Established Patient

	Code	History	Exam	Dec.	Time	
___	99211	Minimal	Minimal	Minimal	5 min.	___
X	99212	Prob. Foc.	Prob. Foc.	Straight	10min.	1
___	99213	Ex. Prob. Foc.	Ex. Prob. Foc.	Low	15 min.	___
___	99214	Detail	Detail	Mod.	25 min.	___
___	99215	Comp.	Comp.	High	40 min.	___

C. HOSPITAL CARE Dx Units

	Dx	Units	Code	
1. Initial Hospital Care (30 min)	___	___	99221	___
2. Subsequent Care	___	___	99231	___
3. Critical Care (30-74 min)	___	___	99291	___
4. each additional 30 min.	___	___	99292	___
5. Discharge Services	___	___	99238	___
6. Emergency Room	___	___	99282	___

D. NURSING HOME CARE Dx Units

	Dx	Units	Code	
Initial Care - New Pt.				
1. Expanded	___	___	99322	___
2. Detailed	___	___	99323	___
Subsequent Care - Estab. Pt.				
3. Problem Focused	___	___	99307	___
4. Expanded	___	___	99308	___
5. Detailed	___	___	99309	___
5. Comprehensive	___	___	99310	___

E. PROCEDURES

	Dx	Code	
1. Arthrocentesis, Small Jt.	___	20600	___
2. Colonoscopy	___	45378	___
3. EKG w/interpretation	___	93000	___
4. X-Ray Chest, PA/LAT	___	71020	___

F. LAB

	Dx	Code	
1. Blood Sugar	___	82947	___
2. CBC w/differential	___	85031	___
3. Cholesterol	___	82465	___
4. Comprehensive Metabolic Panel	___	80053	___
5. ESR	___	85651	___
6. Hematocrit	___	85014	___
7. Mono Screen	___	86308	___
8. Pap Smear	___	88150	___
9. Potassium	___	84132	___
10. Preg. Test, Quantitative	___	84702	___
11. Routine Venipuncture	___	36415	___

F. Cont'd

	Dx	Units	
12. Strep Screen	___	87081	___
13. UA, Routine w/Micro	___	81000	___
14. UA, Routine w/o Micro	___	81002	___
15. Uric Acid	___	84550	___
16. VDRL	___	86592	___
17. Wet Prep	___	82710	___
18. ___	___	___	___

G. INJECTIONS

	Dx	Code	
1. Influenza Virus Vaccine	___	90658	___
2. Pneumoccoccal Vaccine	___	90772	___
3. Tetanus Toxoids	___	90703	___
4. Therapeutic Subcut/IM	___	90732	___
5. Vaccine Administration	___	90471	___
6. Vaccine - each additional	___	90472	___

H. MISCELLANEOUS

1. ___
2. ___

AMOUNT PAID $ 10.00

ck# 8755

Mark diagnosis with (1=Primary, 2=Secondary, 3=Tertiary)

DIAGNOSIS NOT LISTED BELOW ______

DIAGNOSIS	ICD-9-CM 1, 2, 3	
Abdominal Pain	789.0_	___
Allergic Rhinitis, Unspec.	477.9	___
Angina Pectoris, Unspec.	413.9	___
Anemia, Iron Deficiency, Unspec.	280.9	___
Anemia, NOS	285.9	___
Anemia, Pernicious	281.0	___
Asthma w/ Exacerbation	493.92	___
Asthmatic Bronchitis, Unspec.	493.90	___
Atrial Fibrillation	427.31	___
Atypical Chest Pain, Unspec.	786.59	___
Bronchiolitis, due to RSV	466.11	___
Bronchitis, Acute	466.0	___
Bronchitis, NOS	490	___
Cardiac Arrest	427.5	___
Cardiopulmonary Disease, Chronic, Unspec.	416.9	___
Cellulitis, NOS	682.9	___
Congestive Heart Failure, Unspec.	428.0	___
Contact Dermatitis NOS	692.9	___
COPD NOS	496	___
CVA, Acute, NOS	434.91	___
CVA, Old or Healed	438.9	___
Degenerative Arthritis (Specify Site) ___	715.9	___
Dehydration	276.51	___
Depression, NOS	311	___
Diabetes Mellitus, Type II Controlled	250.00	___
Diabetes Mellitus, Type II Controlled	250.02	___
Drug Reaction, NOS	995.29	___
Dysuria	788.1	___
Eczema, NOS	692.2	___
Edema	782.3	___
Fever, Unknown Origin	780.6	___
Gastritis, Acute w/o Hemorrhage	535.00	___
Gastroenteritis, NOS	558.9	___
Gastroesophageal Reflux	530.81	___
Hepatitis A, Infectious	070.1	___
Hypercholesterolemia, Pure	272.0	___
Hypertension, Unspec.	401.9	___
Hypoglycemia NOS	251.2	___
Hypokalemia	276.8	___
Impetigo	684	1
Lymphadenitis, Unspec.	289.3	___
Mononucleosis	075	___
Myocardial Infarction, Acute, NOS	410.9	___
Organic Brain Syndrome	310.9	___
Otitis Externa, Acute NOS	380.10	___
Otitis Media, Acute NOS	382.9	___
Peptic Ulcer Disease	536.9	___
Peripheral Vascular Disease NOS	443.9	___
Pharyngitis, Acute	462	___
Pneumonia, Organism Unspec.	486	___
Prostatitis, NOS	601.9	___
PVC	427.69	___
Rash, Non Specific	782.1	___
Seizure Disorder NOS	780.39	___
Serous Otitis Media, Chronic, Unspec.	381.10	___
Sinusitis, Acute NOS	461.9	___
Tonsillitis, Acute	463.	___
Upper Respiratory Infection, Acute NOS	465.9	___
Urinary Tract Infection, Unspec.	599.0	___
Urticaria, Unspec.	708.9	___
Vertigo, NOS	780.4	___
Viral Infection NOS	079.99	___
Weakness, Generalized	780.79	___
Weight Loss, Abnormal	783.21	___

ABN: I UNDERSTAND THAT MEDICARE PROBABLY WILL NOT COVER THE SERVICES LISTED BELOW

A. ______ B. ______ C. ______

Date ______ Patient Signature ______

Doctor's Signature L.D. Heath MD

RETURN: ______ Days ______ Weeks 1 Months

DOUGLASVILLE MEDICINE ASSOCIATES
5076 BRAND BLVD., SUITE 401
DOUGLASVILLE, NY 01234
PHONE No. (123) 456-7890

☒ L.D. HEATH, M.D. NPI# 9995010111
☐ D.J. SCHWARTZ, M.D. NPI# 9995020212

EIN# 00-1234560

REF# 122949 SB (05 07 09) TO REORDER CALL INHEALTH RECORD SYSTEMS 800-477-7374

Used with permission. InHealth Record Systems, Inc. 5076 Winters Chapel Road, Atlanta, GA 30360, 800-477-7374. http://www.inhealthrecords.com

PLEASE RETURN THIS FORM TO RECEPTIONIST

NAME Ybarra, Elane

Receipt No: 3001

PLACE OF SERVICE:
(X) OFFICE
( ) NEW YORK COUNTY HOSPITAL
( ) COMMUNITY GENERAL HOSPITAL
( ) RETIREMENT INN NURSING HOME
( ) ______

DATE OF SERVICE 10/21/2013

A. OFFICE VISITS - New Patient

	Code	History	Exam	Dec.	Time	
___	99201	Prob. Foc.	Prob. Foc.	Straight	10 min.	___
___	99202	Ex. Prob. Foc.	Ex. Prob. Foc.	Straight	20 min.	___
___	99203	Detail	Detail	Low	30 min.	___
___	99204	Comp.	Comp.	Mod.	45 min.	___
___	99205	Comp.	Comp.	High	60 min.	___

B. OFFICE VISIT - Established Patient

	Code	History	Exam	Dec.	Time	
___	99211	Minimal	Minimal	Minimal	5 min.	___
___	99212	Prob. Foc.	Prob. Foc.	Straight	10min.	___
___	99213	Ex. Prob. Foc.	Ex. Prob. Foc.	Low	15 min.	___
X	99214	Detail	Detail	Mod.	25 min.	1, 2
___	99215	Comp.	Comp.	High	40 min.	___

C. HOSPITAL CARE

	Dx	Units	Code	
1. Initial Hospital Care (30 min)	___	___	99221	___
2. Subsequent Care	___	___	99231	___
3. Critical Care (30-74 min)	___	___	99291	___
4. each additional 30 min.	___	___	99292	___
5. Discharge Services	___	___	99238	___
6. Emergency Room	___	___	99282	___

D. NURSING HOME CARE

	Dx	Units	Code	
Initial Care - New Pt.				
1. Expanded	___	___	99322	___
2. Detailed	___	___	99323	___
Subsequent Care - Estab. Pt.				
3. Problem Focused	___	___	99307	___
4. Expanded	___	___	99308	___
5. Detailed	___	___	99309	___
5. Comprehensive	___	___	99310	___

E. PROCEDURES

		Code	
1. Arthrocentesis, Small Jt.	___	20600	___
2. Colonoscopy	___	45378	___
3. EKG w/interpretation	___	93000	___
4. X-Ray Chest, PA/LAT	___	71020	___

F. LAB

		Code	
1. Blood Sugar	___	82947	___
2. CBC w/differential	___	85031	___
3. Cholesterol	___	82465	___
4. Comprehensive Metabolic Panel	___	80053	___
5. ESR	___	85651	___
6. Hematocrit	___	85014	___
7. Mono Screen	___	86308	___
8. Pap Smear	___	88150	___
9. Potassium	___	84132	___
10. Preg. Test, Quantitative	___	84702	___
11. Routine Venipuncture	___	36415	___

F. Cont'd

	Dx	Code	Units
12. Strep Screen	___	87081	___
13. UA, Routine w/Micro	___	81000	___
14. UA, Routine w/o Micro	___	81002	___
15. Uric Acid	___	84550	___
16. VDRL	___	86592	___
17. Wet Prep	___	82710	___
18. ______	___	___	___

G. INJECTIONS

		Code	
1. Influenza Virus Vaccine	___	90658	___
2. Pneumoccocal Vaccine	___	90772	___
3. Tetanus Toxoids	___	90703	___
4. Therapeutic Subcut/IM	___	90732	___
5. Vaccine Administration	___	90471	___
6. Vaccine - each additional	___	90472	___

H. MISCELLANEOUS

1. ______ ___ ___
2. ______ ___ ___

AMOUNT PAID $ Ø

Mark diagnosis with (1=Primary, 2=Secondary, 3=Tertiary)

DIAGNOSIS NOT LISTED BELOW ______

DIAGNOSIS	ICD-9-CM	1, 2, 3
Abdominal Pain	789.0_	
Allergic Rhinitis, Unspec.	477.9	
Angina Pectoris, Unspec.	413.9	
Anemia, Iron Deficiency, Unspec.	280.9	
Anemia, NOS	285.9	
Anemia, Pernicious	281.0	
Asthma w/ Exacerbation	493.92	
Asthmatic Bronchitis, Unspec.	493.90	
Atrial Fibrillation	427.31	
Atypical Chest Pain, Unspec.	786.59	
Bronchiolitis, due to RSV	466.11	
Bronchitis, Acute	466.0	
Bronchitis, NOS	490	
Cardiac Arrest	427.5	
Cardiopulmonary Disease, Chronic, Unspec.	416.9	
Cellulitis, NOS	682.9	
Congestive Heart Failure, Unspec.	428.0	
Contact Dermatitis NOS	692.9	
COPD NOS	496	
CVA, Acute, NOS	434.91	
CVA, Old or Healed	438.9	
Degenerative Arthritis (Specify Site)	715.9	
Dehydration	276.51	
Depression, NOS	311	
Diabetes Mellitus, Type II Controlled	250.00	
Diabetes Mellitus, Type II Controlled	250.02	
Drug Reaction, NOS	995.29	
Dysuria	788.1	
Eczema, NOS	692.2	
Edema	782.3	
Fever, Unknown Origin	780.6	
Gastritis, Acute w/o Hemorrhage	535.00	
Gastroenteritis, NOS	558.9	
Gastroesophageal Reflux	530.81	2
Hepatitis A, Infectious	070.1	
Hypercholesterolemia, Pure	272.0	
Hypertension, Unspec.	401.9	
Hypoglycemia NOS	251.2	
Hypokalemia	276.8	
Impetigo	684	
Lymphadenitis, Unspec.	289.3	
Mononucleosis	075	
Myocardial Infarction, Acute, NOS	410.9	
Organic Brain Syndrome	310.9	
Otitis Externa, Acute NOS	380.10	
Otitis Media, Acute NOS	382.9	
Peptic Ulcer Disease	536.9	
Peripheral Vascular Disease NOS	443.9	
Pharyngitis, Acute	462	
Pneumonia, Organism Unspec.	486	
Prostatitis, NOS	601.9	
PVC	427.69	
Rash, Non Specific	782.1	
Seizure Disorder NOS	780.39	
Serous Otitis Media, Chronic, Unspec.	381.10	
Sinusitis, Acute NOS	461.9	
Tonsillitis, Acute	463.	1
Upper Respiratory Infection, Acute NOS	465.9	
Urinary Tract Infection, Unspec.	599.0	
Urticaria, Unspec.	708.9	
Vertigo, NOS	780.4	
Viral Infection NOS	079.99	
Weakness, Generalized	780.79	
Weight Loss, Abnormal	783.21	

ABN: I UNDERSTAND THAT MEDICARE PROBABLY WILL NOT COVER THE SERVICES LISTED BELOW

A. ______ B. ______ C. ______

Date ______ Patient Signature ______

Doctor's Signature D.J. Schwartz, MD

RETURN: ______ Days 3 Weeks ______ Months

DOUGLASVILLE MEDICINE ASSOCIATES
5076 BRAND BLVD., SUITE 401
DOUGLASVILLE, NY 01234
PHONE No. (123) 456-7890

☐ L.D. HEATH, M.D. NPI# 9995010111
☒ D.J. SCHWARTZ, M.D. NPI# 9995020212
EIN# 00-1234560

REF# 122949 SB (05 07 09) TO REORDER CALL INHEALTH RECORD SYSTEMS 800-477-7374

JOB SKILL 7-1
Prepare Appointment Sheets

Name ______________________ Date ____________ Score ________

Performance Objective

Task: Set up three appointment pages, labeling each and blocking segments of time.

Conditions: Three appointment records, Forms 10, 11, and 12; pen or pencil. Refer to Procedure 7-1 in the *textbook* for step-by-step directions.

Standards: Complete all steps listed in this skill in ________ minutes with a minimum score of ________. (Time element and accuracy criteria may be given by instructor.)

Time: **Start:** __________ **Completed:** __________ **Total:** __________ minutes

Scoring: One point for each step performed satisfactorily unless otherwise listed or weighted by instructor.

Directions with Performance Evaluation Checklist

1st Attempt	2nd Attempt	3rd Attempt	
____	____	____	Gather materials (equipment and supplies) listed under "Conditions."
____/6	____/6	____/6	1. Set up three appointment sheets for Dr. Gerald Practon (left column) and Dr. Fran Practon (right column).
____/2	____/2	____/2	2. Label the first sheet Monday, October 27, 20XX.
____/2	____/2	____/2	3. Label the second sheet Tuesday, October 28, 20XX.
____/2	____/2	____/2	4. Label the third sheet Wednesday, October 29, 20XX.
____/6	____/6	____/6	5. Refer to the Office Hours section of Office Policies in Part III of this *Workbook* to determine when the physicians are in the office. Circle the opening and closing hours of the office for each day.
____/9	____/9	____/9	6. Block off all periods when the physicians are not in the office, i.e., lunch hours, afternoons off, and surgery/hospital responsibility time.
____/2	____/2	____/2	7. Record Dr. G. Practon's plans to visit Donald Pierce at the hospital at 9:00 a.m. on Tuesday morning and at noon on Wednesday.
____/2	____/2	____/2	8. Record Dr. F. Practon's 1-hour dental appointment with Dr. Bryce Crowe at 2:30 p.m. on Wednesday. She will need to leave the office at 2:15 p.m.
____/9	____/9	____/9	9. Indicate which appointment times are reserved for unscheduled patients (work-ins, emergencies, and so forth).
____	____	____	Complete within specified time.
____/42	____/42	____/42	**Total points earned** (To obtain a percentage score, divide the total points earned by the number of points possible.)

Comments:

Evaluator's Signature: ______________________ **Need to Repeat:** __________

National Curriculum Competency: CAAHEP: Psychomotor: V.P.1	ABHES: 8.c

JOB SKILL 7-2
Schedule Appointments

Name ______________________________ Date ______________ Score ________

Performance Objective

Task: Record patient appointments accurately using acceptable abbreviations on appointment sheets. Adjust to individual patient preferences, medical needs, and unexpected changes.

Conditions: Use the three appointment scheduling sheets from Job Skill 7-1 (Forms 10, 11, and 12), *Workbook* Table 7-1 for patient list and appointment reference information, and *textbook* Table 7-1 also found in Part IV of this *Workbook* (Abbreviation Tables) if you need help decoding appointment and patient care abbreviations. The Office Policy Appointment section may be found in Part III of the *Workbook* and step-by-step directions are in *textbook* Procedure 7-2. Use pen or pencil.

Standards: Complete all steps listed in this skill in ________ minutes with a minimum score of ________. (Time element and accuracy criteria may be given by instructor.)

Time: **Start:** ____________ **Completed:** ____________ **Total:** ____________ minutes

Scoring: One point for each step performed satisfactorily unless otherwise listed or weighted by instructor.

Directions with Performance Evaluation Checklist

All patients are established unless otherwise indicated. An asterisk (*) by a patient's name indicates a patient of Dr. Fran Practon; all others are patients of Dr. Gerald Practon. Refer to the Appointment section of Office Policies to determine the amount of time for each appointment. Schedule an appointment for each patient appearing in this exercise. It may help to use a ruler as you go down the list of names in *Workbook* Table 7-1 and check them off as you schedule.

1st Attempt	2nd Attempt	3rd Attempt	
_____	_____	_____	Gather materials (equipment and supplies) listed under "Conditions."
____/5	____/5	____/5	1. Schedule an appointment for *Melissa Jones.
____/5	____/5	____/5	2. Schedule an appointment for *Marsha MacFadden.
____/5	____/5	____/5	3. Schedule an appointment for Wendy Snow.
____/5	____/5	____/5	4. Schedule an appointment for Phyllis Dayton.
____/5	____/5	____/5	5. Schedule an appointment for *Rebecca Martinez.
____/5	____/5	____/5	6. Schedule an appointment for Jane Call.
____/5	____/5	____/5	7. Schedule an appointment for *Mary Fay Jeffers.
____/5	____/5	____/5	8. Schedule an appointment for *Philip Stevenson Jr.
____/5	____/5	____/5	9. Schedule an appointment for *Shirley Van Alystine.
____/5	____/5	____/5	10. Schedule an appointment for Courtney Pierce.
____/5	____/5	____/5	11. Schedule an appointment for Paul Stone.
____/5	____/5	____/5	12. Schedule an appointment for *Alan Becker.
____/5	____/5	____/5	13. Schedule an appointment for *Marguerite Houston.
____/5	____/5	____/5	14. Schedule an appointment for *Paul Frenzel.
____/5	____/5	____/5	15. Schedule an appointment for Elizabeth Montgomery, RN.

JOB SKILL 7-2 *(continued)*

____/5	____/5	____/5	16. Schedule an appointment for Lu Chung.
____/5	____/5	____/5	17. Schedule an appointment for Jerry Calhoun.
____/5	____/5	____/5	18. Schedule an appointment for Cathy Martinez.
____/5	____/5	____/5	19. Schedule an appointment for Lloyd Wix.
____/5	____/5	____/5	20. Schedule an appointment for Bruce Jeffers.
____/5	____/5	____/5	21. Schedule an appointment for *Ashley Jones.
____/5	____/5	____/5	22. Schedule an appointment for *David Martinez.
____/5	____/5	____/5	23. Schedule an appointment for Carl Freeburg.
____/5	____/5	____/5	24. Schedule an appointment for *Anne Rule.
____/5	____/5	____/5	25. Schedule an appointment for Charles Jones.
____/5	____/5	____/5	26. Schedule an appointment for Robert LaRue.
____/5	____/5	____/5	27. Schedule an appointment for *Phyllis Sperry.
____/5	____/5	____/5	28. Schedule an appointment for Sylvia Cone.
____/5	____/5	____/5	29. Schedule an appointment for *Pat Wochesky.
____/5	____/5	____/5	30. Schedule an appointment for Sheila Haley.
____/5	____/5	____/5	31. Schedule an appointment for Frank Elder.
____/5	____/5	____/5	32. Schedule an appointment for *Donald Eggert.
______	______	______	Complete within specified time.
___/162	___/162	___/162	**Total points earned** (To obtain a percentage score, divide the total points earned by the number of points possible.)

TABLE 7-1
Information Necessary for the Student to Prepare Appointment Schedules for Drs. Fran T. Practon and Gerald M. Practon

Name	Phone Number	Complaint or Procedure	Appointment Preference
*Melissa Jones	487–6650	Pap, estrogen inj.	Tues. p.m.
*Marsha MacFadden	487–0027	ECG, ltd. ov	Tues. a.m.
Wendy Snow	765–6626	Cast ck, leg	Mon.
Phyllis Dayton	411–2244	Pap, limited exam	Mon.
*Rebecca Martinez	765–0008	Measles inj.	Wed.
Jane Call	678–0134	Smallpox vac.	Wed.
*Mary Fay Jeffers	486–2468	MMR	Mon. after school
*Philip Stevenson Jr.	457–1133	BP, UA ltd. exam	Mon.
*Shirley Van Alystine	678–4421	IUD, BP	Tues.
Courtney Pierce	765–9077	Fever, cough	Tues. p.m.
Paul Stone	411–7206	F/U	Late Tues.
*Alan Becker	486–9993	Face infection, ltd. exam	Mon.
*Marguerite Houston	678–7892	Inj. for allergy	Tues. around 3:00 p.m.
*Paul Frenzel	765–8897	Dressing change	Early Wed. a.m.
Elizabeth Montgomery, RN	411–0068	BP	Tues. a.m. (see F. P.?)
Lu Chung	678–4455	Allergy complaint	Mon.
Jerry Calhoun	678–8771	N/P, CPX, CBC	Late as possible Tues.
Cathy Martinez	765–0008	Excise lesion on back	Wed.
Lloyd Wix	678–5529	Consult	Tues. 10:30 a.m.—must see G. P. (Wed.?)
Bruce Jeffers	486–2468	Remove glass from eye	Early Wed.
*Ashley Jones	487–6650	Suture removal	Mon. after 2:30 p.m.
*David Martinez	765–0008	Remove splinter from leg	Wed. a.m.
Carl Freeburg	486–0011	Aspirate left elbow	Late Wed.
*Anne Rule	457–9001	N/P, CPX	Mon. a.m.
Charles Jones	487–6650	Audiogram, ear lavage	Mon. p.m.
Robert LaRue	487–3355	Brief OV, VDRL	Must have Tues. a.m. (see F. P.?)
*Phyllis Sperry	678–1162	N/P, CPX	Tues. p.m.
Sylvia Cone	411–8215	HA, N/P	Wed. after lunch
*Pat Wochesky	765–3446	New OB	Wed. a.m.
Sheila Haley	678–6669	Tetanus	Wed. a.m.
Frank Elder	486–0918	N/P, pain in side, BUN, CBC	Mon.
*Donald Eggert	765–3145	Sore elbow, ltd. exam	Early Mon. p.m.

*Asterisks indicate Dr. Fran T. Practon's patients.

Comments:

Evaluator's Signature: ______________________________ **Need to Repeat:** ____________

National Curriculum Competency: CAAHEP: Psychomotor: V.P.1	ABHES: 8.c

JOB SKILL 7-3
Prepare an Appointment Reference Sheet

Name ______________________________ Date ____________ Score ________

Performance Objective

Task: Key or type the names of patients who are to be seen by the physician on a given day for a reference sheet. Make a photocopy of the appointment sheet for comparison or to use as an alternative reference.

Conditions: One sheet of white paper, computer or word processor, and photocopy machine.

Standards: Complete all steps listed in this skill in ________ minutes with a minimum score of ________. (Time element and accuracy criteria may be given by instructor.)

Time: **Start:** ____________ **Completed:** ____________ **Total:** ____________ minutes

Scoring: One point for each step performed satisfactorily unless otherwise listed or weighted by instructor.

Directions with Performance Evaluation Checklist

1st Attempt	2nd Attempt	3rd Attempt	
_______	_______	_______	Gather materials (equipment and supplies) listed under "Conditions."
_______	_______	_______	1. Locate information from Dr. Gerald Practon's schedule for Day 3 listed in Job Skills 7-1 and 7-2.
_____/3	_____/3	_____/3	2. Center and boldface the following information as the title for the appointment reference sheet: Dr. Gerald Practon, Wednesday, October 29, 20XX.
_____/3	_____/3	_____/3	3. Make three columns and title them in capital letters: TIME, NAME, REASON FOR VISIT.
____/15	____/15	____/15	4. Abstract information and key a single-spaced list of appointment times, patient names (last name first), and reason for visit to let Dr. G. Practon know who is expected the morning of Wednesday, October 29, 20XX.
_______	_______	_______	5. Photocopy the appointment page for Wednesday, October 29, 20XX, and compare it with the typed list. Additional copies would generally be made for office staff.
_______	_______	_______	Complete within specified time.
____/25	____/25	____/25	**Total points earned** (To obtain a percentage score, divide the total points earned by the number of points possible.)

Comments:

Evaluator's Signature: ______________________________ **Need to Repeat:** ____________

National Curriculum Competency: CAAHEP: Psychomotor: V.P.1	ABHES: 8.c

JOB SKILL 7-4
Complete Appointment Cards

Name ______________________________ Date ____________ Score ________

Performance Objective

Task: Write accurate and legible appointment cards.

Conditions: Use appointment cards (Form 13) and pen or pencil.

Standards: Complete all steps listed in this skill in _______ minutes with a minimum score of ________. (Time element and accuracy criteria may be given by instructor.)

Time: **Start:** _____________ **Completed:** _____________ **Total:** _____________ minutes

Scoring: One point for each step performed satisfactorily unless otherwise listed or weighted by instructor.

Directions with Performance Evaluation Checklist

Write the patient's name at the top of the card, check the correct physician, circle the day of the week, and write the appointment date and time for the following patients. *Indicates patient of Fran Practon, MD.

1st Attempt	2nd Attempt	3rd Attempt	
_______	_______	_______	Gather materials (equipment and supplies) listed under "Conditions."
_____/5	_____/5	_____/5	1. Charles Jones, Wednesday, October 29, at 2:00 p.m.
_____/5	_____/5	_____/5	2. *Marguerite Houston, Tuesday, November 12, at 3:00 p.m.
_____/5	_____/5	_____/5	3. Carl Freeburg, Wednesday, November 6, at 2:45 p.m.
_____/5	_____/5	_____/5	4. *Pat Wochesky, Monday, December 2, at 9:00 a.m.
_______	_______	_______	Complete within specified time.
____/22	____/22	____/22	**Total points earned** (To obtain a percentage score, divide the total points earned by the number of points possible.)

Comments:

Evaluator's Signature: ________________________________ **Need to Repeat:** ______________

National Curriculum Competency: CAAHEP: Psychomotor: V.P.1	ABHES: 8.c

JOB SKILL 7-5

Abstract Information and Complete a Hospital/Surgery Scheduling Form

Name ____ Date ______________ Score _______

Performance Objective

Task: Review a patient's medical record and then abstract and key or type the required information on the hospital/surgery scheduling form.

Conditions: Wayne G. Weather's patient information (*Workbook* Figure 7-1), one hospital/surgery scheduling form (Form 14), pen or pencil, and correction fluid. Refer to Procedure 7-4 in the *textbook* for step-by-step directions.

Standards: Complete all steps listed in this skill in _______ minutes with a minimum score of ________. (Time element and accuracy criteria may be given by instructor.)

Time: **Start:** ____________ **Completed:** ____________ **Total:** ____________ minutes

Scoring: One point for each step performed satisfactorily unless otherwise listed or weighted by instructor.

Directions with Performance Evaluation Checklist

Using Mr. Weather's "Patient Information for Medical Records" found in *Workbook* Figure 7-1, abstract data to complete the hospital/surgical scheduling form. Use the following additional information: Mr. Weather was referred to Dr. Gerald Practon by Dr. Mary Hill and is to be admitted to College Hospital for a 33-day stay on Tuesday, October 28, 20XX, at 5:30 a.m. His diagnosis is lumbar herniated nucleus pulposus, and a second opinion is not required. His preadmission testing of CBC, EKG, and chest x-ray was performed on October 27, 20XX. He has not been previously hospitalized. Mr. Weather is a smoker and prefers a ward room. The elective lumbar (L4-L5) laminectomy is scheduled for Tuesday, October 28, 20XX, at 7:30 a.m. Preadmission operation instructions as well as insurance and financial arrangements have been discussed.

Dr. Clarence Cutler will be the assistant surgeon and Dr. Harold Barker will give general anesthesia. The surgery, scheduled by hospital employee Robert Slye, should take approximately 1 hour to complete. Kevin Raye of Aetna Casualty & Security Company provided the authorization number, 8036981, and the scheduling was completed and reported to the patient on October 24. Susan Smith at the referring physician's office has been notified and all arrangements have been posted in the appointment book.

1st Attempt	2nd Attempt	3rd Attempt	
_______	_______	_______	Gather materials (equipment and supplies) listed under "Conditions."
_______	_______	_______	1. Section 1: Indicate patient name.
_______	_______	_______	2. Section 1: Indicate procedure.
_______	_______	_______	3. Section 1: Indicate status of surgery.
_______	_______	_______	4. Section 1: Indicate diagnosis.
_______	_______	_______	5. Section 1: Indicate facility.
_______	_______	_______	6. Section 1: Indicate admitting status.
_______	_______	_______	7. Section 1: Indicate preferred assistant surgeon.
_______	_______	_______	8. Section 1: Indicate preferred anesthesiologist.
_______	_______	_______	9. Section 1: Indicate referring physician.
____/3	____/3	____/3	10. Section 2: Indicate patient's age, date of birth, smoking status.
_______	_______	_______	11. Section 2: Indicate type of room preferred.
____/2	____/2	____/2	12. Section 2: Indicate telephone numbers.

JOB SKILL 7-5 *(continued)*

____/2	____/2	____/2	13. Section 2: Indicate insurance information.
______	______	______	14. Section 2: Indicate second opinion requirements.
____/3	____/3	____/3	15. Section 2: Indicate emergency contact.
______	______	______	16. Section 2: Indicate previous admitting information.
____/3	____/3	____/3	17. Section 2: Indicate preadmission testing.
______	______	______	18. Section 2: Indicate admission procedures reported.
______	______	______	19. Section 2: Indicate instructions given to patient.
______	______	______	20. Section 2: Indicate insurance/financial discussion.
____/2	____/2	____/2	21. Section 3: Indicate operating room reservation.
______	______	______	22. Section 3: Indicate hospital surgical scheduling person.
______	______	______	23. Section 3: Indicate assistant surgeon notified.
______	______	______	24. Section 3: Indicate anesthesiologist notified.
______	______	______	25. Section 3: Indicate referring physician notified.
______	______	______	26. Section 3: Indicate admission and preadmission tests confirmed.
______	______	______	27. Section 3: Indicate prior authorization obtained.
______	______	______	28. Section 3: Indicate appointment book data posted.
______	______	______	29. Section 3: Indicate patient advised.
______	______	______	30. Section 3: Indicate H & P done.
____/2	____/2	____/2	31. Section 3: Indicate name of office scheduler and date scheduled.
______	______	______	Complete within specified time.
___/43	___/43	___/43	**Total points earned** (To obtain a percentage score, divide the total points earned by the number of points possible.)

Comments:

Evaluator's Signature: ______________________________ **Need to Repeat:** ____________

National Curriculum Competency: CAAHEP: Psychomotor: V.P.2	ABHES: 8.f

FIGURE 7-1

PATIENT INFORMATION FOR MEDICAL RECORDS *(Please Print)* **DATE:** 10/24/XX

PATIENT	(MR.) MRS. MISS	LAST NAME: Weather	FIRST NAME: Wayne	MIDDLE: G

PATIENT ADDRESS	STREET	CITY	STATE	ZIP	HOME PHONE
→	6304 Fracture Road	Woodland Hills,	XY	12345	555/965-2110

SOCIAL SECURITY NUMBER	DATE OF BIRTH	AGE	DRIVER'S LICENSE NO.
→ XXX-XX-5334	1-6-43		G-0073-121

PATIENT EMPLOYER	OCCUPATION
→ Bu T. Floor Coverings	carpet layer

EMPLOYER'S ADDRESS	STREET	CITY	STATE	ZIP	BUS PHONE
→	3100 Rug Street,	Woodland Hills,	XY	12345	555/861-0122

SPOUSE'S NAME	MARITAL STATUS	REFERRED BY
→ Nancy B. Weather	(M) S D W SEP.	Employer

SPOUSE'S EMPLOYER	STREET	CITY	STATE	ZIP	BUS. PHONE
Superior Optical Co.	25 E. Main St.,	Woodland Hills,	XY	12345-0000	555/761-0811

IN CASE OF EMERGENCY CONTACT: NAME	ADDRESS	CITY	STATE	ZIP	TELEPHONE
Jolly B. Rosen (stepbrother)	3641 Hope St,	Woodland Hills,	XY	12345	555/876-6025

MEDICAL INSURANCE INFORMATION

COMPANY	POLICY NUMBER
Aetna Casualty and Security Co. 2412 Wilshire Blvd., Woodland Hills, XY 12345-0000	
N/A	3201

IF SOMEONE OTHER THAN PATIENT IS RESPONSIBLE FOR PAYMENT PLEASE COMPLETE THIS SECTION

RESPONSIBLE PARTY	MR. MRS. MISS	LAST NAME	FIRST NAME	MIDDLE	RELATION
ADDRESS →	STREET	CITY	STATE	ZIP	TELEPHONE
OCCUPATION →		EMPLOYED BY			
EMPLOYER'S ADDRESS →	STREET	CITY	STATE	ZIP	BUS. PHONE

I hereby authorize Dr. Gerald Practon to furnish to the above insurance company(s) or to a designated attorney, all information which said insurance company(s) or attorney may request. I hereby assign to Dr. Gerald Practon all money to which I am entitled for medical and/or surgical expense relative to the service rendered by him, but not to exceed my indebtedness to said physician and/or surgeon. It is understood that any money received from the above named insurance company, over and above my indebtedness will be refunded to me when my bill is paid in full. I understand I am financially responsible to said doctor(s) for charges not covered by this assignment. I further agree in the event of non-payment, to bear the cost of collection, and/or Court cost and reasonable legal fees should this be required.

INSURED OR GUARDIAN SIGNATURE ______

Wayne G. Weather
PATIENT'S SIGNATURE

58-8409 © 1976 BIBBERO SYSTEMS, INC., SAN FRANCISCO

Courtesy of Bibbero Systems, Inc., Petaluma, CA. Phone: 800-242-2376; Fax: 800-242-9330; Web site: http://www.bibbero.com.

JOB SKILL 7-6
Transfer Surgery Scheduling Information to a Form Letter

Name ____ Date ______________ Score _______

Performance Objective

Task: Use surgical scheduling information and fill in a form letter to be mailed to persons involved in the procedure.

Conditions: Use hospital/surgery scheduling form (Form 14) for reference. Duplicate form letter (Form 15) using photocopy machine.

Standards: Complete all steps listed in this skill in _______ minutes with a minimum score of ________. (Time element and accuracy criteria may be given by instructor.)

Time: **Start:** ____________ **Completed:** ____________ **Total:** ____________ minutes

Scoring: One point for each step performed satisfactorily unless otherwise listed or weighted by instructor.

Directions with Performance Evaluation Checklist

October 24, 20XX: You have completed all the surgical scheduling arrangements for Mr. Wayne Weather. The next step is to complete the surgical form letter and photocopy it. One copy will be sent to the patient and one will be retained in Dr. Practon's files.

1st Attempt	2nd Attempt	3rd Attempt	
______	______	______	Gather materials (equipment and supplies) listed under "Conditions."
______	______	______	1. Read the surgical scheduling form letter to determine what information needs to be abstracted from the hospital/surgery scheduling form (Form 14).
____/4	____/4	____/4	2. Fill in the date and complete the inside address.
___/10	___/10	___/10	3. Fill in the information in the body of the letter.
____/4	____/4	____/4	4. Sign the letter and fill in the information for the physicians involved.
______	______	______	Complete within specified time.
___/21	___/21	___/21	**Total points earned** (To obtain a percentage score, divide the total points earned by the number of points possible.)

Comments:

Evaluator's Signature: ______________________________________ **Need to Repeat:** ______________

National Curriculum Competency: CAAHEP: Psychomotor: V.P.2	ABHES: 8.f

JOB SKILL 7-7
Complete Requisition Forms for Outpatient Diagnostic Tests

Name ______________________________ Date ____________ Score ________

Performance Objective

Task: Handwrite information on requisition forms to be given to patients to have outpatient diagnostic tests performed.

Conditions: Use Laboratory Requisition (Form 16) and X-Ray Request (Form 17) and pen. Refer to Procedure 7-5 in the *textbook* for step-by-step directions. Refer to Medical Practice Reference Material (Part III of the *Workbook*) for physician data.

Standards: Complete all steps listed in this skill in _______ minutes with a minimum score of ________. (Time element and accuracy criteria may be given by instructor.)

Time: **Start:** ____________ **Completed:** ____________ **Total:** ____________ minutes

Scoring: One point for each step performed satisfactorily unless otherwise listed or weighted by instructor.

Directions with Performance Evaluation Checklist

Read the following case scenario, abstract information, and complete two requisition forms.

An HMO patient, Ted N. Thatcher, comes to the office complaining of neck and right shoulder pain. After an examination, Dr. Fran Practon orders fasting laboratory tests (arthritis profile, uric acid, and urinalysis). Comprehensive cervical spine x-rays and a complete shoulder series are scheduled for March 4, 20XX, at 11:00 a.m. Diagnosis is acute cervical arthritis (*ICD-10-CM* code M43.02) and shoulder pain (*ICD-10-CM* code M25.511). Patient to return in 1 week.

Mr. Thatcher's Social Security number is XXX-XX-9509; birthdate: 5/8/82; new address: 870 N. Seacrest St., Woodland Hills, XY 12345-0846; telephone number: (555) 987-4589; insurance: HMO Net, 4390 Main Street, Woodland Hills, XY 12345-0846, policy no. 459-0987-0. For this particular managed care plan, the outside services that Dr. Practon ordered do not require preauthorization. Today's date: February 28, 20XX.

1st Attempt	2nd Attempt	3rd Attempt	
______	______	______	Gather materials (equipment and supplies) listed under "Conditions."
______	______	______	1. Highlight what type of diagnostic tests are to be performed. ____________
______	______	______	2. Note the date the patient has agreed upon. ____________
______	______	______	3. Write the name of the insurance carrier. ____________
______	______	______	4. Telephone the diagnostic facility (ABC Radiology) and schedule the tests. Note the time the tests are scheduled. ____________
___/20	___/20	___/20	5. Abstract information from the case scenario and fill in the Laboratory Requisition form; hand the form to the patient and record the information in the chart.
___/15	___/15	___/15	6. Abstract information from the case scenario and fill in the X-Ray Request form; hand to the patient and record information in the chart.
______	______	______	Complete within specified time.
___/41	___/41	___/41	**Total points earned** (To obtain a percentage score, divide the total points earned by the number of points possible.)

JOB SKILL 7-7 *(continued)*

Comments:

Evaluator's Signature: ______________________________ **Need to Repeat:** ____________

National Curriculum Competency: CAAHEP: Psychomotor: V.P.2	ABHES: 8.c

CHAPTER **8**

Filing Procedures

OBJECTIVES

After completing the exercises, the student will be able to:

1. Enhance knowledge of medical terminology, interpret abbreviations, and accurately spell medical words.
2. Determine filing units (Job Skill 8-1).
3. Index and file names alphabetically (Job Skill 8-2).
4. File patient and business names alphabetically (Job Skill 8-3).
5. Index names on file folder labels and arrange file cards in alphabetical order (Job Skill 8-4).
6. Color-code file cards (Job Skill 8-5).

FOCUS ON CERTIFICATION*

CMA Content Summary

- Needs, purposes, and terminology of filing systems
- Alphabetic, numeric, and subject filing
- Color-code, tickler, electronic data processing, and cross-reference files
- Storing, protecting, and transferring files
- Retaining and purging files (statute of limitations)
- Scanning equipment

*This *Workbook* and the accompanying *textbook* meet the entry-level administrative and general competencies for the CMA outlined by the AAMA Examination Content Outline and Occupational Analysis and for the RMA and CMAS outlined by the AMT Competencies, Construction Parameters, and Examination Specifications (see Competency Grid in Appendix B of the *textbook*).

RMA Content Summary

- Prepare patient record (by filing information)
- Manage patient medical record system
- File patient and physician communication in chart
- File materials according to proper system (chronological, alphabetical, subject)
- Protect, store, and maintain medical records according to proper conventions and HIPAA privacy regulations

CMAS Content Summary

- Manage documents and patient charts using paper methods
- File records alphabetically, numerically, by subject, and by color
- Employ indexing rules
- Arrange contents of patient charts in appropriate order
- Document and file laboratory results and patient communication in charts
- Store, protect, retain, and destroy records appropriately
- Perform daily chart management
- Observe and maintain confidentiality of records, charts, and test results

STOP AND THINK CASE SCENARIOS AND EXAM-STYLE REVIEW QUESTIONS

Refer to the end of Chapter 8 in the *textbook.*

Abbreviation and Spelling Review

Read the following patient's chart note and write the meanings for the abbreviations listed below the note. To decode any abbreviations you do not understand or that appear unfamiliar to you, refer to the list of abbreviations in Part IV of this *Workbook.* Step-by-step directions for this exercise are found in Procedure 1-1 of Chapter 1 in the *textbook.* Medical terms in the chart note are italicized; study them for spelling. Use your medical dictionary to look up their definitions. Your instructor may give a spelling and definition test that includes these words and abbreviations.

DATE	PROGRESS
12-3-20XX	Doris A Waxman PC: occipital headaches PX: HEENT No *diplopia,* no *tinnitus.* See PI TPR neg. CV: no chest pain, palpitation, *orthopnea, dyspnea* or exertion or *hemoptysis.* GI: one episode of *emesis* last night. Some belching & intolerance to fried foods. RUQ abdom pain; no *hematemesis* or *melena.* GU: no frequency or *dysuria.* GYN: no abnormal bleeding. Ordered *oral cholecystography.* Dx: rule out GB disease.
	Fran Practon, MD
	Fran Practon, MD

PC	______________	GI	______________
PX	______________	RUQ	______________
HEENT	______________	abdom	______________
PI	______________	GU	______________
TPR	______________	GYN	______________
neg.	______________	Dx	______________
CV	______________	GB	______________

Review Questions

Review the objectives, glossary, and chapter information before completing the following review questions.

1. Why is it important for all members of the office staff to follow a general office filing system and obey filing rules? ______
2. When choosing a medical filing system, what must be considered?
   a. ______
   b. ______
   c. ______
   d. ______
   e. ______
   f. ______
3. Name three advantages of using an alphabetical color-coded file system.
   a. ______
   b. ______
   c. ______
4. Name several types of information that may be filed in a subject file.
   a. ______
   b. ______
   c. ______
   d. ______
5. Why is numerical filing considered an indirect method? ______
   ______
   ______
6. Where are numerical filing systems primarily used? ______
   ______
7. In a chronological filing system, numbers are used based on ______.
8. Managing files so that information is not lost in a computerized system requires ______.
9. What is the purpose of a tickler file? ______
10. A person's first name is also called the ______ and the last name is the ______.
11. A married woman may legally write her name three different ways. Give three examples of the way a name can be written.
    a. ______
    b. ______
    c. ______

12. What considerations should be made when selecting filing equipment?

 a. ______________________________

 b. ______________________________

 c. ______________________________

 d. ______________________________

 e. ______________________________

13. Name two purposes served by file guides.

 a. ______________________________

 b. ______________________________

14. What steps would you take when a patient's chart cannot be located?

 a. ______________________________

 b. ______________________________

 c. ______________________________

 d. ______________________________

 e. ______________________________

 f. ______________________________

 g. ______________________________

 h. ______________________________

15. To purge files, what two procedures can solve the problem of determining when to transfer patient files from active to inactive status?

 a. ______________________________

 b. ______________________________

16. Name three space-saving, quick, and easy retrieval methods for storing large volumes of medical records.

 a. ______________________________

 b. ______________________________

 c. ______________________________

Critical Thinking Exercises

1. State at least two circumstances that might require cross-referencing of names in alphabetical files.

 a. ______________________________

 b. ______________________________

JOB SKILL 8-1
Determine Filing Units

Name ____ Date ______________ Score _______

Performance Objective

Task: Designate filing units so that names can be filed alphabetically in an office file.

Conditions: Assemble 50 names and pen or pencil. Refer in the *textbook* to alphabetical filing rules used for indexing and Procedure 8-4 for step-by-step directions.

Standards: Complete all steps listed in this skill in _______ minutes with a minimum score of ________. (Time element and accuracy criteria may be given by instructor.)

Time: **Start:** ____________ **Completed:** ____________ **Total:** ____________ minutes

Scoring: One point for each step performed satisfactorily unless otherwise listed or weighted by instructor.

Directions with Performance Evaluation Checklist

Study each name and designate units using pen or pencil to underline. Use one line for the first unit, two lines for the second unit, three lines for the third unit, and four lines for the fourth unit. Study the example below before beginning.

EXAMPLE

1st Attempt	2nd Attempt	3rd Attempt	
			Underline each unit of name: A. Marsha Moore
_______	_______	_______	Gather materials (equipment and supplies) listed under "Conditions."
_______	_______	_______	1. Underline each unit of name: Rebecca Rodene Rochester.
_______	_______	_______	2. Underline each unit of name: Wm. John Taylor Kelly.
_______	_______	_______	3. Underline each unit of name: Jamie Trethorn.
_______	_______	_______	4. Underline each unit of name: Dan A. DeLeon.
_______	_______	_______	5. Underline each unit of name: E. Mary LeVan.
_______	_______	_______	6. Underline each unit of name: Amy Kay M'Oeters.
_______	_______	_______	7. Underline each unit of name: Shelby C. St. John.
_______	_______	_______	8. Underline each unit of name: Robert F. MacGregor.
_______	_______	_______	9. Underline each unit of name: S. J. VanderLinder.
_______	_______	_______	10. Underline each unit of name: Kelly Saint Thomas.
_______	_______	_______	11. Underline each unit of name: Priscilla Ruby DuMont.
_______	_______	_______	12. Underline each unit of name: Peter deWinter.
_______	_______	_______	13. Underline each unit of name: Sister Mary Beth.
_______	_______	_______	14. Underline each unit of name: Mayor Bill A. King.
_______	_______	_______	15. Underline each unit of name: Dr. John J. Jackson.
_______	_______	_______	16. Underline each unit of name: Mary-Kay deVille.
_______	_______	_______	17. Underline each unit of name: Sji Mulzono.
_______	_______	_______	18. Underline each unit of name: Mark Philip-DeGeer.
_______	_______	_______	19. Underline each unit of name: Pope John Paul.
_______	_______	_______	20. Underline each unit of name: Maj. Steve Royal Smith.

JOB SKILL 8-1 *(continued)*

_______ _______ _______ 21. Underline each unit of name: Mrs. Noreen J. Cline.
_______ _______ _______ 22. Underline each unit of name: Charles T. Lloyd Jr.
_______ _______ _______ 23. Underline each unit of name: Charles T. Lloyd II.
_______ _______ _______ 24. Underline each unit of name: Peter L. Morrison, MD.
_______ _______ _______ 25. Underline each unit of name: Sarah May Dennis-Brit.
_______ _______ _______ 26. Underline each unit of name: C. Ngyume.
_______ _______ _______ 27. Underline each unit of name: Paul Wm. SeValle.
_______ _______ _______ 28. Underline each unit of name: Foster Memorial Community Hospital.
_______ _______ _______ 29. Underline each unit of name: Ft. Benning Convalescent Home.
_______ _______ _______ 30. Underline each unit of name: A-1 Pharmacy.
_______ _______ _______ 31. Underline each unit of name: American Medical Corp.
_______ _______ _______ 32. Underline each unit of name: Dr. Spock's Clinic.
_______ _______ _______ 33. Underline each unit of name: St. Jude's Hospital.
_______ _______ _______ 34. Underline each unit of name: Russ Wilder Ambulance Service.
_______ _______ _______ 35. Underline each unit of name: Mt. Blanc Druggist.
_______ _______ _______ 36. Underline each unit of name: Century 21 Medical Supply.
_______ _______ _______ 37. Underline each unit of name: College of St. Catherine.
_______ _______ _______ 38. Underline each unit of name: Washington School, St. Paul, MN.
_______ _______ _______ 39. Underline each unit of name: Mary Cain Pharmacy, Waco, TX.
_______ _______ _______ 40. Underline each unit of name: Mary Cain Pharmacy, Inc.
_______ _______ _______ 41. Underline each unit of name: Riverside County Public Library.
_______ _______ _______ 42. Underline each unit of name: St. Joseph's Community Hospital, Austin, TX.
_______ _______ _______ 43. Underline each unit of name: University of California–Los Angeles.
_______ _______ _______ 44. Underline each unit of name: University of California–Davis.
_______ _______ _______ 45. Underline each unit of name: St. Louis Publications.
_______ _______ _______ 46. Underline each unit of name: Father Buechner.
_______ _______ _______ 47. Underline each unit of name: Sister Sue Ellen.
_______ _______ _______ 48. Underline each unit of name: C. R. Toll.
_______ _______ _______ 49. Underline each unit of name: Rebecca Toll (Mrs. John).
_______ _______ _______ 50. Underline each unit of name: Mrs. John A. Peterson.
_______ _______ _______ Complete within specified time.
____/52 ____/52 ____/52 **Total points earned** (To obtain a percentage score, divide the total points earned by the number of points possible.)

Comments:

Evaluator's Signature: ______________________________ **Need to Repeat:** ______________

National Curriculum Competency: CAAHEP: Cognitive: V.C.9; Psychomotor: V.P.8	ABHES: 8.a, b

JOB SKILL 8-2
Index and File Names Alphabetically

Name ______________________________ Date ______________ Score ________

Performance Objective

Task: Demonstrate a knowledge of standardized alphabetizing rules to competently file and retrieve medical records; apply this knowledge as you alphabetize names for class discussion.

Conditions: Assemble 18 groups of names and pen or pencil. Refer in the *textbook* to alphabetical filing rules used for indexing and Procedure 8-4 for step-by-step directions.

Standards: Complete all steps listed in this skill in _______ minutes with a minimum score of ________. (Time element and accuracy criteria may be given by instructor.)

Time: **Start:** ____________ **Completed:** ____________ **Total:** ____________ minutes

Scoring: One point for each step performed satisfactorily unless otherwise listed or weighted by instructor.

Directions with Performance Evaluation Checklist

Underline the first, second, and third units of each name to show proper indexing order, placing one line under the surname, two lines under the given name, and three lines under the third name or initial. Alphabetize each group of three names, writing the corresponding letters, in order, in the answer column.

EXAMPLE

Units underlined: (a) J. T. Jefferson (b) John Thompson (c) Mrs. T. J. Brown (Marsha)

Units in correct order: (a) Jefferson, J. T. (b) Thompson, John (c) Brown, Marsha (Mrs. T. J.)

Correct filing order: c a b (c) Brown, Marsha (Mrs. T. J.) (a) Jefferson, J. T. (b) Thompson, John

1st Attempt	2nd Attempt	3rd Attempt		
______	______	______		Gather materials (equipment and supplies) listed under "Conditions."
____/3	____/3	____/3	1. ______	(a) Henrietta S. Lamar (b) Greta Lee Mason (c) Mary Lou LaMotte
____/3	____/3	____/3	2. ______	(a) Raymond Lorenzana (b) R. Lorenzo (c) Tony Lorenzen
____/3	____/3	____/3	3. ______	(a) Roger N. Stephens (b) Garland N. St. John (c) Robert Sprague
____/3	____/3	____/3	4. ______	(a) Walter E. Johnston (b) Willard L. Johnson (c) Geo. W. Johnstone
____/3	____/3	____/3	5. ______	(a) Hugh M. MacAdoo (b) Bruce T. McCall (c) Robert A. Macall
____/3	____/3	____/3	6. ______	(a) Lt. Margaret Kim (b) Margaret LaForgeaus (c) Mrs. M. LeMaster (Loretta)
____/3	____/3	____/3	7. ______	(a) H. King IV (b) H. M. King Jr. (c) Mrs. H. M. King (Alice)
____/3	____/3	____/3	8. ______	(a) Mrs. Tina Simmons (Leonard) (b) Richard K. Simmons (c) R. K. Simons-Steele
____/3	____/3	____/3	9. ______	(a) J. W. Winn, MD, 1404 Rosealea Rd., Cleveland, Ohio (b) James W. Winn, 1203 Venetta Drive, Cleveland, Ohio (c) J. W. Winn, 18 Maple St., Cleveland, Ohio
____/3	____/3	____/3	10. ______	(a) Mary Sue Shelton (b) Martha Lee Shelton-Alston (c) Sheila-Lynn Alston (Mrs. Shelton A.)
____/3	____/3	____/3	11. ______	(a) Willard Champs, 1072 Main St. (b) Willard Champs, 290 Main St. (c) Wilfred Champs, 10234 Main St.
____/3	____/3	____/3	12. ______	(a) Jas. E. McBean (b) J. L. MacBeen (c) Jason McBean

JOB SKILL 8-2 *(continued)*

____/3	____/3	____/3	13. ______	(a) W. L. Arthur-Davis (b) Carolyn Archer (Mrs. David) (c) Sister Arletta-Marie
____/3	____/3	____/3	14. ______	(a) Grace Ayers (b) A. Joseph Almonzaz (c) Mrs. Anthony Ayers (Gloria)
____/3	____/3	____/3	15. ______	(a) Norman Gilliam (b) N. Gilliam (c) Mrs. N. R. Gilliam (Norma)
____/3	____/3	____/3	16. ______	(a) Matthew Kuboushek (b) Toshi Kubota (c) I. M. Kuchenberg
____/3	____/3	____/3	17. ______	(a) Dr. Vincent DeLucca (b) Victoria Deems (c) Dr. Carl Deams Jr.
____/3	____/3	____/3	18. ______	(a) Mrs. Loretta Maggio (b) Bokker T. Magallon Sr. (c) B. L. Magill, Rev.
______	______	______	Complete within specified time.	
____/56	____/56	____/56	**Total points earned** (To obtain a percentage score, divide the total points earned by the number of points possible.)	

Comments:

Evaluator's Signature: ______________________________ **Need to Repeat:** ______________

National Curriculum Competency: CAAHEP: Cognitive: V.C.9, 10; Psychomotor: V.P.3, 8	ABHES: 8.a, b

JOB SKILL 8-3
File Patient and Business Names Alphabetically

Name ______________________________ Date ______________ Score ________

Performance Objective

Task: Sort patient names and business names in alphabetical order according to standardized alphabetical filing rules. **Note: This is an advanced exercise.**

Conditions: Assemble 10 groups of names and pen or pencil. Refer in the *textbook* to alphabetical filing rules used for indexing and Procedure 8-4 for step-by-step directions.

Standards: Complete all steps listed in this skill in _______ minutes with a minimum score of ________. (Time element and accuracy criteria may be given by instructor.)

Time: **Start:** ____________ **Completed:** ____________ **Total:** ____________ minutes

Scoring: One point for each step performed satisfactorily unless otherwise listed or weighted by instructor.

Directions with Performance Evaluation Checklist

After each group of four names, indicate by letter the order in which the names would be arranged in a file.

1st Attempt	2nd Attempt	3rd Attempt		
______	______	______		Gather materials (equipment and supplies) listed under "Conditions."
____/4	____/4	____/4	1. ______	a. Mrs. Allene Baker
				b. A. Baker
				c. A. Barker, MD
				d. Dr. Barker
____/4	____/4	____/4	2. ______	a. The Apple Advertising Co.
				b. Apple-Cornwall, Inc.
				c. Appling Health Care
				d. Allan Applesey Corp.
____/4	____/4	____/4	3. ______	a. Brother Brian Advertising
				b. The Bonita Rehab Facility
				c. B and B Clinic
				d. Bonita Rd. Care
____/4	____/4	____/4	4. ______	a. Larue-McGuire Canyon Hospital
				b. Los Angeles Community Care
				c. Laruem Medical Clinic
				d. Las Robles Medical Center
____/4	____/4	____/4	5. ______	a. Fortieth St. Convalescent Center
				b. The Forrest Hospital
				c. The Frew-Forrest Medical Group
				d. Forrest Medical Facility
____/4	____/4	____/4	6. ______	a. Professor Sam A. Zimmer
				b. Zimmer-Kliev Agency
				c. Prof. A. Zimmer
				d. Z and Z Druggists

JOB SKILL 8-3 *(continued)*

____/4 ____/4 ____/4 7. ______ a. Robin Persy-Doerr
b. Philip Persico Retirement Care
c. Poinsettia Residential Care
d. Persicona-Philips Mortuary

____/4 ____/4 ____/4 8. ______ a. Mcdonald, Calvin
b. MacDonald, Carl, MD
c. Macdonald, C. A.
d. Dr. McDermott

____/4 ____/4 ____/4 9. ______ a. Tyler-Hill Medical Assn
b. Mark Tyler-Hill Mortuary
c. The Pleasant Hills Pharmacy
d. Phyllis G. Hills

____/4 ____/4 ____/4 10. ______ a. Kevin St. Mann Jr.
b. Chauncey A. Southern
c. Kevin St. Mann
d. Southwest St. Pharmaceuticals

______ ______ ______ Complete within specified time.

____/42 ____/42 ____/42 **Total points earned** (To obtain a percentage score, divide the total points earned by the number of points possible.)

Comments:

Evaluator's Signature: ______________________ **Need to Repeat:** ____________

National Curriculum Competency: CAAHEP: Cognitive: V.C.9, 10; Psychomotor: V.P.8	ABHES: 8.a, b

JOB SKILL 8-4
Index Names on File Folder Labels and Arrange File Cards in Alphabetical Order

Name ______________________________ Date ____________ Score ________

Performance Objective

Task: Key names on file labels uniformly in correct indexing order. Affix labels to file cards or type names on file cards and alphabetize.

Conditions: Use Forms 18, 19, and 20, sixty file folder labels (optional), and sixty 3″ by 5″ index cards (or slips of paper). Refer in the *textbook* to alphabetical filing rules used for indexing and Procedure 8-4 for step-by-step directions.

Standards: Complete all steps listed in this skill in ______ minutes with a minimum score of ______. (Time element and accuracy criteria may be given by instructor.)

Time: **Start:** __________ **Completed:** __________ **Total:** __________ minutes

Scoring: One point for each step performed satisfactorily unless otherwise listed or weighted by instructor.

Directions with Performance Evaluation Checklist

Dr. Practon has asked you to key or type patient names appearing on Forms 18, 19, and 20 on file folder labels, as if they were to be attached to folder tabs, in proper indexing order. These can be printed neatly by hand using the forms provided; typed using a typewriter; or keyed and printed from a computer on actual file folder labels. Affix labels to, or type names at the top right of index cards and arrange in alphabetical order. These may be spread out on your desk, or a small recipe box may be used for sorting. Note: There are several options for completing this job skill. Please read through all the steps prior to starting and determine if you will be using the worksheet (forms) provided for file labels or actual file folder labels and index cards.

1st Attempt	2nd Attempt	3rd Attempt	
______	______	______	Gather materials (equipment and supplies) listed under "Conditions."
___/30	___/30	___/30	1. Use the labels on Forms 18, 19, and 20 as a worksheet and write (in pencil) each patient's name in the correct indexing order. Check with the instructor if you have problems determining units and indexing sequence. If you are not using actual file folder labels for this job skill, you may use a blank sheet of paper for the worksheet and these labels (which will be cut up into slips of paper for alphabetizing) for printing or typing patient names.
______	______	______	2. Use blank labels marked "X" at the end of Form 20 for any names that need to be cross-referenced; these may vary per student.
___/30	___/30	___/30	3. Key or type names uniformly on file folder labels in indexing order starting at the left margin. At the right margin, key or type the reference number that appears by the patient's name as if it were an account number.

EXAMPLE—FILE LABEL

McDougall, Walter Louis	Acct. #1

___/30	___/30	___/30	4. Affix labels to index cards (top right), or key/type each name and number at the top of a card.

JOB SKILL 8-4 *(continued)*

___/30 ___/30 ___/30 5. Alphabetize all cards or slips.

___/10 ___/10 ___/10 6. Complete an answer sheet by either listing the account numbers in the order they were filed or keying each name in the sequence you have determined.

EXAMPLE—ANSWER SHEET

34. Albert, Frank
17. *Benjamin, Thomas
57. Bennett, C. Richard

___ ___ ___ Complete within specified time.

___/133 ___/133 ___/133 **Total points earned** (To obtain a percentage score, divide the total points earned by the number of points possible.)

Comments:

Evaluator's Signature: ____________ **Need to Repeat:** ________

National Curriculum Competency: CAAHEP: Cognitive: V.C.9, 10; Psychomotor: V.P.8	ABHES: 8.a, b

JOB SKILL 8-5
Color-Code File Cards

Name ______________________________ Date ______________ Score ________

Performance Objective

Task: Color-code 60 file cards.

Conditions: Use file index cards from Job Skill 8-4 and highlight pens (orange, red, green, blue, violet).

Standards: Complete all steps listed in this skill in ________ minutes with a minimum score of ________. (Time element and accuracy criteria may be given by instructor.)

Time: **Start:** ____________ **Completed:** ____________ **Total:** ____________ minutes

Scoring: One point for each step performed satisfactorily unless otherwise listed or weighted by instructor.

Directions with Performance Evaluation Checklist

Dr. Practon may ask you to add color to the medical office filing system, or he may already use Remington's Variadex color-coding system. When a file is placed in a cabinet or drawer, or a card in a box, alphabetical dividers will indicate the first letter of the first filing unit. Then, the names are filed according to the color code of the ***second*** letter of the last name.

1st Attempt	2nd Attempt	3rd Attempt	
______	______	______	Gather materials (equipment and supplies) listed under "Conditions."
___/60	___/60	___/60	1. Highlight the top edge of each 3″ by 5″ index card by color coding the ***second*** letter in the first unit of each name. Use the color guide in the following box. To help you remember the five divisions of the alphabetical system, notice that the first letter of each of the five groups is a vowel except for the last group, which begins with the letter "r."

If the second letter of the patient's surname is:	the tab guide color is:
a, b, c, or d	orange
e, f, g, or h	red
i, j, k, l, m, or n	green
o, p, or q	blue
r, s, t, u, v, w, x, y, or z	violet

______	______	______	Complete within specified time.
___/62	___/62	___/62	**Total points earned** (To obtain a percentage score, divide the total points earned by the number of points possible.)

JOB SKILL 8-5 *(continued)*

Comments:

Evaluator's Signature: ______________________________ **Need to Repeat:** ____________

National Curriculum Competency: CAAHEP: Cognitive: V.C.9, 10; Psychomotor: V.P.8	ABHES: 8.a, b

CHAPTER 9

Medical Records

OBJECTIVES

After completing the exercises, the student will be able to:

1. Write meanings for chart note abbreviations.
2. Enhance spelling skills by learning new medical words.
3. Prepare a patient record and insert progress notes (Job Skill 9-1).
4. Prepare a patient record and format chart notes (Job Skill 9-2).
5. Correct a patient record (Job Skill 9-3).
6. Abstract from a medical record (Job Skill 9-4).
7. Prepare a history and physical (H & P) report (Job Skill 9-5).
8. Record test results on a flow sheet (Job Skill 9-6).

FOCUS ON CERTIFICATION*

CMA Content Summary

- Documentation and reporting
- Medical records
- Patient activity and care
- Medical record ownership
- Formats (chart notes)
- Records management
- Paper and electronic records
- Organization of patient records
- Problem- and source-oriented records
- Collecting information
- Making corrections
- Components of a patient history

*This *Workbook* and the accompanying *textbook* meet the entry-level administrative and general competencies for the CMA outlined by the AAMA Examination Content Outline and Occupational Analysis and for the RMA and CMAS outlined by the AMT Competencies, Construction Parameters, and Examination Specifications (see Competency Grid in Appendix B of the *textbook*.).

- Equipment operation (computer)
- Storage devices
- Computer applications (word processing, database, security/passwords, patient data)

RMA Content Summary

- Understand and utilize proper documentation
- Prepare patient record
- Records and chart management
- Record diagnostic test results in patient chart
- Problem-oriented medical records
- Prepare and release private health information
- Identify and employ proper documentation procedures
- Adhere to standard charting guidelines
- Identify and understand application of basic software and operating systems
- Recognize software application for patient record maintenance
- Encryption, passwords, access restrictions, and activity logs
- Obtain patient history employing appropriate terminology and abbreviations
- Differentiate between subjective and objective information
- Understand and employ SOAP and POMR charting systems

CMAS Content Summary

- Demonstrate knowledge and manage patient medical records
- Manage documents and patient charts using paper methods
- Manage documents and patient charts using computerized methods
- Arrange contents of charts in proper order
- Document and file laboratory results and patient communication in charts
- Perform corrects and additions to charts
- Transfer files
- Perform daily chart management
- Prepare charts for external review and audits
- Observe and maintain confidentiality of records, charts, and test results

STOP AND THINK CASE SCENARIOS AND EXAM-STYLE REVIEW QUESTIONS

Refer to the end of Chapter 9 in the *textbook*.

Abbreviation and Spelling Review

Read the following patient's chart note and write the meanings for the abbreviations listed following the note. To decode any abbreviations you do not understand or that appear unfamiliar to you, refer to the list of abbreviations in Part IV of this *Workbook*. Step-by-step directions for this exercise are in Procedure 1-1 of Chapter 1 in the *textbook*. Medical terms in the chart note are italicized; study them for spelling. Use your medical dictionary to look up their definitions. Your instructor may give a spelling and definition test that includes these words and abbreviations.

Elizabeth A. Warner

November 16, 20XX CC: *constipation, rectal* bleeding & pain after BM. CPX reveals int & ext *hemorrhoids*. BP 150/95. *Sigmoidoscopy* to 15 cm. Rx: adv hospitalization for removal of hemorrhoids. Dg: bleeding hemorrhoids, int & ext; anal *fistula*; HBP.

Gerald Practon, MD

Gerald Practon, MD

CC ______ cm ______

BM ______ Rx ______

CPX ______ adv ______

int ______ Dg ______

ext ______ HBP ______

BP ______

Review Questions

Review the objectives, glossary, and chapter information before completing the following review questions.

1. List five reasons for keeping medical records.
   a. ______
   b. ______
   c. ______
   d. ______
   e. ______
2. List some of the disadvantages of a paper-based medical record system.
   a. ______
   b. ______
   c. ______
   d. ______
   e. ______
   f. ______
3. What equipment is necessary to digitize medical records when converting from a paper-based system to an electronic-based system? ______
4. Why are flow sheets, charts, and graphs used in the medical record? ______
5. Name five advantages of using a medical record organizational system such as the problem-oriented medical record (POMR).
   a. ______
   b. ______
   c. ______
   d. ______
   e. ______

6. Match the physician titles in the left column with the definitions in the right column and insert the correct letter in the blank space.

_________ attending physician
_________ consulting physician
_________ ordering physician
_________ referring physician
_________ treating or performing physician

a. provider who sends the patient for testing
b. provider whose opinion is requested
c. medical staff member who is legally responsible for care of patient
d. provider who renders service to patient
e. provider directing selection, preparation, or administration of tests, medication, or treatment

7. Since all documenters must sign their name to the portions of the medical record that they documented, when can initials legally be used? ____
____
____

8. List what the abbreviations stand for in the following chart format and briefly describe each term.

a. S: ____
b. O: ____
c. A: ____
d. P: ____

9. Using the documentation guidelines, state briefly what is said about the following.

a. patient encounters: ____
b. the assessment: ____
c. abbreviations: ____
d. diagnostic and ancillary services: __________________________________
e. risk factors: ____
f. procedure and diagnostic codes: ____________________________________
g. staff members assisting physician: __________________________________
h. patient education and instructions: _________________________________

10. List items that should be documented in the medical record for skin lacerations and lesions.

a. ____
b. ____
c. ____
d. ____
e. ____

11. List the four basic elements of a patient history and their abbreviations.

a. ____
b. ____
c. ____
d. ____

12. If a patient is seen in the office, a history and physical is dictated, and then the patient is admitted to the hospital, can the dictated history and physical be used for the hospital documentation? ___________

____

____

13. Name ways in which the physician collects objective data.

    a. ____

    b. ____

    c. ____

    d. ____

14. Is there a difference between a chart note and a progress note? If yes, state the difference. ___________

____

15. State types of patient encounters and common medical events that require charting on a medical record.

    a. ____

    b. ____

    c. ____

    d. ____

    e. ____

    f. ____

    g. ____

    h. ____

    i. ____

    j. ____

Critical Thinking Exercise

1. The following phrases appeared on a history and physical. Place an ***S*** after those that are *subjective* and an ***O*** after those considered *objective*.

    a. Patient complains of feeling faint ______________

    b. BP 120/80 ______________

    c. Headache ______________

    d. Skin shows no rashes ______________

    e. Patient denies chest pain ______________

    f. Mother L & W ______________

    g. No inguinal hernia ______________

    h. Heart tones normal ______________

    i. No masses palpable ______________

j. Patient had an episode of nausea ____________

k. Patient feels lethargic ____________

l. Temperature 101.1 F ____________

m. Blood in stool ____________

n. Stomachache ____________

o. Leg cramping ____________

p. Blurred vision ____________

q. Vision 20/40 R. eye ____________

r. HCT 40% ____________

s. Pap smear class II ____________

t. Heel pain ____________

u. Lump in left breast ____________

v. Joint stiffness ____________

w. X-ray showed fracture R. ulna ____________

x. Urinalysis negative ____________

y. Acne ____________

z. Patient feels tired all the time ____________

2. Pair with another student and role-play the following scenarios to practice documentation skills. Use the date, Friday, July 30, 20XX, and correct abbreviations.

   a. **Participants—two students: Patient and receptionist**
   An established patient presents at the reception desk of Practon Medical Group with no appointment. He or she just walked in and wants to be seen as soon as possible. The schedule is busy so the receptionist asks the office manager what to do. The office manager advises the receptionist to take the chief complaint and vital signs.

   Patient: Make up a reason for being there and communicate it to the receptionist.

   Your blood pressure is 180/92 and your weight is 185 pounds.

   Receptionist: Record the chief complaint and vital signs.

   ____

   ____

   ____

   b. **Participants—two students: Dr. Practon and medical assistant**
   Dr. Practon has had a busy morning and is ready to go to a lunch meeting. He has just finished dictating and approaches the medical assistant with all the morning charts. He asks the assistant to schedule the following tests for the patients who have been seen. Schedule all tests and procedures (making up the dates and times), then document them in the patients' medical records. Use critical thinking skills to instruct the patient according to each test or procedure protocol.

   1. **Patient A:** Magnetic resonance imaging of the brain at College Hospital for headaches and visual changes—sometime next week.

      ____

      ____

      ____

2. **Patient B:** Pulmonary function test at College Hospital for asthma—sometime next week.

3. **Patient C:** Mammogram at the Women's Clinic for breast screening—no hurry.

4. **Patient D:** Blood culture at College Hospital for unresolved fever of unknown origin, lethargy, and malaise—immediately.

5. **Patient E:** Chest x-ray at College Hospital for chest congestion, rule out pneumonia—as soon as possible.

6. **Patient F:** Five-hour glucose tolerance test at College Hospital for elevated fasting blood sugar and frequency of urination—sometime next week.

JOB SKILL 9-1
Prepare a Patient Record and Insert Progress Notes

Name ______________________________ Date ______________ Score ________

Performance Objective

Task: Key a patient record form with demographic information and progress notes; type a file card and file folder label.

Conditions: Computer, electronic typewriter, or word processor; one file folder, one file folder label, one patient record (Form 21), and one 3″ by 5″ file card.

Standards: Complete all steps listed in this skill in _______ minutes with a minimum score of _______. (Time element and accuracy criteria may be given by instructor.)

Time: **Start:** ____________ **Completed:** ____________ **Total:** ____________ minutes

Scoring: One point for each step performed satisfactorily unless otherwise listed or weighted by instructor.

Directions with Performance Evaluation Checklist

Today is October 24, 20XX, and new patient Wayne G. Weather has come in as an emergency case; he was hurt on the job and has an injury to his lower back. He completed the patient information form (see Figure 7-1 in *Workbook* Job Skill 7-5). Complete the demographic information on the patient record form (21), file folder label, and file card. His wife, Nancy Weather, is a receptionist. His patient record number is 1180, which is keyed in the right corner of the record, file card, and file label. Use the detailed information listed in the directions to Job Skill 7-5 pertaining to Mr. Weather's condition, and enter the progress notes for today and the day of his hospital admit.

1st Attempt	2nd Attempt	3rd Attempt	
______	______	______	Gather materials (equipment and supplies) listed under "Conditions."
____/2	____/2	____/2	1. Complete the file folder label with patient name and medical record number; affix to the file folder.
____/2	____/2	____/2	2. Complete the file card with patient name and medical record number.
____/25	____/25	____/25	3. Key the patient record number and demographic information on the top portion of the patient record.
____/15	____/15	____/15	4. Key the progress note for 10/24/20XX noting emergency office visit, on-the-job injury, diagnosis, surgical scheduling information, and preadmission testing.
____/5	____/5	____/5	5. Key the note for 10/28/20XX regarding hospital admit.
____/4	____/4	____/4	6. Proofread the form, checking capitalization, punctuation, spelling, and spacing.
____/2	____/2	____/2	7. Finalize the record for the correct physician's signature.
______	______	______	Complete within specified time.
____/57	____/57	____/57	**Total points earned** (To obtain a percentage score, divide the total points earned by the number of points possible.)

JOB SKILL 9-1 *(continued)*

Comments:

Evaluator's Signature: ______________________________ **Need to Repeat:** ____________

National Curriculum Competency: CAAHEP: Psychomotor: IX.P.7	ABHES: 8.b

JOB SKILL 9-2
Prepare a Patient Record and Format Chart Notes

Name ______________________________ Date ______________ Score ________

Performance Objective

Task: Format and key a patient record, label a file folder, and type a file card.

Conditions: Computer, electronic typewriter, or word processor; one file folder, one file label, one patient record (Form 22), and one 3″ by 5″ file card. Refer to Figure 9-7 in the *textbook* for a chart note format example.

Standards: Complete all steps listed in this skill in _______ minutes with a minimum score of _______. (Time element and accuracy criteria may be given by instructor.)

Time: **Start:** ____________ **Completed:** ____________ **Total:** ____________ minutes

Scoring: One point for each step performed satisfactorily unless otherwise listed or weighted by instructor.

Directions with Performance Evaluation Checklist

You will be preparing a patient record, filling in the top portion with demographic information and the bottom portion with progress notes. Refer to Figure 9-7 in the *textbook* for an example of the charting format using the chief complaint (CC), physical examination (PE), diagnosis (DX), and treatment plan (Plan) as headings for the appropriate lines.

1st Attempt	2nd Attempt	3rd Attempt	
_______	_______	_______	Gather materials (equipment and supplies) listed under "Conditions."
_____/2	_____/2	_____/2	1. Use the name Krista Lee Carlisle and medical record number 1181. Complete a file folder label; affix to file folder.
_____/2	_____/2	_____/2	2. Type a 3″ by 5″ file card with patient name and medical record number at top right.
____/25	____/25	____/25	3. Complete the top portion of the medical record (Form 22) for Krista Carlisle using your own personal information, or interview a person in class or someone at home to obtain this information (address, telephone number, insurance name, and so forth).
_____/5	_____/5	_____/5	4. Complete the bottom portion of the medical record using the data found in *Workbook* Figure 9-1. Use a format similar to that found in *textbook* Figure 9-7 and abbreviate medical terms when appropriate.
____/10	____/10	____/10	5. Make a separate entry for Dr. Fran Practon's examination on October 25, 20XX.
____/10	____/10	____/10	6. Make a separate entry for the follow-up visit on October 28, 20XX.
____/10	____/10	____/10	7. Make a separate entry for the follow-up visit on November 15, 20XX.
_____/4	_____/4	_____/4	8. Make a separate entry for the canceled appointment.
_______	_______	_______	Complete within specified time.
____/70	____/70	____/70	**Total points earned** (To obtain a percentage score, divide the total points earned by the number of points possible.)

JOB SKILL 9-2 *(continued)*

FIGURE 9-1

10/25/XX Height 5'10" Weight 222 pounds. Blood pressure 140/60. Chief complaint: Patient complained of several weeks' history of fatigue, lack of appetite, and headache; has lost approximately 8 pounds since October 1, 20XX, denies smoking. Averages three beers a day. On examination liver appears somewhat enlarged, tender on palpitation. All other systems appear normal. No apparent jaundice. Urinalysis findings: dark amber urine, bilirubinemia and proteinuria 2+. Patient sent to laboratory for blood workup; complete blood count, chemistry panel, liver panel, hepatitis panel. Diagnosis: hepatomegaly, rule out hepatitis. Patient instructed to adhere to strict bed rest, low-fat, high-carbohydrate diet. Disability for 2 weeks; instructions given. Return to the office in three days. Call sooner if symptoms increase, Tylenol tablets every 4 to 6 hours for headache.

Fran Practon, MD

Fran Practon, MD

10/28/XX Weight: 220 pounds. Blood pressure 128/64. Chief complaint: Follow-up visit for laboratory results. Definitive diagnosis: hepatitis A. All other laboratory results normal. Patient to increase disability to 8 weeks, mild activity as tolerated. Instructions to use no alcohol, continue same diet, fluids as tolerated. Tylenol as needed. Call office immediately if unable to tolerate fluids or diet. Return to office in 1 week.

Fran Practon, MD

Fran Practon, MD

11/15/XX Weight: 224 pounds. Blood pressure 130/66. Chief complaint: Follow-up visit. Patient states "Is feeling much better," tolerating diet and fluids, good weight gain; urinalysis: clear yellow urine, protein-trace, Vital signs normal. On examination, no tenderness on palpitation of abdomen. Patient to follow up in 2 weeks. Continue modified activity as tolerated. Call if symptoms increase.

Fran Practon, MD

Fran Practon, MD

12/03/XX Pt called to cancel appointment (3:00 p.m.); did not reschedule.

Margaret Dun, MA

Marqaret Dun, MA

Comments:

Evaluator's Signature: ______________________ **Need to Repeat:** ____________

National Curriculum Competency: CAAHEP: Psychomotor: IX.P.7	ABHES 8.b

JOB SKILL 9-3
Correct a Patient Record

Name ______________________________ Date ______________ Score ________

Performance Objective

Task: Make a correction on a patient record.

Conditions: Use the patient medical record for Krista Lee Carlisle (No. 1181 from Job Skill 9-2). Refer to Procedure 9-3 in the *textbook* for step-by-step directions.

Standards: Complete all steps listed in this skill in _______ minutes with a minimum score of _______. (Time element and accuracy criteria may be given by instructor.)

Time: **Start:** ____________ **Completed:** ____________ **Total:** ____________ minutes

Scoring: One point for each step performed satisfactorily unless otherwise listed or weighted by instructor.

Directions with Performance Evaluation Checklist

On October 28, 20XX, Dr. Fran Practon indicated the patient would be disabled for eight weeks. On November 15, she realized she should have indicated the disability for six weeks. Correct the medical record.

1st Attempt	2nd Attempt	3rd Attempt	
_______	_______	_______	Gather materials (equipment and supplies) listed under "Conditions."
____/2	____/2	____/2	1. Make the necessary change on the patient record by crossing out the incorrect entry ("~~X 8 weeks~~").
____/2	____/2	____/2	2. Handwrite, in ink, the correct entry above the words "~~X 8 weeks~~."
____/4	____/4	____/4	3. In the margin, write the word "correction," your initials, and the date you are making the correction.
_______	_______	_______	Complete within specified time.
____/10	____/10	____/10	**Total points earned** (To obtain a percentage score, divide the total points earned by the number of points possible.)

Comments:

Evaluator's Signature: ______________________________ **Need to Repeat:** ______________

National Curriculum Competency: CAAHEP: Psychomotor: IX.P.7	ABHES: 8.a, b

JOB SKILL 9-4
Abstract from a Medical Record

Name ______________________________ Date ______________ Score ________

Performance Objective

Task: Abstract information from a patient record to answer questions and fill in a medical record abstract form.

Conditions: Use patient medical record No. 1181 for Krista Lee Carlisle from Job Skill 9-2, pen or pencil, and the medical record abstract (Form 23). Refer to Procedure 9-4 in the *textbook* for step-by-step directions.

Standards: Complete all steps listed in this skill in _______ minutes with a minimum score of ________. (Time element and accuracy criteria may be given by instructor.)

Time: **Start:** _____________ **Completed:** _____________ **Total:** _____________ minutes

Scoring: One point for each step performed satisfactorily unless otherwise listed or weighted by instructor.

Directions with Performance Evaluation Checklist

1st Attempt	2nd Attempt	3rd Attempt	
_______	_______	_______	Gather materials (equipment and supplies) listed under "Conditions."
____/25	____/25	____/25	1. Abstract information from the medical record (No. 1181) and answer each question on the abstract form; complete the form.
_______	_______	_______	Complete within specified time.
____/27	____/27	____/27	**Total points earned** (To obtain a percentage score, divide the total points earned by the number of points possible.)

Comments:

Evaluator's Signature: ______________________________ **Need to Repeat:** ______________

National Curriculum Competency: CAAHEP: Cognitive: IV.C.12; Psychomotor: IX.P.3	ABHES: 8.b, jj

JOB SKILL 9-5
Prepare a History and Physical (H & P) Report

Name ______________________________ Date ______________ Score ________

Performance Objective

Task: Complete a patient record with demographic information, key a history and physical report, prepare a file folder with file label, type a 3″ by 5″ file card, and make a photocopy of the H & P report.

Conditions: Computer, electronic typewriter, or word processor; photocopy machine; patient record (Form 24); patient information form for Sun Low Chung (Figure 9-2); history and physical data (Figure 9-3); one file folder, one file folder label, one file card (3″ by 5″), and two sheets of 8½″ by 11″ white paper. Refer to *textbook* Figures 9-6A and 9-6B for history and physical format examples.

Standards: Complete all steps listed in this skill in ________ minutes with a minimum score of ________. (Time element and accuracy criteria may be given by instructor.)

Time: **Start:** ____________ **Completed:** ____________ **Total:** ____________ minutes

Scoring: One point for each step performed satisfactorily unless otherwise listed or weighted by instructor.

Directions with Performance Evaluation Checklist

You will be completing the demographic information on a patient record for Sun Low Chung and keying the history and physical examination in report form on separate paper.

1st Attempt	2nd Attempt	3rd Attempt	
______	______	______	Gather materials (equipment and supplies) listed under "Conditions."
______	______	______	1. Prepare a file folder label for Sun Low Chung with medical record No. 1182; affix to the file folder.
______	______	______	2. Prepare a 3″ by 5″ file card for Sun Low Chung.
____/20	____/20	____/20	3. Use Sun Low Chung's patient information form (*Workbook* Figure 9-2) to key his patient record number and demographic information on the top portion of the patient record (Form 24).
______	______	______	4. Read the H & P in *Workbook* Figure 9-3.
____/3	____/3	____/3	5. Highlight the proper headings and subheadings that will be used when keying the data in a history and physical examination format (see *textbook* Figures 9-6A and 9-6B for examples).
______	______	______	6. Insert patient name and medical record number, then date the report using current dates as dictated and transcribed dates.
______	______	______	7. Key in full block style.
______	______	______	8. Set margins so they are even, equal, and of correct size.
____/20	____/20	____/20	9. Key data in using proper history and physical format. Note: You will not be using the bottom portion of the patient record (Form 24) for this patient because a complete H & P report is being prepared for the medical record; reference it in the area of the progress notes.
____/15	____/15	____/15	10. Insert main topic headings and correct paragraphing.
____/7	____/7	____/7	11. Insert subtopic headings.

JOB SKILL 9-5 *(continued)*

____/4	____/4	____/4	12. Insert capitalization, punctuation, tab stops, and correct spacing.
____/4	____/4	____/4	13. Insert page 2 heading.
____/3	____/3	____/3	14. Place a signature line at the end of H & P; Dr. Gerald Practon is the physician.
______	______	______	15. Insert the typist's identifying signoff data for the H & P.
____/2	____/2	____/2	16. Proofread the report for spelling and typographical errors on screen or while the H & P remains in the computer or word processor.
____/2	____/2	____/2	17. Finalize the document for the physician to review and sign.
______	______	______	18. Make a photocopy of the completed H & P report.
______	______	______	Complete within specified time.
____/10	____/10	____/10	**Total points earned** (To obtain a percentage score, divide the total points earned by the number of points possible.)

Comments:

Evaluator's Signature: ______________________________ **Need to Repeat:** ____________

National Curriculum Competency: CAAHEP: Cognitive: IV.C.12; Psychomotor: IV.P.1, 3 ABHES: 8.b, jj

JOB SKILL 9-5 *(continued)*

FIGURE 9-2

PATIENT INFORMATION FOR MEDICAL RECORDS *(Please Print)* DATE: 10/25/XX

PATIENT	(MR.) MRS. MISS	LAST NAME	FIRST NAME	MIDDLE
		Chung	Sun	Low

PATIENT ADDRESS	STREET	CITY	STATE	ZIP	HOME PHONE
→	2375 Laney Street	Woodland Hills,	XY	12345	555/278-6135

SOCIAL SECURITY NUMBER	DATE OF BIRTH	AGE	DRIVER'S LICENSE NO.
→ XXX-XX-6712	5-20-45		6-0065-178

PATIENT EMPLOYER	OCCUPATION
→ Civil Service Maintenance	Mechanic

EMPLOYER'S ADDRESS	STREET	CITY	STATE	ZIP	BUS PHONE
→	742 Redwood Highway,	Port Davis,	XY	12346	555/271-4811

SPOUSE'S NAME	MARITAL STATUS	REFERRED BY
→ Song Su Chung	(M) S D W SEP.	Employer

SPOUSE'S EMPLOYER	STREET	CITY	STATE	ZIP	BUS. PHONE
Best Market	214 Main Street,	Woodland Hills,	XY	12345	555/279-4827

IN CASE OF EMERGENCY CONTACT:	NAME	ADDRESS	CITY	STATE	ZIP	TELEPHONE
	Pat Chung (brother)	2851 Laney St,	Woodland Hills,	XY	12345	555/278-7812

MEDICAL INSURANCE INFORMATION

COMPANY	POLICY NUMBER
Blue Shield 2751 Courntney St., Woodland Hills, XY 12345	
COMPANY	POLICY NUMBER
	27894B
COMPANY	POLICY NUMBER

IF SOMEONE OTHER THAN PATIENT IS RESPONSIBLE FOR PAYMENT PLEASE COMPLETE THIS SECTION

RESPONSIBLE PARTY	MR. MRS. MISS	LAST NAME	FIRST NAME	MIDDLE	RELATION

ADDRESS	STREET	CITY	STATE	ZIP	TELEPHONE
→					

OCCUPATION	EMPLOYED BY
→	

EMPLOYER'S ADDRESS	STREET	CITY	STATE	ZIP	BUS. PHONE
→					

I hereby authorize Dr. Gerald Praston to furnish to the above insurance company(s) or to a designated attorney, all information which said insurance company(s) or attorney may request. I hereby assign to Dr. Gerald Praston all money to which I am entitled for medical and/or surgical expense relative to the service rendered by him, but not to exceed my indebtedness to said physician and/or surgeon. It is understood that any money received from the above named insurance company, over and above my indebtedness will be refunded to me when my bill is paid in full. I understand I am financially responsible to said doctor(s) for charges not covered by this assignment. I further agree in the event of non-payment, to bear the cost of collection, and/or Court cost and reasonable legal fees should this be required.

Sun Low Chung
INSURED OR GUARDIAN SIGNATURE

Sun Low Chung
PATIENT'S SIGNATURE

Courtesy of Bibbero Systems, Inc., Petaluma, CA. Phone: 800-242-2376; Fax: 800-242-9330; Web site: http://www.bibbero.com.

JOB SKILL 9-5 *(continued)*

FIGURE 9-3

Sun Low Chung

History. Chief complaint. Palpitations for 1 week. Present illness. This patient has had known hypertension for 4 years. He has been taking Serpasil 0.25 mg daily. About 1 month ago, the medication was changed to Dyazide 250 mg, one tablet per day. Since that time, the patient has felt more nervous and anxious, with occasional chest tightness. One week ago the patient noted some skipped heartbeats occurring in the evening. There were no other associated symptoms and no history of paroxysmal nocturnal dyspnea, orthopnea, or ankle edema. Palpitation subsided spontaneously but recurred the following night, with a fast throbbing sensation in his right ear. He was seen by Dr. Chan 2 weeks later and had a chest x-ray and cardiac enzymes done. These were normal values. An electrocardiogram showed normal sinus rhythm, with nonspecific ST abnormalities. He experiences palpitations in the evening. The patient has been asked to avoid any strenuous exercise and to stay at home until he is seen by the undersigned physician. Past history. The patient was born in Hankow, China, but has lived in the United States since 1952. He has worked in the Air Force and airplane industry but lately is working for civil service at Port Davis. He has been subjected to some work pressure recently. There was no history of coronary artery disease, heart murmurs, rheumatic fever, or joint problems in childhood. Malaria in his youth in China. Hypothyroidism diagnosed about 10 years ago, and he has been on thyroid 1 grain q.d. Operations none. Allergies none. Medication as stated above, and Valium 5 milligrams one b.i.d. to t.i.d. p.r.n., Thyroid 1 grain q.d. Social history. The patient smoked one pack of cigarettes per day for 10 years but has discontinued for about 15 years. He does not drink. He consumes about two cups of coffee per day and very little tea. The family history. Most of the family members were separated during the war, and their health conditions are not known. Mother died from an unknown illness at the age of 35. The patient has two children, 36 and 27, both in good health. No known diabetes, hypertension, or heart problems in the family. The review of systems. General. No recent weight gain or weight loss. No unusual fatigue. No recent fevers. The patient has myopia in both eyes. Glasses have not been checked for the past 5 years, and distant vision is not good. EENT. Negative. CR. As in PI. No history of hemoptysis or chronic cough. Gl. Negative. GU. Nocturia once a night for many years. NP. No history of headache, syncope, or light-headedness. No history of paralysis. MS. No history of joint problems. Physical examination. General. This patient is an elderly Asian male in no acute distress. Blood pressure in right arm 148 over 80 and left arm 138 over 88. Pulse 80 and regular. Respirations 18. Height 5 feet, 7 inches. Weight 176 1/4 pounds. The patient is afebrile. HEENT. Not pale or cyanotic. Tympanic membranes intact. Fundus normal in the left; right cannot be visualized because of question of early cataract or marked refractive error. Neck. Supple. No jugular venous pulse, thyromegaly, or lymphadenopathy. Carotid upstrokes normal. Chest. Point of maximum, impulse in the fifth intercostal space in the mid-clavicular line. S1, S2 normal. A soft S4 was heard. No S3. No murmurs. Lungs clear. Abdomen. Soft, nontender. No hepatosplenomegaly. No masses felt. No abdominal bruits. Musculoskeletal. Bilateral hallux valgus. No edema or clubbing. All peripheral pulses normal and equal. Neurological. No gross abnormalities. Diagnosis. 1. Palpitations, probably premature ventricular contractions. Rule out coronary artery disease. Rule out malignant arrhythmias. 2. History of hypertension. 3. History of hypothyroidism. Therapeutic Plan. 1. Review old records. 2. Tumor skin test. 3. EKG with 12-hour Hotter monitor. 4. Measure blood pressure once a week x 3 weeks. Decide whether long-term hypertensive medication is necessary. 5. Ophthalmology consult.

JOB SKILL 9-6
Record Test Results on a Flow Sheet

Name ______________________________ Date ______________ Score ________

Performance Objective

Task: Record laboratory test results for triglycerides, cholesterol, and glucose on a patient flow sheet.

Conditions: Test results (Figure 9-4), flow sheet (Form 25), and pen. Refer to *textbook* Example 9–2 for a completed flow sheet form.

Standards: Complete all steps listed in this job skill in ________ minutes with a minimum score of ________. (Time element and accuracy criteria may be given by instructor.)

Time: **Start:** ______________ **Completed:** ______________ **Total:** ______________ minutes

Scoring: One point for each step performed satisfactorily unless otherwise listed or weighted by instructor.

Directions with Performance Evaluation Checklist

Record test results for patient Richard Freeman on a flow sheet.

1st Attempt	2nd Attempt	3rd Attempt	
_______	_______	_______	Gather materials (equipment and supplies) listed under "Conditions."
_____/2	_____/2	_____/2	1. Record the date of the laboratory report on Richard Freeman's flow sheet.
_____/2	_____/2	_____/2	2. Record his triglycerides on the flow sheet.
_____/2	_____/2	_____/2	3. Record his total cholesterol on the flow sheet.
_____/2	_____/2	_____/2	4. Record his HDL cholesterol on the flow sheet.
_____/2	_____/2	_____/2	5. Record his LDL cholesterol on the flow sheet.
_____/2	_____/2	_____/2	6. Record his cholesterol/high-density lipoprotein cardiac risk ratio on the flow sheet.
_____/2	_____/2	_____/2	7. Record his fasting glucose on the flow sheet.
_____/2	_____/2	_____/2	8. Distinguish between normal and abnormal test results and list any that were out of range, indicating if they were high or low. ________________ ____
_______	_______	_______	Complete within specified time.
____/18	____/18	____/18	**Total points earned** (To obtain a percentage score, divide the total points earned by the number of points possible.)

Comments:

Evaluator's Signature: ________________________________ **Need to Repeat:** ______________

National Curriculum Competency: CAAHEP: Psychomotor: II.P.2; Affective: II.A.2	ABHES: 8.a, b

JOB SKILL 9-6 *(continued)*

FIGURE 9-4

LABORATORY REPORT

PRACTON MEDICAL GROUP, INC.
4567 BROAD AVENUE
WOODLAND HILLS, XY 12345-4700

PATIENT NAME	PATIENT ID	ROOM NO	AGE	SEX	PHYSICIAN
FREEMAN, RICHARD E	08051944RF		64	M	Practon, Gerald M

PAGE	REQUISITION NO.	ACCESSION NO.	LAB REF. #	COLLECTION DATE & TIME	LOG-IN DATE	REPORT DATE	& TIME
1	0013188	EN77346IN		072120XX 1044	07212009		4:25PM

REMARKS
FASTING

PACIFIC TIME

REPORT STATUS FINAL TEST	RESULT IN RANGE	RESULT OUT OF RANGE	UNITS	REFERENCE RANGE	SITE CODE
rth: 08/05					
Patient Phone:(555)487-7892					
GLUCOSE		171 H	mg/dL	65-99	EN
				FASTING REFERENCE INTERVAL	
LIPID PANEL					
TRIGLYCERIDES	127		mg/dL	<150	EN
CHOLESTEROL, TOTAL	156		mg/dL	125-200	EN
HDL CHOLESTEROL	40		mg/dL	> OR = 40	EN
LDL CHOLESTEROL	91		mg/dL (CALC)	<130	EN
DESIRABLE RANGE <100 MG/DL FOR PATIENTS WITH CHD OR DIABETES AND <70 MG/DL FOR DIABETIC PATIENTS WITH KNOWN HEART DISEASE.					
CHOL/HDLC RATIO	3.9		(CALC)	< OR = 5.0	EN

CHAPTER 10

Drug and Prescription Records

OBJECTIVES

After completing the exercises, the student will be able to:

1. Enhance knowledge of medical terminology, interpret abbreviations, and accurately spell medical words.
2. Spell drug names (Job Skill 10-1).
3. Determine the correct spelling of drug names (Job Skill 10-2).
4. Use a *Physicians' Desk Reference* (*PDR*) (Job Skill 10-3).
5. Translate prescriptions (Job Skill 10-4).
6. Record prescription refills in medical records (Job Skill 10-5).
7. Write a prescription (Job Skill 10-6).
8. Interpret a medication log (Job Skill 10-7).
9. Record on a medication schedule (Job Skill 10-8).

FOCUS ON CERTIFICATION*

CMA Content Summary

- Documentation reporting
- Food and Drug Administration
- Drug Enforcement Administration (DEA)
- Disposal of biohazardous material
- Classes of drugs
- Drug action/uses

*This *Workbook* and the accompanying *textbook* meet the entry-level administrative and general competencies for the CMA outlined by the AAMA Examination Content Outline and Occupational Analysis and for the RMA and CMAS outlined by the AMT Competencies, Construction Parameters, and Examination Specifications (see Competency Grid in Appendix B of the *textbook*).

- Side effects/adverse reactions
- Substance abuse
- Prescription safekeeping
- Medication recordkeeping
- Control substance guidelines
- Immunizations
- Commonly used medications

RMA Content Summary

- Determine terminology association with pharmacology
- Identify and define common prescription abbreviations
- Identify and define drug schedules and legal prescription requirements
- Understand procedures for completing prescriptions
- Identify and perform proper documentation of medication transactions
- Identify Drug Enforcement Administration regulations for ordering, dispensing, prescribing, storing, and documenting regulated drugs
- Identify and define drug categories
- Identify commonly used drugs
- Identify and describe routes of administration for parenteral, rectal, topical, vaginal, sublingual, oral, inhalation, and instillation drugs
- Demonstrate ability to use drug references (*PDR*)

CMAS Content Summary

- Understand basic pharmacological concepts and terminology
- Chart patient information

STOP AND THINK CASE SCENARIOS AND EXAM-STYLE REVIEW QUESTIONS

Refer to the end of Chapter 10 in the *textbook*.

Abbreviation and Spelling Review

Read the following patient's chart note and write the meanings for the abbreviations listed following the note. To decode any abbreviations you do not understand or that appear unfamiliar to you, refer to the list of abbreviations in Part IV of this *Workbook*. Step-by-step directions for this exercise are found in Procedure 1-1 of Chapter 1 in the *textbook*. Medical terms in the chart note are italicized; study them for spelling. Use your medical dictionary to look up their definitions. Your instructor may give a spelling and definition test that includes these words and abbreviations.

Lillian M. Chan

February 17, 20XX, OB case. LMP 12-14-20XX. Pt had D & C in 20XX following *spontaneous abortion*. First child delivered by C-section. Ordered CBC, UA, and WR. Pt to ret in 1 mo.

Fran Practon, MD

Fran Practon, MD

OB	______________	CBC	______________
LMP	______________	UA	______________
Pt	______________	WR	______________
D & C	______________	ret	______________
C-section	______________	mo	______________

Review Questions

Review the objectives, glossary, and chapter information before completing the following review questions.

1. Match the law or agency in the right column with the description in the left column by writing the correct letters in the blanks.

________	Law requiring transfer tax for those who sold marijuana.	a. Harrison Narcotic Act
________	Federal law that requires the pharmaceutical industry to maintain physical security and strict recordkeeping for scheduled drugs.	b. Volstead Act
________	First law to control the prescription, sale, and possession of narcotic drugs.	c. Marijuana Tax Act
________	Organization that regulates the manufacturing and dispensing of dangerous and potentially abused drugs.	d. Food, Drug, and Cosmetic Act
________	Law that prohibited the manufacture, transportation, and sale of beverages containing more than 0.5% alcohol.	e. Controlled Substances Act
________	Agency that determines the safety of drugs before it permits them to be marketed.	f. Food and Drug Administration
________	First law that required the labeling of drugs with directions for safe use.	g. Drug Enforcement Administration

2. Where must the physician register for a narcotic license and when must the license be renewed?

____

3. Refer to *textbook* Table 10-1, Five Schedules of Controlled Substances, and answer the following questions:

   a. On which schedule(s) may prescriptions be written by the health care worker?

   ____

   b. On which schedule(s) will the medical assistant most likely be handling triplicate forms for the doctor?

   ____

   c. On which schedule(s) do drugs have the most potential for abuse?

   ____

4. Name and define the three types of drug names.

   a. ____

   b. ____

   c. ____

5. Define *generic drug:* ______________________________

____

6. In the *Physicians' Desk Reference* (*PDR*), which section is used most frequently by the medical assistant?

____

7. Name and define the four components of a prescription.

 a. ______________________________
 b. ______________________________
 c. ______________________________
 d. ______________________________

8. Match the drug route in the right column with the correct definition in the left column by writing the correct letters in the blanks.

________	medication administered into a joint	a. ophthalmic
________	medication administered through the ear	b. otic
________	medication absorbed through the skin using a patch	c. endotracheal
________	medication placed between the cheek and gum	d. intra-articular
________	medication administered to the eye	e. buccal
________	medication placed under the tongue	f. sublingual
________	medication administered through the trachea	g. transdermal

9. Write the abbreviation or symbol for the following pharmaceutical terms.

 a. after meals ______________________________
 b. drops ______________________________
 c. every morning ______________________________
 d. every two hours______________________________
 e. intramuscular ______________________________
 f. when necessary ______________________________

10. Name several ways the medical assistant can instruct the patient about drug dosages to be sure the patient understands the directions.

 a. ______________________________
 b. ______________________________
 c. ______________________________
 d. ______________________________
 e. ______________________________

11. Name three important items to include when instructions are given to patients taking antibiotics.

 a. ______________________________
 b. ______________________________
 c. ______________________________

12. Match the drug categories in the right column with the definitions in the left column by writing the correct letters in the blanks.

________	drug that causes general or local loss of sensation to pain and touch	a. narcotic
________	drug that decreases congestion	b. antiemetic
________	drug that exerts a tranquilizing effect	c. stimulant
________	drug that increases excretion of urine	d. diuretic
________	drug that relieves pain and produces sleep	e. coagulant
________	drug that causes blood to clot	f. sedative
________	drug that relieves vomiting	g. hemostatic
________	drug that increases activity in the body or any of its organs	h. anesthetic
________	drug used to check bleeding	i. antitussive
________	drug used to relieve cough	j. decongestant

13. Name three ways a medical assistant can track a patient's drug use habits.

a. ____________________

b. ____________________

c. ____________________

14. Name five ways to protect prescription pads from being misused.

a. ____________________

b. ____________________

c. ____________________

d. ____________________

e. ____________________

15. Name some common side effects associated with medications.

a. ____________	g. ____________
b. ____________	h. ____________
c. ____________	i. ____________
d. ____________	j. ____________
e. ____________	k. ____________
f. ____________	l. ____________

16. If the patient does not have any known allergies, what is the abbreviation listed on the "alert tag" on the front of the patient's chart? ____________________

____

____

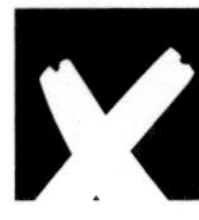

Critical Thinking Exercises

1. If a pharmacist calls the office and the physician approves a refill on Mr. Hamilton's prescription, what administrative task should the medical assistant then perform (list details)?

____

____

____

____

2. Mrs. Schwartz telephones and says that the doctor prescribed Hytrin, but she cannot remember why. With the physician's permission, you would tell her that the medication is being prescribed for her:

   a. headaches
   b. hypertension
   c. nerves
   d. hypotension

   (Find the answer in the *Physicians' Desk Reference* or other drug reference book.)

3. Rewrite the following statements as they would appear on a prescription, using Latin abbreviations.

   a. Proventil (albuterol) inhaler, one hundred milligrams per five milliliters, one or two inhalations every four hours whenever necessary.

   ____

   b. Cardizem CD (diltiazem HCl) capsules, 180 milligrams, number one hundred, once a day before meals, and one before bedtime.

   ____

   c. Lanoxin (digoxin) tablets, zero point one hundred and twenty-five milligrams, number sixty, one every day.

   ____

   d. Vantin (cefpodoxime proxetil) tablets, two hundred milligrams, number twenty-eight, one by mouth, every twelve hours for fourteen days.

   ____

JOB SKILL 10-1
Spell Drug Names

Name ______________________________ Date ____________ Score ______

Performance Objective

Task: Correctly spell brand or generic drug names.

Conditions: Use the 10 drug names listed next to each step, a computer or word processor, and a drug reference book such as the *Physicians' Desk Reference (PDR), Instant Drug Index, Hospital Formulary,* or *Pharmaceutical Terminology.* Refer to Procedure 10-1 in the *textbook* for step-by-step directions.

Standards: Complete all steps listed in this skill in ______ minutes with a minimum score of ______. (Time element and accuracy criteria may be given by instructor.)

Time: **Start:** __________ **Completed:** __________ **Total:** __________ minutes

Scoring: One point for each step performed satisfactorily unless otherwise listed or weighted by instructor.

Directions with Performance Evaluation Checklist

Dr. Practon has dictated 10 drug names for several patients, and you have written them phonetically. Find the correct spelling for each drug. Be sure to begin all brand names with a capital letter and all generic names with a lowercase letter.

1st Attempt	2nd Attempt	3rd Attempt	
______	______	______	Gather materials (equipment and supplies) listed under "Conditions."
____/3	____/3	____/3	1. Spell **CAR-de-zem** ______________________
____/3	____/3	____/3	2. Spell **di-ah-BEN-eze** ______________________
____/3	____/3	____/3	3. Spell **FEE-a-sol** ______________________
____/3	____/3	____/3	4. Spell **NAP-ro-sin** ______________________
____/3	____/3	____/3	5. Spell **LIP-a-tour** ______________________
____/3	____/3	____/3	6. Spell **LAY-six** ______________________
____/3	____/3	____/3	7. Spell **eye-bu-PRO-fen** ______________________
____/3	____/3	____/3	8. Spell **die-AS-a-pam** ______________________
____/3	____/3	____/3	9. Spell **TEN-or-min** ______________________
____/3	____/3	____/3	10. Spell **aug-MEN-tin** ______________________
______	______	______	Complete within specified time.
___/32	___/32	___/32	**Total points earned** (To obtain a percentage score, divide the total points earned by the number of points possible.)

JOB SKILL 10-1 *(continued)*

Comments:

Evaluator's Signature: ______________________ **Need to Repeat:** ____________

National Curriculum Competency: ABHES: 6b

JOB SKILL 10-2
Determine the Correct Spelling of Drug Names

Name ______________________________ Date ______________ Score ________

Performance Objective

Task: Determine the correct spellings for brand, generic, or over-the-counter drug names.

Conditions: Use the 10 sentences in the steps below, each has two spellings of a medication; a pen or pencil; and a drug reference book such as the *Physicians' Desk Reference (PDR), Instant Drug Index, Hospital Formulary,* or *Pharmaceutical Terminology.* Refer to Procedure 10-1 in the *textbook* for step-by-step directions. For over-the-counter drugs, use your common knowledge, an over-the-counter drug book, or visit a local drug store to locate the medication on the shelf.

Standards: Complete all steps listed in this skill in _______ minutes with a minimum score of ________. (Time element and accuracy criteria may be given by instructor.)

Time: **Start:** ____________ **Completed:** ____________ **Total:** ____________ minutes

Scoring: One point for each step performed satisfactorily unless otherwise listed or weighted by instructor.

Directions with Performance Evaluation Checklist

Read the following sentences and circle the correct spelling from each pair of generic or brand-name medications. These sentences contain some frequently misspelled drug names.

1st Attempt	2nd Attempt	3rd Attempt	
______	______	______	Gather materials (equipment and supplies) listed under "Conditions."
____/3	____/3	____/3	1. Dr. Practon's last chart note on Mr. Hoy Cho states, "advised the patient to take (a) Aspirin, (b) aspirin, 1 tab b.i.d."
____/3	____/3	____/3	2. After Ray Nunez suffered a mild heart attack, the physician prescribed a (a) nitroglycerin, (b) nitroglycerine patch daily.
____/3	____/3	____/3	3. Maria Sanchez telephones stating she has a cold and wants to know if it is all right to take (a) Contac, (b) Contact, an over-the-counter drug.
____/3	____/3	____/3	4. Mrs. Hatakeyama's allergy is easily treated with (a) Actafed, (b) Actifed.
____/3	____/3	____/3	5. Rosaria LaMaccia suffered a mild respiratory infection and Dr. Practon gave her a prescription for (a) Ceclor, (b) Seklor.
____/3	____/3	____/3	6. The patient is complaining of muscle spasms in the lumbar region, so a prescription for (a) Flexeril, (b) Flexoril is given.
____/3	____/3	____/3	7. Fayetta Brown's diagnosis is duodenal ulcer, so she is given a prescription for (a) Bentil, (b) Bentyl.
____/3	____/3	____/3	8. A year ago Mae James had a urinary tract infection and was prescribed (a) Ceptra, (b) Septra.
____/3	____/3	____/3	9. Ventricular arrhythmias are diagnosed in Cameron Lesser's case, so (a) Quiniglute, (b) Quinaglute is given.
____/3	____/3	____/3	10. After the death of her spouse, Danielle La Fleur became depressed and Dr. Practon prescribed (a) amatriptyline, (b) amitriptyline.

JOB SKILL 10-2 *(continued)*

_______ _______ _______ Complete within specified time.

____/32 ____/32 ____/32 **Total points earned** (To obtain a percentage score, divide the total points earned by the number of points possible.)

Comments:

Evaluator's Signature: ______________________________ **Need to Repeat:** ____________

National Curriculum Competency: ABHES: 6b

JOB SKILL 10-3
Use the *Physicians' Desk Reference (PDR)*

Name ______________________________ Date ____________ Score ______

Performance Objective

Task: Identify medication in the correct section of the *Physicians' Desk Reference (PDR).*

Conditions: *Physician's Desk Reference* (or Figure 10-3 in *textbook*); pen or pencil. Refer to Procedure 10-1 in the *textbook* for step-by-step directions.

Standards: Complete all steps listed in this skill in ______ minutes with a minimum score of ______. (Time element and accuracy criteria may be given by instructor.)

Time: **Start:** __________ **Completed:** __________ **Total:** __________ minutes

Scoring: One point for each step performed satisfactorily unless otherwise listed or weighted by instructor.

Directions with Performance Evaluation Checklist

Dr. Practon has just received a prothrombin time report on Mrs. Darcuiel. He asks you to call the patient and verify her present dosage of Coumadin before he makes an adjustment. When you call the patient, she states she put all the pills in a medication container and no longer remembers her dosage. She says it is the only medication she is taking and it is ***blue***. Refer to the *PDR* or Figure 10-3 in the *textbook* to determine how many milligrams she is taking.

1st Attempt	2nd Attempt	3rd Attempt	
______	______	______	Gather materials (equipment and supplies) listed under "Conditions."
____/5	____/5	____/5	1. Dosage Mrs. Darcuiel is taking: ______________________
____/3	____/3	____/3	2. In which section of the *PDR* did you find the information? __________
______	______	______	Complete within specified time.
____/10	____/10	____/10	**Total points earned** (To obtain a percentage score, divide the total points earned by the number of points possible.)

Comments:

Evaluator's Signature: ______________________________ **Need to Repeat:** __________

National Curriculum Competency: ABHES: 6b

JOB SKILL 10-4
Translate Prescriptions

Name ____ Date ______________ Score _______

Performance Objective

Task: Translate prescriptions from Latin into common English.

Conditions: Nine written prescriptions, one sheet of plain paper, and pen or pencil. Refer to Procedure 10-2 in the *textbook* for step-by-step directions.

Standards: Complete all steps listed in this skill in _______ minutes with a minimum score of ________. (Time element and accuracy criteria may be given by instructor.)

Time: **Start:** _____________ **Completed:** _____________ **Total:** _____________ minutes

Scoring: One point for each step performed satisfactorily unless otherwise listed or weighted by instructor.

Directions with Performance Evaluation Checklist

Translate the nine prescriptions in *Workbook* Figure 10-1 into common English by referring to *textbook* Table 10-3, Common Prescription Abbreviations and Symbols. Refer to Procedure 10-2 in the *textbook* for step-by-step instructions.

EXAMPLE:

Valium 10 mg
#21
Sig.: t̄ p.o. t.i.d.

Translation: Valium, ten milligrams, number twenty-one, one by mouth three times a day.

1st Attempt	2nd Attempt	3rd Attempt	
_______	_______	_______	Gather materials (equipment and supplies) listed under "Conditions."
_____/5	_____/5	_____/5	1. Translate prescription for Tagamet.
_____/5	_____/5	_____/5	2. Translate prescription for Darvocet.
_____/5	_____/5	_____/5	3. Translate prescription for Diovan.
_____/5	_____/5	_____/5	4. Translate prescription for Tenormin.
_____/5	_____/5	_____/5	5. Translate prescription for Robitussin.
_____/5	_____/5	_____/5	6. Translate prescription for Isordil.
_____/5	_____/5	_____/5	7. Translate prescription for Compazine.
_____/5	_____/5	_____/5	8. Translate prescription for Vanceril.
_____/5	_____/5	_____/5	9. Translate prescription for Timoptic Solution.

JOB SKILL 10-4 *(continued)*

_______ _______ _______ Complete within specified time.

____/47 ____/47 ____/47 **Total points earned** (To obtain a percentage score, divide the total points earned by the number of points possible.)

Comments:

FIGURE 10-1

1 Tagamet 400 mg
#30
Sig.: ṫ p.o. h.s.

2 Darvocet N-100
#60 Tabs
Sig.: ṫṫ every 4h.
p.r.n. pain

3 Diovan HCT
160mg/12.5mg
#100
sig.: ṫ p.o. every day

4 Tenormin 50 mg
#100
ṫ every day

5 Robitussin DAC
4 oz. bottle
2 tsp every 4h. p.r.n.
cough

6 Isordil
(isosorbide dinitrate)
20 mg
#30
ṫ p.o every 12°

7 Compazine
25 mg suppositories
#14
ṫ rectally b.i.d.
p.r.n. vomiting

8 Vanceril Inhalation Aerosol
42 mcg
#1 bottle
2 inhalations q.i.d
p.r.n. asthma

9 Timoptic Solution
0.25%
1 bottle
ṫ gt. each eye b.i.d.

Evaluator's Signature: ______________________ **Need to Repeat:** __________

National Curriculum Competency: ABHES: 6c

JOB SKILL 10-5
Record Prescription Refills in Medical Records

Name ______________________________ Date ______________ Score ________

Performance Objective

Task: Record four prescription refills in patient medical records.

Conditions: Four large file folder labels (Form 26) and pen. Use (1) medical record for Wayne[LP5] G. Weather completed in Job Skill 7-5 and Job Skill 9-1; (2) medical record for Krista Lee Carlisle completed in Job Skill 9-2; and (3) medical record for Sun Low Chung completed in Job Skill 9-5. Refer to Procedure 10-3 in the *textbook* for step-by-step directions. Use pharmaceutical abbreviations and symbols found in *textbook* Table 10-3, Common Prescription Abbreviations and Symbols, or Part IV of this *Workbook*.

Standards: Complete all steps listed in this skill in ________ minutes with a minimum score of ________. (Time element and accuracy criteria may be given by instructor.)

Time: **Start:** ____________ **Completed:** ____________ **Total:** ____________ minutes

Scoring: One point for each step performed satisfactorily unless otherwise listed or weighted by instructor.

Directions with Performance Evaluation Checklist

Read the following scenarios and abstract the prescription information. Record each transaction on a label, use the current date, initial it, and then secure the label in the patient's medical record.

1st Attempt	2nd Attempt	3rd Attempt	
_______	_______	_______	Gather materials (equipment and supplies) listed under "Conditions."
____/10	____/10	____/10	1. Record: The ABC Pharmacy calls about a prescription for Wayne G. Weather. Dr. Practon approves a refill for Darvocet N-100, number twenty, one tablet every four hours whenever necessary for pain.
____/10	____/10	____/10	2. Record: The Dalton Pharmacy calls about Krista Lee Carlisle. The pharmacist asks if a refill on Sonata, ten-milligram capsules, number ten, one by mouth at bedtime, can be approved. Dr. Practon approves.
____/10	____/10	____/10	3. Record: The Georgetown Pharmacy calls regarding Sun Low Chung. He has a urinary tract infection again and would like a refill on his Bactrim, double strength, number twenty-eight, one by mouth two times a day for fourteen days. Dr. Practon approves.
____/10	____/10	____/10	4. Record: Two days later, Sun Low Chung calls Dr. Practon reporting an adverse reaction to the Bactrim. Dr. Practon calls the Main Street Pharmacy to order Macrodantin, one-hundred milligram capsules, number forty, one by mouth four times a day with milk or meals for ten days.
_____/4	_____/4	_____/4	5. Secure prescription documentation (on labels) in correct medical records.
_______	_______	_______	Complete within specified time.
____/46	____/46	____/46	**Total points earned** (To obtain a percentage score, divide the total points earned by the number of points possible.)

JOB SKILL 10-5 *(continued)*

Comments:

Evaluator's Signature: ______________________ **Need to Repeat:** __________

National Curriculum Competency: CAAHEP: Psychomotor: IX.P.7	ABHES: 6c

JOB SKILL 10-6
Write a Prescription

Name ____ Date ______________ Score _______

Performance Objective

Task: Write a prescription.

Conditions: In some regions, medical assistants may be allowed to write prescriptions for patients; the physician must sign all originals. This exercise is designed to help understand the different components of a prescription form and the abbreviations used. Use one prescription (Form 27) and refer to *textbook* Figure 10-5 for a visual example. Refer to *textbook* Table 10-3, Common Prescription Abbreviations and Symbols, or the list of abbreviations in Part IV of this *Workbook.*

Standards: Complete all steps listed in this skill in _______ minutes with a minimum score of ________. (Time element and accuracy criteria may be given by instructor.)

Time: **Start:** ____________ **Completed:** ____________ **Total:** ____________ minutes

Scoring: One point for each step performed satisfactorily unless otherwise listed or weighted by instructor.

Directions with Performance Evaluation Checklist

Read the following scenario and write a prescription using today's date:

Felisha Weiss, 456 Los Angeles Avenue, Woodland Hills, XY 12345, needs prophylactic treatment for migraine headache syndrome. She will be given verapamil, one hundred eighty milligrams, sustained release, number one hundred and twenty tablets. Directions are to take one by mouth every morning; she may have two refills.

1st Attempt	2nd Attempt	3rd Attempt	
_______	_______	_______	Gather materials (equipment and supplies) listed under "Conditions."
_____/5	_____/5	_____/5	1. Complete patient demographic information and enter today's date.
_____/4	_____/4	_____/4	2. Complete inscription.
_____/2	_____/2	_____/2	3. Complete subscription.
_____/4	_____/4	_____/4	4. Complete signature.
_______	_______	_______	5. Indicate number of refills.
_______	_______	_______	6. Proofread form prior to physician's signature.
_______	_______	_______	Complete within specified time.
____/19	____/19	____/19	**Total points earned** (To obtain a percentage score, divide the total points earned by the number of points possible.)

JOB SKILL 10-6 *(continued)*

Comments:

Evaluator's Signature: ____ **Need to Repeat:** ________________

National Curriculum Competency: ABHES: 6c, d, e

JOB SKILL 10-7
Interpret a Medication Log

Name ______________________________ Date ______________ Score ________

Performance Objective

Task: Study the medication log and determine the drug use habits of a patient.

Conditions: Refer to the medication log (*Workbook* Figure 10-2) and use a pen or pencil. See Procedure 10-3 in the *textbook* for step-by-step directions.

Standards: Complete all steps listed in this skill in _______ minutes with a minimum score of ________. (Time element and accuracy criteria may be given by instructor.)

Time: **Start:** ____________ **Completed:** ____________ **Total:** ____________ minutes

Scoring: One point for each step performed satisfactorily unless otherwise listed or weighted by instructor.

Directions with Performance Evaluation Checklist

It is November 17, current year, and Mary Beth Foley calls to request a refill on her Glucotrol. Study the medication log and answer the following questions.

1st Attempt	2nd Attempt	3rd Attempt	
_______	_______	_______	Gather materials (equipment and supplies) listed under "Conditions."
_____/2	_____/2	_____/2	1. Has Mary Beth Foley been prescribed the medication? YES NO
_____/2	_____/2	_____/2	2. How many days has it been since she got her last refill? ________ days
_____/2	_____/2	_____/2	3. Is it time to refill the medication? YES NO
_____/2	_____/2	_____/2	4. When may she call for the next refill? ____________________________
_______	_______	_______	Complete within specified time.
____/10	____/10	____/10	**Total points earned** (To obtain a percentage score, divide the total points earned by the number of points possible.)

Comments:

Evaluator's Signature: ______________________________ **Need to Repeat:** ______________

National Curriculum Competency: CAAHEP: Psychomotor: IV.P.8	ABHES: 6c

JOB SKILL 10-7 *(continued)*

FIGURE 10-2

MEDICATION LOG

PATIENT NAME: FOLEY, Mary Beth **DATE OF BIRTH:** 9-30-52

ALLERGIES: NKA

DATE	MEDICATIONS	DOSE	#	INSTRUCTIONS (SIG)	PRN REG	TEL WRIT	PHARMACY	DR. SIG.
8/5/XX	Amitriptyline	100 mg	90	i p.o. h.s.	R	T	ABC Pharm	GMP
9/23/XX	Glucotrol	10 mg	30	i p.o. a.c./a.m.	R	T	ABC Pharm	GMP
9/23/XX	Verapamil SR	240 mg	30	i p.o. q.a.m.	R	T	ABC Pharm	GMP
10/7/XX	Glucotrol	10 mg	90	i p.o. a.c./a.m.	R	W	mail order pharmacy	GMP
10/7/XX	Tetracycline	250 mg	30	i p.o. T.I.D. p.r.n. yellow sputum	P	T	ABC Pharm	GMP
10/16/XX	Verapamil SR	240 mg	90	i p.o. q.a.m.	R	W	mail order pharmacy	GMP
10/28/XX	Amitriptyline	100 mg	90	i p.o. h.s.	R	T	ABC Pharm	GMP

JOB SKILL 10-8
Record on a Medication Schedule

Name ______________________________ Date ____________ Score ______

Performance Objective

Task: Record medication name, dosage, and instructions on a medication schedule.

Conditions: Medication schedule (Form 28) and a pen or pencil. Refer to *textbook* Figure 10-6 for a visual example.

Standards: Complete all steps listed in this skill in ______ minutes with a minimum score of ______. (Time element and accuracy criteria may be given by instructor.)

Time: **Start:** __________ **Completed:** __________ **Total:** __________ minutes

Scoring: One point for each step performed satisfactorily unless otherwise listed or weighted by instructor.

Directions with Performance Evaluation Checklist

Mr. Delbert Silva has just seen Dr. Fran Practon. She has prescribed Paxil for his depression. The dosage is 20 milligrams every morning. He is very confused, and Dr. Practon would like you to record all of his prescription information on a medication schedule for him. There is information in his chart indicating he is also taking Sinemet 20/250 milligrams for his Parkinson's disease. He takes two tablets four times a day. He is also on Lopressor, 100 milligrams twice a day, for his hypertension. You have verified that Mr. Silva is still on these medications. Please set up and fill out the medication schedule for Mr. Silva.

1st Attempt	2nd Attempt	3rd Attempt	
______	______	______	Gather materials (equipment and supplies) listed under "Conditions."
____/2	____/2	____/2	1. Fill in patient name and physician name.
____/4	____/4	____/4	2. Set up schedule for "a.m.," "NOON," "p.m.," and "BED."
____/4	____/4	____/4	3. Record information for Paxil medication.
____/8	____/8	____/8	4. Record information for Sinemet medication.
____/5	____/5	____/5	5. Record information for Lopressor medication.
______	______	______	6. Proofread schedule prior to giving it to the patient.
______	______	______	Complete within specified time.
____/26	____/26	____/26	**Total points earned** (To obtain a percentage score, divide the total points earned by the number of points possible.)

JOB SKILL 10-8 *(continued)*

Comments:

Evaluator's Signature: ________________________ **Need to Repeat:** ____________

National Curriculum Competency: CAAHEP: Psychomotor: IV.P.8	ABHES: 6c

CHAPTER 11

Written Correspondence

OBJECTIVES

After completing the exercises, the student will be able to:

1. Enhance knowledge of medical terminology, interpret abbreviations, and accurately spell medical words.
2. Spell medical words (Job Skill 11-1).
3. Key a letter of withdrawal (Job Skill 11-2).
4. Edit written communication (Job Skill 11-3).
5. Compose and key a letter for a failed appointment (Job Skill 11-4).
6. Compose and key a letter for an initial visit (Job Skill 11-5).
7. Compose and key a letter to another physician (Job Skill 11-6).
8. Compose and key a letter requesting payment (Job Skill 11-7).
9. Key two interoffice memorandums (Job Skill 11-8).
10. Abstract information from a medical record; compose and key a letter (Job Skill 11-9).
11. Key a two-page letter (Job Skill 11-10).

FOCUS ON CERTIFICATION*

CMA Content Summary

- Medical terminology
- Spelling
- Data entry
- Reports
- Documents
- Correspondence
- Letters
- Memos
- Messages
- Fundamental writing skills
- Sentence structure
- Grammar
- Punctuation
- Keyboard fundamentals
- Formats (letters, memos, reports)
- Proofreading
- Making corrections from rough draft
- Computer storage devices
- Word processing applications
- Report generation

RMA Content Summary

- Medical terminology (word definitions, spelling)
- Apply proper written communication to instruct patients
- Understand and correctly apply terminology associated with secretarial duties
- Compose correspondence employing acceptable business format
- Employ effective written communication skills adhering to ethics and laws of confidentiality
- Transcription and dictation

CMAS Content Summary

- Medical terminology
- Employ effective written communication
- Format business documents and correspondence appropriately
- Possess fundamental knowledge of word processing

STOP AND THINK CASE SCENARIOS AND EXAM-STYLE REVIEW QUESTIONS

Refer to the end of Chapter 11 in the *textbook*.

Abbreviation and Spelling Review

Read the following patient's chart note and write the meanings for the abbreviations listed below the note. To decode any abbreviations you do not understand or that appear unfamiliar to you, refer to the list of abbreviations in Part IV of this *Workbook*. Step-by-step directions for this exercise are in Procedure 1-1 of Chapter 1 in the *textbook*. Medical terms in the chart note are italicized; study them for spelling. Use your medical dictionary to look up their definitions. Your instructor may give a spelling and definition test that includes these words and abbreviations.

*This *Workbook* and the accompanying *textbook* meet the entry-level administrative and general competencies for the CMA outlined by the AAMA Examination Content Outline and Occupational Analysis and for the RMA and CMAS outlined by the AMT Competencies, Construction Parameters, and Examination Specifications (see Competency Grid in Appendix B of the *textbook*).

DATE	PROGRESS
1-3-20XX	Maria K Morgan CC: Pt complains of back pain, *nausea, dysuria,* & *oliguria* of 1 wk. PH: *Congenital stricture* rt. *ureter* at *ureterovesical junction.* UA: Occ WBC, occ epith., pH 7, alb 1, sugar O. Dr. Woodman's summary rev. Dilat to K35 c̄ Brev sodium, ordered IVP. *Unilateral nephrectomy* may be indicated. Dx: possible *urinary calculi.* RTO 1 wk. for UA & possible Dilat.
	Gerald Practon, MD Gerald Practon, MD

CC ____________________
pt ____________________
wk ____________________
PH ____________________
UA ____________________
occ ____________________
WBC ____________________
epith. ____________________
pH ____________________
alb ____________________
rev ____________________
dilat ____________________
K35 ____________________
c̄ ____________________
Brev ____________________
IVP ____________________
Dx ____________________
RTO ____________________

Review Questions

Review the objectives, glossary, and chapter information before completing the following review questions.

1. How should a letter of an official or legal nature be sent when there is a need to expedite it? ____________________
2. Why would a computerized medical office have a typewriter or word processor? ____________________
3. When keying a letter on a computer, what type of software would you use? ____________________
4. List three flaws that would make a letter unmailable.
   a. ____________________
   b. ____________________
   c. ____________________
5. Which style is the least personal of the various letter formats? ____________________
6. Which two punctuation styles are most commonly used? Briefly describe each.
   a. ____________________
   b. ____________________
7. What are the typical default settings for right and left margins? ____________________

8. Name three devices you could use to arouse the reader's interest in the first paragraph of a letter you are writing for the physician.

   a. ______________________________

   b. ______________________________

   c. ______________________________

9. Explain the following text-editing features of electronic word processors.

   a. Directional keys ______________________________

   b. Function keys ______________________________

   c. Memory functions ______________________________

   d. Tool features ______________________________

   ____

   e. Edit features ______________________________

   ____

   f. Printing feature ______________________________

   ____

   g. Format functions ______________________________

   ____

   ____

10. When checking for layout or format prior to printing, what software program option would you use to view an entire page of a document? ______________________________

    ____

11. Transcription needs in the physician's office will be based on the following factors:

    a. ______________________________

    b. ______________________________

    c. ______________________________

    d. ______________________________

12. What procedure should be followed when the transcriptionist cannot understand a word or phrase of a physician's dictation? ______________________________

    ____

13. The following are three methods the physician may use to create letters. Briefly describe the physician's and medical transcriber's roles when using these methods.

    a. Dictation equipment: ______________________________

    ____

    ____

    b. Voice-activated software: ______________________________

    ____

    ____

c. Remote device (PDA): ______________________________

____

____

14. List five ways to increase the productivity of photocopy machines.

a. ______________________________

b. ______________________________

c. ______________________________

d. ______________________________

e. ______________________________

Critical Thinking Exercises

1. The following examples are parts of a letter. Read each example, and then identify and name the part of the letter.

a. Attn: Philip Kellogg, MD

____

b. Re: *Administrative Medical Assisting*, 7th edition

____

c. P.S. Please call me if you need directions.

____

d. Sincerely,

____

e. Arthur Miller, MD
2300 Broad Avenue
Woodland Hills, XY 12345-4700

____

f. Dear Dr. Rogers:

____

g. CC: Bernice Brantley, MD

____

h. Enc. (3)

____

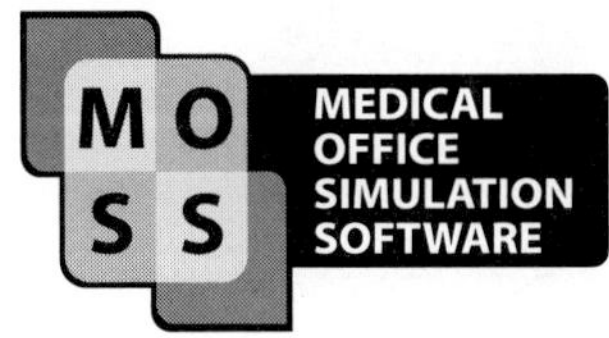

Computer Competency

Today's Date Is Monday, 10/23/2013

Simulation: You are the administrative medical assistant for the doctors of Douglasville Medicine Associates. One of your responsibilities is to transcribe written correspondence dictated by the physicians. **You will need to reference the**

MOSS Source Documents (Dictated Letters) found at the end of this section to complete the exercises. Alternatively, these are available as Audio Files in Chapter 11 Resources on the Premium Web site at http://www.cengagebrain.com.

1. Written Correspondence: Patient Lagasse

The office manager has dropped off a dictation tape in the in-box with correspondence to be transcribed today. Using the *Correspondence* feature in MOSS, transcribe the document, being sure to format the letter properly. Pay special attention to spelling, grammar, and punctuation. All transcribed documents will be placed on the physician's desk for signature. The mailing envelope should also be prepared and be attached to any document that is to be mailed.

A. After setting up the transcription equipment and inserting the tape, click on the *Billing* drop-down menu option in MOSS and click on *Patient Ledger*.

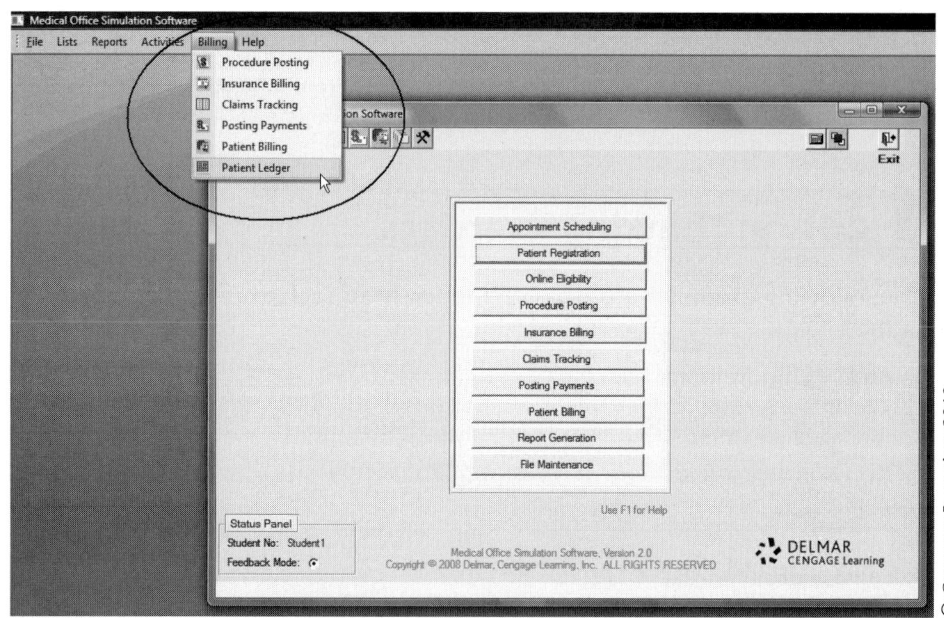

© Cengage Learning 2013

B. Select Patient Lagasse from the *Patient Account* list and click on *View*. This will display the patient's ledger.

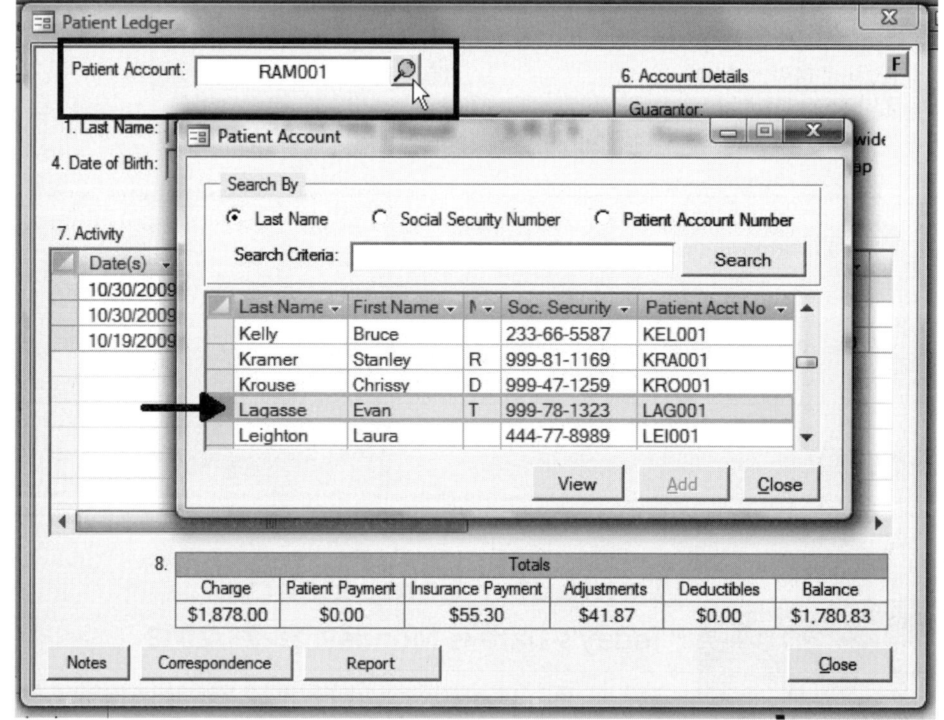

© Cengage Learning 2013

C. At the bottom left of the ledger screen, click on the *Correspondence* button.

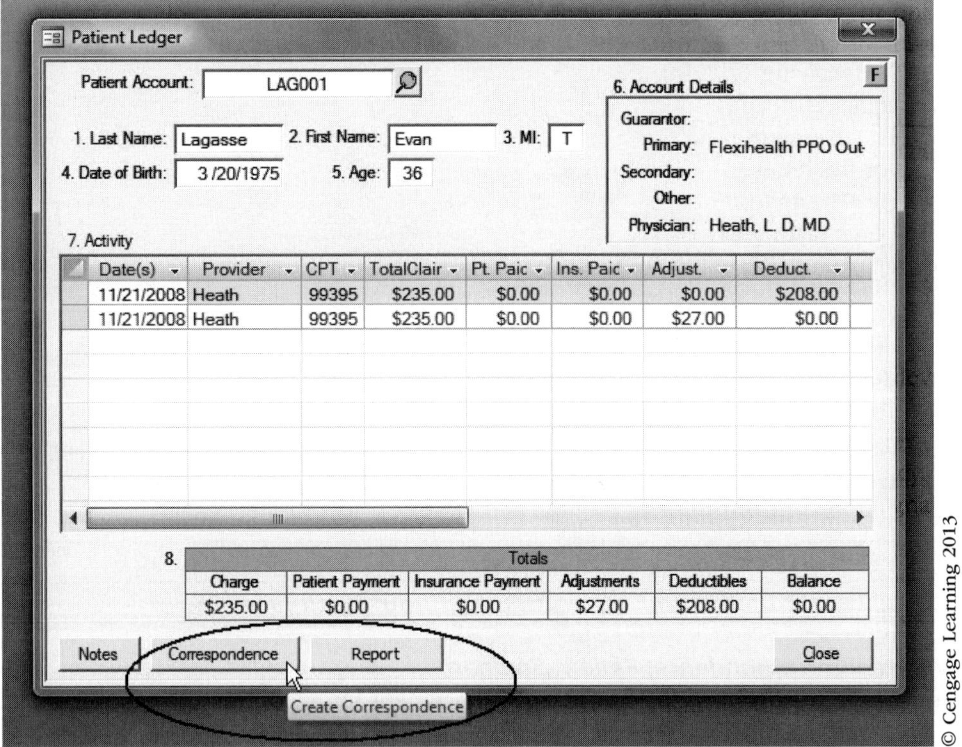

© Cengage Learning 2013

D. The *Output To* dialog box will open. Select a location to save your letter and name it as follows: **lagasse_letter_yourlastname** Click *OK* to save the letter.

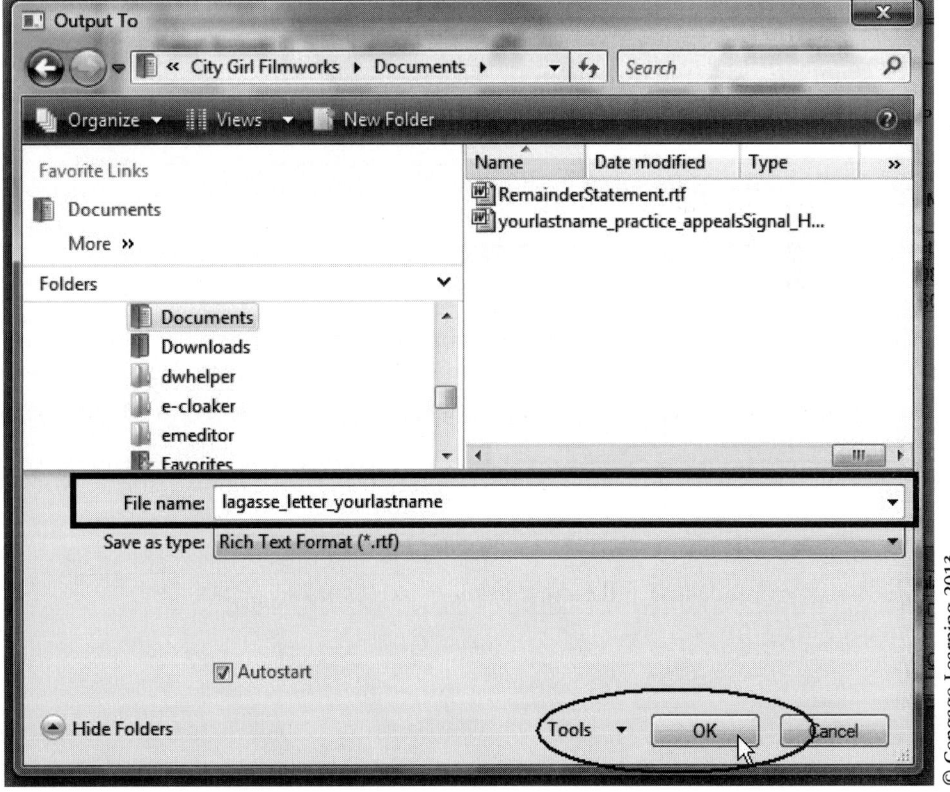

© Cengage Learning 2013

E. After a short pause, the letterhead for Douglasville Medicine Associates opens. Change the date of the letter to 10/23/2013 and put your own last name in the *Student No.* field.

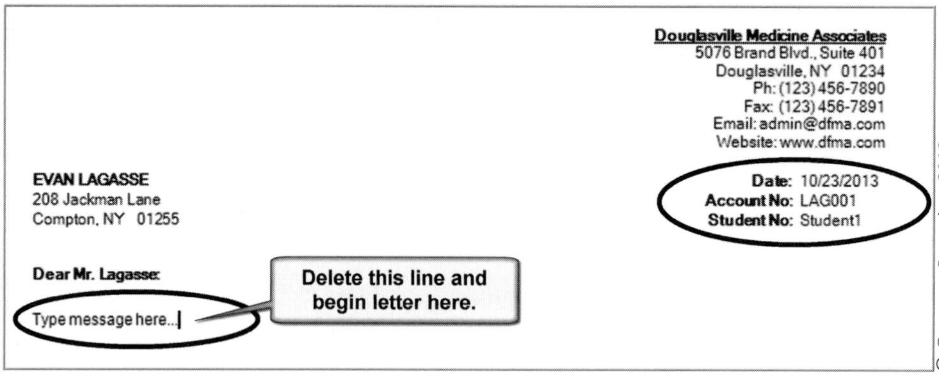

Douglasville Medicine Associates
5076 Brand Blvd., Suite 401
Douglasville, NY 01234
Ph: (123) 456-7890
Fax: (123) 456-7891
Email: admin@dfma.com
Website: www.dfma.com

EVAN LAGASSE
208 Jackman Lane
Compton, NY 01255

Date: 10/23/2013
Account No: LAG001
Student No: Student1

Dear Mr. Lagasse:

Type message here...|

Delete this line and begin letter here.

© Cengage Learning 2013

With the cursor, click at *Type Message Here* and delete that line. Start the body of the letter at that location.

F. Transcribe (type) the physician's dictation as shown on the source document **(Source Documents: Dictated Letters).**

G. When complete, save the document in your word processing software.

H. Print the letter so the physician may sign it. Prepare a mailing envelope.

I. Close the word processor and return to the *Main Menu* in MOSS.

2. Written Correspondence: Patient Shuman

Using the skills just learned, complete the document found on the tape for Alan Shuman.

A. Click on the *Billing* drop-down menu option in MOSS and open the *Patient Ledger* for Alan Shuman. Click on *Correspondence*, and then open and save a practice letterhead as previously learned.

B. Transcribe (type) the physician's dictation as shown on the source document **(Source Documents: Dictated Letters).**

C. When complete, save the document by clicking on the *Save* button on the word processor.

D. Print the letter so the physician may sign it, and turn in a copy to your instructor. Prepare a mailing envelope.

E. Close the word processor and return to the *Main Menu* in MOSS.

3. Written Correspondence: Patient Yamagata

Using the skills just learned, complete the document found on the tape for Naomi Yamagata.

A. Click on the *Billing* drop-down menu option in MOSS and open the *Patient Ledger* for Naomi Yamagata. Click on *Correspondence*, and then open and save a practice letterhead as previously learned.

B. Transcribe (type) the physician's dictation as shown on the source document **(Source Documents: Dictated Letters).**

C. When complete, save the document by clicking on the *Save* button on the word processor.

D. Print the letter so the physician may sign it, and turn in a copy to your instructor. Prepare a mailing envelope.

E. Close the word processor and return to the *Main Menu* in MOSS.

4. Written Correspondence: Patient Altizer

Using the skills just learned, complete the document found on the tape for Luke Altizer.

A. Click on the *Billing* drop-down menu option in MOSS and open the *Patient Ledger* for Luke Altizer. Click on *Correspondence*, and then open and save a practice letterhead as previously learned.

B. This correspondence is being sent to another physician regarding the patient.

Change the name and address of the recipient to that of Dr. Jennings, as dictated by the physician on the source document **(Source Documents: Dictated Letters).**

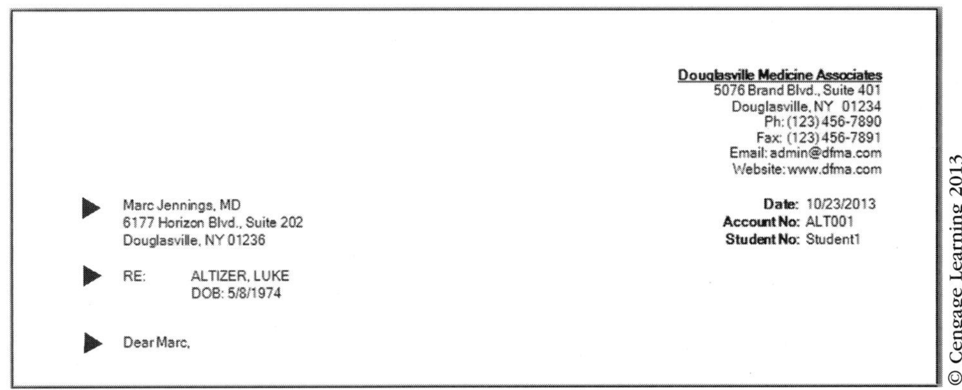
Douglasville Medicine Associates
5076 Brand Blvd., Suite 401
Douglasville, NY 01234
Ph: (123) 456-7890
Fax: (123) 456-7891
Email: admin@dfma.com
Website: www.dfma.com

Date: 10/23/2013
Account No: ALT001
Student No: Student1

Marc Jennings, MD
6177 Horizon Blvd., Suite 202
Douglasville, NY 01236

RE: ALTIZER, LUKE
DOB: 5/8/1974

Dear Marc,

C. Insert a reference line before the salutation that includes the patient's name (last name first) and date of birth (DOB).

D. Change the salutation as required by the dictation.

E. Transcribe (type) the physician's dictation of the letter as shown on the source document **(Source Documents: Dictated Letters).**

F. When complete, save the letter by clicking on the *Save* button on the word processor.

G. Print the letter so the physician may sign it, and turn in a copy to your instructor. Prepare a mailing envelope.

Computer Competency Source Documents: Dictated Letters

Note: These dictated letters are also available as audio files (mp3 format) on the Premium Website.

Patient: Evan Lagasse

Physician: L.D. Heath, M.D.

Dictated Correspondence:

this is a collections letter to...patient evan lagasse…l a g a s s e…two zero eight…jackman lane…compton new york…zero one two five five…dear mr lagasse…the billing manager for douglasville medicine associates has brought your… past due account to my attention….make that your severely past due account…to my attention…your insurance plan, flexihealth p p o…applied the charges for services received on… november eleventh…two thousand and twelve…to your annual deductible…the amount due is…two hundred and eight dollars…(new paragraph)…as you know…deductibles are due…from the insured…over the past year…our billing department…has sent letters and placed phone calls…in an attempt to collect this past due amount…unfortunately they have not been able to resolve this matter with you…(new paragraph)…i have asked my billing manager to hold any action…on your account…for five business days…please contact our office to make a payment within…five days of receipt of this letter…and bring your account current…we can also set up a payment plan…to further assist you…(new paragraph)…i would prefer to avoid assigning your account to a collections agency…and look forward to hearing from you…thank you for your cooperation with this matter…sincerely yours…l d heath…m d…(be sure to flag this file…if there is no response…authorize sending the account to our collections agency)…

Patient: Alan Shuman

Physician: L.D. Heath, M.D.

Dictated Correspondence:

please send this letter to…mr alan shuman…look up his address in our records…dear mr shuman…upon reviewing our records…i am concerned that i have not seen you in the office for your annual examination…for over a year…it is important…that you have a c t scan once a year…to monitor your abdominal…aortic…aneurysm…(do not abbreviate the diagnosis)…it is imperative that your condition be monitored regularly…so that you may continue to enjoy…good health without complications...it is important that your aneurysm be checked for size…and any critical changes that may require…medical attention...(new paragraph)…if you have not scheduled an annual examination…with a physician… in the past year…I strongly recommend that you call my office…and schedule an appointment…at your earliest convenience…at this time…I suggest a repeat c t scan of the abdomen…an electrocardiogram…a stress test and a complete physical…including blood work…(new paragraph)…your health is of great concern to me…I look forward to seeing you in my office soon…should you have any questions…do not hesitate calling me at four five six…seven eight nine zero…sincerely yours…l d heath…m d…(please be sure to flag mr shuman's record…alert me when he has made an appointment…or if he has not responded within two weeks)…

Patient: Naomi Yamagata

Physician: D.J. Schwartz , M.D.

Dictated Correspondence:

send this letter to…patient…naomi y a m a g a t a…two one six eight…greely avenue…douglasville new york…zero one two three five…subject…bone density d x a… (capital d x a in parenthesis) …scan…dear ms yamagata…your insurance plan…signal h m o…has sent me a list of patients…from our practice…that have been recommended to have a… d x a…in the coming year…signal hmo is recommending that you…have this test within the next twelve months…this is due to…the fact you have…undergone a medically necessary… total hysterectomy…at an early age…combined with a history…of anorexia nervosa…for this reason…as a preventative measure…and to obtain a baseline…i strongly support the recommendation of your insurance plan…the bone density scan is a…painless and quick procedure…which can be completed in less than…twenty minutes…i encourage you to call our office…and obtain the names of the… facilities in your plan network…we will provide the necessary authorization…once you have selected a convenient location…do not hesitate to call my office…should you have any questions…or concerns…you may also speak to my medical assistant…renee gallager…at four five six…seven eight nine zero for assistance…best regards to you and your family…d j schwartz…m d…(signal h m o…sent brochures explaining this procedure…please enclose one…it is called…what is a bone density scan…thank you)…

Patient: Luke Altizer

Physician: Greg Wallace, M.D.

Dictated Correspondence:

send this letter to doctor marc jennings...six one seven seven horizon boulevard...douglasville... new york...suite two zero two...zip code zero one two three six...in reference to luke altizer...date of birth may eighth...nineteen hundred and seventy four...dear marc...thank you for referring luke altizer to my office...i saw mr altizer in consultation on...october fifteen at quali-care during pulmonary clinic...he brought x rays from your office with him...mr altizer presents with a consistent cough...phlegm production...and a low grade fever...his history is well documented in your records and will not be provided here...on physical examination...the patient is a well nourished...well developed black male...in his mid to late thirties...He presents with significant rales and rhonchi...on auscultation...breath sounds were moderately diminished...on the...left side...because of a history of...chronic bronchitis...and persistent cough in the past year...i have ordered a computed tomography scan...of the chest...i have strongly suggested...to the patient...that he stop smoking...he stated trying several cessation....programs without success...based on several weeks of prednisone usage...at different times...over the past two years...to keep his breathing comfortable...i feel it is prudent to investigate further...with a scan...a sputum sample...was taken and sent to the laboratory... also of interest are an...immunoglobulin e... (capital i lowercase g capital e)...of more than...fourteen hundred nanograms per milliliter...and complete blood count shows...a marked increase in...eosinophils...given the latter I have...recommended he also consult...with an allergy immunologist...after the computed tomography scan is taken...i will follow up with...mr altizer in two weeks and have...placed him back on prednisone sixty milligrams...daily...for seven days...and will start to wean him...down over the following...weeks...hopefully he will realize...some relief with his dyspnea...until these tests are completed...he should be encouraged to...continue trying to stop smoking...i will keep you informed...of his progress...sincerely yours greg...wallace...m d...(enclosures to send...our recent laboratory results)...

JOB SKILL 11-1
Spell Medical Words

Name ______________________________ Date ____________ Score ________

Performance Objective

Task: Identify correctly spelled medical terms.

Conditions: Pen or pencil.

Standards: Complete all steps listed in this skill in ________ minutes with a minimum score of ________. (Time element and accuracy criteria may be given by instructor.)

Time: **Start:** ____________ **Completed:** ____________ **Total:** ____________ minutes

Scoring: One point for each step performed satisfactorily unless otherwise listed or weighted by instructor.

Directions with Performance Evaluation Checklist

Select and circle the correctly spelled medical word from the choices given.

1st Attempt	2nd Attempt	3rd Attempt			
______	______	______	Gather materials (equipment and supplies) listed under "Conditions."		
______	______	______	1. conchiousness	consciousness	consceousness
______	______	______	2. exhaustion	exsaustion	exhausion
______	______	______	3. theraputic	therapuetic	therapeutic
______	______	______	4. antidiarrheal	antidiarrhial	antidiarheal
______	______	______	5. neurolysis	nuerolysis	neurolosis
______	______	______	6. medisinal	medicinal	medicenal
______	______	______	7. roentegenogram	rentegenogram	roentgenogram
______	______	______	8. kinesiology	kenesiology	kenisiology
______	______	______	9. pharmasuetical	pharmaceutical	pharmaceutical
______	______	______	10. humeris	humerus	humerous
______	______	______	11. esophaglagia	esophagalgia	esopagalgia
______	______	______	12. critereon	criterion	creiterion
______	______	______	13. cauterisation	caterization	cauterization
______	______	______	14. methastasize	metastasize	metasthasize
______	______	______	15. spontaneous	spontenous	spontaneous
______	______	______	16. capitation	captation	capitasion
______	______	______	17. pancretectomy	pancraetectomy	pancreatectomy
______	______	______	18. indemity	endemnity	indemnity
______	______	______	19. negoteable	negotiable	negotable

JOB SKILL 11-1 *(continued)*

______	______	______	20. intemperance	intemperance	intemparance
______	______	______	21. ajudicate	adjudicate	adgudicate
______	______	______	22. cursor	curser	courser
______	______	______	23. stethoscope	steathescope	stethescrope
______	______	______	24. purelent	purulent	peurulent
______	______	______	25. ausculation	auscultation	auscultasion
______	______	______	Complete within specified time.		
____/27	____/27	____/27	**Total points earned** (To obtain a percentage score, divide the total points earned by the number of points possible.)		

Comments:

Evaluator's Signature: ______________________________ **Need to Repeat:** ____________

National Curriculum Competency: CAAHEP: Cognitive: IV.C.8	ABHES: 3.a, b, c, d; 8.jj

JOB SKILL 11-2
Key a Letter of Withdrawal

Name ______________________ Date ____________ Score ________

Performance Objective

Task: Key a letter of withdrawal for the physician's signature.

Conditions: Letterhead for Practon Medical Group, Inc., formatted in a word processing program, or one sheet of letterhead (Form 29). Refer to *textbook* Figure 11-3 and Figure 11-4 for format. Refer to Figure 3-11 in *textbook* Chapter 3 for an example and Procedure 11-1 in the *textbook* for step-by-step directions.

Standards: Complete all steps listed in this skill in ________ minutes with a minimum score of ________. (Time element and accuracy criteria may be given by instructor.)

Time: **Start:** ____________ **Completed:** ____________ **Total:** ____________ minutes

Scoring: One point for each step performed satisfactorily unless otherwise listed or weighted by instructor.

Directions with Performance Evaluation Checklist

Mrs. Stanfield refused to follow the treatment prescribed by Dr. Gerald Practon, and he has asked you to type a letter of withdrawal on his letterhead. Follow the steps below to complete this job skill.

1st Attempt	2nd Attempt	3rd Attempt	
______	______	______	Gather materials (equipment and supplies) listed under "Conditions."
______	______	______	1. Format letterhead or use Form 29.
______	______	______	2. Use the current date.
______	______	______	3. Address the letter to Constance M. Stanfield, 2090 Hope Street, Woodland Hills, XY 12345.
______	______	______	4. Use the correct salutation.
______	______	______	5. Key in full block style.
______	______	______	6. Use open punctuation.
______	______	______	7. Use even and equal left and right margins.
______	______	______	8. Place the letter on stationery with correct spacing.
____/10	____/10	____/10	9. Compose an appropriate letter with wording that is legally correct.
______	______	______	10. Check paragraphing and punctuation.
____/2	____/2	____/2	11. Place the complimentary close and signature line in the appropriate place.
______	______	______	12. Key reference initials.
______	______	______	13. Key an enclosure notation.
______	______	______	14. Proofread for spelling and typographical errors while on-screen or in the typewriter.

JOB SKILL 11-2 *(continued)*

______ ______ ______ 15. Correct, print, and proofread again.

______ ______ ______ 16. Correct all errors and ready for the physician's signature.

______ ______ ______ Complete within specified time.

____/28 ____/28 ____/28 **Total points earned** (To obtain a percentage score, divide the total points earned by the number of points possible.)

Comments:

Evaluator's Signature: ____________________________ **Need to Repeat:** ____________

National Curriculum Competency: CAAHEP: Cognitive: IV.C.8; Psychomotor: IV.P.10	ABHES: 7.a, b; 8.jj

JOB SKILL 11-3
Edit Written Communication

Name ______________________________ Date ______________ Score ________

Performance Objective

Task:	Edit sentences for improvement.
Conditions:	Assemble 20 sentences and pen or pencil.
Standards:	Complete all steps listed in this skill in _______ minutes with a minimum score of _______. (Time element and accuracy criteria may be given by instructor.)
Time:	**Start:** ____________ **Completed:** ____________ **Total:** ____________ minutes
Scoring:	One point for each step performed satisfactorily unless otherwise listed or weighted by instructor.

Directions with Performance Evaluation Checklist

Read each of the following sentences and edit to eliminate words, change the sequence of words, and eliminate redundant phrases.

1st Attempt	2nd Attempt	3rd Attempt	
_______	_______	_______	Gather materials (equipment and supplies) listed under "Conditions."
_______	_______	_______	1. Mrs. Benson just recovered from an attack of pneumonia.
_______	_______	_______	2. The letter arrived at a time when we were busy.
_______	_______	_______	3. During the year of 20XX the unpaid accounts were numerous.
_______	_______	_______	4. If the population, as in the general case, increases, we'll plan on expanding our practice.
_______	_______	_______	5. The water is for drinking purposes only.
_______	_______	_______	6. The close proximity of the police department scared the thief.
_______	_______	_______	7. It costs the sum of 20 dollars.
_______	_______	_______	8. The young secretary has a beautiful future before her.
_______	_______	_______	9. The wreck occurred at the corner of Fourth and Rampart Streets.
_______	_______	_______	10. The color of the prize rose was dark red.
_______	_______	_______	11. We are now engaged in building a new medical office.
_______	_______	_______	12. Somebody or other must assume the responsibility.
_______	_______	_______	13. The file is made out of steel.
_______	_______	_______	14. There is much construction in the city of Ventura.
_______	_______	_______	15. It happened at the hour of midnight.
_______	_______	_______	16. The package should be there in three weeks' time.
_______	_______	_______	17. We will ship the office supplies at a later date.
_______	_______	_______	18. The character of the road was smooth.

JOB SKILL 11-3 *(continued)*

_______	_______	_______	19. The physician spoke at a meeting held in Miami Beach.
_______	_______	_______	20. The patient appeared for her appointment at the hour of 2:30 p.m.
_______	_______	_______	Complete within specified time.
____/22	____/22	____/22	**Total points earned** (To obtain a percentage score, divide the total points earned by the number of points possible.)

Comments:

Evaluator's Signature: ________________________________ **Need to Repeat:** ____________

National Curriculum Competency: CAAHEP: Cognitive: IV.C.8; Psychomotor: IV.P.10	ABHES: 7.a, b; 8.jj

JOB SKILL 11-4
Compose and Key a Letter for a Failed Appointment

Name ______________________________ Date ______________ Score ________

Performance Objective

Task: Compose and key an original letter dealing with a failed appointment.

Conditions: Letterhead for Practon Medical Group, Inc., formatted in a word processing program, or one sheet of letterhead (Form 30) and dictionary. Refer to *textbook* Figure 11-3 and Figure 11-4 for format. Refer to Procedure 11-1 in the *textbook* for step-by-step directions.

Standards: Complete all steps listed in this skill in ________ minutes with a minimum score of ________. (Time element and accuracy criteria may be given by instructor.)

Time: **Start:** ____________ **Completed:** ____________ **Total:** ____________ minutes

Scoring: One point for each step performed satisfactorily unless otherwise listed or weighted by instructor.

Directions with Performance Evaluation Checklist

Margaret B. Hanson (Mrs. C. L.) of 2319 Warren Street, Woodland Hills, XY 12345 calls on September 20 to make a 4 p.m. appointment for her 18-year-old son, James P. Hanson, on September 25. The patient does not show (DNS) for the appointment. Write a letter to Mrs. Hanson with a reference line notifying her about her son's failure to keep his appointment. Remember that this is a legal document that must be prepared for Dr. Fran Practon's signature. Key this letter in full block style with mixed punctuation; assume a file copy will be made.

1st Attempt	2nd Attempt	3rd Attempt	
______	______	______	Gather materials (equipment and supplies) listed under "Conditions."
______	______	______	1. Design letterhead or use Form 30.
______	______	______	2. Date the letter using the current date.
______	______	______	3. Key the inside address.
______	______	______	4. Key an appropriate salutation.
______	______	______	5. Key the reference or subject line.
______	______	______	6. Use full block style.
______	______	______	7. Use mixed punctuation.
______	______	______	8. Center the letter with even margins.
____/5	____/5	____/5	9. Mention the failed appointment with date and time in the body of the letter in a clear, concise manner.
______	______	______	10. Insert proper paragraphing.
____/2	____/2	____/2	11. Key an appropriate complimentary close and signature line.
______	______	______	12. Insert proper reference initials.
______	______	______	13. Proofread while the document is on-screen or in the typewriter for spelling, punctuation, capitalization, and typing errors.
______	______	______	14. Correct, print, and proofread again.
______	______	______	15. Make corrections and ready for the physician's signature.

JOB SKILL 11-4 *(continued)*

______	______	______	Complete within specified time.
____/22	____/22	____/22	**Total points earned** (To obtain a percentage score, divide the total points earned by the number of points possible.)

Comments:

Evaluator's Signature: ______________________________ **Need to Repeat:** ____________

National Curriculum Competency: CAAHEP: Cognitive: IV.C.8; Psychomotor: IV.P.10	ABHES: 7.a, b; 8.jj

JOB SKILL 11-5
Compose and Key a Letter for an Initial Visit

Name ______________________________ Date ______________ Score ________

Performance Objective

Task: Compose and key an original letter to a new patient explaining procedures for the initial visit and requesting insurance information.

Conditions: Letterhead for Practon Medical Group, Inc., formatted in a word processing program, or one sheet of letterhead (Form 31) and a dictionary. Refer to *textbook* Figure 11-3 and Figure 11-4 for format. Refer to Procedure 11-1 in the *textbook* for step-by-step directions.

Standards: Complete all steps listed in this skill in _______ minutes with a minimum score of _______. (Time element and accuracy criteria may be given by instructor.)

Time: **Start:** ____________ **Completed:** ____________ **Total:** ____________ minutes

Scoring: One point for each step performed satisfactorily unless otherwise listed or weighted by instructor.

Directions with Performance Evaluation Checklist

You are an administrative medical assistant. Write a letter over your own signature to Raymond E. Stokes Jr., 4053 Magnolia Boulevard, Woodland Hills, XY 12345. Remind him of his appointment with Dr. Fran Practon at 2:30 p.m. on Thursday, October 2, (current year). Inform him that the fee for an initial office visit is approximately $70.92. Suggest that he bring all insurance information if he has insurance coverage. Use full block style with mixed punctuation.

1st Attempt	2nd Attempt	3rd Attempt	
_______	_______	_______	Gather materials (equipment and supplies) listed under "Conditions."
_______	_______	_______	1. Design letterhead or use Form 31.
_______	_______	_______	2. Date the letter using the current date.
_______	_______	_______	3. Key the inside address.
_______	_______	_______	4. Key an appropriate salutation.
_______	_______	_______	5. Key a reference or subject line.
_______	_______	_______	6. Use full block style.
_______	_______	_______	7. Use mixed punctuation.
_______	_______	_______	8. Center the letter with even margins.
_____/5	_____/5	_____/5	9. Mention the appointment time, date, fee, and insurance coverage information in the body of the letter.
_______	_______	_______	10. Insert proper paragraphing.
_____/2	_____/2	_____/2	11. Key an appropriate complimentary close and signature line.
_______	_______	_______	12. Insert proper reference initials.
_______	_______	_______	13. Proofread while the document is on-screen or in the typewriter for spelling, punctuation, capitalization, and typing errors.
_______	_______	_______	14. Correct, print, and proofread again.
_______	_______	_______	15. Make corrections and sign.

JOB SKILL 11-5 *(continued)*

_______	_______	_______	Complete within specified time.
____/22	____/22	____/22	**Total points earned** (To obtain a percentage score, divide the total points earned by the number of points possible.)

Comments:

Evaluator's Signature: ______________________________ **Need to Repeat:** __________

National Curriculum Competency: CAAHEP: Cognitive: IV.C.8; Psychomotor: IV.P.10	ABHES: 7.a, b; 8.jj

JOB SKILL 11-6
Compose and Key a Letter to Another Physician

Name ______________________________ Date ______________ Score ________

Performance Objective

Task: Compose and key an original letter referring a patient to another physician.

Conditions: Letterhead for Practon Medical Group, Inc., formatted in a word processing program, or one sheet of letterhead (Form 32) and dictionary. Refer to *textbook* Figure 11-3 and Figure 11-4 for format. Refer to Procedure 11-1 in the *textbook* for step-by-step directions.

Standards: Complete all steps listed in this skill in ________ minutes with a minimum score of ________. (Time element and accuracy criteria may be given by instructor.)

Time: **Start:** ____________ **Completed:** ____________ **Total:** ____________ minutes

Scoring: One point for each step performed satisfactorily unless otherwise listed or weighted by instructor.

Directions with Performance Evaluation Checklist

Write a letter to Dr. Manuel Madero-Gonzales, Av. Mexico 131, Parque San Andreas, Mexico 21, D.F., referring Dr. Fran Practon's patient, Mr. Hector Gutierrez, who may need medical attention while vacationing in Mexico from September 30 through October 21, 20XX. He has been treated for infectious hepatitis, and his recent laboratory studies and clinical evaluations were within normal limits; assume you are enclosing copies of the most recent laboratory report and clinical evaluation. Tell Dr. Madero-Gonzales that you have instructed Mr. Gutierrez to contact him if any medical problems develop during his three-week stay. Use modified block style and open punctuation; make a copy to mail to the patient.

1st Attempt	2nd Attempt	3rd Attempt	
______	______	______	Gather materials (equipment and supplies) listed under "Conditions."
______	______	______	1. Design letterhead or use Form 32.
______	______	______	2. Date the letter using the current date.
______	______	______	3. Key the inside address.
______	______	______	4. Key an appropriate salutation.
______	______	______	5. Key the reference or subject line.
______	______	______	6. Use modified block style.
______	______	______	7. Use open punctuation.
______	______	______	8. Center the letter with even margins.
____/5	____/5	____/5	9. Mention the enclosed clinical evaluation in the body of the letter.
______	______	______	10. Insert proper paragraphing.
____/2	____/2	____/2	11. Key the appropriate complimentary close and signature line.
______	______	______	12. Insert proper reference initials.
______	______	______	13. Key the enclosure notation.
______	______	______	14. Key the copy notation.
______	______	______	15. Proofread while the document is on-screen or in the typewriter for spelling, punctuation, capitalization, and typing errors.

JOB SKILL 11-6 *(continued)*

_______ _______ _______ 16. Correct, print, and proofread again.

_______ _______ _______ 17. Make corrections and prepare for the physician's signature.

_______ _______ _______ 18. Make a copy to mail to the patient.

_______ _______ _______ Complete within specified time.

____/25 ____/25 ____/25 **Total points earned** (To obtain a percentage score, divide the total points earned by the number of points possible.)

Comments:

Evaluator's Signature: ____ **Need to Repeat:** ________________

National Curriculum Competency: CAAHEP: Cognitive: IV.C.8; Psychomotor: IV.P.10	ABHES: 7.a, b; 8.jj

JOB SKILL 11-7
Compose and Key a Letter Requesting Payment

Name ______________________________ Date ______________ Score ________

Performance Objective

Task: Compose and key a letter requesting payment on an overdue bill.

Conditions: Letterhead for Practon Medical Group, Inc., formatted in a word processing program, or one sheet of letterhead (Form 33) and a dictionary. Refer to *textbook* Figure 11-3 and Figure 11-4 for format. Refer to Procedure 11-1 in the *textbook* for step-by-step directions.

Standards: Complete all steps listed in this skill in ________ minutes with a minimum score of ________. (Time element and accuracy criteria may be given by instructor.)

Time: **Start:** ______________ **Completed:** ______________ **Total:** ______________ minutes

Scoring: One point for each step performed satisfactorily unless otherwise listed or weighted by instructor.

Directions with Performance Evaluation Checklist

When checking the financial records, you find that Christine LaMairre (Mrs. C. J.), 247 South Lincoln Boulevard, Apartment 5, Topanga, XY 12345, has not paid her bill for three months. She was seen for a consultation and complete physical examination; the fee was $70.92. She has no insurance coverage. Write a firm letter requesting payment by a specific date so it is not necessary to turn her account over to a collection agency. Enclose a copy of the current statement. Compose and key an original letter over Dr. Gerald Practon's signature in modified block style with open punctuation; assume a file copy of the letter will be made.

1st Attempt	2nd Attempt	3rd Attempt	
_______	_______	_______	Gather materials (equipment and supplies) listed under "Conditions."
_______	_______	_______	1. Design letterhead or use Form 33.
_______	_______	_______	2. Date the letter using the current date.
_______	_______	_______	3. Key the inside address.
_______	_______	_______	4. Key an appropriate salutation.
_______	_______	_______	5. Key the reference or subject line.
_______	_______	_______	6. Use modified block style.
_______	_______	_______	7. Use open punctuation.
_______	_______	_______	8. Center the letter with even margins.
_____/5	_____/5	_____/5	9. Request payment, stating the amount owed in the body of the letter using firm language.
_______	_______	_______	10. Insert proper paragraphing.
_____/2	_____/2	_____/2	11. Key an appropriate complimentary close and signature line.
_______	_______	_______	12. Insert proper reference initials.
_______	_______	_______	13. Key the enclosure notation.
_______	_______	_______	14. Proofread while the document is on-screen or in the typewriter for spelling, punctuation, capitalization, and typing errors.
_______	_______	_______	15. Correct, print, and proofread again.
_______	_______	_______	16. Make corrections and prepare for the physician's signature.

JOB SKILL 11-7 *(continued)*

_______	_______	_______	17. Make a file copy.
_______	_______	_______	Complete within specified time.
____/24	____/24	____/24	**Total points earned** (To obtain a percentage score, divide the total points earned by the number of points possible.)

Comments:

Evaluator's Signature: ________________________________ **Need to Repeat:** ____________

National Curriculum Competency: CAAHEP: Cognitive: IV.C.8; Psychomotor: IV.P.10	ABHES: 7.a, b; 8.jj

JOB SKILL 11-8
Key Two Interoffice Memorandums

Name ______________________________ Date ______________ Score ________

Performance Objective

Task: Key two interoffice memorandums from handwritten notes.

Conditions: Use two interoffice memos (Forms 34 and 35) and handwritten notes (*Workbook* Figure 11-1 and Figure 11-2). See *textbook* Figure 11-6 for an example.

Standards: Complete all steps listed in this skill in _______ minutes with a minimum score of _______. (Time element and accuracy criteria may be given by instructor.)

Time: **Start:** ____________ **Completed:** ____________ **Total:** ____________ minutes

Scoring: One point for each step performed satisfactorily unless otherwise listed or weighted by instructor.

Directions with Performance Evaluation Checklist

Scenario A: Dr. Gerald Practon has written a note and asked you to key a memorandum to Dr. Yong Hall. Abstract information from his handwritten note and key the message accurately on an interoffice memo. Use guide words such as those found on Form 34.
Scenario B: Dr. Fran Practon has written you a note (*Workbook* Figure 11-2) asking you to key a memorandum to Cathy Crowe, RPT. Dr. Practon will take it to the hospital and place it in Cathy's box. Key the appropriate memo.

1st Attempt	2nd Attempt	3rd Attempt	
_____	_____	_____	Gather materials (equipment and supplies) listed under "Conditions."
_____/2	_____/2	_____/2	1. Read each note before beginning to compose the memos.
_____/2	_____/2	_____/2	2. Prepare a rough draft of each memo.
_____/2	_____/2	_____/2	3. Align and key memo headings (or use those on Forms 34 and 35).
_____/2	_____/2	_____/2	4. Fill in spaces after each guide word with appropriate data.
_____/2	_____/2	_____/2	5. Choose appropriate information for the subject heading.
____/10	____/10	____/10	6. Write a concise message using appropriate sentence structure.
_____/2	_____/2	_____/2	7. Include all relevant information.
_____/2	_____/2	_____/2	8. Proofread the memos while the documents are on-screen for spelling, punctuation, capitalization, and typing errors.
_____/2	_____/2	_____/2	9. Print hard copies.
_____	_____	_____	Complete within specified time.
____/28	____/28	____/28	**Total points earned** (To obtain a percentage score, divide the total points earned by the number of points possible.)

Comments:

Evaluator's Signature: ______________________________ **Need to Repeat:** ____________

National Curriculum Competency: CAAHEP: Cognitive: IV.C.8; Psychomotor: IV.P.10	ABHES: 7.a, b; 8.jj

JOB SKILL 11-8 *(continued)*

FIGURE 11-1

From the Desk of... G. P.

3-22

Jean:

Ask Dr. Hall if he saw article "Evaluation of Biofeedback Training + Its Effects upon pt's with Tension Headaches" - Jan, 20XX. AMA Journal by Dr. Hugh James, pgs 21-25 - relevant to his research: very informative!

G. P.

P.S. Does he need a reprint?

FIGURE 11-2

From the Desk of... Fran

3-22

J:-

Please type a memo so I can take it to the hospital today to Cathy Crowe, RPT. Tell her we haven't rec'd copy of muscle strength Evaluation form for pt. Eric Willard. I desperately need it by 24th before I see Eric.

Thanks!

F.P.

JOB SKILL 11-9
Abstract Information from a Medical Record; Compose and Key a Letter

Name ______________________________ Date ____________ Score ________

Performance Objective

Task: Abstract patient information from a chart note, then key a letter to a referring physician.

Conditions: Letterhead for Practon Medical Group, Inc., formatted in a word processing program, or one sheet of letterhead (Form 36) and a dictionary. Refer to *textbook* Figure 11-3 and Figure 11-4 for format. Refer to *textbook* Procedure 11-1 for step-by-step directions.

Standards: Complete all steps listed in this skill in ________ minutes with a minimum score of ________. (Time element and accuracy criteria may be given by instructor.)

Time: **Start:** ____________ **Completed:** ____________ **Total:** ____________ minutes

Scoring: One point for each step performed satisfactorily unless otherwise listed or weighted by instructor.

Directions with Performance Evaluation Checklist

Dr. Fran Practon has asked you to review the chart notes of Ben Olman (*Workbook* Figure 11-3) and send a letter, dated March 22, 20XX, to the referring physician outlining the treatment since the last letter. Use full block style with mixed punctuation and key the letter for the physician's signature.

1st Attempt	2nd Attempt	3rd Attempt	
______	______	______	Gather materials (equipment and supplies) listed under "Conditions."
______	______	______	1. Design letterhead or use Form 36.
______	______	______	2. Date the letter.
______	______	______	3. Key the inside address.
______	______	______	4. Key an appropriate salutation.
______	______	______	5. Key the reference or subject line.
______	______	______	6. Use full block style.
______	______	______	7. Use mixed punctuation.
______	______	______	8. Center the letter with even margins.
____/3	____/3	____/3	9. Include the patient's name and the purpose of the letter at the beginning of the letter.
____/10	____/10	____/10	10. Include all dates and medical information since the previous letter.
______	______	______	11. Insert proper paragraphing.
____/2	____/2	____/2	12. Key an appropriate closing sentence.
____/2	____/2	____/2	13. Key an appropriate complimentary close and signature line.
______	______	______	14. Insert proper reference initials.
______	______	______	15. Proofread while the document is on-screen or in the typewriter for spelling, punctuation, capitalization, and typing errors.
______	______	______	16. Correct, print, and proofread again.
______	______	______	17. Make corrections and prepare for the physician's signature.

JOB SKILL 11-9 *(continued)*

______ ______ ______ Complete within specified time.

___/32 ___/32 ___/32 **Total points earned** (To obtain a percentage score, divide the total points earned by the number of points possible.)

FIGURE 11-3

DATE	PROGRESS Olman, Ben A.
2/3/XX	Pt moved recently to area and was referred to me by Dr. Ann Coleman, 4021 Indiana Ave, Ste 2, Pacific Palisades, CA 90272. States he has a long HX of tonsillitis. Pt seen in ofc complaining of chills, sore throat since January 26.Temp. 102.6° F. CPX shows tonsils that appear enlarged & red. Throat culture taken. llf Fran Practon, MD
2/5/XX	Pt improved. Tonsils appear less swollen. Throat culture neg. for strep. Continue penicillin Rx for 10 days p.o. t.i.d. Call if not improved. llf Fran Practon, MD
2/20/XX	Pt comes in again with severe sore throat. Began 3 days after penicillin was dc. Malaise. Temp 101.4° F. Tonsil culture taken and await results before prescribing antibiotic. Ret 3 days. llf Fran Practon, MD
2/23/XX	Pt presents with acute sore throat, red & inflamed. Temp 102.4° F. Adv tonsillectomy after acute phase subsides. Rx antibiotic, Suprax, 20 mg q. 12 h. llf Fran Practon, MD
2/23/XX	Letter mailed to Dr. Coleman.
3/2/XX	Pt RTO. Throat improved. Scheduled T & A at College Hospital for 3/15/XX. llf Fran Practon, MD
3/15/XX	Pt adm to outpatient surgery at College Hospital. T & A with disc. same day. llf
3/21/XX	PO; no complaints. Temp 98.4° F. To retn p.r.n. llf Fran Practon, MD

Comments:

Evaluator's Signature: ____________________ **Need to Repeat:** ________

National Curriculum Competency: CAAHEP: Cognitive: IV.C.8; Psychomotor: IV.P.10 ABHES: 7.a, b; 8.jj

JOB SKILL 11-10
Key a Two-Page Letter

Name ______________________________ Date ______________ Score ________

Performance Objective

Task: Key a two-page letter using an appropriate second-page heading.

Conditions: Letterhead for Practon Medical Group, Inc., formatted in a word processing program, or one sheet of letterhead (Form 37) and a dictionary. Refer to *textbook* Figure 11-3 and Figure 11-4 for format and Example 11-21 for a second-page heading. Refer to Procedure 11-1 in the *textbook* for step-by-step directions.

Standards: Complete all steps listed in this skill in _______ minutes with a minimum score of _______. (Time element and accuracy criteria may be given by instructor.)

Time: **Start:** ____________ **Completed:** ____________ **Total:** ____________ minutes

Scoring: One point for each step performed satisfactorily unless otherwise listed or weighted by instructor.

Directions with Performance Evaluation Checklist

Using the current date, format and key a two-page letter to the attention of the education chair of your local county medical society; use their address. The subject for the letter is "Work Experience for the Medical Office Student," and the text, written by Dr. Gerald Practon, is found in *Workbook* Figure 11-4. Set 1½-inch margins, use full block style with open punctuation, determine paragraphing, and make capitalization corrections as required.

1st Attempt	2nd Attempt	3rd Attempt	
______	______	______	Gather materials (equipment and supplies) listed under "Conditions."
______	______	______	1. Design letterhead or use Form 37 and one sheet of plain paper for the second page.
______	______	______	2. Date the letter using the current date.
______	______	______	3. Key the inside address.
______	______	______	4. Include the attention line.
______	______	______	5. Key an appropriate salutation.
______	______	______	6. Key the reference or subject line.
______	______	______	7. Use full block style.
______	______	______	8. Use open punctuation.
______	______	______	9. Center the letter using 1½-inch margins.
____/6	____/6	____/6	10. Insert proper paragraphing.
______	______	______	11. Make necessary capitalization corrections.
______	______	______	12. Choose the appropriate line to end page 1.
____/3	____/3	____/3	13. Insert a second-page heading.
____/5	____/5	____/5	14. Key all information accurately.
______	______	______	15. Key an appropriate concluding sentence.
____/2	____/2	____/2	16. Key an appropriate complimentary close and signature line.

JOB SKILL 11-10 *(continued)*

_______ _______ _______ 17. Insert proper reference initials.

_______ _______ _______ 18. Proofread while the document is on-screen or in the typewriter for spelling, punctuation, capitalization, and typing errors.

_______ _______ _______ 19. Correct, print, and proofread again.

_______ _______ _______ 20. Make corrections and prepare for the physician's signature.

_______ _______ _______ Complete within specified time.

____/34 ____/34 ____/34 **Total points earned** (To obtain a percentage score, divide the total points earned by the number of points possible.)

FIGURE 11-4

In reply to your request for information on work experience, I am enclosing a summary of the material I have found for your group, and I hope it answers some of your questions. Physicians, administrators, educational and medical associations, and officials of school districts have expressed increased interest in the value of on-the-job training and career-related work-study programs for their medical office students. Some colleges have instituted major curriculum changes to provide for internships and hospital work-study assignments. As a result of this interest, employers, including medical agencies, as well as federal agencies, are being asked to support the objectives of this new educational concept by providing new training opportunities for medical office students. Many agencies have inquired as to the role that they may play in making medical facilities available and in providing training to support these work-study medical programs. These inquiries have requested clarification in three general program areas: (1) programs established through legislation; (2) part-time, intermittent, or temporary employment; and (3) the selective exposure of students, in a nonpaid status, to learning projects related to educational objectives. Agencies are now providing and are encouraged to expand work-study opportunities for students and enrollees in programs authorized by legislation. Such legislation includes the Higher Education, Vocational Education Training, Economic Opportunity, and Social Security acts. Under these programs, students receive stipends form financial grants provided by statute. Similar support is urged for part-time, intermittent, and cyclic employment programs for students. Hospital programs such as cooperative work-study, summer and vacation employment, and part-time employment during the school year offer agencies an excellent opportunity to make significant contributions through medical-related assignments. These programs are also in keeping with federal long-range recruitment objectives. I hope this summarizes for your group the information you requested. If I can be of any further assistance in setting up the program in your area, please feel free to contact me.

Comments:

Evaluator's Signature: ______________________________ **Need to Repeat:** ______________

National Curriculum Competency: CAAHEP: Cognitive: IV.C.8; Psychomotor: IV.P.10	ABHES: 7.a, b; 8.jj

CHAPTER 12

Processing Mail and Telecommunications

OBJECTIVES

After completing the exercises, the student will be able to:

1. Enhance knowledge of medical terminology, interpret abbreviations, and accurately spell medical words.
2. Process incoming mail (Job Skill 12-1).
3. Annotate mail (Job Skill 12-2).
4. Classify outgoing mail (Job Skill 12-3).
5. Address envelopes for OCR scanning (Job Skill 12-4).
6. Complete a mail-order form for postal supplies (Job Skill 12-5).
7. Compose a letter and prepare an envelope for Certified Mail (Job Skill 12-6).
8. Prepare a cover sheet for fax transmission (Job Skill 12-7).
9. Key and fold an original letter; address a small envelope for Certified Mail, Return Receipt requested (Job Skill 12-8).
10. Key and fold an original letter; address a large envelope for Certified Mail, Return Receipt requested (Job Skill 12-9).

FOCUS ON CERTIFICATION*

CMA Content Summary

- Modalities for incoming and outgoing mail
- Prioritizing incoming and outgoing mail
- Keyboard fundamentals and functions (envelopes)
- Equipment operation (computer, fax machine)
- Computer applications (electronic mail)
- Screening and processing mail
- U.S. Postal Service classifications and types of mail services
- Postal machine/meter
- Processing incoming mail
- Preparing outgoing mail (labels, OCR)

RMA Content Summary

- Compose correspondence employing acceptable business format
- Employ effective written communication skills adhering to ethics and laws of confidentiality
- Identify and understand application of basic software

CMAS Content Summary

- Process incoming and outgoing mail
- Possess fundamental knowledge of word processing
- Employ e-mail applications

STOP AND THINK CASE SCENARIOS AND EXAM-STYLE REVIEW QUESTIONS

Refer to the end of Chapter 12 in the *textbook.*

Abbreviation and Spelling Review

Read the following patients' chart notes and write the meanings for the abbreviations listed following the notes. To decode any abbreviations you do not understand or that appear unfamiliar to you, refer to the list of abbreviations in Part IV of this *Workbook*. Step-by-step directions for this exercise are found in Procedure 1-1 of Chapter 1 in the *textbook*. Medical terms in the chart note are italicized; study them for spelling. Use your medical dictionary to look up their definitions. Your instructor may give a spelling and definition test that includes these words and abbreviations.

Stephen L. Boasberg

January 17, 20XX OC: Biopsy report pos. for CA of *prostate*. TURP & *bilateral orchiectomy, scrotal.* Adm to hosp in 2 days. Est. TD: 6 wks. Adv dc pain medication in 3 days.

Fran Practon, MD

Fran Practon, MD

*This *Workbook* and the accompanying *textbook* meet the entry-level administrative and general competencies for the CMA outlined by the AAMA Examination Content Outline and Occupational Analysis and for the RMA and CMAS outlined by the AMT Competencies, Construction Parameters, and Examination Specifications (see Competency Grid in Appendix B of the *textbook*).

OC	______	est.	______
pos.	______	TD	______
CA	______	wks	______
TURP	______	adv	______
adm	______	dc	______
hosp	______		

Terence O. Williams

January 17, 20XX Sunday, 4 a.m. pt seen in ER complaining of pain, R ear, abt 3 days, PX revealed fluid & pus. Temp. 100°F.

Fran Practon, MD

Fran Practon, MD

a.m.	______	abt	______
pt	______	PX	______
ER	______	temp.	______
R	______	F	______

Review Questions

Review the objectives, glossary, and chapter information before completing the following review questions.

1. According to the U.S. Postal Service, the *domestic mail* zone includes ______

   ______
2. OCR stands for ______
3. List three advantages of using a postage meter.
   a. ______
   b. ______
   c. ______
4. Name three ways in which postage stamps can be obtained.
   a. ______
   b. ______
   c. ______
5. List the items that should be available when opening mail.
   a. ______
   b. ______
   c. ______
   d. ______
   e. ______
   f. ______

6. Why should all incoming correspondence be dated? ______________________________

____

7. Generally, a letter marked ______________________ or ______________________ is not opened by the medical assistant.

8. Parcel post is also known as ______________________________ mail.

9. The most expedient way to send a letter that weighs under 13 ounces is ______________________,

and the most expedient way to send a letter that weighs over 13 ounces is ______________________.

10. The fastest and most reliable delivery service offered by the U.S. Postal Service, which guarantees a

delivery date and time (next day, second day), is called ______________________________

11. OCR envelope guidelines require keying the attention line ______________________________

____

12. Name four service endorsements that can be placed on envelopes to notify the U.S. Postal Service of action to take when a piece of mail is undeliverable as addressed.

a. ______________________________

b. ______________________________

c. ______________________________

d. ______________________________

13. A type of mail service that electronically sends, receives, stores, and forwards messages in digital form

over telecommunication lines is known as ______________________________

14. An e-mail business communication should follow the format of a ______________________________

15. Answer "True" or "False" to the following statements.

a. __________ Informal salutations may be used with e-mail.

b. __________ Informal complementary closings may be used with e-mail.

c. __________ Pronouns are recommended in the composition of all e-mails.

d. __________ It is all right to forward chain letters via office e-mail as long as it is done quickly.

e. __________ E-mail attachments should never be sent with office e-mail.

f. __________ Even though HIPAA does not directly address e-mail in its standards, both the privacy and security rules apply.

g. __________ A secure messaging service allows e-mail to be encrypted.

h. __________ It is recommended that you check your e-mail box at work every hour.

16. Describe three situations in which the physician might use facsimile (fax) transmission from the office.

a. ______________________________

b. ______________________________

c. ______________________________

17. What method of mailing should be used to send a patient chart to a lawyer for use in a malpractice

court hearing? ______________________________

18. List six legal requirements that apply when faxing confidential medical records.

a. ______________________________

b. ______________________________

c. ______________________________

d. ______________________________

e. ______________________________

f. ______________________________

Critical Thinking Exercises

1. Select the best statement regarding composing e-mail messages and comment on your answers.
   a. There is no need to worry about typographical or spelling errors.
   b. It is *important* to proofread for spelling and accuracy.
   c. It is permissible to use abbreviations because the recipient will understand what you mean.

____

____

____

2. Select the best statement regarding answering e-mail messages and comment on your answers.
   a. Respond as soon as possible, but after you finish the task you are doing.
   b. Answer immediately.
   c. Print the message, put it in your inbox with other fax and telephone requests, and answer when convenient.
   d. Always acknowledge that the message has been received.

____

____

____

3. Respond to the following statements regarding the insertion of your telephone number on e-mail messages.
   a. It is not necessary because you reply directly to the sender of the message.
   b. Always include it.
   c. It depends on the preference of the employer or individual sending the message.

____

____

____

4. Select the best statement regarding printing e-mail messages and comment on your answers.
   a. If the message is important or if a hardcopy record is needed, then print the message.
   b. Always print the message.
   c. Never print the message.

____

____

____

5. Read the following scenario, then search each Internet site for the shipping companies listed and compare what it would cost to send a package by (1) United States Postal Service, (2) United Parcel Service, and (3) Federal Express. Refer to the *Resources* section at the end of *textbook* Chapter 12 for Web site addresses.

   Scenario: You are working for Practon Medical Group, Inc., and have been asked to mail a package that is 18 inches long by 4 inches high by 10 inches wide; it weighs 2 pounds, and needs to arrive by tomorrow (anytime). You are mailing it from Clifton Park, New York 12065, to Ventura, California 93003.

   List the cost of each company and determine which is the most reasonable:

   a. USPS:

   ____

   ____

   b. UPS:

   ____

   ____

   c. FedEx:

   ____

   ____

JOB SKILL 12-1
Process Incoming Mail

Name ______________________________ Date ______________ Score ________

Performance Objective

Task: Sort and process incoming mail; determine the disbursement and action for each communication.

Conditions: List of incoming mail, *Workbook* Figure 12-1, pen or pencil.

Standards: Complete all steps listed in this skill in _______ minutes with a minimum score of ________. (Time element and accuracy criteria may be given by instructor.)

Time: **Start**: ____________ **Completed**: ____________ **Total**: ____________ minutes

Scoring: One point for each step performed satisfactorily unless otherwise listed or weighted by instructor.

Directions with Performance Evaluation Checklist

You will be opening today's mail and determining what action needs to take place for each piece. Some of the mail will be placed on the physician's desk; please designate its importance by indicating "top," "middle," or "bottom" of the mail stack. You may need to read and annotate some mail, route mail to other office workers, pull a patient's chart and possiably place the chart on the physician's desk (if the office does not use EMRs), record items on a calendar (physician or medical assistant), or set up a file folder. All money received needs to be posted or recorded on the patient's ledger or account, the daysheet or journal, and the bank deposit (you can simply check "record payment") and then put in a safe place (locked drawer or safe). You will need to verify the address on all checks received against the office records to make sure each address is current. You have the ability to write checks if an invoice needs to be paid and you may simply file or discard an item.

Study the following list of mail items and use critical thinking skills to determine what action needs to be taken. Refer to the headings in *Workbook* Figure 12-1 and indicate with a checkmark (✓) how each piece of mail is to be handled (check all that apply).

1st Attempt	2nd Attempt	3rd Attempt	
_______	_______	_______	Gather materials (equipment and supplies) listed under "Conditions."
_______	_______	_______	1. Letter and check from a patient.
_______	_______	_______	2. Announcement of a medical society meeting.
_______	_______	_______	3. Advertisement for an x-ray machine.
_______	_______	_______	4. Mail-order gardening catalog.
_______	_______	_______	5. Letter from patient, Mr. C. J. Conway.
_______	_______	_______	6. Check from patient Mr. Bill Owen.
_______	_______	_______	7. Advertisement about a new tranquilizer drug.
_______	_______	_______	8. *Journal of the American Medical Association* (current issue).
_______	_______	_______	9. A request for a reprint of an article written by Dr. Practon.
_______	_______	_______	10. Letter marked "Personal" to Dr. Fran Practon.
_______	_______	_______	11. A drug sample.
_______	_______	_______	12. Letter referring a patient to Dr. Gerald Practon.
_______	_______	_______	13. A piece of pornographic literature.

JOB SKILL 12-1 *(continued)*

______	______	______	14. Letter announcing an evening professional meeting in 2 months.
______	______	______	15. License tax-due notice.
______	______	______	16. Charity solicitation letter.
______	______	______	17. Insurance query about patient Mrs. Dorothy Ranger.
______	______	______	18. Medicare payment for patient Beth Cook.
______	______	______	19. Lab test results on patient Mary Murdock.
______	______	______	20. Consultant report on patient Bill McKean.
______	______	______	21. Check from Aetna Insurance Company for service rendered to Samantha Boatman.
______	______	______	22. Prudential insurance form on patient Tom Patten.
______	______	______	23. Invoice from V. Mueller Supply Company.
______	______	______	24. Letter from patient Clarice Stark without date or return address (these do appear on the envelope).
______	______	______	25. Letter from Dr. Lees concerning a research project.
______	______	______	26. Letter about cancellation of appointment by a patient who is on vacation.
______	______	______	27. *Time* magazine.
______	______	______	28. Mutual funds investment letter.
______	______	______	29. Local medical society agenda for monthly meeting.
______	______	______	30. Ad for new filing equipment.
______	______	______	31. Mail-order medical instrument catalog.
______	______	______	32. Gift parcel from Mrs. Gaspar Whelan (patient).
______	______	______	33. Letter notifying Dr. Fran Practon of the death of a colleague.
______	______	______	34. Telegram from Dr. Perry Cardi congratulating Dr. Gerald Practon on his election as vice president of the local medical society.
______	______	______	35. Personal letter, opened by mistake.
______	______	______	Complete within specified time.
____/37	____/37	____/37	**Total points earned** (To obtain a percentage score, divide the total points earned by the number of points possible.)

Comments:

Evaluator's Signature: ______________________________ **Need to Repeat:** ____________

National Curriculum Competency: ABHES: 8.a, hh, ii, jj

FIGURE 12-1

No.	Importance of Mail Piece			Read Mail	Annotate	Route Mail to:	Pull Patient Chart	Place Chart on MD Desk	Record on Calendar (MD/MA) or Appt Book	Setup File	Record Payment	Place Money in Secure Place	Verify Address on Check	Write Check	F=File D=Discard
	Top	Middle	Bottom												
1															
2															
3															
4															
5															
6															
7															
8															
9															
10															
11															
12															
13															
14															
15															
16															
17															
18															
19															

(*Continues*)

FIGURE 12-1 (*Continued*)

No.	Importance of Mail Piece			Read Mail	Annotate	Route Mail to:	Pull Patient Chart	Place Chart on MD Desk	Record on Calendar (MD/MA) or Appt Book	Setup File	Record Payment	Place Money in Secure Place	Verify Address on Check	Write Check	F=File D=Discard
	Top	Middle	Bottom												
20															
21															
22															
23															
24															
25															
26															
27															
28															
29															
30															
31															
32															
33															
34															
35															

JOB SKILL 12-2
Annotate Mail

Name ______________________________ Date ______________ Score ________

Performance Objective

Task: Read a letter, annotate significant words or phrases, and make comments in the margin concerning the action to be taken.

Conditions: Use the letter in *Workbook* Figure 12-2 for reference and a highlighter or colored pen. Refer to *textbook* Procedure 12-3 for step-by-step directions.

Standards: Complete all steps listed in this skill in _______ minutes with a minimum score of _________. (Time element and accuracy criteria may be given by instructor.)

Time: **Start**: _____________ **Completed**: _____________ **Total**: _____________ minutes

Scoring: One point for each step performed satisfactorily unless otherwise listed or weighted by instructor.

Directions with Performance Evaluation Checklist

Read the letter from Mr. Glen Marchall (*Workbook* Figure 12-2) that arrived today. Note significant words or phrases by highlighting them or by underlining with colored pen. Annotate any action requirements in the right margin using colored pen.

1st Attempt	2nd Attempt	3rd Attempt	
_______	_______	_______	Gather materials (equipment and supplies) listed under "Conditions."
____/10	____/10	____/10	1. Underline important words or phrases.
_____/5	_____/5	_____/5	2. Annotate action areas of letter.
_______	_______	_______	Complete within specified time.
____/17	____/17	____/17	**Total points earned** (To obtain a percentage score, divide the total points earned by the number of points possible.)

Comments:

Evaluator's Signature: ______________________________ **Need to Repeat:** ____________

National Curriculum Competency: ABHES: 8.a, hh, ii, jj

JOB SKILL 12-2 *(continued)*

FIGURE 12-2

MARCHALL RENTS
23990 WEST VALLEY ROAD
SEPULVEDA, XY 93087

December 2, 20XX

Gerald Practon, MD
4567 Broad Avenue
Woodland Hills, XY 12345

Dear Dr. Practon:

We have recently opened a medical equipment rental-sales company in your area and are anxious for members of the medical profession to know of our specialized home-care equipment.

Our staff is highly trained to help you determine and meet the precise requirements for each patient's comfort and safety. We handle only the best equipment—from oxygen equipment to wheelchairs, hospital beds, and patient lifts—and we are on 24-hour call.

Our salesman will be in your area around January 13, so we are contacting you to see if we can set up an appointment for him to show and demonstrate pieces of equipment.

We will follow this communication with a personal telephone call to determine a date that is satisfactory. We hope that we can meet with you soon and work as a team to help satisfy your patients' needs.

Sincerely,

Glen Marchall

Mr. Glen Marchall
President

GM:jf

JOB SKILL 12-3
Classify Outgoing Mail

Name ______________________________ Date ______________ Score ________

Performance Objective

Task: Identify classes of mail.

Conditions: Use list of outgoing mail and pen or pencil. Refer to *Mail Classifications* in the *Handling Outgoing Mail* section and Procedure 12-4 in the *textbook* for help.

Standards: Complete all steps listed in this skill in ________ minutes with a minimum score of ________. (Time element and accuracy criteria may be given by instructor.)

Time: **Start**: ____________ **Completed**: ____________ **Total**: ____________ minutes

Scoring: One point for each step performed satisfactorily unless otherwise listed or weighted by instructor.

Directions with Performance Evaluation Checklist

You will be mailing various pieces and types of mail for the physicians, and it will be helpful if you can determine classifications before going to the post office. After each piece of mail, indicate the appropriate classification or special services used.

1st Attempt	2nd Attempt	3rd Attempt	
______	______	______	Gather materials (equipment and supplies) listed under "Conditions."
______	______	______	1. Income tax forms mailed on deadline date ____________
______	______	______	2. Proof that estimated income tax form was mailed by deadline ____________
______	______	______	3. Prescription ____________
______	______	______	4. Postal card ____________
______	______	______	5. Photograph ____________
______	______	______	6. Medical pamphlet ____________
______	______	______	7. Newspaper ____________
______	______	______	8. Bound 28-page manuscript ____________
______	______	______	9. Unsealed circular weighing 12 ounces ____________
______	______	______	10. Green diamond border envelope to enclose an item weighing more than 2 pounds ____________
______	______	______	11. U.S. treasury bond ____________
______	______	______	12. X-rays with letter ____________
______	______	______	13. Cultured pearl necklace ____________
______	______	______	14. Sealed dental catalog ____________
______	______	______	15. Monthly statement ____________
______	______	______	16. Letter with check enclosed ____________
______	______	______	17. Laboratory report ____________
______	______	______	18. Package weighing 36 pounds ____________

JOB SKILL 12-3 *(continued)*

______ ______ ______ 19. Fastest delivery for a medical tape ____________

______ ______ ______ 20. Important item to be delivered within 24 hours; it is Saturday noon ____________

______ ______ ______ 21. A final collection letter from medical office ____________

______ ______ ______ 22. Thirty-page book with advertising ____________

______ ______ ______ 23. Medical society journal ____________

______ ______ ______ Complete within specified time.

___/25 ___/25 ___/25 **Total points earned** (To obtain a percentage score, divide the total points earned by the number of points possible.)

Comments:

Evaluator's Signature: ____________________ **Need to Repeat:** __________

National Curriculum Competency: ABHES: 8.a, hh, ii, jj

JOB SKILL 12-4
Address Envelopes for OCR Scanning

Name ______________________________ Date ____________ Score ______

Performance Objective

Task: Address small envelopes for OCR scanning using acceptable abbreviations and correct ZIP codes.

Conditions: Three number 6 envelopes or Forms 38 and 39. Use the format recommended for OCR processing found in *textbook* Table 12-2 and Figure 12-6. See *textbook* Table 12-3 for address abbreviations, and refer to *Workbook* Figure 12-3 for those that cannot be abbreviated to 13 positions. Refer to *textbook* Table 12-4 for two-letter state abbreviations and *Workbook* Figure 12-3 for ZIP codes from the National ZIP Code directory.

Standards: Complete all steps listed in this skill in ______ minutes with a minimum score of ______. (Time element and accuracy criteria may be given by instructor.)

Time: **Start**: __________ **Completed**: __________ **Total**: __________ minutes

Scoring: One point for each step performed satisfactorily unless otherwise listed or weighted by instructor.

Directions with Performance Evaluation Checklist

Dr. Fran Practon has three letters that need to be mailed immediately. Key the three addresses listed below on number 6 envelopes using standard abbreviations and ZIP codes. If using real envelopes, key Dr. Practon's office address (see *Workbook* Part III) in the upper left corner of each envelope.

1. Mr. and Mrs. Arthur L. Duncally
   Post Office Box 286
   West Boothbay Harbor, Maine
2. Coastal Community Hospital
   8900 West Elvingston Drive
   Brooklyn-Curtis Bay, Maryland
   Attn: Elizabeth Collingswood, MD
3. Mr. Randolph G. Greenworthy Jr.
   49021 67th Avenue North
   Apartment 8
   Washington Grove, Maryland

1st Attempt	2nd Attempt	3rd Attempt	
_____	_____	_____	Gather materials (equipment and supplies) listed under "Conditions."
____/9	____/9	____/9	1. Key return address if not using Forms 37 and 38.
____/9	____/9	____/9	2. Key addresses for three envelopes.
____/9	____/9	____/9	3. Use OCR format.
____/9	____/9	____/9	4. Look up and use abbreviations.
____/3	____/3	____/3	5. Look up and key correct ZIP codes.
_____	_____	_____	6. Place attention line in correct position.
_____	_____	_____	7. Proofread for typographical, spelling, and spacing errors.
_____	_____	_____	Complete within specified time.
___/43	___/43	___/43	**Total points earned** (To obtain a percentage score, divide the total points earned by the number of points possible.)

JOB SKILL 12-4 *(continued)*

FIGURE 12-3

MAINE

04006-0000	Biddeford Pool	BIDDEFRD POOL
04625-0000	Cranberry Isles	CRANBERRY IS
04021-0000	Cumberland Center	CUMBRLND CTR
04426-0000	Dover-Foxcroft	DOVR FOXCROFT
04940-0000	Farmington Falls	FARMINGTN FLS
04575-0000	West Boothbay Harbor	W BOOTHBY HBR

MARYLAND

21005-0000	Aberdeen Proving Ground	ABRDN PRV GRD
20331-0000	Andrews Air Force Hospital	ANDRS AF HOSP
21225-0000	Brooklyn-Curtis Bay	BKLYN CTS BAY
20622-0000	Charlotte Hall	CHARLOTE HALL
20732-0000	Chesapeake Beach	CHESAPKE BCH
20904-0000	Ednor Cloverly	EDNR CLOVERLY
21713-0000	Fahrney Keedy Memorial Home	FHRN MEM HOME
20755-0000	Fort George G. Meade	FT MEADE
21240-0000	Friendship Airport	FRNDSHP ARPRT
21078-0000	Havre de Grace	HVRE DE GRACE
20014-0000	National Naval Medical Center	NAVAL MED CTR
20390-0000	Naval Air Facility	NAV AIR FACIL
20678-0000	Prince Frederick	PRNC FREDERCK
20788-0000	Prince Georges Plaza	PRNC GEO PLZ
21152-0000	Sparks Glencoe	SPRKS GLENCOE
21784-0000	Springfield State Hospital	SPRINFLD HOSP
20390-0000	U.S. Naval Communications Center	NAV COMMS CTR
20880-0000	Washington Grove	WASHINGTN GRV

Comments:

Evaluator's Signature: ______________________ **Need to Repeat:** __________

National Curriculum Competency: ABHES: 8.a, hh, ii, jj

JOB SKILL 12-5
Complete a Mail-Order Form for Postal Supplies

Name ______________________________ Date ____________ Score ________

Performance Objective

Task: Complete a mail-order form for postal supplies and compute the total amount owed.

Conditions: Use Form 40 and pen.

Standards: Complete all steps listed in this skill in ________ minutes with a minimum score of ________. (Time element and accuracy criteria may be given by instructor.)

Time: **Start**: ____________ **Completed**: ____________ **Total**: ____________ minutes

Scoring: One point for each step performed satisfactorily unless otherwise listed or weighted by instructor.

Directions with Performance Evaluation Checklist

Complete in ink the mail-order form for stamps. For each item ordered, list the quantity and multiply it by the price to obtain the cost, and then add all figures in the "cost" column to determine the total cost of the order. A check would ordinarily be made out to the U.S. Postmaster and enclosed with the order; however, since check writing is discussed in a future chapter, a check will not be written for this exercise.

1st Attempt	2nd Attempt	3rd Attempt	
______	______	______	Gather materials (equipment and supplies) listed under "Conditions."
____/5	____/5	____/5	1. Print the medical practice's telephone number, name, and complete address.
____/3	____/3	____/3	2. Order five roles of 45-cent stamps; 100 in each roll.
____/3	____/3	____/3	3. Order one sets of 1-cent stamps (20 stamps per set).
____/2	____/2	____/2	4. Order one book of "Forever Stamps," which can be used for first-class mail regardless of future postal rate increases.
____/3	____/3	____/3	5. Order forty 2-cent stamps for extra postage.
____/3	____/3	____/3	6. Order two hundred 20-cent additional ounce stamps for first-class postage (20 stamps per set).
______	______	______	7. Compute the total cost and insert.
______	______	______	Complete within specified time.
____/22	____/22	____/22	**Total points earned** (To obtain a percentage score, divide the total points earned by the number of points possible.)

Comments:

Evaluator's Signature: ______________________________ **Need to Repeat:** ____________

National Curriculum Competency: ABHES: 8.a, hh, ii, jj

JOB SKILL 12-6
Compose a Letter and Prepare an Envelope for Certified Mail

Name ______________________ Date ____________ Score ______

Performance Objective

Task: Compose and key a letter in a specified format; address and prepare a large envelope for OCR processing as Certified Mail.

Conditions: One letterhead (create on a word-processing program or use Form 41), one number 10 envelope or Form 42 (see *textbook* Figure 12-6), a Certified Mail form or Form 43 (see *textbook* Figure 12-4 and Figure 12-5), and pen. Refer to *textbook* Procedures 12-5 and 12-6 for step-by-step directions.

Standards: Complete all steps listed in this skill in _______ minutes with a minimum score of ________. (Time element and accuracy criteria may be given by instructor.)

Time: **Start**: ____________ **Completed**: ____________ **Total**: ____________ minutes

Scoring: One point for each step performed satisfactorily unless otherwise listed or weighted by instructor.

Directions with Performance Evaluation Checklist

Mrs. Jane K. Call of 199 Eisenhower Boulevard, Apartment 17-J, Canoga Park, XY 12345-0001, telephoned yesterday stating that she wanted no further treatment from Dr. Gerald Practon. Write a letter to confirm this discharge by the patient stating that Dr. Practon feels further treatment is necessary and recommends that she contact the Valley Medical Society at (555) 659-2234 to obtain the name of another physician. See *textbook* Figure 3-13 in Chapter 3 for help with letter composition. Read through and follow the format specifications listed below for the letter, envelope, and certification form.

1st Attempt	2nd Attempt	3rd Attempt	
_______	_______	_______	Gather materials (equipment and supplies) listed under "Conditions."

LETTER

_______	_______	_______	1. Use Practon letterhead.
_______	_______	_______	2. Use modified block style.
_______	_______	_______	3. Use mixed punctuation.
_______	_______	_______	4. Use current date.
_______	_______	_______	5. Center letter with even margins.
_______	_______	_______	6. Key inside address.
_______	_______	_______	7. Key appropriate salutation.
_______	_______	_______	8. Mention patient name and purpose of letter at beginning.
_______	_______	_______	9. Compose appropriate letter with wording that is legally correct.
_______	_______	_______	10. Insert proper paragraphing.
_______	_______	_______	11. Key complementary closing line in correct position.
_______	_______	_______	12. Key signature line.
_______	_______	_______	13. Key reference initials.

JOB SKILL 12-6 *(continued)*

______	______	______	14. Proofread letter while the document is on screen or in typewriter for typographical, spelling, punctuation, and capitalization errors.
______	______	______	15. Correct errors.
______	______	______	16. Print letter and proofread again.
______	______	______	17. Present letter ready for physician to read and sign.

ENVELOPE

____/8	____/8	____/8	18. Key large envelope in OCR format with no errors.
______	______	______	19. Determine the correct postage via the Internet or by calling your local post office and write the amount where the stamp would be placed on the envelope.

CERTIFICATION FORM

____/5	____/5	____/5	20. Complete data on front of certification form.
____/5	____/5	____/5	21. Complete data on back of certification form.
____/5	____/5	____/5	22. Complete Domestic Return Receipt for Certified Mail.
______	______	______	23. Fold letter correctly and insert in envelope; do not seal.
______	______	______	Complete within specified time.
___/44	___/44	___/44	**Total points earned** (To obtain a percentage score, divide the total points earned by the number of points possible.)

Comments:

Evaluator's Signature: ______________________ **Need to Repeat:** ____________

National Curriculum Competency: CAAHEP: Cognitive: IV.C.8; Psychomotor: IV.P.10 ABHES: 8.a, hh, ii, jj

JOB SKILL 12-7
Prepare a Cover Sheet for Fax Transmission

Name ______________________________ Date ______________ Score ________

Performance Objective

Task: Prepare a transmission slip to accompany a message for fax communication.

Conditions: Fax transmittal (Form 44) and computer or typewriter. Refer to *textbook* Procedure 12-9 for step-by-step directions and Figure 12-12 for a visual example of a cover sheet.

Standards: Complete all steps listed in this skill in _______ minutes with a minimum score of ________. (Time element and accuracy criteria may be given by instructor.)

Time: **Start**: ____________ **Completed**: ____________ **Total**: ____________ minutes

Scoring: One point for each step performed satisfactorily unless otherwise listed or weighted by instructor.

Directions with Performance Evaluation Checklist

Dr. Fran Practon is scheduled to speak at the Massachusetts American Women's Medical Association convention on November 20 in Boston. She asks you to prepare a fax cover sheet to accompany a two-page letter she will write for fax transmission. The fax will be directed to Dr. Elmo Reardon, 891 So. Revere Way, Boston, MA 02100; fax number: (555) 326-9923; phone number: (555) 326-9921. Abstract the necessary information and complete the fax cover sheet dated November 13, current year.

1st Attempt	2nd Attempt	3rd Attempt	
_______	_______	_______	Gather materials (equipment and supplies) listed under "Conditions."
_____/8	_____/8	_____/8	1. Complete the top portion of the fax cover sheet.
_______	_______	_______	2. Indicate number of pages sent.
_____/3	_____/3	_____/3	3. Write in the "Remarks" section of the fax sheet requesting prompt confirmation of fax receipt by fax or telephone.
_______	_______	_______	4. List student name as contact.
_______	_______	_______	Complete within specified time.
____/15	____/15	____/15	**Total points earned** (To obtain a percentage score, divide the total points earned by the number of points possible.)

Comments:

Evaluator's Signature: ______________________________ **Need to Repeat:** ______________

National Curriculum Competency: ABHES: 8.a, hh, ii, jj

JOB SKILL 12-8
Key and Fold an Original Letter; Address a Small Envelope for Certified Mail, Return Receipt Requested

Name ______________________________ Date ____________ Score ________

Performance Objective

Task: Key a letter using specified format, prepare an envelope for OCR processing, fold and insert the letter into the envelope, and attach special mailing forms.

Conditions: One letterhead (create on a word-processing program or use Form 45), one number 6 envelope or Form 46 (see *textbook* Figure 12-6), a Certified Mail form or Form 47 (see *textbook* Figure 12-4 and Figure 12-5), and pen. Refer to *textbook* Procedures 12-5 and 12-6 for step-by-step directions.

Standards: Complete all steps listed in this skill in _______ minutes with a minimum score of ________. (Time element and accuracy criteria may be given by instructor.)

Time: **Start:** ____________ **Completed:** ____________ **Total:** ____________ minutes

Scoring: One point for each step performed satisfactorily unless otherwise listed or weighted by instructor.

Directions with Performance Evaluation Checklist

Mr. Henry J. Stone, One April Circle, Pacoima, XY 91331-0000, has had surgery and is negligent about following Dr. Gerald Practon's advice; he is at risk of having further injury. Compose an appropriate letter to Mr. Stone advising him of Dr. Practon's withdrawal from the case as of 30 days from the date of this letter. Refer to *textbook* Figure 3-11 in Chapter 3 for help with letter composition. Read and follow the format specifications listed below for the letter, envelope, and certification form.

1st Attempt	2nd Attempt	3rd Attempt	
______	______	______	Gather materials (equipment and supplies) listed under "Conditions."
LETTER			
______	______	______	1. Use Practon letterhead.
______	______	______	2. Use full block style.
______	______	______	3. Use mixed punctuation.
______	______	______	4. Use current date.
______	______	______	5. Center letter with even margins.
______	______	______	6. Key inside address.
______	______	______	7. Key appropriate salutation.
______	______	______	8. Compose letter of withdrawal with wording that is legally correct.
______	______	______	9. Insert proper paragraphing.
______	______	______	10. Key complementary closing line in correct position.
______	______	______	11. Key signature line.
______	______	______	12. Key reference initials.
______	______	______	13. Proofread letter while the document is on screen or in typewriter for typographical, spelling, punctuation, and capitalization errors.

JOB SKILL 12-8 *(continued)*

______	______	______	14. Correct errors.
______	______	______	15. Print letter and proofread again.
______	______	______	16. Present letter ready for physician to read and sign.

ENVELOPE

____/8	____/8	____/8	17. Key small envelope in OCR format with no errors.
______	______	______	18. Determine the correct postage via the Internet or by calling your local post office and write the amount where the stamp would be placed on the envelope.

CERTIFICATION FORM

____/5	____/5	____/5	19. Complete data on front of certification form.
____/5	____/5	____/5	20. Complete data on back of form.
____/5	____/5	____/5	21. Complete Domestic Return Receipt for Certified Mail.
______	______	______	22. Fold letter correctly and insert in envelope; do not seal.
______	______	______	Complete within specified time.
____/43	____/43	____/43	**Total points earned** (To obtain a percentage score, divide the total points earned by the number of points possible.)

Comments:

Evaluator's Signature: ______________________________ **Need to Repeat:** ____________

National Curriculum Competency: CAAHEP: Cognitive: IV.C.8; Psychomotor: IV.P.10	ABHES: 8.a, hh, ii, jj

JOB SKILL 12-9

Key and Fold an Original Letter; Address a Large Envelope for Certified Mail, Return Receipt Requested

Name ______________________________ Date ______________ Score ________

Performance Objective

Task: Key a letter, prepare a large envelope for OCR processing, fold and insert the letter into the envelope, and attach special mailing forms.

Conditions: One letterhead (create on a word-processing program or use Form 48), one number 10 envelope or Form 49 (see *textbook* Figure 12-6), a Certified Mail form or Form 50 (see *textbook* Figure 12-4 and Figure 12-5), and pen. Refer to *textbook* Procedures 12-5 and 12-6 for step-by-step directions.

Standards: Complete all steps listed in this skill in _______ minutes with a minimum score of ________. (Time element and accuracy criteria may be given by instructor.)

Time: **Start**: ____________ **Completed:** ____________ **Total***:* ____________ minutes

Scoring: One point for each step performed satisfactorily unless otherwise listed or weighted by instructor.

Directions with Performance Evaluation Checklist

Miss Henrietta M. Marskovskie of 4311 Eberly Street, Woodland Hills, XY 12345-4700, was referred to Practon Medical Group by Dr. Ambrose Kistler, 698 Madison Way, Gretna, NE 54321-0009, when she relocated to Woodland Hills. Dr. Gerald Practon went to medical school at the University of Omaha, Nebraska, with Dr. Kistler. Dr. Kistler and his wife, Julie, share the Practon's love for the game of golf; they have played many rounds together. Dr. Practon would like you to write a letter acknowledging this kind referral, and he will edit it prior to its finalization. He saw the patient yesterday and will be taking over her care. She is being treated for renal disease, which is now under control; the patient is doing well and looks very healthy. She is thrilled to be in her new home and close to her grandchildren. Write a friendly referral thank-you letter under Dr. Gerald Practon's signature.

1st Attempt	2nd Attempt	3rd Attempt	
_______	_______	_______	Gather materials (equipment and supplies) listed under "Conditions."

LETTER

_______	_______	_______	1. Use Practon letterhead.
_______	_______	_______	2. Use modified block style.
_______	_______	_______	3. Use mixed punctuation.
_______	_______	_______	4. Use current date.
_______	_______	_______	5. Center letter with even margins.
_______	_______	_______	6. Key inside address.
_______	_______	_______	7. Key appropriate salutation.
_______	_______	_______	8. Compose a friendly letter thanking Dr. Kistler for the referral.
_______	_______	_______	9. Insert proper paragraphing.
_______	_______	_______	10. Key complementary closing line in correct position.
_______	_______	_______	11. Key signature line.
_______	_______	_______	12. Key reference initials.

JOB SKILL 12-9 *(continued)*

_______	_______	_______	13. Proofread letter while the document is on screen or in typewriter for typographical, spelling, punctuation, and capitalization errors.
_______	_______	_______	14. Correct errors.
_______	_______	_______	15. Print letter and proofread again.
_______	_______	_______	16. Present letter ready for physician to read and edit.
_______	_______	_______	17. Incorporate any changes into the letter, print, and present for signature.

ENVELOPE

_____/8	_____/8	_____/8	18. Key large envelope in OCR format with no errors.
_______	_______	_______	19. Determine the correct postage via the Internet or by calling your local post office and write the amount where the stamp would be placed on the envelope.

CERTIFICATION FORM

_____/5	_____/5	_____/5	20. Complete data on front of certification form.
_____/5	_____/5	_____/5	21. Complete data on back of certification form.
_____/5	_____/5	_____/5	22. Complete Domestic Return Receipt for Certified Mail.
_______	_______	_______	23. Fold letter correctly and insert in envelope; do not seal.
_______	_______	_______	Complete within specified time.
____/44	____/44	____/44	**Total points earned** (To obtain a percentage score, divide the total points earned by the number of points possible.)

Comments:

Evaluator's Signature: ______________________________ **Need to Repeat:** ______________

National Curriculum Competency: CAAHEP: Cognitive: IV.C.8; Psychomotor: IV.P.10	ABHES: 8.a, hh, ii, jj

CHAPTER 13

Fees, Credit, and Collection

OBJECTIVES

After completing the exercises, the student will be able to:

1. Enhance knowledge of medical terminology, interpret abbreviations, and accurately spell medical words.
2. Role-play collection scenarios (Job Skill 13-1).
3. Use a calculator (Job Skill 13-2).
4. Complete and post on a ledger card: charges, payments, a returned check, and a check from a collection agency (Job Skill 13-3).
5. Complete cash receipts (Job Skill 13-4).
6. Compose a collection letter, prepare an envelope and ledger, and post transactions (Job Skill 13-5).
7. Complete a financial agreement (Job Skill 13-6).

FOCUS ON CERTIFICATION*

CMA Content Summary

- Charges, payments, and adjustments
- Reconciling payments
- Fee schedules (methods for establishing)
- Contracted fees
- Accounts receivable
- Billing procedures (itemization/billing cycles)
- Aging/collection procedures
- Collection agencies
- Consumer protection acts
- Processing accounts receivable

*This *Workbook* and the accompanying *textbook* meet the entry-level administrative and general competencies for the CMA outlined by the AAMA Examination Content Outline and Occupational Analysis and for the RMA and CMAS outlined by the AMT Competencies, Construction Parameters, and Examination Specifications (see Competency Grid in Appendix B of the *textbook*).

RMA Content Summary

- Process insurance payments and contractual write-off amounts
- Generate aging reports
- Maintain and explain fee schedules
- Collect and post payments
- Manage patient ledgers and accounts
- Understand and prepare Truth in Lending Statements
- Prepare and mail itemized statements
- Understand and employ available billing methods
- Understand and employ billing cycles
- Collections
- Prepare aging reports and identify delinquent accounts
- Perform skip tracing
- Understand application of the Fair Debt Collection Practices Act
- Identify and understand bankruptcy and small claims procedures
- Understand and perform appropriate collection procedures
- Financial mathematics
- Understand and perform appropriate calculations related to patient and practice accounts

CMAS Content Summary

- Perform financial computations
- Manage accounts receivable
- Understand professional fee structures
- Understand physician/practice owner compensation provisions
- Understand credit arrangements
- Manage patient accounts/ledgers
- Manage patient billing (methods, cycle billing procedures)
- Manage collections in compliance with state and federal regulations

STOP AND THINK CASE SCENARIOS AND EXAM-STYLE REVIEW QUESTIONS

Refer to the end of Chapter 13 in the *textbook*.

Abbreviation and Spelling Review

Read the following patient's chart note and write the meanings for the abbreviations listed following the note. To decode any abbreviations you do not understand or that appear unfamiliar to you, refer to the list of abbreviations in Part IV of this *Workbook*. Step-by-step directions for this exercise are found in Procedure 1-1 of Chapter 1 in the *textbook*. Medical terms in the chart note are italicized; study them for spelling. Use your medical dictionary to look up their definitions. Your instructor may give a spelling and definition test that includes these words and abbreviations.

> Robert M Feldman-Pt seen for *bronchial asthma*, ASHD, HBP & *sebaceous cyst*. ECG ordered stat. Lab & x-rays ordered. Comp PX to be done on Friday. PTR next wk for I & D of sebaceous cyst of ® *axilla*.
>
> Fran Practon, MD
>
> Fran Practon, MD

pt	______	comp	______
ASHD	______	PX	______
HBP	______	PTR	______
ECG	______	wk	______
stat.	______	I & D	______
lab	______	®	______

Review Questions

Review the objectives, glossary, and chapter information before completing the following review questions.

1. Match the terms in the right column with the definitions in the left column by writing the letters in the blanks.

______	analysis of accounts receivable showing 30, 60, 90, and 120 days' delinquency	a. garnishment
______	a legal proceeding in which money (salary) and property are attached so they can be used to pay a debt	b. credit
______	a list of the physician's procedures, services, and fees	c. open accounts
______	a message to remind a patient about delinquent payment	d. dun
______	record of business transactions on the books that represents an unsecured	e. skip
______	accounts receivable where credit has been extended without a formal written contract	f. aging account
______	to trust in an individual's integrity to meet financial obligations	g. fee schedule
______	a debtor who moves and does not leave a forwarding address	

2. Name three reasons why a patient registration (information) form is valuable for the collection process.

   a. ______

   b. ______

   c. ______

3. How often should a patient information form be updated? ______

4. The job of discussing and collecting fees is usually relegated to the ______

5. Name four factors involved in establishing fees for a physician.

   a. ______

   b. ______

   c. ______

   d. ______

6. For states that allow multiple fee schedules, a medical practice may have separate fee schedules for what type of programs or plans?

   a. ______

   b. ______

   c. ______

   d. ______

7. To increase the percentage of patients who pay their bills and for good public relations, how should a medical assistant approach a patient?

   a. ______

   b. ______

   c. ______

   d. ______

   e. ______

8. When is a managed care copayment usually collected? ______

9. Name several things to look for in a deadbeat patient.

   a. ______

   b. ______

   c. ______

   d. ______

   e. ______

   f. ______

   g. ______

   h. ______

10. When is the best time to collect for an office visit and why? ______

    ______

    ______

11. What are some names used for the form that serves as a combination bill, insurance form, and routing document?

    a. ______

    b. ______

    c. ______

    d. ______

    e. ______

    f. ______

    g. ______

    h. ______

    i. ______

12. Explain cycle billing. ______

    ______

    ______

13. Name four advantages of using a billing service.

    a. ______

    b. ______

    c. ______

    d. ______

14. If a patient is called about a delinquent bill at 10 p.m., what federal law is being violated? ___________

____

15. If credit is refused to a patient, what federal legislation must be complied with? ___________

____

16. If, in an obstetrical case, a patient is asked for monthly payments before delivery of the baby, what form must be completed, signed, and given to the patient? ___________

    If there are fewer than ___________ payment installments, this form is not necessary.

17. If interest is charged on a monthly billing statement, what law requires the disclosure of these costs before the time of service? ___________

____

18. Which law states the requirements and limitations for the patient and the medical practice when a complaint is registered about a billing statement error? ___________

____

19. Name the time limit for collection on an open account in your state. ___________

20. Explain aging an account and state why it is necessary. ___________

____

____

21. An itemized billing statement is usually sent every ___________ days, and when an account becomes delinquent a ___________ message is sent to prompt payment.

22. What is the average time frame for turning an account over to a collection agency? ___________

____

23. If a physician asks you to file a claim in small-claims court, where would you go to get the form and detailed information about the process? ___________

____

____

24. Define wage garnishment: ___________

____

25. Name two types of bankruptcy.

    a. ___________

    b. ___________

Critical Thinking Exercises

1. Mr. Hernandez starts an argument with you about the physician's fee. What would be your response?

____

____

____

____

2. Dr. Practon expects you to ask patients to pay at the time of their office visits. Mr. Owen passes your desk without stopping after seeing the doctor. What would you say?

____

____

____

____

3. What are the most important precautions to take in case a patient becomes a *skip* and you have to conduct a *trace*? ____

____

____

____

____

JOB SKILL 13-1
Role-Play Collection Scenarios

Name ______________________________ Date ______________ Score ________

Performance Objective

Task: State how you would handle fee collection in 20 scenarios illustrated in this exercise.

Conditions: Practon Medical Group, Inc., office policy and fee schedule (Part III of this *Workbook*), two sheets of plain bond paper, pencil or pen, and computer or typewriter.

Standards: Complete all steps listed in this skill in _______ minutes with a minimum score of ________. (Time element and accuracy criteria may be given by instructor.)

Time: **Start:** ____________ **Completed:** ____________ **Total:** ____________ minutes

Scoring: One point for each step performed satisfactorily unless otherwise listed or weighted by instructor.

Directions with Performance Evaluation Checklist

Refer to Part III at the end of the *Workbook*, Appendix for Practon Medical Group, Inc., and read about "Office Policies," "Payment Policies and Health Insurance Protocol," and the "Fee Schedule." Then study the fee schedule to familiarize yourself with how it is set up. There are main headings (in capital letters) and subheadings to help you find various types of services. The columns under the headings include (1) procedure codes, (2) levels of service or description of procedures, (3) mock fees (used by private payers or private insurance companies), (4) Medicare participating provider fees, (5) Medicare nonparticipating provider fees, and (6) Medicare limiting charges. After reading this section, state how you would handle each of the following collection situations.

1st Attempt	2nd Attempt	3rd Attempt	
_______	_______	_______	Gather materials (equipment and supplies) listed under "Conditions."
_____/5	_____/5	_____/5	1. A new private pay patient, Anne Rule, calls for an appointment for Monday morning. It is your office policy to collect the physician's fee at the time of the first visit. Convey this information during your conversation.
_____/5	_____/5	_____/5	2. An established patient, Sylvia Cone, came in on Wednesday for a Level IV examination. She calls today and says she is not going to pay the bill because she is not satisfied with the treatment. She says, "Go ahead and send my account to a collection agency. I'll call my attorney. I can make trouble for you and Dr. Practon." Prepare your response.
_____/5	_____/5	_____/5	3. Mrs. Katrina Frenzel calls to ask you about the bill she just received for her son, Paul, who recently made his first visit to the office. She thinks the bill for $132.28 is "very high" and wonders if there is a mistake because the fee seems out of line. She says she has recently moved into this area. Prepare your response and state what action you would take.
_____/5	_____/5	_____/5	4. Today you call Miss Wendy Snow about her account, which is overdue. You have sent her two statements, telephoned her, and finally sent a letter asking her to call the office about the $80 she owes. She has not responded. According to your records, she was seen on November 2, she lives at home with her parents, and she has health insurance but has not paid the deductible. Prepare questions you would ask her.

JOB SKILL 13-1 (*continued*)

_____/5 _____/5 _____/5 5. Recently, Dr. Gerald Practon performed a two-hour operation and billed the patient his standard fee, which is what physicians generally charge in your region. However, the patient's husband considers the fee exorbitant and has paid only part of it. What action would you take, and how would you collect the outstanding amount?

_____/5 _____/5 _____/5 6. Last week, Dr. Fran Practon made a lengthy long-distance telephone call to check on a postoperative patient who had complicated major surgery. Should you bill the patient for the telephone charges? Explain your answer.

_____/5 _____/5 _____/5 7. Recently, a patient whose account you have turned over to a collection agency saw you in the supermarket and mentioned that she would be telephoning for an appointment soon. Before making the appointment, you notify Dr. Practon of this circumstance. He insists she pay what she owes, and requires any future bills be paid in cash. Is this ethical? Explain your answer.

_____/5 _____/5 _____/5 8. You routinely bill Dr. Practon's patients the amount that appears on the established fee schedule. In reviewing an account, Dr. Practon finds that a certain patient has been charged more than was intended. The patient makes no complaint and pays the bill in full. What action would you take?

_____/5 _____/5 _____/5 9. Sister Mary Benedict Ramer, a new patient, is seen in consultation. She gives you her insurance card and asks whether she will be given a discount because she is a member of the clergy. How would you respond?

_____/5 _____/5 _____/5 10. Dr. Practon's fee for an appendectomy is $568.36 (CPT code 44950). Mr. Jefferson's hospital stay for his appendectomy was unusually troublesome. His first symptoms appeared after midnight, and he was admitted to the hospital as an emergency patient. A decision to operate immediately was postponed by Dr. Practon when the patient began to improve; however, he had several abnormal laboratory results. During the following night, the patient's condition worsened, and the appendectomy was performed, thereby interrupting Dr. Practon's sleep for a second night. After the operation, the patient had a bad case of postanesthesia nausea and was quite demanding while in the hospital. Would Dr. Practon be justified in charging him extra because he was "a lot of trouble"? Explain.

_____/5 _____/5 _____/5 11. You send a bill for $1,500 to Mrs. Jamison for major surgery. She tells you that the physician told her in a presurgery conversation that the charge would be "about $1,300." Dr. Practon says he does not remember quoting the figure to her. If the usual charge is $1,500 for this procedure, what should you do about the bill? Explain.

_____/5 _____/5 _____/5 12. Mr. French calls in complaining about an overdue refund. He, as well as the insurance company, paid for a procedure, and he is owed a return of his payment. You have been swamped with billing and reply that the statements come first and when you can "get to it" you will mail the refund. What is the proper procedure in this instance? Describe.

_____/5 _____/5 _____/5 13. Patient Joanie Franklin comes in to see Dr. Practon for an initial visit. When asked about insurance coverage, she states, "According to our divorce settlement, my husband's insurance should be billed first." How would you respond?

_____/5 _____/5 _____/5 14. An established patient telephones and says, "The letter I received from the insurance company said you charged too much." How would you respond?

_____/5 _____/5 _____/5 15. New patient Bill Songer comes in to see Dr. Gerald Practon. He says, "My wife handles all the bills, so you will have to call her." How would you reply?

_____/5 _____/5 _____/5 16. An established patient was seen by Dr. Fran Practon and returned the following week to have a treadmill test. His insurance was billed; however, the explanation of benefits was sent to the patient denying payment for the test. The patient came in and stated, "My insurance should have covered that service." What questions would you ask and what action would you take?

_____/5 _____/5 _____/5 17. You call patient Mary Edwards regarding an overdue account and reach an answering machine—the patient is not home. What will you do?

_____/5 _____/5 _____/5 18. A patient who has not seen Dr. Practon in a long time comes in for an office visit. Upon leaving, the patient states, "My attorney told me not to pay the bill." What would you say and what question(s) would you ask?

_____/5 _____/5 _____/5 19. A longstanding patient owes over $500, which is now past due. She calls stating, "I have just declared bankruptcy." How would you respond?

_____/5 _____/5 _____/5 20. You are calling Jana Lynn Rose about an overdue account. Her spouse answers the phone and states that the patient is deceased. How would you respond?

_______ _______ _______ Complete within specified time.

___/102 ___/102 ___/102 **Total points earned** (To obtain a percentage score, divide the total points earned by the number of points possible.)

Comments:

Evaluator's Signature: ____ **Need to Repeat:** ________________

National Curriculum Competency: CAAHEP: Cognitive: VI.C.9, 11, 12; Psychomotor: VI.P.2.c; Affective:VI.A.1	ABHES: 8.i, v

JOB SKILL 13-2
Use a Calculator

Name ________________________________ Date ______________ Score ________

Performance Objective

Task: Compute charges, payments, and adjustments on a ledger card using a calculator and determine a running balance.

Conditions: Use calculator, adding machine, or computer calculator; pen or pencil; and ledger card (Form 51). Refer to Procedures 13-2 and 13-3 in the *textbook* for step-by-step directions.

Standards: Complete all steps listed in this skill in ________ minutes with a minimum score of ________. (Time element and accuracy criteria may be given by instructor.)

Time: **Start:** ____________ **Completed:** ____________ **Total:** ____________ minutes

Scoring: One point for each step performed satisfactorily unless otherwise listed or weighted by instructor.

Directions with Performance Evaluation Checklist

Using a calculator, practice touch operation by moving your fingers correctly from the home row to other numbered keys as shown in the illustration. Set up a ledger card for the patient, and add charges and subtract payments and adjustments line by line to determine a running balance.

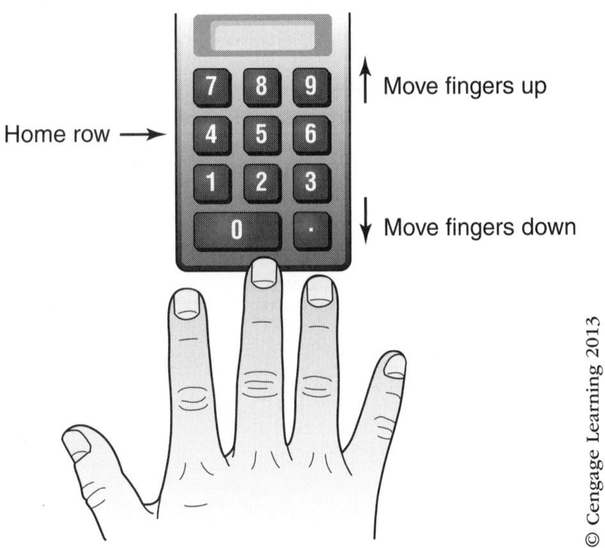

1st Attempt	2nd Attempt	3rd Attempt	
______	______	______	Gather materials (equipment and supplies) listed under "Conditions."
____/8	____/8	____/8	1. Set up a ledger card by inserting the following information for patient John Dearborn (DOB 9/30/50), 112 South Fifth Street, Woodland Hills, XY 12345; home telephone number: (555) 486-0943; work telephone number: (555) 486-5098; insured with Aetna Casualty, policy No. 12345 AET.
____/2	____/2	____/2	2. Starting from the top of the ledger card, add the balance forward and the charge from Line 1, and insert the total in the balance column on the right.
____/2	____/2	____/2	3. Add the charge from Line 2, and insert the total in the balance column.
____/2	____/2	____/2	4. Add the charge from Line 3, and insert the total in the balance column.
____/2	____/2	____/2	5. Add the charge from Line 4, and insert the total in the balance column.

JOB SKILL 13-2 *(continued)*

____/2 ____/2 ____/2 6. Add the charge from Line 5, and insert the total in the balance column.

____ ____ ____ 7. Bring down the balance from Line 5 to Line 6 in the balance column. *Rationale: When a line is used for notations only, the balance should always be brought forward to the next line.*

____/2 ____/2 ____/2 8. Add the charge from Line 7, and insert the total in the balance column.

____/2 ____/2 ____/2 9. Add the charge from Line 8, and insert the total in the balance column.

____/2 ____/2 ____/2 10. Subtract the payment from Line 9, and insert the total in the balance column.

____/2 ____/2 ____/2 11. Subtract the payment from Line 10, and insert the total in the balance column.

____/2 ____/2 ____/2 12. Subtract the adjustment from Line 11, and insert the total in the balance column.

____ ____ ____ 13. Bring down the balance from Line 11 to Line 12 in the balance column.

____/2 ____/2 ____/2 14. Subtract the payment from Line 13, and insert the total in the balance column.

____/2 ____/2 ____/2 15. Subtract the payment from Line 14, and insert the total in the balance column.

____/2 ____/2 ____/2 16. Subtract the adjustment from Line 15, and insert the total in the balance column.

____ ____ ____ 17. Circle the running balance on the ledger that appears in Line 15 (keep the calculator tape when applicable).

____ ____ ____ Complete within specified time.

____/39 ____/39 ____/39 **Total points earned** (To obtain a percentage score, divide the total points earned by the number of points possible.)

Comments:

Evaluator's Signature: ______________________ **Need to Repeat:** ____________

National Curriculum Competency: CAAHEP: Cognitive: II.C.1	ABHES: 6.a, 8.a, w

JOB SKILL 13-3

Complete and Post on a Ledger Card: Charges, Payments, a Returned Check, and a Check from a Collection Agency

Name ______________________________ Date ____________ Score ________

Performance Objective

Task: Prepare a ledger card: post charges, payments, a returned check for NSF, and a check from a collection agency, making correct notations and calculating a running balance.

Conditions: Use calculator, adding machine, or computer calculator; pen or pencil; and ledger card (Form 52). Refer to Procedures 13-2 and 13-3 in the *textbook* for step-by-step directions. See *textbook* Example 13-5 and Figure 13-4 for posting illustrations. Refer to the fee schedule in Part III of this *Workbook* for procedure (*CPT*) codes and mock fees.

Standards: Complete all steps listed in this skill in _______ minutes with a minimum score of ________. (Time element and accuracy criteria may be given by instructor.)

Time: **Start:** ____________ **Completed:** ____________ **Total:** ____________ minutes

Scoring: One point for each step performed satisfactorily unless otherwise listed or weighted by instructor.

Directions with Performance Evaluation Checklist

Set up a ledger card for the patient. Post entries line by line, adding all charges and subtracting all payments and adjustments to determine a running balance.

1st Attempt	2nd Attempt	3rd Attempt	
______	______	______	Gather materials (equipment and supplies) listed under "Conditions."
_____8	_____/8	_____/8	1. Set up a ledger card for established patient Helen Rice (DOB 1/17/58), 212 Hemmingway Road, Woodland Hills, XY 12345; home telephone number: (555) 486-7721; work telephone number: (555) 486-3333; insured with QRS Insurance Company, policy No. QRS 212345-678.
______	______	______	2. Enter balance forward of $360.00.
_____/5	_____/5	_____/5	3. Enter the charge for a Level IV office visit on 3/16/XX with proper reference and description; compute a running balance.
_____/4	_____/4	_____/4	4. Enter a notation that the insurance company was billed on 3/17/XX for these services and bring down the balance.
_____/5	_____/5	_____/5	5. Post the patient payment (check No. 987) on 3/20/XX in the amount of $360 for amount owed; compute a running balance.
_____/5	_____/5	_____/5	6. The bank calls, stating check No. 987 is being returned for nonsufficient funds (NSF). Post a reversal of the payment and calculate a new running balance. The patient is called and asked to bring in cash or a money order within three days.
_____/5	_____/5	_____/5	7. On 3/30/XX, you receive notification from the insurance company that the patient no longer has insurance coverage. Bill the patient for the entire balance and make a notation on the ledger; bring down the running balance.
_____/5	_____/5	_____/5	8. On 4/30/XX, you send a second statement to the patient indicating "Account is overdue, please play balance." Make an entry on the ledger and bring down the running balance.

JOB SKILL 13-3 (*continued*)

_____/5 _____/5 _____/5 9. On 5/30/XX, you send a third statement to the patient indicating "If payment is not received in five days, your account will be sent to a collection agency." Bring down the running balance.

_____/3 _____/3 _____/3 10. On 6/5/XX, you send the account to the Collect 4U Agency. Make a notation on the ledger; adjust the entire balance (subtract it from the running balance), circle it, and post a zero balance.

_____/6 _____/6 _____/6 11. On 7/15/XX, the patient pays the collection agency $200. The agency sends check No. 9876543 to the office. Post the agency check on the patient's ledger, reverse the adjustment by $200, and indicate account closed.

_______ _______ _______ Complete within specified time.

____/54 ____/54 ____/54 **Total points earned** (To obtain a percentage score, divide the total points earned by the number of points possible.)

Comments:

Evaluator's Signature: ______________________________ **Need to Repeat:** ______________

National Curriculum Competency: CAAHEP: Cognitive: VI.C.10; Psychomotor: VI.P.2.d, e, g, h ABHES: 8.i, k, m, n, p, q, v

JOB SKILL 13-4
Complete Cash Receipts

Name ______________________________ Date ______________ Score ________

Performance Objective

Task: Complete four cash receipt forms.

Conditions: Use one sheet of cash receipts (Form 53), photocopy machine, and pen. Refer to the Fee Schedule in Part III and Abbreviations (Table 7-1 and Table 15-2) in Part IV of this *Workbook.*

Standards: Complete all steps listed in this skill in _______ minutes with a minimum score of ________. (Time element and accuracy criteria may be given by instructor.)

Time: **Start:** ____________ **Completed:** ____________ **Total:** ____________ minutes

Scoring: One point for each step performed satisfactorily unless otherwise listed or weighted by instructor.

Directions with Performance Evaluation Checklist

The following patients have paid in full for professional services. Post all entries and make a copy of each receipt for Dr. Practon's file (which you can keep for your records). Give the original receipts to the instructor for grading; these originals in a real situation would be given to the patient for his or her records.

1st Attempt	2nd Attempt	3rd Attempt	
______	______	______	Gather materials (equipment and supplies) listed under "Conditions."
______	______	______	1. Use February 16 of the current year as the date of service and posting date.
______	______	______	2. The first patient is Ms. Beth T. Hobson; record the last name first.
______	______	______	3. Refer to the number in the bottom right corner of the receipt to use for the "reference" column.
____/3	____/3	____/3	4. The first patient, Beth Hobson, is established and has a Level I office visit and therapeutic estrogen injection. Charge separately for the office visit, administration of the injection (intramuscular), and the drug (supply). Use correct abbreviations to list the description. She has no previous balance.
____/2	____/2	____/2	5. She pays in full by cash. Post the charges and add to the previous balance, list payments or adjustments and subtract from the previous balance, then calculate and post the current balance.
______	______	______	6. Indicate in "Other" area if the payment is by cash, or list check and check number.
____/10	____/10	____/10	7. Follow steps 2 through 6 to post and produce a cash receipt for new patient Henry P. Morgan. He has a Level IV examination and pays in cash.
____/10	____/10	____/10	8. Follow steps 2 through 6 to post and produce a cash receipt for a Level II office consultation for Mrs. Harriet F. Garber. She pays in cash.
____/10	____/10	____/10	9. Follow steps 2 through 6 to post and produce a cash receipt for established patient Miss Carole V. Putnam. She has a Level III office visit and a two-view x-ray of her right wrist. Previous balance $50; she pays the account in full with check No. 4706.
______	______	______	Complete within specified time.
____/41	____/41	____/41	**Total points earned** (To obtain a percentage score, divide the total points earned by the number of points possible.)

JOB SKILL 13-4 *(continued)*

Comments:

Evaluator's Signature: ________________________ **Need to Repeat:** ____________

National Curriculum Competency: CAAHEP: Psychomotor: VI.P.2	ABHES: 8.a

JOB SKILL 13-5

Compose a Collection Letter, Prepare an Envelope and Ledger, and Post Transactions

Name ______________________________ Date ______________ Score ________

Performance Objective

Task: Compose a collection letter, address an envelope, and complete a ledger card. Make notations on the ledger and make a photocopy of the letter and ledger.

Conditions: One letterhead (Form 54), one number 10 envelope (Form 55), and one ledger card (Form 56). Refer to step-by-step directions in Chapter 11 of the *textbook* (Procedure 11-1) for written correspondence and Chapter 13 (Procedure 13-3) for posting on an account. Refer to Procedure 12-6 in Chapter 12 in the *textbook* for instruction on addressing a business envelope and Figure 12-6 for an illustration.

Standards: Complete all steps listed in this skill in ________ minutes with a minimum score of ________. (Time element and accuracy criteria may be given by instructor.)

Time: **Start:** ____________ **Completed:** ____________ **Total:** ____________ minutes

Scoring: One point for each step performed satisfactorily unless otherwise listed or weighted by instructor.

Directions with Performance Evaluation Checklist

1st Attempt	2nd Attempt	3rd Attempt	
______	______	______	Gather materials (equipment and supplies) listed under "Conditions."

LEDGER

____/8	____/8	____/8	1. Prepare a ledger card for Mrs. Mae Van Alystine (DOB 4/12/56) of 2381 Maple Street, Woodland Hills, XY 12345; home telephone number: (555) 421-8700. She is insured with Mutual Insurance Company, policy number J148, and employed by TBC Import Company, work telephone number: (555) 421-0707.
____/10	____/10	____/10	2. On July 10, current year, she is a new patient and has a 30-minute office visit (Level III) and an intrauterine device inserted (58300). Post both charges, listing *CPT* code numbers in the "reference" column, and calculate a running balance.
____/4	____/4	____/4	3. Indicate on the ledger that the insurance company is billed on the same day services are rendered; bring forward the balance owed.
____/4	____/4	____/4	4. On July 25 the insurance company denies payment because the visit was for a contraceptive device. Indicate that the patient is billed on the ledger card.
____/4	____/4	____/4	5. The patient is billed a second time on August 25; indicate this on the ledger card and bring forward the balance owed.
____/4	____/4	____/4	6. The patient is billed a third time on September 25; indicate this on the ledger card and bring forward the balance owed.
____/4	____/4	____/4	7. Compose a rough draft of a collection letter (letter No. 1) to be sent on October 25 with a copy of the ledger (statement); indicate this on the ledger card, and bring forward the balance owed.

JOB SKILL 13-5 *(continued)*

LETTER

____/8	____/8	____/8	8. Use letterhead to produce a collection letter, centered on the page with full block style, even and equal margins, consistent punctuation, and appropriate paragraphing, capitalization, and abbreviations.
____	____	____	9. Date the letter October 25 of the current year.
____/3	____/3	____/3	10. Use proper address format for the inside address.
____	____	____	11. Place a salutation identifying the person to whom the letter is being written.
____	____	____	12. Include a reference line indicating the date of service and charges.
____/5	____/5	____/5	13. In the body of the letter, state the reason for the letter and indicate the expected response.
____/2	____/2	____/2	14. Place a complimentary close and signature line.
____	____	____	15. Insert the proper enclosure notation.
____	____	____	16. Proofread for spelling and typographical errors while the letter remains on the computer screen or in the typewriter.
____	____	____	17. Make corrections, proof again, and prepare a final copy for signature.

ENVELOPE

____/5	____/5	____/5	18. Prepare the envelope using the U.S. Postal Service's approved format.
____	____	____	19. Copy the letter, ledger card, and envelope.
____	____	____	20. Attach the original letter and ledger card to the envelope.
____	____	____	Complete within specified time.
____/71	____/71	____/71	**Total points earned** (To obtain a percentage score, divide the total points earned by the number of points possible.)

Comments:

Evaluator's Signature: ______________________ **Need to Repeat:** __________

National Curriculum Competency: CAAHEP: I Psychomotor: VI.P.2.c	ABHES: 8.a, i, k, jj

JOB SKILL 13-6
Complete a Financial Agreement

Name ______________________________ Date ______________ Score ________

Performance Objective

Task: Fill in a financial agreement with a schedule of payments.

Conditions: Financial Agreement (Form 58), calculator, and pen or pencil. Refer in the *textbook* to Figure 13-8 for a visual example and Procedure 13-5 for step-by-step directions.

Standards: Complete all steps listed in this skill in _______ minutes with a minimum score of _______. (Time element and accuracy criteria may be given by instructor.)

Time: **Start:** ____________ **Completed:** ____________ **Total:** ____________ minutes

Scoring: One point for each step performed satisfactorily unless otherwise listed or weighted by instructor.

Directions with Performance Evaluation Checklist

Mr. Biederman has received an itemization of all charges that are now overdue. He has no insurance and has agreed to a payment plan; there will be no financial charge.

1st Attempt	2nd Attempt	3rd Attempt	
_______	_______	_______	Gather materials (equipment and supplies) listed under "Conditions."
_____/2	_____/2	_____/2	1. Enter patient's name, Alan Biederman, and telephone number, (555) 486-9093, on the financial agreement form.
_____/9	_____/9	_____/9	2. Mr. Biederman has incurred $3,000 for medical services with Dr. Gerald Practon and has agreed to pay $600 as a down payment. Determine the unpaid balance and fill in Sections 1 through 9 on the agreement form.
_____/8	_____/8	_____/8	3. Mr. Biederman agrees to pay $200 on the first of every month starting August 1 (current year). Calculate the amount and number of monthly payments and fill in the lower section of the form.
_______	_______	_______	4. Have Mr. Biederman sign and date the form; it is July 1 (current year).
_____/3	_____/3	_____/3	5. On the Schedule of Payment, fill in the total amount owed, the down payment (DP), and the balance owed in the top right portion of the form.
____/24	____/24	____/24	6. Complete the Schedule of Payment by filling in all dates and the amount of each installment payment.
_______	_______	_______	7. Present the form to Dr. Practon for his signature.
_______	_______	_______	Complete within specified time.
____/50	____/50	____/50	**Total points earned** (To obtain a percentage score, divide the total points earned by the number of points possible.)

JOB SKILL 13-5 *(continued)*

Comments:

Evaluator's Signature: ______________________________ **Need to Repeat:** ______________

National Curriculum Competency: CAAHEP: Cognitive: VI.C.9; Psychomotor: VI.P.2	ABHES: 8.a,i, k

CHAPTER 14

Banking

OBJECTIVES

After completing the exercises, the student will be able to:

1. Enhance knowledge of medical terminology, interpret abbreviations, and accurately spell medical words.
2. Prepare a bank deposit (Job Skill 14-1).
3. Write checks (Job Skill 14-2).
4. Endorse a check (Job Skill 14-3).
5. Inspect a check (Job Skill 14-4).
6. Post a payment to a ledger (Job Skill 14-5)
7. Post entries to ledger cards and calculate balances (Job Skill 14-6).
8. Reconcile a bank statement (Job Skill 14-7).

FOCUS ON CERTIFICATION*

CMA Content Summary

- Banking procedures
- Preparing bank deposits

*This *Workbook* and the accompanying *textbook* meet the entry-level administrative and general competencies for the CMA outlined by the AAMA Examination Content Outline and Occupational Analysis and for the RMA and CMAS outlined by the AMT Competencies, Construction Parameters, and Examination Specifications (see Competency Grid in Appendix B of the *textbook*).

RMA Content Summary

- Banking procedures
- Prepare and make bank deposits
- Reconcile bank statements
- Understand check processing procedures and requirements
- Non sufficient funds (NSF)
- Endorsements

CMAS Content Summary

- Understanding banking services and procedures
- Bank accounts
- Lines of credit
- Checking endorsements
- Bank deposits
- Bank reconciliation and statements

STOP AND THINK CASE SCENARIOS AND EXAM-STYLE REVIEW QUESTIONS

Refer to the end of Chapter 14 in the *textbook*.

Abbreviation and Spelling Review

Read the following patient's chart note and write the meanings for the abbreviations listed below the note. To decode any abbreviations you do not understand or that appear unfamiliar to you, refer to the list of abbreviations in Part IV of this *Workbook*. Step-by-step directions for this exercise are found in Procedure 1-1 of Chapter 1 in the *textbook*. Medical terms in the chart note are italicized; study them for spelling. Use your medical dictionary to look up their definitions. Your instructor may give a spelling and definition test that includes these words and abbreviations.

Etta Chan

June 22, 20XX Pt was born with *cystic hydromas* and has had *epileptic seizures* without *vomiting* or *dyspnea*. Pt is on *Dilantin*. Pt is to be started on *phenobarbital* 100 mg t.i.d. i.e., 2 mg/kg per day. Ordered CT scan.

Gerald Practon, MD

Gerald Practon, MD

pt ______________________ i.e. ______________________

mg ______________________ kg ______________________

t.i.d. ______________________ CT ______________________

Note: "i.e." is a Latin abbreviation and may be found in an English dictionary.

Review Questions

Review the objectives, glossary, and chapter information before completing the following review questions.

1. Match the terms in the left column with the definitions in the right column by writing the letters in the blanks.

________	debit	a. a check stub
________	payee	b. deposit or addition to a bank account

_________	voucher	c. the person signing a check to pay out funds from a checking account
_________	ABA number	d. withdrawal or subtraction from a bank account
_________	payer	e. a fee assessed by a bank for processing transactions
_________	credit	f. the person named on a check as the recipient of the amount shown
		g. bank or transit number

2. Write the meanings of these abbreviations.

   a. NSF ____________________

   b. EFTS ____________________

   c. POS ____________________

   d. MICR ____________________

   e. ATM ____________________

3. Name the most common types of checking accounts.

   a. ____________________

   b. ____________________

4. Answer the following questions regarding inspecting a check presented for payment in a physician's office.

   a. What identification should be requested? ____________________

   ____

   b. What should you do if a patient presents an out-of-state check? ____________________

   ____

   c. What do you compare the information on the check to when verifying it? ____________________

   ____

5. What does ABA stand for and what is it used for? ____________________

   ____

   ____

   ____

6. What is the federal act that allows the use of electronic checks? ____________________

   ____

7. When calling the bank to use a pay-by-phone system, you would say, "I would like a ____________________

   ____

8. The following check endorsements are either blank, restrictive, or full. Note next to each statement the type of endorsement.

   a. For deposit only
      Jane Garner ____________________

   b. Ronald P. Yeager ____________________

   c. Pay to the order of
      Stationer's Corporation
      Betty T. White
      Harold M. Jeffers ____________________

9. ATMs are open ____________ hours a day and ____________ days a week; a ____________ card is used for transactions.

10. Explain what procedures you should follow if an error is made in writing or typing a check. ____________

11. Name three options you have when a check is missing the payer's signature.

    a. ____________

    b. ____________

    c. ____________

12. In reconciling the monthly bank statement, refer to *textbook* Example 14-3 and indicate whether to *add* or *subtract* the following from (1) the balance appearing on the bank statement or (2) the balance in the checkbook.

    a. outstanding checks ____________

    b. bank service charges ____________

    c. deposits not shown on the bank statement ____________

13. In adjusting the checkbook balance to obtain a reconciliation with the bank statement, what debits, besides checks, might you list and subtract from the checkbook balance?

    a. ____________

    b. ____________

    c. ____________

14. If an error is found when reconciling a bank statement, what number should be used to divide the amount of the difference by to find out if a transposition error has been made on the check stub register? ____________

Critical Thinking Exercises

1. Compare electronic banking and traditional banking methods and summarize the differences between them.

   Features of electronic banking:

   a. ____________

   b. ____________

   c. ____________

   d. ____________

   Features of traditional banking:

   a. ____________

   b. ____________

2. State why you would choose to bank using either electronic banking or traditional banking.

JOB SKILL 14-1
Prepare a Bank Deposit

Name ______________________________ Date ______________ Score ________

Performance Objective

Task: Record checks on a bank deposit slip and calculate total.

Conditions: Use a deposit slip (Form 59) and pen or pencil. Refer to *textbook* Figure 14-3 for a visual example and *textbook* Procedure 14-1 for step-by-step directions.

Standards: Complete all steps listed in this skill in _______ minutes with a minimum score of ________. (Time element and accuracy criteria may be given by instructor.)

Time: **Start:** ____________ **Completed:** ____________ **Total:** ____________ minutes

Scoring: One point for each step performed satisfactorily unless otherwise listed or weighted by instructor.

Directions with Performance Evaluation Checklist

You open today's mail and find six checks patients have sent to Practon Medical Group, Inc., to pay on their accounts. Record the date and amount of each check on a bank deposit slip, and the ABA routing number, then calculate the amount for deposit.

Keith Austin
7637 Concord Circle
Woodland Hills, XY 12345

16-21/1220

6335

Date *March 24, 20xx*

Pay to the order of *Gerald Practon, MD* $ *36.92*

Thirty six and 92/100 Dollars

Santa Paula Interstate Bank

Memo *insurance balance* *Keith Austin*

Hope Wilburn
PO BOX 309
Woodland Hills, XY 12345

55-60/3222

1226

Date *March 26, 20xx*

Pay to the order of *Fran Practon, MD* $ *250.00*

Two hundred and fifty dollars and no/100 Dollars

Woodland Hills CITI Bank

Memo *April payment installment* *Hope Wilburn*

JOB SKILL 14-1 *(continued)*

Richard Rickman
444 Platte Place
Woodland Hills, XY 12345

154-20/440

410

Date *March 25, 20xx*

Pay to the order of *Practon Medical Group* $ *15.00*

Fifteen and no/100 Dollars

County Bank

Memo *Copay*

R. Rickman

Houshang Hutton
8989 Telegraph Rd
Woodland Hills, XY 12345

90-8030/2000

1229

Date *March 26, 20xx*

Pay to the order of *Practon Medical Group, Inc.* $ *70.65*

Seventy dollars and 65/100 Dollars

Westlake Bank & Trust

Memo *Noncovered services*

Houshang Hutton

Carla M. Gafford
613 Redwood Avenue
Woodland Hills, XY 12345

90-4268/1222

4851

Date *March 25, 20xx*

Pay to the order of *Gerald Practon, MD* $ *500.00*

Five hundred and no/100 Dollars

Intercommercial Bank

Memo *Outpatient surgery deductible*

Carla Gafford

JOB SKILL 14-1 *(continued)*

Dick and Angie Hundley
109 Linden Drive
Woodland Hills, XY 12345

16-24/1220

8203

Date March 26, 20xx

Pay to the order of Dr. Fran Practon $ 124.00

One hundred and twenty four dollars and no/100 Dollars

Hillcrest Bank & Mortgage

Memo Medicare deductible

Angie Hundley

1st Attempt	2nd Attempt	3rd Attempt	
_____	_____	_____	Gather materials (equipment and supplies) listed under "Conditions."
_____	_____	_____	1. Enter the date on the front of the deposit slip; use March 28 (current year).
____/2	____/2	____/2	2. Enter the first check from Keith Austin on the back of the deposit slip, recording the bank ABA number on the left and the amount on the right.
____/2	____/2	____/2	3. Enter the check from Hope Wilburn.
____/2	____/2	____/2	4. Enter the check from Richard Rickman.
____/2	____/2	____/2	5. Enter the check from Houshang Hutton.
____/2	____/2	____/2	6. Enter the check from Carla Gafford.
____/2	____/2	____/2	7. Enter the check from Angie Hundley.
_____	_____	_____	8. Total the amounts from all checks and record.
____/6	____/6	____/6	9. Total the check amounts written on the deposit slip and compare with the total of all checks. If the amounts match, write the total on the back of the deposit slip.
_____	_____	_____	10. Enter total of all checks from the reverse side on the front of the deposit slip.
_____	_____	_____	11. Enter the subtotal.
_____	_____	_____	12. Enter the total of the deposit, referred to as "net deposit."
_____	_____	_____	Complete within specified time.
____/25	____/25	____/25	**Total points earned** (To obtain a percentage score, divide the total points earned by the number of points possible.)

JOB SKILL 14-1 *(continued)*

Comments:

Evaluator's Signature: ______________________ **Need to Repeat:** ____________

National Curriculum Competency: CAAHEP: Cognitive: II.C.1, VI.C.3; Psychomotor: VI.P.1	ABHES: 8.g

JOB SKILL 14-2
Write Checks

Name ______________________________ Date ______________ Score ________

Performance Objective

Task: Handwrite or type two checks.

Conditions: Use two blank checks and two invoices (Form 60) and a pen. Refer to Procedure 14-2 in the *textbook* for step-by-step directions and *textbook* Figures 14-1A and 14-1B for visual illustrations.

Standards: Complete all steps listed in this skill in _______ minutes with a minimum score of _________. (Time element and accuracy criteria may be given by instructor.)

Time: **Start:** ____________ **Completed:** ____________ **Total:** ____________ minutes

Scoring: One point for each step performed satisfactorily unless otherwise listed or weighted by instructor.

Directions with Performance Evaluation Checklist

You have received two invoices for the Practon Medical Group. Handwrite or type two checks for Dr. Practon's signature to pay these bills. Note: The check stub is shown on the face of the check for this exercise but would actually appear as the "stub" shown in *textbook* Figure 14-1B, or as a register with consecutive lines for the date, check number, payee name, amount of check or deposit, and running balance.

1st Attempt	2nd Attempt	3rd Attempt	
_______	_______	_______	Gather materials (equipment and supplies) listed under "Conditions."
_______	_______	_______	1. Date the first check (No. 485) May 27 of the current year.
_____/3	_____/3	_____/3	2. Make the check payable to Stationer's Corporation; include the company's address.
_____/3	_____/3	_____/3	3. Make the check payable for the amount due indicated on the invoice.
_____/3	_____/3	_____/3	4. Insert the balance forward from the checkbook on the check stub; the amount is $9,825.55.
_____/3	_____/3	_____/3	5. Note the date, what the check is for, and the amount on the check stub.
_______	_______	_______	6. Calculate a new balance and record.
_____/3	_____/3	_____/3	7. Bring the balance forward to the next check, No. 486.
_______	_______	_______	8. Date check No. 486 May 27 of the current year.
_____/3	_____/3	_____/3	9. Make the check payable to Randolph Electrical Supply; include the company's address.
_____/3	_____/3	_____/3	10. Make the check payable for the amount due indicated on the invoice.
_____/3	_____/3	_____/3	11. Note the date, what the check is for, and the amount on the check stub.
_______	_______	_______	12. Calculate a new balance and record.
_____/6	_____/6	_____/6	13. Record the date paid, check number, and amount paid on each invoice.
_______	_______	_______	Complete within specified time.
____/36	____/36	____/36	**Total points earned** (To obtain a percentage score, divide the total points earned by the number of points possible.)

JOB SKILL 14-2 *(continued)*

Comments:

Evaluator's Signature: ______________________________ **Need to Repeat:** ______________

National Curriculum Competency: CAAHEP: Cognitive: VI.C.3	ABHES: 8.j

JOB SKILL 14-3
Endorse a Check

Name ______________________ Date __________ Score ______

Performance Objective

Task: Enter a restrictive endorsement on a check in the proper location.

Conditions: Check from patient Jeffrey Brown and pen. Refer to chapter material and Figure 14-2 in the *textbook*.

Standards: Complete all steps listed in this skill in ________ minutes with a minimum score of ________. (Time element and accuracy criteria may be given by instructor.)

Time: **Start:** __________ **Completed:** __________ **Total:** __________ minutes

Scoring: One point for each step performed satisfactorily unless otherwise listed or weighted by instructor.

Directions with Performance Evaluation Checklist

Jeffrey Brown
7827 Minnow Street
Woodland Hills, XY 12345
Phone: 555-482-1976

90-7177/3222 750
7504003778

164

Date June 3, 20XX

Pay to the order of Practon Medical Group, Inc. $ 199.03

One hundred ninety nine and 03/100 Dollars

College National Bank
741 Main Street
Woodland Hills, XY 12345

Memo ______ Jeffrey Brown

⑆322271779⑆0164 ⑈750 4003164⑈

ENDORSE HERE

DO NOT WRITE, STAMP, OR SIGN BELOW THIS LINE
RESERVED FOR FINANCIAL INSTITUTION USE

JOB SKILL 14-3 *(continued)*

1st Attempt	2nd Attempt	3rd Attempt	
_______	_______	_______	Gather materials (equipment and supplies) listed under "Conditions."
____/4	____/4	____/4	1. Enter correct wording for a restrictive endorsement.
____/4	____/4	____/4	2. Place restrictive endorsement in proper location.
_______	_______	_______	Complete within specified time.
____/10	____/10	____/10	**Total points earned** (To obtain a percentage score, divide the total points earned by the number of points possible.)

Comments:

Evaluator's Signature: ______________________________ **Need to Repeat:** ____________

National Curriculum Competency: CAAHEP: Cognitive: VI.C.5	ABHES: 8.d

JOB SKILL 14-4
Inspect a Check

Name ______________________________ Date ______________ Score ________

Performance Objective

Task: Inspect a check and answer questions.

Conditions: Use information given for the case, pen or pencil, and illustration of a handwritten check from Rita Stevens.

Standards: Complete all steps listed in this skill in _______ minutes with a minimum score of ________. (Time element and accuracy criteria may be given by instructor.)

Time: **Start:** ____________ **Completed:** ____________ **Total:** ____________ minutes

Scoring: One point for each step performed satisfactorily unless otherwise listed or weighted by instructor.

Directions with Performance Evaluation Checklist

As you learned after reading Chapter 14 in the *textbook*, a handwritten check has certain requirements that must be met to be valid. An established patient, Rita Stevens, wrote a check for a Level III office visit totaling $40.20 before leaving the office on May 21, 20XX. Inspect the check and answer the following questions.

RITA STEVENS
126 Sunset Lane
Woodland Hills, XY 12345

90-7177/3222 750
7504003778

164

Date May 25, 20XX

Pay to the order of Practon Medical Group, Inc. $ 40.00

Forty and 20/100 Dollars

College National Bank
741 Main Street
Woodland Hills, XY 12345

Memo Level III OV Rita Stevens

⑆322271779⑆0164 ⑈750 4003778⑈

© Cengage Learning 2013

1st Attempt	2nd Attempt	3rd Attempt	
_______	_______	_______	Gather materials (equipment and supplies) listed under "Conditions."
_____/2	_____/2	_____/2	1. What two personal identification items should be obtained from the patient before accepting a check? ______________________
_____/2	_____/2	_____/2	2. Does the check list the complete name, address, and telephone number of the patient? ________ If not, what is missing? ______________
_____/2	_____/2	_____/2	3. Is the check dated correctly? ________ If not, what is the problem? _______
_______	_______	_______	4. Is the check made out to the correct payee? ______________________

JOB SKILL 14-3 (*continued*)

______	______	______	5. Did Mrs. Stevens make the check out for the proper amount? ______________
_____/2	_____/2	_____/2	6. If not, what is the problem? ______________
_____/2	_____/2	_____/2	7. How much will Dr. Practon receive? ______________
______	______	______	8. Is the check signed by Rita Stevens? ______________
______	______	______	Complete within specified time.
____/15	____/15	____/15	**Total points earned** (To obtain a percentage score, divide the total points earned by the number of points possible.)

Comments:

Evaluator's Signature: ______________________________ **Need to Repeat:** ______________

National Curriculum Competency: CAAHEP: Cognitive: VI.C.4	ABHES: 8.a

JOB SKILL 14-5
Post a Payment to a Ledger

Name ______________________ Date ____________ Score ________

Performance Objective

Task: Post a payment received by check to a patient's ledger card.

Conditions: Use the check received from patient Jeffrey Brown in *Workbook* Job Skill 14-3, the ledger card following this exercise, and pen.

Standards: Complete all steps listed in this skill in ________ minutes with a minimum score of ________. (Time element and accuracy criteria may be given by instructor.)

Time: **Start:** ____________ **Completed:** ____________ **Total:** ____________ minutes

Scoring: One point for each step performed satisfactorily unless otherwise listed or weighted by instructor.

Directions with Performance Evaluation Checklist

1st Attempt	2nd Attempt	3rd Attempt	
______	______	______	Gather materials (equipment and supplies) listed under "Conditions."
______	______	______	1. Post the payment using the same date the check was written.
______	______	______	2. Record the check number in the reference column.
____/2	____/2	____/2	3. Use correct abbreviations to describe the payment received on the account.
____/2	____/2	____/2	4. Post the payment in the correct column.
____/2	____/2	____/2	5. Calculate the correct balance and record it in the balance column.
______	______	______	Complete within specified time.
____/10	____/10	____/10	**Total points earned** (To obtain a percentage score, divide the total points earned by the number of points possible.)

Comments:

Evaluator's Signature: ______________________ **Need to Repeat:** ____________

National Curriculum Competency: CAAHEP: Psychomotor: VI.P.2	ABHES: 8.k

JOB SKILL 14-5 *(continued)*

STATEMENT

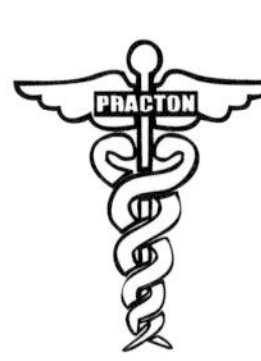

PRACTON MEDICAL GROUP, INC.
4567 Broad Avenue
Woodland Hills, XY 12345-4700
Tel. 555-486-9002
Fax No. 555-488-7815

Mr. Jeffery Brown
230 Main Street
Woodland Hills, XY 12345-0001

DATE	REFERENCE	DESCRIPTION	CHARGES		CREDITS PYMNTS.		CREDITS ADJ.		BALANCE	
1-9-20XX		BALANCE FORWARD →							20	00
1-9-20XX	99213	Level III OV	36	80					56	80
1-10-20XX	1-9-20XX	Medicare billed							56	80
3-5-20XX	1-9-20XX	Medicare pmt			24	99			27	36
4-3-20XX	47600	Cholecystectomy	858	35					885	71
4-5-20XX	4-3-20XX	Medicare billed							885	71
6-2-20XX	4-3-20XX	Medicare pmt			686	68			199	03
——	MEDICARE HAS PAID THEIR PORTION OF THIS CLAIM. THE								199	03
——	BALANCE IS YOUR RESPONSIBILITY. PLEASE REMIT.								199	03

RB40BC-2-96

PLEASE PAY LAST AMOUNT IN BALANCE COLUMN

THIS IS A COPY OF YOUR ACCOUNT AS IT APPEARS ON OUR RECORDS

JOB SKILL 14-6
Post Entries to Ledger Cards and Calculate Balances

Name ______________________________ Date ______________ Score ________

Performance Objective

Task: Post entries to patients' ledger cards and calculate running balances.

Conditions: Use pen or pencil and the five ledger cards shown below. For steps 5 through 9, refer to the mock Fee Schedule in Part III of this *Workbook* for procedure codes and charges (find under section titles, i.e., *Evaluation and Management* for office visits, *Pathology and Laboratory* for lab tests, and *Maternity Care and Delivery* for OB care). Refer to Procedure 13-3 in the *textbook* for step-by-step directions.

Standards: Complete all steps listed in this skill in _______ minutes with a minimum score of ________. (Time element and accuracy criteria may be given by instructor.)

Time: **Start:** ____________ **Completed:** ____________ **Total:** ____________ minutes

Scoring: One point for each step performed satisfactorily unless otherwise listed or weighted by instructor.

Directions with Performance Evaluation Checklist

Complete the following ledger cards, using the current date to post all transactions. Note: Typically, when using a ledger card all transactions that occur on the same day are posted on one line. However, in this exercise, each transaction is posted on a separate line to simplify the learning process and make sure that the addition of charges, subtraction of payments and adjustments, and the running balance are calculated correctly.

1. Elizabeth Hooper

DATE	REFERENCE	DESCRIPTION	CHARGES		CREDITS pymnts		CREDITS Adj		BALANCE	
		BALANCE FORWARD								
6-1-20XX	99203	OV Level III NP	70	92						
6-1-20XX	99000	Handling Pap	5	00						
8-15-20XX	ck# 778	ROA ABC Ins.			69	00				

2. Maria Sanchez

DATE	REFERENCE	DESCRIPTION	CHARGES		CREDITS pymnts		CREDITS Adj		BALANCE	
		BALANCE FORWARD								
7-6-20XX	99244	Consult Level IV	145	05						
7-20-20XX	ck# 432	ROA Pt			25	00				
8-15-20XX	ck# 451	ROA Pt			50	00				
9-18-20XX	ck# 463	ROA Pt			25	00				

JOB SKILL 14-6 *(continued)*

3. Brett Walker

DATE	REFERENCE	DESCRIPTION	CHARGES		CREDITS pymnts		CREDITS Adj		BALANCE	
		BALANCE FORWARD								
7-1-20XX	99203	OV Level III NP	70	92						
7-15-20XX	45308	Proctosigmoidoscopy with removal polyp	135	34						
7-20-20XX	ck 2005	ROA Pt			50	00				
9-1-20XX	Voucher 4006	ROA Blue Cross			165	00				

4. Edna Hargrove

DATE	REFERENCE	DESCRIPTION	CHARGES		CREDITS pymnts		CREDITS Adj		BALANCE	
		BALANCE FORWARD								
8-1-20XX	99213	OV Level III	40	20						
8-1-20XX	58300	IUD insertion	100	00						
8-14-20XX	ck 101	ROA Pt			100	00				

5.–9. Beth Jones

DATE	REFERENCE	DESCRIPTION	CHARGES		CREDITS pymnts		CREDITS Adj		BALANCE	
		BALANCE FORWARD								

JOB SKILL 14-6 *(continued)*

1st Attempt	2nd Attempt	3rd Attempt	
______	______	______	Gather materials (equipment and supplies) listed under "Conditions."
____/8	____/8	____/8	1. Elizabeth Hooper has a small uncollected balance due. Dr. Practon said he wishes to write off the balance. Calculate the running balance and post the adjustment entry.
____/4	____/4	____/4	2. Maria Sanchez was in for a consultation and has made several payments on her account. Calculate each posting entry to determine the running balances.
____/9	____/9	____/9	3. Brett Walker paid on his account and his insurance also paid, resulting in an overpayment. The patient is to receive a refund. Calculate the running balances and post the refund (check 2068) to clear the negative balance.
____/14	____/14	____/14	4. Edna Hargrove issued a check for payment toward her last office visit, but it was returned today by XYZ Bank and marked nonsufficient funds (NSF). Calculate the running balance and post the returned check as well as the $10 bank charge on the ledger card.
____/5	____/5	____/5	5. Beth Jones comes in today for a Level III new patient examination. She is complaining of fatigue, nausea, and dysuria. Post the office visit and calculate the running balance.
____/5	____/5	____/5	6. Dr. Practon feels a laboratory test is needed for Beth (urinalysis, nonautomated without microscopy). Post this service and calculate the running balance.
____/5	____/5	____/5	7. The urinalysis was negative; however, Dr. Practon would like to run a urine pregnancy test. Post this service and calculate a running balance.
____/3	____/3	____/3	8. It is determined that she is pregnant with her first child. The medical assistant discusses maternity care and delivery and advises her of the obstetric fee for a routine vaginal delivery, which includes all antepartum and postpartum visits. The fee is $____________.
____/10	____/10	____/10	9. Her insurance is verified and it is determined that they will pay 85% of Dr. Practon's usual and customary fee for OB care. She pays by check (No. 798) for 15% of the total obstetric fee. Post this payment to her ledger card. Do not post the charge for the OB care; it will be posted at the time of delivery. Her ledger will indicate a negative balance until the obstetric fee is posted.
______	______	______	Complete within specified time.
____/65	____/65	____/65	**Total points earned** (To obtain a percentage score, divide the total points earned by the number of points possible.)

Comments:

Evaluator's Signature: ______________________________ **Need to Repeat:** ____________

National Curriculum Competency: CAAHEP: Psychomotor: VI.P.2.d, e, f, g	ABHES: 8.k, m, n, o, p

JOB SKILL 14-7
Reconcile a Bank Statement

Name ______________________________ Date ______________ Score ________

Performance Objective

Task: Reconcile a bank statement.

Conditions: Use the bank statement shown following this exercise in the *Workbook*, pen or pencil, and bank reconciliation worksheet (Form 61). Refer to Procedure 14-3 in the *textbook* for step-by-step directions.

Standards: Complete all steps listed in this skill in _______ minutes with a minimum score of ________. (Time element and accuracy criteria may be given by instructor.)

Time: **Start:** ____________ **Completed:** ____________ **Total:** ____________ minutes

Scoring: One point for each step performed satisfactorily unless otherwise listed or weighted by instructor.

Directions with Performance Evaluation Checklist

1st Attempt	2nd Attempt	3rd Attempt	
_______	_______	_______	Gather materials (equipment and supplies) listed under "Conditions."
____/10	____/10	____/10	1. You compare and check off each transaction recorded in your checkbook with those listed in this statement and discover the following outstanding checks: No. 318 for $25, No. 337 for $60, No. 338 for $78, No. 340 for $15, and No. 341 for $18.20. Record these on the reconciliation form under "Outstanding Checks."
____/10	____/10	____/10	2. Add the total of outstanding checks and record on the reconciliation form.
_____/4	_____/4	_____/4	3. Assume you made deposits of $3,500 on June 30, 20XX, and $1,800 on July 2, 20XX, which do not show on the statement. Record these on the reconciliation form under "Deposits Not Credited."
_____/4	_____/4	_____/4	4. Add the total of deposits not credited and record on the reconciliation form.
_____/2	_____/2	_____/2	5. Enter the ending statement balance on the reconciliation form.
_____/2	_____/2	_____/2	6. Add the total of the deposits not credited to the ending statement balance and record (making a note of the subtotal).
_____/2	_____/2	_____/2	7. Subtract the total of the outstanding checks from the figure determined in step 6 and record.
_______	_______	_______	8. Verify the adjusted total you determined with the checkbook balance, which is $6,807.89
_______	_______	_______	9. Do these figures match and does the checkbook balance? _________ If not, repeat the above steps, recalculating figures.
_______	_______	_______	Complete within specified time.
____/38	____/38	____/38	**Total points earned** (To obtain a percentage score, divide the total points earned by the number of points possible.)

JOB SKILL 14-7 *(continued)*

COLLEGE NATIONAL BANK
ACCOUNT ACTIVITY

College National Bank
700 West Main Street
Woodland Hills, XY 12345
(800) 540-5060

PRACTON MEDICAL GROUP, INC 140
4567 BROAD AVENUE
WOODLAND HILLS XY 12345

PAGE 1
ITEM COUNT 30

CHECKING — ACCOUNT 12345-6789

SUMMARY

BEGINNING STATEMENT BALANCE ON 20XX	$	633.87
TOTAL OF 4 DEPOSITS/OTHER CREDITS		1414.75
TOTAL OF 15 CHECKS PAID		271.53
5 WITHDRAWALS/OTHER CHARGES		73.00
ENDING STATEMENT BALANCE ON 20XX		1704.09

CHECKS/ WITHDRAWALS/ OTHER CHARGES

CHECKS:

NUMBER	DATE	AMOUNT	NUMBER	DATE	AMOUNT
0317	06-08	17.40	0328	06-10	29.90
1319	05-25	30.00	0329	05-26	32.05
0320	05-30	7.59	0330	06-02	2.75
0321	05-27	9.00	0331	06-02	30.79
0322	05-24	1.00	0332	06-02	11.47
0323	06-03	6.13			
0324	05-30	1.78			
0325	06-02	67.50			
0326	05-25	21.92			
0327	06-03	2.25			

TOTAL OF 15 CHECKS PAID 271.53

WITHDRAWALS/OTHER CHARGES:

DATE	TRANSACTION DESCRIPTION	AMOUNT
06-10	SURGICAL SUPPLY PAYMENT AT ELECTRONIC BANKING	34.30
06-07	STAR FREE PRESS PAYMENT AT ELECTRONIC BANKING	2.00
06-07	MARINER'S MAIL PAYMENT AT ELECTRONIC BANKING	1.00
06-07	CELLULAR ONE PAYMENT AT ELECTRONIC BANKING	16.00
06-03	CLINT PHARMACY PAYMENT AT ELECTRONIC BANKING	19.70

DEPOSITS/ OTHER CREDITS

DEPOSITS:

DATE	TRANSACTION DESCRIPTION	AMOUNT
06-07	BRANCH DEPOSIT	250.24
06-09	BRANCH DEPOSIT	1000.00
06-15	BRANCH DEPOSIT	156.69
06-16	CHECK DEPOSIT AT BANK BY MAIL	7.82

DAILY BALANCES

DATE	BALANCE	DATE	BALANCE	DATE	BALANCE
05-24	632.87	06-02	418.02	06-09	1605.78
05-25	580.95	06-03	389.94	06-10	1573.88
05-26	548.90	06-07	623.18	06-15	1730.57
05-27	539.90	06-08	605.78	06-16	1704.09
05-30	530.53				

Comments:

Evaluator's Signature: ____________________ **Need to Repeat:** __________

National Curriculum Competency: CAAHEP: Cognitive: VI.C.3 ABHES: 8.g

CHAPTER 15

Bookkeeping

OBJECTIVES

After completing the exercises, the student will be able to:

1. Enhance knowledge of medical terminology, interpret abbreviations, and accurately spell medical words.
2. Prepare ledger cards (Job Skill 15-1).
3. Bookkeeping Day 1—Post to patient ledger cards and prepare cash receipts (Job Skill 15-2).
4. Bookkeeping Day 1—Prepare the daily journal (Job Skill 15-3).
5. Bookkeeping Day 1—Post charges, payments, and adjustments using a daily journal (Job Skill 15-4).
6. Bookkeeping Day 1—Balance the daysheet (Job Skill 15-5).
7. Bookkeeping Day 2—Prepare the daily journal (Job Skill 15-6).
8. Bookkeeping Day 2—Post charges, payments, and adjustments to patient ledger cards and to the daily journal; prepare cash receipts and the bank deposit (Job Skill 15-7).
9. Bookkeeping Day 2—Balance the daysheet (Job Skill 15-8).
10. Bookkeeping Day 3—Prepare the daily journal (Job Skill 15-9).
11. Bookkeeping Day 3—Post charges, payments, and adjustments to patient ledger cards and to the daily journal; prepare cash receipts and the bank deposit (Job Skill 15-10).
12. Bookkeeping Day 3—Balance the daysheet (Job Skill 15-11).
13. Bookkeeping Day 4—Set up the daysheet for a new month (Job Skill 15-12).

FOCUS ON CERTIFICATION*

CMA Content Summary

- Bookkeeping principles
- Daily reports, charge slips, receipts, ledgers
- Charges, payments, and adjustments
- Identifying and correcting errors
- Petty cash
- Reconciling third-party payments

RMA Content Summary

- Process insurance payments and contractual write-off amounts
- Understand terminology associated with medical financial bookkeeping
- Collect and post payments
- Manage patient ledgers and accounts
- Employ appropriate accounting procedures (pegboard/double entry, computerized)
- Perform daily balancing procedures
- Prepare monthly trial balance
- Apply accounts receivable principles
- Understand and manage petty cash account
- Understand and maintain disbursement accounts
- Financial mathematics

CMAS Content Summary

- Perform bookkeeping procedures including balancing accounts
- Perform financial computations
- Manage accounts receivable
- Manage patient accounts/ledgers
- Manage petty cash
- Use computer for billing and financial transactions

STOP AND THINK CASE SCENARIOS AND EXAM-STYLE REVIEW QUESTIONS

Refer to the end of Chapter 15 in the *textbook*.

Abbreviation and Spelling Review

Read the following patient's chart note and write the meanings for the abbreviations listed below the note. To decode any abbreviations you do not understand or that appear unfamiliar to you, refer to the list of abbreviations in Part IV of this *Workbook*. Step-by-step directions for this exercise are found in Procedure 1-1 of Chapter 1 in the *textbook*. Medical terms in the chart note are italicized; study them for spelling. Use your medical dictionary to look up their definitions. Your instructor may give a spelling and definition test that includes these words and abbreviations.

Kevin T. Dusseau

June 30, 20XX Pt has off and on problems with eye. Dx: Acute *bacterial conjunctivitis* L eye. Treat R eye at first sign of *symptoms*. Cold compresses L eye ad lib. for comfort. Retn p.r.n.

Fran Practon, MD

Fran Practon, MD

*This *Workbook* and the accompanying *textbook* meet the entry-level administrative and general competencies for the CMA outlined by the AAMA Examination Content Outline and Occupational Analysis and for the RMA and CMAS outlined by the AMT Competencies, Construction Parameters, and Examination Specifications (see Competency Grid in Appendix B of the *textbook*).

Pt ______________________ ad lib. ______________________

Dx ______________________ retn ______________________

L ______________________ p.r.n. ______________________

R ______________________

Review Questions

Review the objectives, glossary, and chapter information before completing the following review questions.

1. Match the terms in the left column with the definitions in the right column and write the letters in the blanks.

________ debit	a. bookkeeping entry that decreases assets and increases earnings
________ post	b. register or checkbook that lists amounts paid out for expenses of the business practice
________ accounts receivable ledger	c. the owner's net worth
________ asset	d. to record a charge, payment, or adjustment on a ledger or account
________ liability	e. register for recording all daily business transactions of patients
________ daysheet	f. that which is owned by the business
________ credit	g. monies that are owed for business expenditures
________ proprietorship	h. record of all patients' outstanding accounts showing how much each one owes for services rendered
________ accounts payable ledger	i. a bookkeeping entry that records increases in assets and expenses and decreases liabilities

2. Name one or more advantages and disadvantages of each of the following accounting systems:

	Advantage	Disadvantage
a. single-entry	______________	______________
b. double-entry	______________	______________
c. pegboard	______________	______________
d. computerized	______________	______________

3. When using a computerized bookkeeping system, you would post charges, payments, and adjustments to a patient ______________; in a manual system, you would post to a ______________.

4. Charges are posted on the date ______________; payments are posted on the date ______________.

5. Circle the correct answer: Charges are (debited/credited) to the account; payments and adjustments are (debited/credited) to the account.

6. Write the bookkeeping term that each abbreviation stands for.

   a. B/F ______________________________

   b. pd ______________________________

   c. adj ______________________________

   d. ROA ______________________________

   e. recd ______________________________

7. On the daysheet, the total of what patients have paid by cash and check must equal the total ______________ for that day.

8. Explain what calculations need to be made to determine the new accounts receivable figure at the end of the month.

   a. ______________________________

   b. ______________________________

   c. ______________________________

9. An amount evenly divisible by ______________ may indicate a transposed figure, and an amount evenly divisible by ______________ may indicate posting to the wrong column.

10. If a posting error occurs when writing 900 for 90, this type of error is called ______________.

11. At the end of the day, to reconcile the cash and change drawer, the ______________ should equal the cash amount on the ______________, and the remaining amount in the change drawer should be the same as the beginning amount.

12. When is the petty cash fund replenished? ______________ or ______________, depending on the demand for funds.

13. When replenishing the petty cash fund, add the ______________ to the ______________ and compare this total to the amount established for the fund; they should equal.

14. Make a list of all forms required when using a pegboard bookkeeping system, and give a brief explanation of the function of each one.

	Form	Function
a.	______________	______________________________
		______________________________
		______________________________
b.	______________	______________________________
		______________________________
		______________________________
c.	______________	______________________________
		______________________________
		______________________________
d.	______________	______________________________
		______________________________
		______________________________

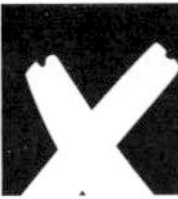

Critical Thinking Exercises

1. Explain the purposes of a cash or change drawer and a petty cash fund, and tell why a medical practice needs both systems in place. ____

____

____

2. Mrs. Landry's account shows a delinquent balance of $30, and Dr. Practon wants the amount written off the books and the account closed. Explain what you would do.

____

____

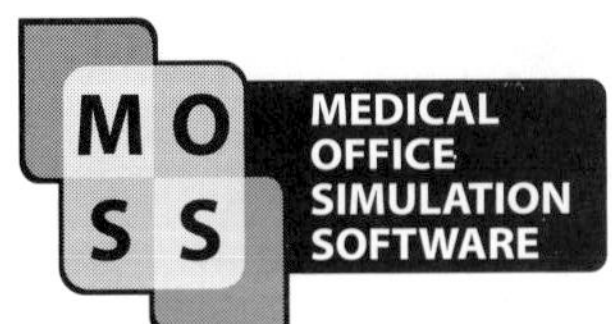

Computer Competency

Today's Date Is Monday, 10/21/2013

Simulation: You are the medical biller for Douglasville Medicine Associates. At the end of each business day, the biller is responsible for posting the procedures for all office services provided to patients that day. **You will need to reference the MOSS Source Documents (Encounter Forms) found at the end of this section *as well as from Chapter 7* to complete the exercises.** *Note: You must complete the prior Computer Competency exercises in this Workbook prior to starting.*

1. Posting Procedures: Patient Albertson

The medical biller will post procedures to each patient account as provided on the encounter form (superbill) that was completed by the doctor and clinical staff. Any payments made at the time of service will also be posted to the patient account where applicable. **Note: The Source Document for this patient is found in the Chapter 7 Source Documents.**

A. Gather the encounter forms (superbills) for the date 10/21/2013 and review each one **(Source Documents: Encounter Forms)**. Circle the information for each of the following on the form:

   Patient name

   Encounter reference number (under patient name)

   Date of service

   Place of service

   Procedure (*CPT*) code(s) for services rendered

   Diagnostic (*ICD*) code(s) for each diagnosis

   Amount paid

   Doctor providing service

B. When all of the encounter forms have been reviewed and the information circled, look at encounter form 2999, Patient Albertson **(Source Documents: Encounter Forms, Chapter 7).**

C. Click on the *Procedure Posting* button from the *Main Menu.*

D. Search for Josephine Albertson, and then click on *Add*, since charges will be added to the patient's account.

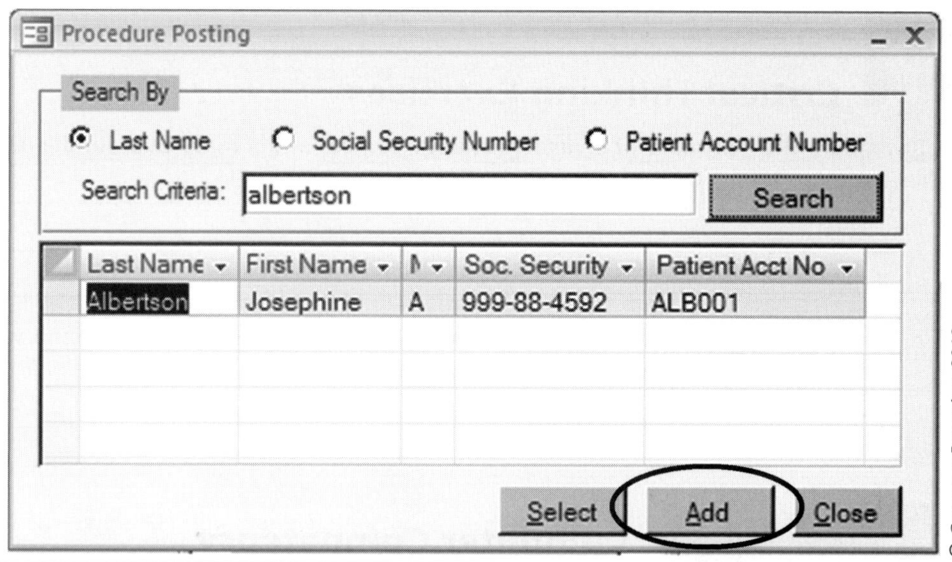

© Cengage Learning 2013

E. Using the information circled on Ms. Albertson's encounter form, complete Fields 1-12 in the top half of the *Procedure Posting* screen. Only input information that is applicable. For example, Fields 4, 6, and 9 do not require any input.

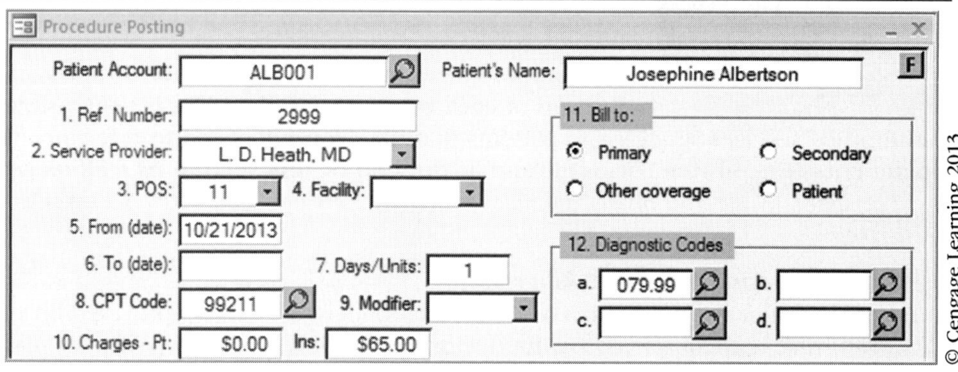

© Cengage Learning 2013

F. Click on the *Post* button to apply the charges to the patient account.

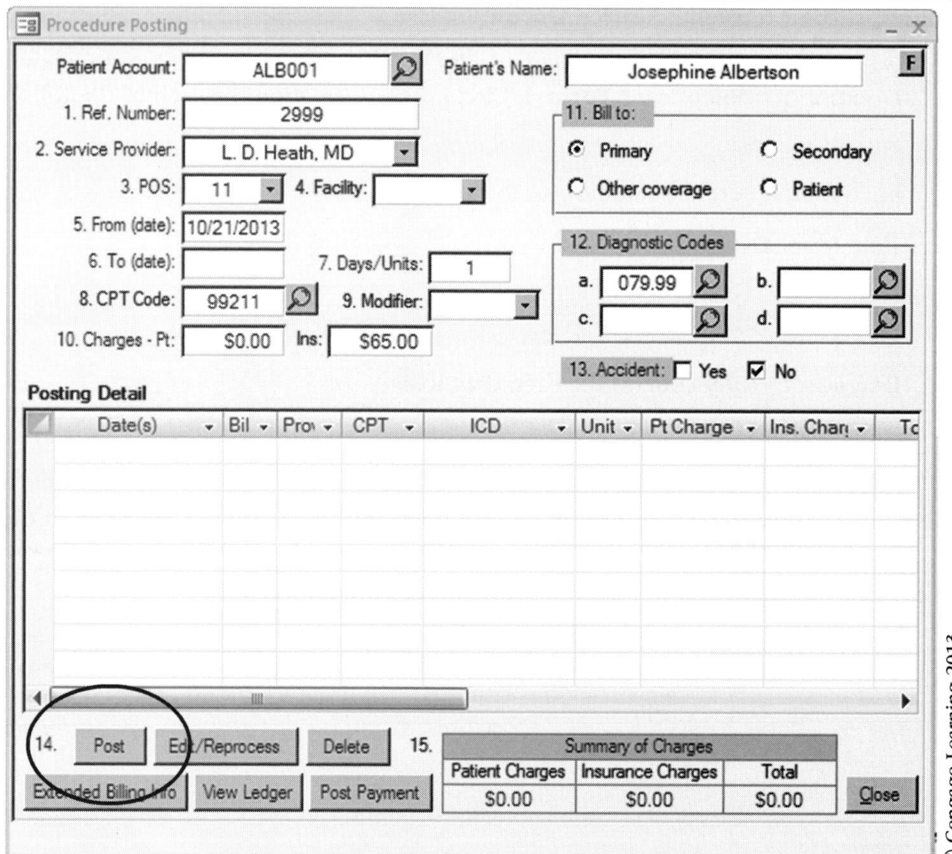

© Cengage Learning 2013

G. The charge is now transferred to the *Posting Detail* area. Review the *Posting Detail* and check your work.

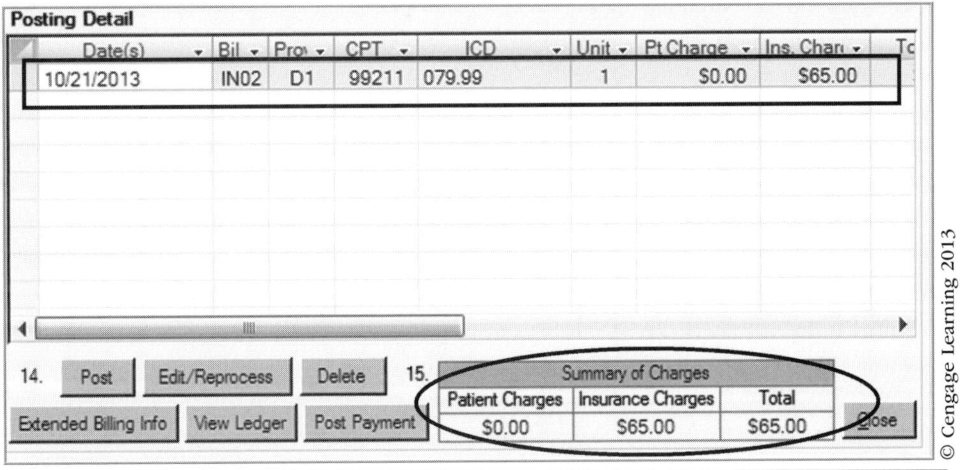

H. Close the *Procedure Posting* screen and return to the patient selection list.

2. Posting Procedures and a Payment: Ryan Ashby

The medical biller will post procedures to Patient Ashby's account as provided on the encounter form (superbill) that was completed by the doctor and clinical staff. The payment made at the time of service will also be posted to the patient account. **Note: The Source Document for this patient is found in the Chapter 7, Source Documents.**

A. Look at the encounter form (superbill) for Patient Ashby, reference number 3000 **(Source Documents: Encounter Forms, Chapter 7).**

B. Click on the *Procedure Posting* button from the *Main Menu.*

C. Search for Ryan Ashby, and then click on *Add*, since charges will be added to the patient's account.

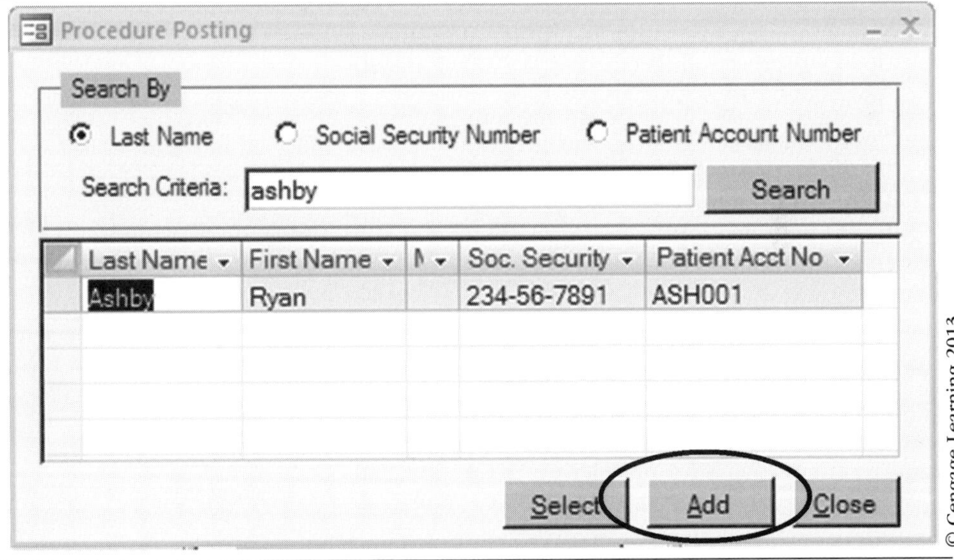

D. Using the information circled on Mr. Ashby's encounter form, complete Fields 1-12 in the top half of the *Procedure Posting* screen. Only input information that is applicable. For example, Fields 4, 6, and 9 do not require any input. Pay special attention that the correct physician is selected as the provider of service.

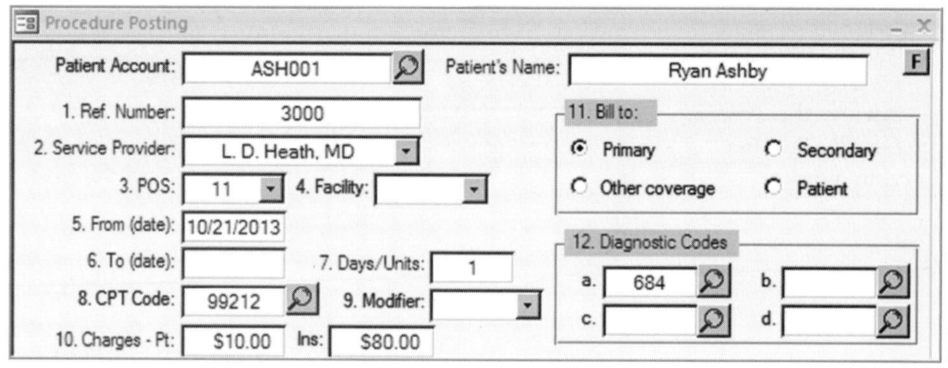

E. Click on the *Post* button to apply the charges to the patient account.

F. Review the *Posting Detail* and check your work.

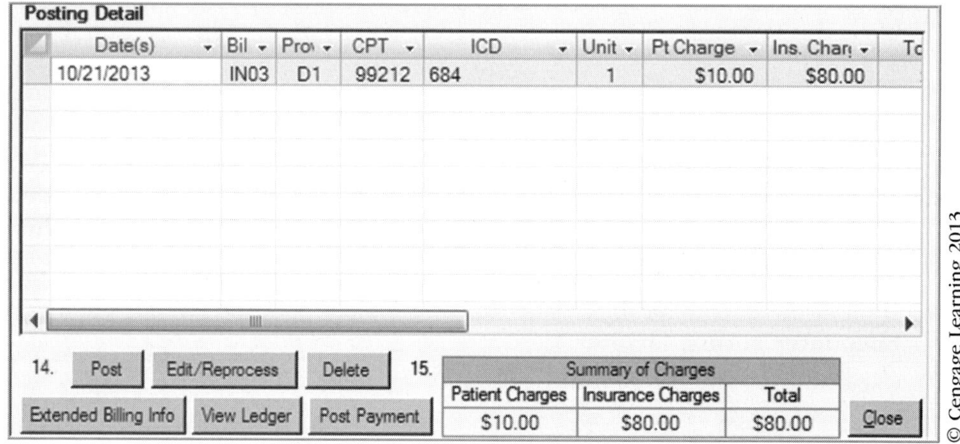

G. Close all screens and return to the *Main Menu*.

H. Click on the *Payment Posting* button on the *Main Menu*. Find Ryan Ashby from the list and click on *Apply Payment*.

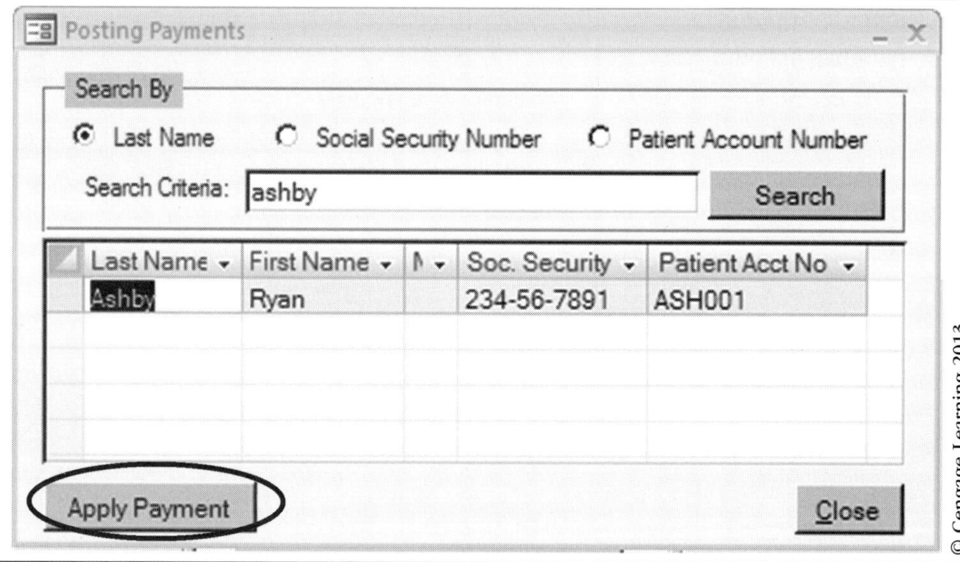

I. Click on the line item in the *Procedure Charge History* area (Field 1), and then click on the *Select/ Edit* button. If done correctly, Field 13 will show the correct *Balance Due*, and the buttons along the bottom will become active. If the *Balance Due* does not appear, the line item has not been selected.

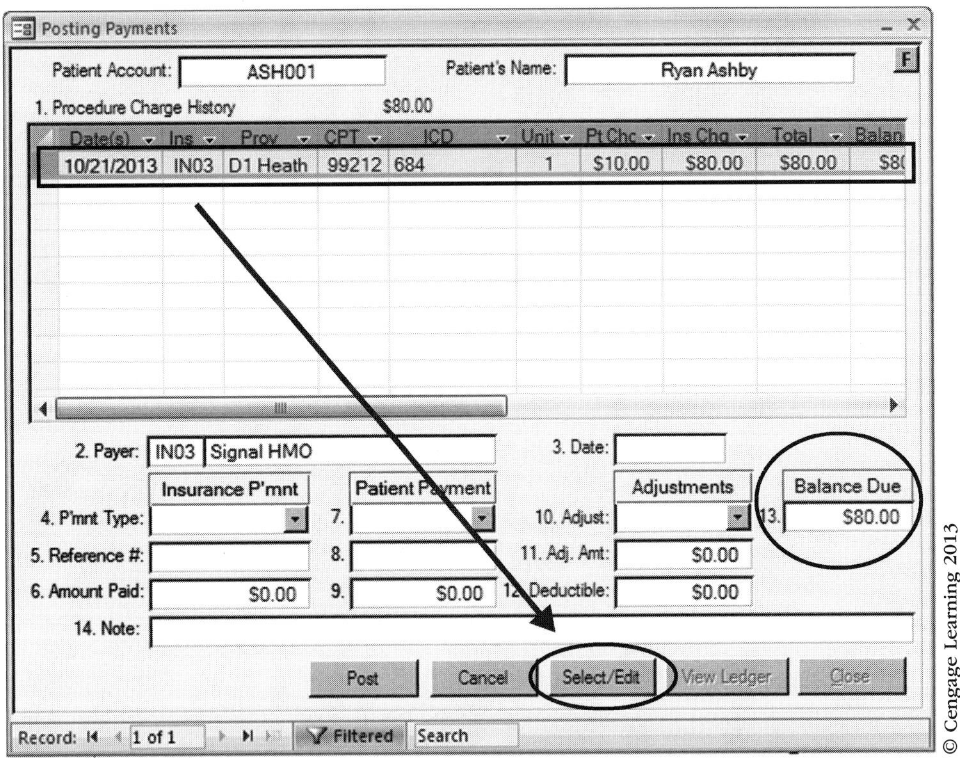

© Cengage Learning 2013

J. Input the date of posting (10/21/2013) and the following patient payment information:

Paid by check (Field 7)

Check number 8755 (Field 8)

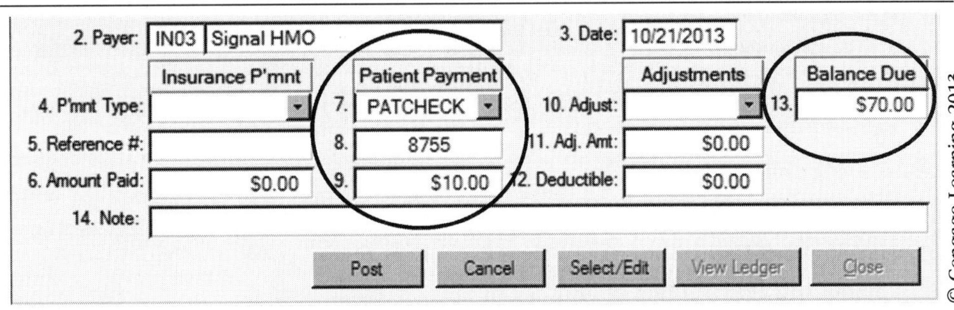

© Cengage Learning 2013

Amount of payment $10.00 (Field 9)

Press *Enter* when finished to update the *Balance Due* (Field 13)

K. Review all entries carefully. When correct, click the *Post* button to apply the payment.

L. Close all screens and return to the *Main Menu* in MOSS.

3. Posting Procedures: Patient Ybarra

The medical biller will post procedures to Patient Ybarra's account as provided on the encounter form (superbill) that was completed by the doctor and clinical staff. **Note: The Source Document for this patient is found in the Chapter 7, Source Documents.**

A. Look at the encounter form (superbill) for Patient Ybarra, reference number 3001 **(Source Documents: Encounter Forms, Chapter 7).**

B. Click on *Procedure Posting*, find Patient Ybarra, and then click the *Add* button.

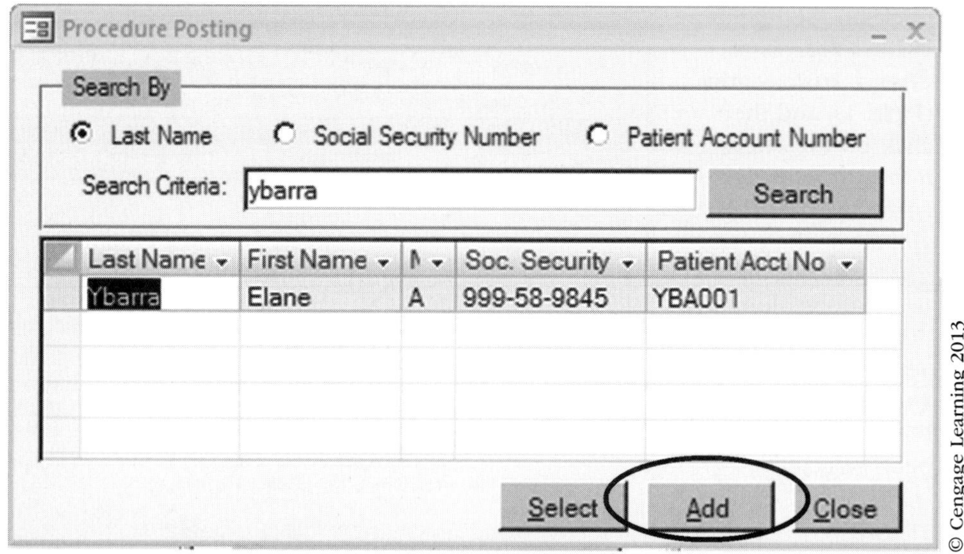

C. Using the information circled on Ms. Ybarra's encounter form, complete Fields 1-12 in the top half of the *Procedure Posting* screen. Only input information that is applicable.

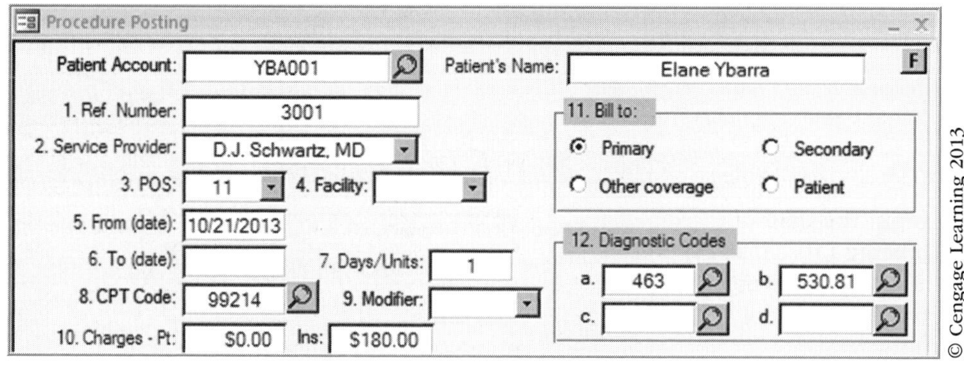

Take note that the patient has two diagnoses to enter.

D. Click on the *Post* button to apply the charges to the patient account.

E. Review the *Posting Detail* and check your work.

F. Close the *Procedure Posting* screen and return to the patient selection list.

4. Posting Procedures and a Payment: Patient Merricks

The medical biller will post procedures to Patient Merricks's account as provided on the encounter form (superbill) that was completed by the doctor and clinical staff. The payment made at the time of service will also be posted to the patient account.

A. Look at the encounter form (superbill) for Patient Merricks, reference number 3002 **(Source Documents: Encounter Forms).**

B. Click on *Procedure Posting*, find Patient Merricks and then click the *Add* button.

C. Using the information circled on Deanna Merricks' encounter form, complete Fields 1-12 in the top half of the *Procedure Posting* screen. Only input information that is applicable.

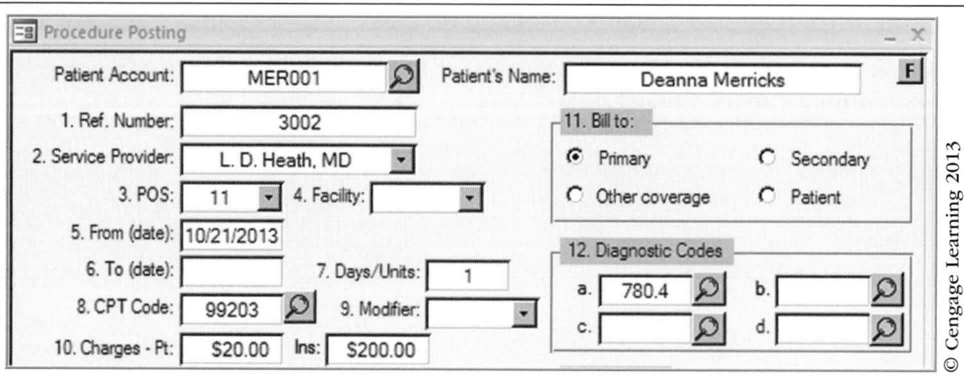

D. Click on the *Post* button to apply the charges to the patient account.

E. Review the *Posting Detail* and check your work.

F. Close all screens and return to the *Main Menu* in MOSS.

G. Click on the *Posting Payments* button and find Deanna Merricks, then click on the *Apply Payment* button.

H. Click on the line item in the *Procedure Charge History* area (Field 1), and then click on the *Select/ Edit* button. Make certain Field 13 shows the correct *Balance Due.*

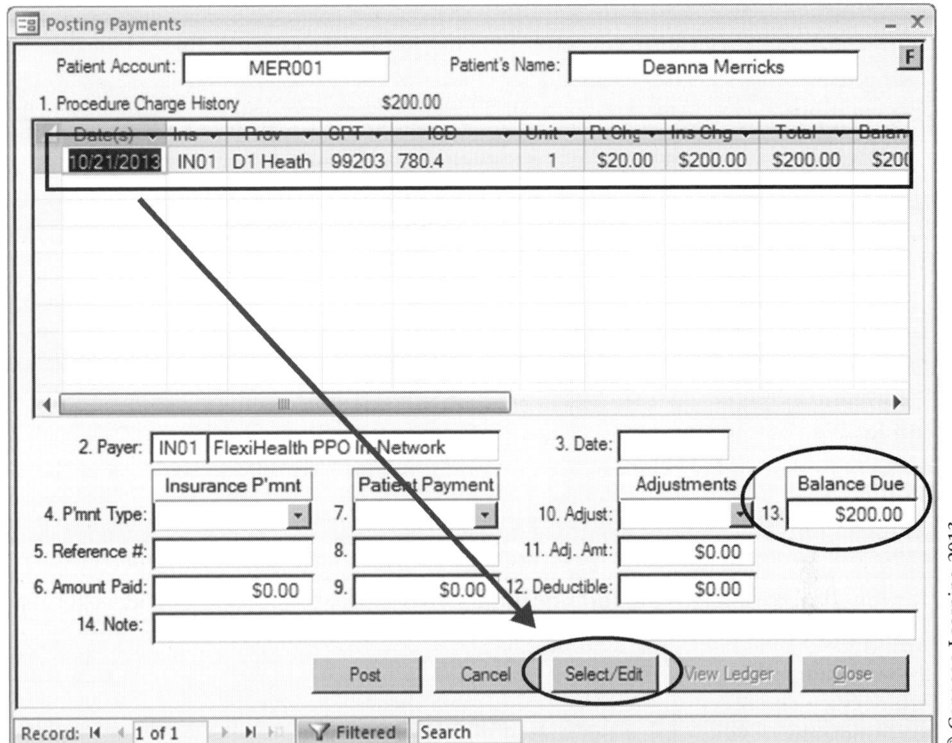

© Cengage Learning 2013

I. Input the date of posting (10/21/2013) and the following patient payment information:

2. Payer: IN01 FlexiHealth PPO In-Network | 3. Date: 10/21/2013 | Insurance P'mnt | Patient Payment | Adjustments | Balance Due | 4. P'mnt Type: | 7. PATCHECK | 10. Adjust: | 13. $180.00 | 5. Reference #: | 8. 325 | 11. Adj. Amt: $0.00 | 6. Amount Paid: $0.00 | 9. $20.00 | 12. Deductible: $0.00 | 14. Note: | Post | Cancel | Select/Edit | View Ledger | Close

© Cengage Learning 2013

Paid by check (Field 7)

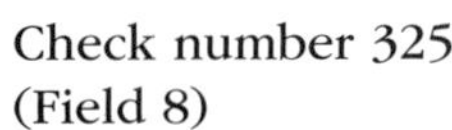

Check number 325 (Field 8)

Amount of payment $20.00 (Field 9)

Press *Enter* when finished to update the *Balance Due* (Field 13)

J. Click the *Post* button to apply the payment.

K. Close all screens and return to the *Main Menu* in MOSS.

5. Posting Procedures: Patient Cartwright

The medical biller will post procedures to Patient Cartwright's account as provided on the encounter form (superbill) that was completed by the doctor and clinical staff.

A. Look at the encounter form (superbill) for Patient Cartwright, reference number 3003 **(Source Documents: Encounter Forms).**

B. Click on *Procedure Posting*, search for Patient Cartwright and then click the *Add* button.

C. Using the information circled on Patient Cartwright's encounter form, complete Fields 1-12 in the top half of the *Procedure Posting* screen. Only input information that is applicable.

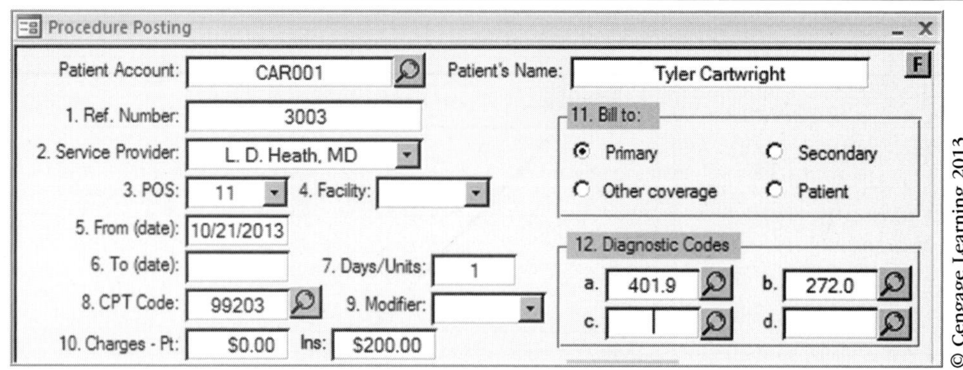

Take note that the patient has two procedures and two diagnoses.

Enter the office visit first.

D. Click on the *Post* button to apply the first charge to the patient account.

E. Review the *Posting Detail* and check your work.

F. Using the same screen, enter the lab service next and click the *Post* button.

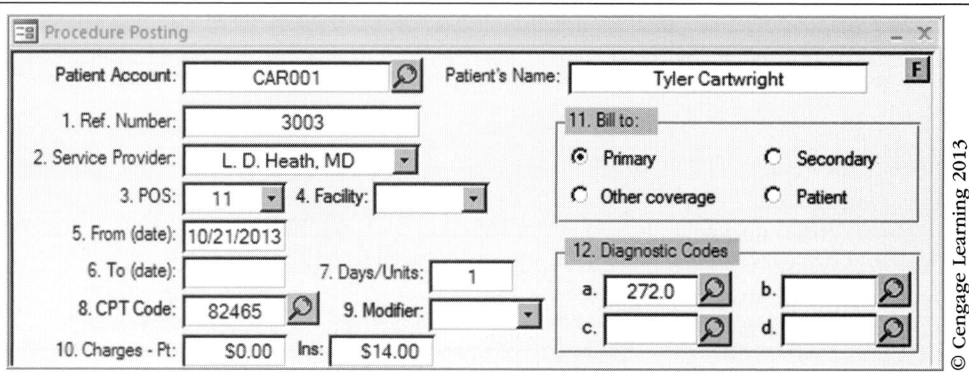

G. Now, highlight the lab charge in the Posting Detail, and click on the *Extended Billing Information* button.

The extended billing information informs the insurance plan (Medicare) where the labs were sent for processing and the total charges for the procedure billed by the physician's office.

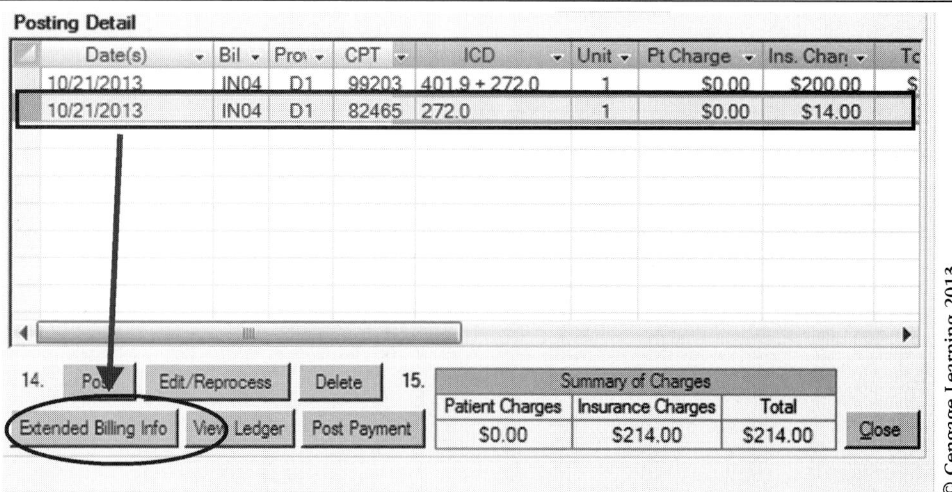

H. The *Extended Billing Information* screen opens. Input data for Fields 7, 8, and 9 as follows:

Field 7: Check the box *Outside Lab.*

Field 8: Enter $14.00 (charges for lab).

Field 9: Select *BioPace Laboratory* from the list (click on magnifying glass).

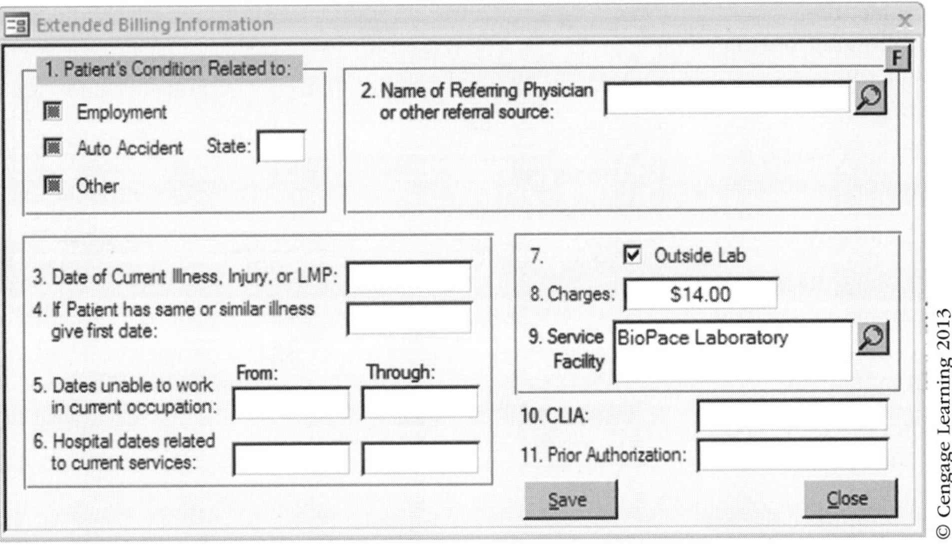

© Cengage Learning 2013

I. Click *Save* in the *Extended Billing* screen. Click *OK* through the confirmation prompt. Click *Close* when finished and return to the *Procedure Posting* screen.

J. Review the *Posting Detail* and check your work.

K. Close the *Procedure Posting* screen and return to the *Main Menu* in MOSS.

Today's Date Is Thursday, 10/31/2013

Simulation: You are the administrative medical assistant for the doctors of Douglasville Medicine Associates. At the end of each month, you are responsible for printing and mailing patient statements and providing dun messages as required.

6. Preparing Patient Statements Using MOSS

The administrative assistant will prepare and mail statements to patients who have had their insurance plans billed for services during the month of October 2013. These plans are pending payment from the primary insurance carrier.

A. Click on the *Patient Billing* button on the *Main Menu* in MOSS.

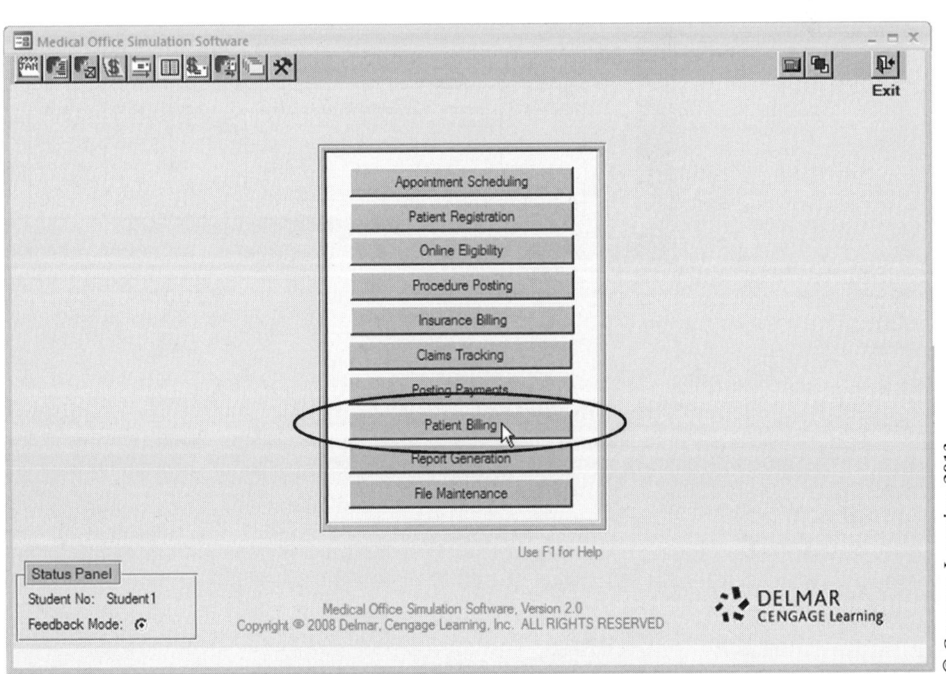

© Cengage Learning 2013

B. Select the following settings for the *Patient Billing* screen.

Field 1: 30-60-90 Standard Statement

Field 2: All

Field 3: Service dates: 10/01/2013 through 10/31/2013

Report Date: 10/31/2013

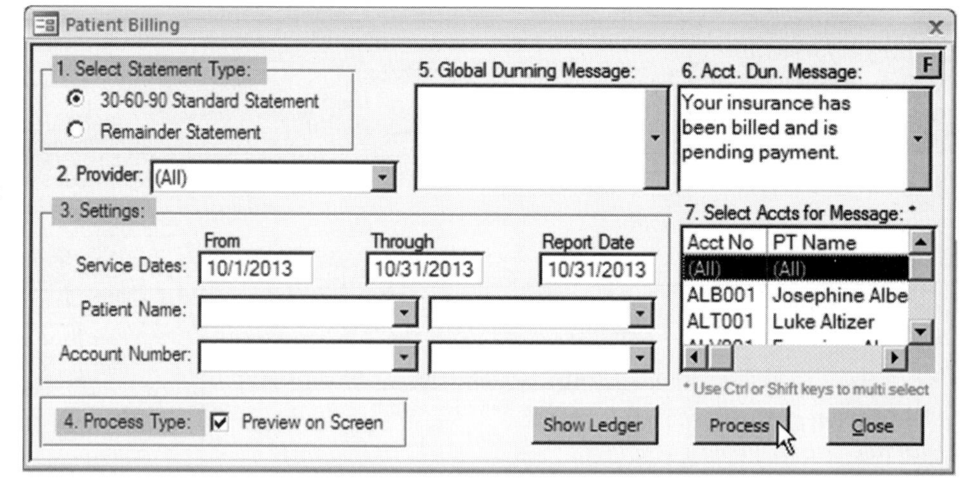

© Cengage Learning 2013

Field 4: Preview on screen

Field 5: Leave blank

Field 6: Type the following dun message in the box: “Your insurance has been billed and is pending payment.”

Field 7: All

C. Click on the *Process* button to view the statements.

Note: Click on the drop down button Size box if a larger viewing size is required.

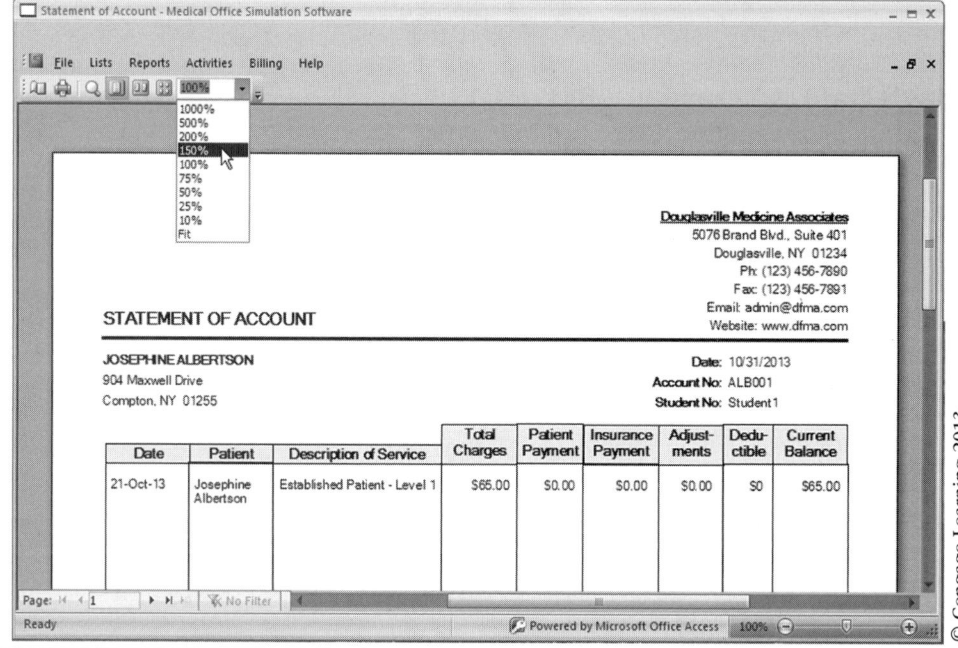

Date	Patient	Description of Service	Total Charges	Patient Payment	Insurance Payment	Adjust-ments	Dedu-ctible	Current Balance
21-Oct-13	Josephine Albertson	Established Patient - Level 1	$65.00	$0.00	$0.00	$0.00	$0	$65.00

© Cengage Learning 2013

D. A total of five statements have been produced. To view each one, use the record bar at the lower left of the screen.

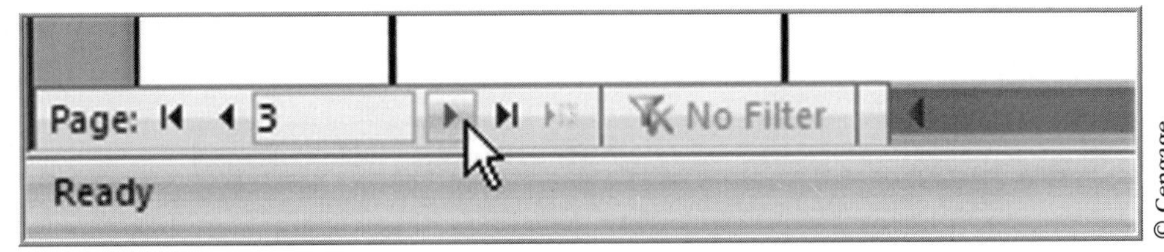

© Cengage Learning 2013

E. Review the balance due from each patient, and check that the dun message is on each statement.

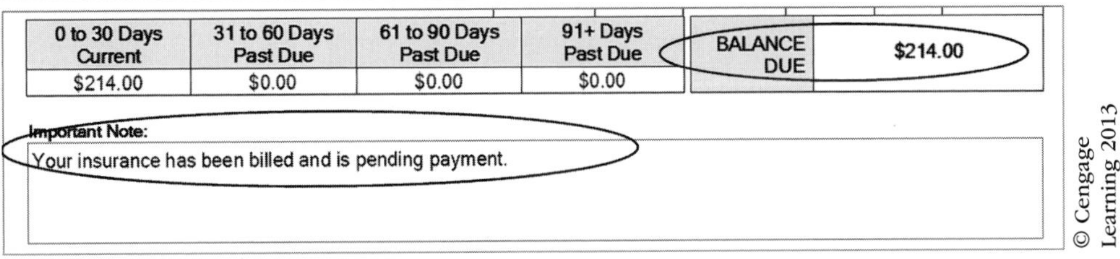

0 to 30 Days Current	31 to 60 Days Past Due	61 to 90 Days Past Due	91+ Days Past Due	BALANCE DUE	$214.00
$214.00	$0.00	$0.00	$0.00		

Important Note:
Your insurance has been billed and is pending payment.

© Cengage Learning 2013

F. Print the statements using the *Print icon* on the upper left screen.

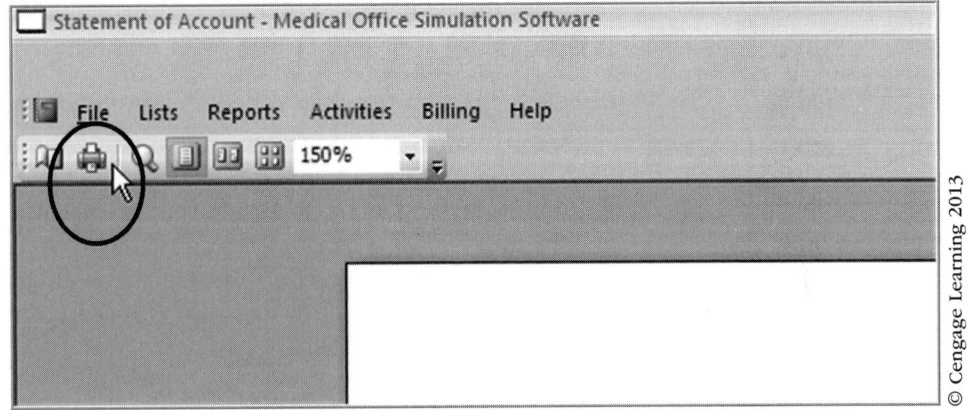

© Cengage Learning 2013

G. Close the statements window, and then close the *Patient Billing* screen and return to the *Main Menu* in MOSS.

Computer Competency Source Documents: Encounter Forms

PLEASE RETURN THIS FORM TO RECEPTIONIST

NAME Deanna Merricks

Receipt No: 3002

PLACE OF SERVICE: (X) OFFICE ( ) NEW YORK COUNTY HOSPITAL ( ) COMMUNITY GENERAL HOSPITAL ( ) RETIREMENT INN NURSING HOME ( ) ______

DATE OF SERVICE 10/21/2013

A. OFFICE VISITS - New Patient

	Code	History	Exam	Dec.	Time	
	99201	Prob. Foc.	Prob. Foc.	Straight	10 min.	
	99202	Ex. Prob. Foc.	Ex. Prob. Foc.	Straight	20 min.	
X	99203	Detail	Detail	Low	30 min.	1
	99204	Comp.	Comp.	Mod.	45 min.	
	99205	Comp.	Comp.	High	60 min.	

B. OFFICE VISIT - Established Patient

	Code	History	Exam	Dec.	Time	
	99211	Minimal	Minimal	Minimal	5 min.	
	99212	Prob. Foc.	Prob. Foc.	Straight	10min.	
	99213	Ex. Prob. Foc.	Ex. Prob. Foc.	Low	15 min.	
	99214	Detail	Detail	Mod.	25 min.	
	99215	Comp.	Comp.	High	40 min.	

C. HOSPITAL CARE

	Dx	Units	Code	
1. Initial Hospital Care (30 min)			99221	
2. Subsequent Care			99231	
3. Critical Care (30-74 min)			99291	
4. each additional 30 min.			99292	
5. Discharge Services			99238	
6. Emergency Room			99282	

D. NURSING HOME CARE

	Dx	Units	Code	
Initial Care - New Pt.				
1. Expanded			99322	
2. Detailed			99323	
Subsequent Care - Estab. Pt.				
3. Problem Focused			99307	
4. Expanded			99308	
5. Detailed			99309	
5. Comprehensive			99310	

E. PROCEDURES

	Dx	Code	
1. Arthrocentesis, Small Jt.		20600	
2. Colonoscopy		45378	
3. EKG w/interpretation		93000	
4. X-Ray Chest, PA/LAT		71020	

F. LAB

	Dx	Code	
1. Blood Sugar		82947	
2. CBC w/differential		85031	
3. Cholesterol		82465	
4. Comprehensive Metabolic Panel		80053	
5. ESR		85651	
6. Hematocrit		85014	
7. Mono Screen		86308	
8. Pap Smear		88150	
9. Potassium		84132	
10. Preg. Test, Quantitative		84702	
11. Routine Venipuncture		36415	

F. Cont'd

	Dx	Units	
12. Strep Screen		87081	
13. UA, Routine w/Micro		81000	
14. UA, Routine w/o Micro		81002	
15. Uric Acid		84550	
16. VDRL		86592	
17. Wet Prep		82710	
18.			

G. INJECTIONS

	Dx	Code	
1. Influenza Virus Vaccine		90658	
2. Pneumococcal Vaccine		90772	
3. Tetanus Toxoids		90703	
4. Therapeutic Subcut/IM		90732	
5. Vaccine Administration		90471	
6. Vaccine - each additional		90472	

H. MISCELLANEOUS

1. ______
2. ______

AMOUNT PAID $ 20.00
ck# 325

Mark diagnosis with (1=Primary, 2=Secondary, 3=Tertiary)

DIAGNOSIS NOT LISTED BELOW ______

DIAGNOSIS	ICD-9-CM	1, 2, 3
Abdominal Pain	789.0_	
Allergic Rhinitis, Unspec.	477.9	
Angina Pectoris, Unspec.	413.9	
Anemia, Iron Deficiency, Unspec.	280.9	
Anemia, NOS	285.9	
Anemia, Pernicious	281.0	
Asthma w/ Exacerbation	493.92	
Asthmatic Bronchitis, Unspec.	493.90	
Atrial Fibrillation	427.31	
Atypical Chest Pain, Unspec.	786.59	
Bronchiolitis, due to RSV	466.11	
Bronchitis, Acute	466.0	
Bronchitis, NOS	490	
Cardiac Arrest	427.5	
Cardiopulmonary Disease, Chronic, Unspec.	416.9	
Cellulitis, NOS	682.9	
Congestive Heart Failure, Unspec.	428.0	
Contact Dermatitis NOS	692.9	
COPD NOS	496	
CVA, Acute, NOS	434.91	
CVA, Old or Healed	438.9	
Degenerative Arthritis (Specify Site) ______	715.9	
Dehydration	276.51	
Depression, NOS	311	
Diabetes Mellitus, Type II Controlled	250.00	
Diabetes Mellitus, Type II Controlled	250.02	
Drug Reaction, NOS	995.29	
Dysuria	788.1	
Eczema, NOS	692.2	
Edema	782.3	
Fever, Unknown Origin	780.6	
Gastritis, Acute w/o Hemorrhage	535.00	
Gastroenteritis, NOS	558.9	
Gastroesophageal Reflux	530.81	
Hepatitis A, Infectious	070.1	
Hypercholesterolemia, Pure	272.0	
Hypertension, Unspec.	401.9	
Hypoglycemia NOS	251.2	
Hypokalemia	276.8	
Impetigo	684	
Lymphadenitis, Unspec.	289.3	
Mononucleosis	075	
Myocardial Infarction, Acute, NOS	410.9	
Organic Brain Syndrome	310.9	
Otitis Externa, Acute NOS	380.10	
Otitis Media, Acute NOS	382.9	
Peptic Ulcer Disease	536.9	
Peripheral Vascular Disease NOS	443.9	
Pharyngitis, Acute	462	
Pneumonia, Organism Unspec.	486	
Prostatitis, NOS	601.9	
PVC	427.69	
Rash, Non Specific	782.1	
Seizure Disorder NOS	780.39	
Serous Otitis Media, Chronic, Unspec.	381.10	
Sinusitis, Acute NOS	461.9	
Tonsillitis, Acute	463.	
Upper Respiratory Infection, Acute NOS	465.9	
Urinary Tract Infection, Unspec.	599.0	
Urticaria, Unspec.	708.9	
Vertigo, NOS	780.4	1
Viral Infection NOS	079.99	
Weakness, Generalized	780.79	
Weight Loss, Abnormal	783.21	

ABN: I UNDERSTAND THAT MEDICARE PROBABLY WILL NOT COVER THE SERVICES LISTED BELOW

A. ______ B. ______ C. ______

Date ______ Patient Signature ______

Doctor's Signature L.D. Heath, MD

RETURN: ______ Days ______ Weeks PRN Months

DOUGLASVILLE MEDICINE ASSOCIATES
5076 BRAND BLVD., SUITE 401
DOUGLASVILLE, NY 01234
PHONE No. (123) 456-7890

☒ L.D. HEATH, M.D. NPI# 9995010111
☐ D.J. SCHWARTZ, M.D. NPI# 9995020212
EIN# 00-1234560

REF# 122949 SB (05 07 09) TO REORDER CALL INHEALTH RECORD SYSTEMS 800-477-7374

Used with permission. InHealth Record Systems, Inc. 5076 Winters Chapel Road, Atlanta, GA 30360, 800-477-7374. http://www.inhealthrecords.com

PLEASE RETURN THIS FORM TO RECEPTIONIST

NAME Tyler Cartwright

Receipt No: 3003

PLACE OF SERVICE:
(X) OFFICE
( ) NEW YORK COUNTY HOSPITAL
( ) COMMUNITY GENERAL HOSPITAL
( ) RETIREMENT INN NURSING HOME
( ) ____

DATE OF SERVICE 10/21/2013

A. OFFICE VISITS - New Patient

	Code	History	Exam	Dec.	Time	
	99201	Prob. Foc.	Prob. Foc.	Straight	10 min.	
	99202	Ex. Prob. Foc.	Ex. Prob. Foc.	Straight	20 min.	
X	99203	Detail	Detail	Low	30 min.	1, 2
	99204	Comp.	Comp.	Mod.	45 min.	
	99205	Comp.	Comp.	High	60 min.	

B. OFFICE VISIT - Established Patient

	Code	History	Exam	Dec.	Time	
	99211	Minimal	Minimal	Minimal	5 min.	
	99212	Prob. Foc.	Prob. Foc.	Straight	10min.	
	99213	Ex. Prob. Foc.	Ex. Prob. Foc.	Low	15 min.	
	99214	Detail	Detail	Mod.	25 min.	
	99215	Comp.	Comp.	High	40 min.	

C. HOSPITAL CARE

	Dx	Units	Code	
1. Initial Hospital Care (30 min)			99221	
2. Subsequent Care			99231	
3. Critical Care (30-74 min)			99291	
4. each additional 30 min.			99292	
5. Discharge Services			99238	
6. Emergency Room			99282	

D. NURSING HOME CARE

	Dx	Units	Code	
Initial Care - New Pt.				
1. Expanded			99322	
2. Detailed			99323	
Subsequent Care - Estab. Pt.				
3. Problem Focused			99307	
4. Expanded			99308	
5. Detailed			99309	
5. Comprehensive			99310	

E. PROCEDURES

	Dx	Code	Units
1. Arthrocentesis, Small Jt.		20600	
2. Colonoscopy		45378	
3. EKG w/interpretation		93000	
4. X-Ray Chest, PA/LAT		71020	

F. LAB

	Dx	Code	Units
1. Blood Sugar		82947	
2. CBC w/differential		85031	
3. Cholesterol	2	82465	X
4. Comprehensive Metabolic Panel		80053	
5. ESR		85651	
6. Hematocrit		85014	
7. Mono Screen		86308	
8. Pap Smear		88150	
9. Potassium		84132	
10. Preg. Test, Quantitative		84702	
11. Routine Venipuncture		36415	

F. Cont'd

	Dx	Code	Units
12. Strep Screen		87081	
13. UA, Routine w/Micro		81000	
14. UA, Routine w/o Micro		81002	
15. Uric Acid		84550	
16. VDRL		86592	
17. Wet Prep		82710	
18.			

G. INJECTIONS

	Dx	Code	Units
1. Influenza Virus Vaccine		90658	
2. Pneumococcal Vaccine		90772	
3. Tetanus Toxoids		90703	
4. Therapeutic Subcut/IM		90732	
5. Vaccine Administration		90471	
6. Vaccine - each additional		90472	

H. MISCELLANEOUS

1. ____
2. ____

AMOUNT PAID $ Ø

Mark diagnosis with (1=Primary, 2=Secondary, 3=Tertiary)

DIAGNOSIS NOT LISTED BELOW ____

DIAGNOSIS	ICD-9-CM	1, 2, 3
Abdominal Pain	789.0_	
Allergic Rhinitis, Unspec.	477.9	
Angina Pectoris, Unspec.	413.9	
Anemia, Iron Deficiency, Unspec.	280.9	
Anemia, NOS	285.9	
Anemia, Pernicious	281.0	
Asthma w/ Exacerbation	493.92	
Asthmatic Bronchitis, Unspec.	493.90	
Atrial Fibrillation	427.31	
Atypical Chest Pain, Unspec.	786.59	
Bronchiolitis, due to RSV	466.11	
Bronchitis, Acute	466.0	
Bronchitis, NOS	490	
Cardiac Arrest	427.5	
Cardiopulmonary Disease, Chronic, Unspec.	416.9	
Cellulitis, NOS	682.9	
Congestive Heart Failure, Unspec.	428.0	
Contact Dermatitis NOS	692.9	
COPD NOS	496	
CVA, Acute, NOS	434.91	
CVA, Old or Healed	438.9	
Degenerative Arthritis (Specify Site) ____	715.9	
Dehydration	276.51	
Depression, NOS	311	
Diabetes Mellitus, Type II Controlled	250.00	
Diabetes Mellitus, Type II Controlled	250.02	
Drug Reaction, NOS	995.29	
Dysuria	788.1	
Eczema, NOS	692.2	
Edema	782.3	
Fever, Unknown Origin	780.6	
Gastritis, Acute w/o Hemorrhage	535.00	
Gastroenteritis, NOS	558.9	
Gastroesophageal Reflux	530.81	
Hepatitis A, Infectious	070.1	
Hypercholesterolemia, Pure	272.0	2
Hypertension, Unspec.	401.9	1
Hypoglycemia NOS	251.2	
Hypokalemia	276.8	
Impetigo	684	
Lymphadenitis, Unspec.	289.3	
Mononucleosis	075	
Myocardial Infarction, Acute, NOS	410.9	
Organic Brain Syndrome	310.9	
Otitis Externa, Acute NOS	380.10	
Otitis Media, Acute NOS	382.9	
Peptic Ulcer Disease	536.9	
Peripheral Vascular Disease NOS	443.9	
Pharyngitis, Acute	462	
Pneumonia, Organism Unspec.	486	
Prostatitis, NOS	601.9	
PVC	427.69	
Rash, Non Specific	782.1	
Seizure Disorder NOS	780.39	
Serous Otitis Media, Chronic, Unspec.	381.10	
Sinusitis, Acute NOS	461.9	
Tonsillitis, Acute	463.	
Upper Respiratory Infection, Acute NOS	465.9	
Urinary Tract Infection, Unspec.	599.0	
Urticaria, Unspec.	708.9	
Vertigo, NOS	780.4	
Viral Infection NOS	079.99	
Weakness, Generalized	780.79	
Weight Loss, Abnormal	783.21	

ABN: I UNDERSTAND THAT MEDICARE PROBABLY WILL NOT COVER THE SERVICES LISTED BELOW

A. ____ B. ____ C. ____

Date ____ Patient Signature ____

Doctor's Signature L. D. Heath

RETURN: ____ Days ____ Weeks PRN ____ Months

DOUGLASVILLE MEDICINE ASSOCIATES
5076 BRAND BLVD., SUITE 401
DOUGLASVILLE, NY 01234
PHONE No. (123) 456-7890

☒ L.D. HEATH, M.D. NPI# 9995010111
☐ D.J. SCHWARTZ, M.D. NPI# 9995020212
EIN# 00-1234560

REF# 122949 SB (05 07 09) TO REORDER CALL INHEALTH RECORD SYSTEMS 800-477-7374

Used with permission. InHealth Record Systems, Inc. 5076 Winters Chapel Road, Atlanta, GA 30360, 800-477-7374. http://www.inhealthrecords.com

BOOKKEEPING JOB SKILLS 15-1 THROUGH 15-12

Job Skills 15-1 through 15-12 take you through step-by-step procedures to gain experience in bookkeeping practices. Although these job skills utilize the pegboard bookkeeping system, the concepts learned apply to computerized bookkeeping and will help you understand posting steps needed in both systems and computations automatically done in computerized systems. Job Skills 15-2 through 15-5 (Day 1), 15-6 through 15-8 (Day 2), and 15-9 through 15-11 (Day 3) may be assigned individually; however, they must be done in order. Instead, the instructor may choose to assign these job skills as three projects to be done in class or as homework. Each grouping represents a different day in the medical practice that requires various posting, calculating, and balancing of financial records. Job Skill 15-1 involves setting up 28 ledger cards that will be used in the rest of the job skills. Job Skill 15-12 involves setting up a daysheet for a new month. You will also be looking up procedure (*CPT*) codes and using the fee schedule found in Part III of this *Workbook*. The selection of codes are arranged according to sections found in the 2012 *Current Procedural Terminology** code book. Locate the section and subsection as indicated, then find the description. Last, determine the patient's insurance and locate the fee according to the insurance type and categories listed. With each job skill, read it entirely before beginning.

*2012 Current Procedural Terminology © *2011 American Medical Association. All rights reserved.*

JOB SKILL 15-1
Prepare Ledger Cards

Name ______________________________ Date ____________ Score ________

Performance Objective

Task: Insert demographic information and post a balance forward to set up 28 ledger cards and arrange them in alphabetical sequence. These will be used for future job skills in this chapter.

Conditions: Use 14 sheets of ledger cards (Forms 62 through 75) for a total of 28 ledgers and typewriter or pen.

Standards: Complete all steps listed in this skill in ________ minutes with a minimum score of ________. (Time element and accuracy criteria may be given by instructor.)

Time: **Start:** ____________ **Completed:** ____________ **Total:** ____________ minutes

Scoring: One point for each step performed satisfactorily unless otherwise listed or weighted by instructor.

Directions with Performance Evaluation Checklist

Set up ledger cards for the following patients by typing or filling in their names, addresses, telephone numbers, dates of birth (DOB), and insurance information; each member of a family has a separate ledger. Indicate the current year in the first "DATE" column and post a balance forward on each ledger card as indicated. NOTE: If completing only Day 1 due to time constraints (Job Skills 15-2 through 15-5), you will set up 10 ledgers for patients listed in Steps 1, 3, 4, 5, 6, 7, 9, 10, 26, and 28.

1st Attempt	2nd Attempt	3rd Attempt	
______	______	______	Gather materials (equipment and supplies) listed under "Conditions."
___/10	___/10	___/10	1. Set up a ledger card for Mary Lou Chaney 4902 Saviers Road Woodland Hills, XY 12345-0000 Tel: 555-490-8755—home Tel: 555-490-5578—work DOB: 7/30/50 Ins: South West Ins. ID # 459-08-7655 Previous balance: new pt
___/10	___/10	___/10	2. Set up a ledger card for Russell P. Smith 2336 East Manly Street Woodland Hills, XY 12345-0000 Tel: 555-786-0123—home Tel: 555-786-3210—work DOB: 5/6/56 Ins: Blue Cross/Blue Shield Cert. # 58557AT Group # T84 Previous balance: zero
___/10	___/10	___/10	3. Set up a ledger card for Jody F. Swinney 4300 Saunders Road Woodland Hills, XY 12345-0000 Tel: 555-908-6605—home DOB: 1/16/64 Ins: Aetna Casualty Company Policy # 7821-11 Previous balance: $25.00

JOB SKILL 15-1 *(continued)*

____/10 ____/10 ____/10 4. Set up a ledger card for Miss Adrienne Cane
6502 North J Street
Woodland Hills, XY 12345-0000
Tel: 555-498-2110—home
DOB: 7/29/46
Ins: R. L. Kautz & Company
Policy # 7821-1KBM
Previous balance: $85.00

____/10 ____/10 ____/10 5. Set up a ledger card for Mark B. Hanson
2560 South M Street
Woodland Hills, XY 12345-0000
Tel: 555-980-2210—home
Tel: 555-980-0122—work
DOB: 6/22/49
Ins: Prudential Insurance Co.
Policy # 4579
Previous balance: zero

____/10 ____/10 ____/10 6. Set up a ledger card for Robert T. Jenner
1300 Hampshire Road
Woodland Hills, XY 12345-0000
Tel: 555-986-6790—home
Tel: 555-986-0976—work
DOB: 2/28/68
Ins: Guarantee Insurance Company
Policy # 67021
Previous balance: zero

____/10 ____/10 ____/10 7. Set up a ledger card for Harold B. Mason
6107 Harcourt Street
Woodland Hills, XY 12345-0000
Tel: 555-615-0123—home
Tel: 555-615-3201—work
DOB: 8/20/46
Ins: Allstate Insurance Company
Policy # 7632111 BA
Previous balance: zero

____/10 ____/10 ____/10 8. Set up a ledger card for J. B. Haupman
15761 Dickens Street
Woodland Hills, XY 12345-0000
Tel: 555-457-0561—home
DOB: 7/23/28
Ins: Medicare
Medicare ID # XXX-XX-0988A
Previous balance: $1,466.56

____/10 ____/10 ____/10 9. Set up a ledger card for Mrs. Betty K. Lawson
6400 Best Way
Woodland Hills, XY 12345-0000
Tel: 555-450-9533—home
DOB: 1/27/69
Ins: TRICARE Extra ID # 5430982XX
Previous balance: zero

JOB SKILL 15-1 *(continued)*

____/10 ____/10 ____/10 10. Set up a ledger card for Miss Carol M. Wolf
2765 Honey Lane Street
Woodland Hills, XY 12345-0000
Tel: 555-892-0651—home
DOB: 8/25/76
Ins: Blue Cross/Blue Shield
Cert. # 76502 AT
Group # T85
Previous balance: zero

____/10 ____/10 ____/10 11. Set up a ledger card for Margaret Jenkins, RN
5692 Rose Avenue
Woodland Hills, XY 12345-0000
Tel: 555-760-3211—home
Tel: 555-760-1123—work
DOB: 6/29/70
Ins: Blue Cross/Blue Shield
Cert. # 65923AT
Group # T76
Previous balance: new pt

____/10 ____/10 ____/10 12. Set up a ledger card for Roger T. Simpson
792 Baker Street
Woodland Hills, XY 12345-0000
Tel: 555-549-0879—home
Tel: 555-549-9780—work
DOB: 11/2/52
Ins: Farmers Insurance Group
Policy # 56892
Previous balance: $45.00

____/10 ____/10 ____/10 13. Set up a ledger card for Joan Gomez
4391 Wooden Street
Woodland Hills, XY 12345-0000
Tel: 555-459-2399—home
Tel: 555-459-9932—work
DOB: 3/15/47
Ins: Fremont Indemnity Company
Policy # 56702111
Previous balance: $60.00

____/10 ____/10 ____/10 14. Set up a ledger card for Maria Bargioni
4892 Simpson Street
Woodland Hills, XY 12345-0000
Tel: 555-549-2344—home
Tel: 555-549-4432—work
DOB: 4/5/76
Ins: Fireman's Fund Insurance Companies
Policy # 568 MB 2111
Previous balance: $25.00

JOB SKILL 15-1 *(continued)*

____/10 ____/10 ____/10 15. Set up a ledger card for Jack J. Johnson
5490 Olive Mill Road
Woodland Hills, XY 12345-0000
Tel: 555-857-9920—home
DOB: 5/27/59
Ins: Medicaid
Insurance ID # 458962016
Previous balance: zero

____/10 ____/10 ____/10 16. Set up a ledger card for Lois A. Conrad
8920 Canton Street
Woodland Hills, XY 12345-0000
Tel: 555-569-2201—home
Tel: 555-569-1022—work
DOB: 5/8/55
Ins: Gates, McDonald & Company
Policy # 4591 XT
Previous balance: $31.50

____/10 ____/10 ____/10 17. Set up a ledger card for Miss Marylou Conrad, c/o Lois Conrad
8920 Canton Street
Woodland Hills, XY 12345-0000
Tel: 555-569-2201—home
DOB: 4/22/95
Ins: Gates, McDonald & Company
Policy # 4591 XT
Previous balance: zero

____/10 ____/10 ____/10 18. Set up a ledger card for Hannah F. Riley
459 Fifth Avenue
Woodland Hills, XY 12345-0000
Tel: 555-789-2201—home
Tel: 555-789-1022—work
DOB: 10/8/62
Ins: Hartford Insurance Group
Policy # 5601221
Previous balance: zero

____/10 ____/10 ____/10 19. Set up a ledger card for Stephen B. Riley Jr.
459 Fifth Avenue
Woodland Hills, XY 12345-0000
Tel: 555-789-2201—home
Tel: 555-789-1022—work
DOB: 6/29/62
Ins: Hartford Insurance Group
Policy # 5601221
Previous balance: new pt

____/10 ____/10 ____/10 20. Set up a ledger card for Rosa K. Okida
7900 Shatto Place
Woodland Hills, XY 12345-0000
Tel: 555-420-1121—home
Tel: 555-420-1211—work
DOB: 11/2/58
Ins: Home Insurance Company
Policy # 789-1191-21K
Previous balance: $201.00

JOB SKILL 15-1 *(continued)*

____/10 ____/10 ____/10 21. Set up a ledger card for Howard S. Chan
3200 Shaw Avenue
Woodland Hills, XY 12345-0000
Tel: 555-660-3211—home
Tel: 555-660-1123—work
DOB: 8/3/58
Ins: Imperial Insurance Company
Policy # 21019KBM
Previous balance: zero

____/10 ____/10 ____/10 22. Set up a ledger card for Rachel T. O'Brien
5598 East 17 Street
Woodland Hills, XY 12345-0000
Tel: 555-566-2199—home
Tel: 555-566-9912—work
DOB: 3/19/68
Ins: North America Health Net POS
Policy # 54901
Previous balance: $50.00

____/10 ____/10 ____/10 23. Set up a ledger card for Martin P. Owens
430 Herndon Place
Woodland Hills, XY 12345-0000
Tel: 555-542-2232—home
Tel: 555-542-2322—work
DOB: 12/3/73
Ins: John Deere Insurance Company
Policy # 67401 J
Previous balance: $25.00

____/10 ____/10 ____/10 24. Set up a ledger card for Joseph C. Smith
P.O. Box 4301
Woodland Hills, XY 12345-0000
Tel: 555-549-1124—home
Tel: 555-549-4211—work
DOB: 6/20/73
Ins: Home Insurance Company
Policy # 589102K
Previous balance: new pt

____/10 ____/10 ____/10 25. Set up a ledger card for Kathryn L. Hope
6680 Bascom Road
Woodland Hills, XY 12345-0000
Tel: 555-210-9980—home
Tel: 555-210-0899—work
DOB: 8/14/60
Ins: Met Life HMO
Policy # 8921
Previous balance: zero

JOB SKILL 15-1 *(continued)*

____/10 ____/10 ____/10 26. Set up a ledger card for Russell O. Smith
459 University Avenue
Woodland Hills, XY 12345-0000
Tel: 555-129-1980—home
Tel: 555-129-0891—work
DOB: 2/15/65
Ins: International Insurance Company
Policy # 8901
Previous balance: new pt

____/10 ____/10 ____/10 27. Set up a ledger card for Charlotte J. Brown
769 Sky Park Circle
Woodland Hills, XY 12345-0000
Tel: 555-780-2341—home
Tel: 555-780-1432—work
DOB: 9/5/66
Ins: Kemper Insurance Company
Policy # 5769
Previous balance: $35.00

____/3 ____/3 ____/3 28. Set up a ledger card with the heading "Miscellaneous Other Income" to be used to record charges and payments for lectures, published articles, and other miscellaneous items; previous balance zero.

____/28 ____/28 ____/28 29. Cut ledger cards apart and arrange them in alphabetical sequence with the "Miscellaneous Other Income" ledger at the end of the file.

_______ _______ _______ Complete within specified time.

___/303 ___/303 ___/303 **Total points earned** (To obtain a percentage score, divide the total points earned by the number of points possible.)

Comments:

Evaluator's Signature: ______________________________ **Need to Repeat:** ______________

National Curriculum Competency: CAAHEP: Cognitive: II.C.1, V.C.10	ABHES: 8.k

JOB SKILL 15-2
Bookkeeping Day 1—Post to Patient Ledger Cards and Prepare Cash Receipts

Name ______________________________ Date ______________ Score ________

Performance Objective

Task: Post charges and payments to patient ledger cards, calculate running balances, and prepare cash receipts.

Conditions: Select ledger cards, which have been alphabetized, from Job Skill 15-1. Use five checks received by Practon Medical Group (Forms 76 and 77), cash receipts (Form 78), calculator, and pencil. Refer to *textbook* Figure 15-2A and Figure 15-5 for posting illustrations and Figure 15-6 for a cash receipt example.

Standards: Complete all steps listed in this skill in _______ minutes with a minimum score of ________. (Time element and accuracy criteria may be given by instructor.)

Time: **Start:** ____________ **Completed:** ____________ **Total:** ____________ minutes

Scoring: One point for each step performed satisfactorily unless otherwise listed or weighted by instructor.

Directions with Performance Evaluation Checklist

It is June 28, current year. Pull ledger cards for patients who are on today's schedule (they are highlighted in step-by-step instructions in **boldface**). Post all charges (line by line), referring to the "Mock Fee Schedule" (Figure A-1 in Part III of this *Workbook*) to obtain fees; calculate a running balance for each line of posting. For all commercial (private) insurance programs, Medicaid, and TRICARE, use figures from the "Mock Fees." Cut checks apart and post all payments after charges have been posted; calculate balance due. Complete a receipt for all patients who paid cash using Form 78.

1st Attempt	2nd Attempt	3rd Attempt	
______	______	______	Gather materials (equipment and supplies) listed under "Conditions."
____/20	____/20	____/20	1. Post charges for patient **Mark B. Hanson**. Est Pt OV Level II (E/M Section) Post cash payment (patient paid in full); indicate receipt number in reference column. Complete cash receipt No. 147 (see Form 78).
____/5	____/5	____/5	2. Post charges for patient **Russell O. Smith**. NP Office Consult Level III (E/M Section)
____/20	____/20	____/20	3. Post charges for patient **Betty K. Lawson**. Est Pt Level I OV (E/M Section) Therapeutic injection (IM—Medicine Section) Vitamin B12 (medication supply—Special Services and Reports); fee $9. Post copayment received by check (see Form 77).
____/10	____/10	____/10	4. Post charges for patient **Jody F. Swinney**. Est Pt Level II OV (E/M Section) Post copayment received by check (see Form 77).
____/30	____/30	____/30	5. Post charges for patient **Mary Lou Chaney**. NP Level IV OV (E/M Section) UA (nonautomated with microscopy—Laboratory Section) Comprehensive audiometry (Medicine Section)

JOB SKILL 15-2 *(continued)*

Post cash payment (patient paid in full) and indicate receipt number in reference column.
Complete cash receipt No. 148 (see Form 78).

___/15 ___/15 ___/15 6. Post charges for patient **Carol M. Wolf**.
Est Pt Level I OV (E/M Section)
DPT Immunization Injection (vaccine product—Medicine Section)
Immunization administration (DPT—Medicine Section); fee $2.50

___/10 ___/10 ___/10 7. Post charges for patient **Harold B. Mason**.
Est Pt Level II OV (E/M Section)
ECG (Medicine Section)

___/5 ___/5 ___/5 8. Post charges for patient **Robert T. Jenner**.
Initial hospital care (30 minutes, Level I—E/M Section)

INCOMING MAIL: Several checks have been received in the mail today (see Form 76). Some will be posted to the "Miscellaneous Other Income" account. When payments are posted to this account, post the charges at the same time the check is received; this is standard office protocol.

___/6 ___/6 ___/6 9. Post check from ***Family Health Magazine*** for article written by Dr. Gerald Practon.

___/6 ___/6 ___/6 10. Post check from **Colony Boys School** for lecture by Dr. Fran Practon.

___/5 ___/5 ___/5 11. Post personal check from patient **Adrienne Cane**; payment on account.

___ ___ ___ Complete within specified time.

___/134 ___/134 ___/134 **Total points earned** (To obtain a percentage score, divide the total points earned by the number of points possible.)

Comments:

Evaluator's Signature: ________________ **Need to Repeat:** ________

National Curriculum Competency: CAAHEP: Cognitive: VI.P.2	ABHES: 8.k

JOB SKILL 15-3
Bookkeeping Day 1—Prepare the Daily Journal

Name ______________________________ Date ______________ Score ________

Performance Objective

Task: Set up the daily journal by inserting figures from the previous day's totals.

Conditions: Daily journal—Day 1 (Form 79) and pencil. You may want to use a photocopy machine to enlarge this to legal size to ease handwritten entries. See the daily journal posting illustration in *textbook* Figure 15-5 and step-by-step directions in *textbook* Procedure 15-1.

Standards: Complete all steps listed in this skill in _______ minutes with a minimum score of ________. (Time element and accuracy criteria may be given by instructor.)

Time: **Start:** ____________ **Completed:** ____________ **Total:** ____________ minutes

Scoring: One point for each step performed satisfactorily unless otherwise listed or weighted by instructor.

Directions with Performance Evaluation Checklist

1st Attempt	2nd Attempt	3rd Attempt	
_____	_____	_____	Gather materials (equipment and supplies) listed under "Conditions."
____/2	____/2	____/2	1. It is June 28, current year. Enter this date on the top of the daysheet and in the "Record of Deposits" area and use it for all transactions that will occur today.
____/2	____/2	____/2	2. All transactions for June 28, 20XX, will fit on one daysheet; label it page 1 of 1.
____/2	____/2	____/2	3. Insert the daily journal (daysheet) previous page total ($14,336.60) for Column A from the previous day, June 27, 20XX.
____/2	____/2	____/2	4. Insert the daily journal previous page total ($8,592.41) for Column B-1 from the previous day, June 27, 20XX.
____/2	____/2	____/2	5. Insert the daily journal previous page total ($450.00) for Column B-2 from the previous day, June 27, 20XX.
____/2	____/2	____/2	6. Insert the daily journal previous page total ($1,387.56) for Column C from the previous day, June 27, 20XX.
____/2	____/2	____/2	7. Insert the daily journal previous page total ($980.00) for Column D from the previous day, June 27, 20XX.
____/2	____/2	____/2	8. Enter the "Accounts Receivable Control," "Previous Day's Total" figure: $30,526.32.
____/2	____/2	____/2	9. Enter "Accounts Receivable Proof," "First of Month" figure: $25,232.13.
____/2	____/2	____/2	10. Enter the "Beginning Cash On Hand" figure: $50.00.
____/2	____/2	____/2	11. Insert your name at the bottom of the daysheet in the "Prepared by" area.
_____	_____	_____	Complete within specified time.
____24	____24	____24	**Total points earned** (To obtain a percentage score, divide the total points earned by the number of points possible.)

JOB SKILL 15-3 *(continued)*

Comments:

Evaluator's Signature: ______________________ **Need to Repeat:** ____________

National Curriculum Competency: CAAHEP: Psychomotor: VI.P.2	ABHES: 8.a, h

JOB SKILL 15-4
Bookkeeping Day 1—Post Charges, Payments, and Adjustments Using a Daily Journal

Name ______________________________ Date ______________ Score ________

Performance Objective

Task: Post charges, payments, and adjustments on the daily journal; record payments on the bank deposit slip and in the cash control section; endorse checks and prepare the bank deposit.

Conditions: Ledgers used in Job Skill 15-2, daysheet prepared in Job Skill 15-3, checks (Forms 76 and 77) used in Job Skill 15-2, number 10 envelope, calculator, and pencil. Refer to *textbook* Procedure 15-1 for step-by-step directions.

Standards: Complete all steps listed in this skill in _______ minutes with a minimum score of ________. (Time element and accuracy criteria may be given by instructor.)

Time: **Start:** ____________ **Completed:** ____________ **Total:** ____________ minutes

Scoring: One point for each step performed satisfactorily unless otherwise listed or weighted by instructor.

Directions with Performance Evaluation Checklist

Daily Journal Instructions

Post all charges, payments, and adjustments for each patient seen on a *single line* of the daysheet. Specific instructions follow:

COLUMNS:

Date: Enter date of posting in first column (e.g., 6/28/20XX).

Reference: This column may be used for various references. For this exercise, all charges and payments for each patient's professional services taking place today will be posted on **one line**; use this column to enter the patient's check number when payment is received (e.g., ck 123).

Description: Enter *CPT* code numbers for all professional services rendered. Enter "Miscellaneous Other Income" to designate the ledger you are posting to for checks received from other sources.

Charges: List **total** charge for **all** professional services rendered by each patient.

Credits—Payments: List payment amount.

Credits—Adjustments: List the amount to be written off the account.

Balance: Add the previous balance to charges and subtract credits (payments and adjustments) to obtain the current balance.

Previous Balance: Obtain and enter the amount extended from each patient's ledger card.

Name: Enter last name, first name, and middle initial.

Numbered Lines: Each line is numbered for reference to help with posting accuracy.

Receipt Number: Enter the number from the cash receipt.

RECORD OF DEPOSITS: Make a photocopy of the "Record of Deposit" section of the daysheet to use as a bank deposit slip. At the top of the *deposit slip*, insert the name of the bank (The First National Bank) and checking account number (12345-6789).

Date: Enter the current date on top of the daily journal form.

ABA: Enter the bank ABA number listed on check.

Cash: Enter amount of cash payment.

Checks: Enter amount of check payment.

BUSINESS ANALYSIS SUMMARY: Label and enter the copayment amount in Column 1; other columns may be used for various entries depending on the needs of the office.

JOB SKILL 15-4 *(continued)*

For posting information, refer to the ledgers used to post current charges and payments in Job Skill 15-2. In a pegboard bookkeeping system, journal entries will be automatically posted as they are written on ledgers by means of NCR paper. In a computerized system, journal entries will be automatically posted as they are input into the patient's account.

1st Attempt	2nd Attempt	3rd Attempt	
______	______	______	Gather materials (equipment and supplies) listed under "Conditions."
____/7	____/7	____/7	1. Post charge and payment for **Mark B. Hanson**.
____/5	____/5	____/5	2. Post charge for **Russell O. Smith**.
____/10	____/10	____/10	3. Post charges and copayment for **Betty K. Lawson**.
____/10	____/10	____/10	4. Post charge and copayment for **Jody F. Swinney**.
____/7	____/7	____/7	5. Post charges and payment for **Mary Lou Chaney**.
____/5	____/5	____/5	6. Post charges for **Carol M. Wolf**.
____/5	____/5	____/5	7. Post charges for **Harold B. Mason**.
____/5	____/5	____/5	8. Post charge for **Robert T. Jenner**.
____/8	____/8	____/8	9. Post check (and charge) from ***Family Health Magazine***.
____/8	____/8	____/8	10. Post check (and charge) from **Colony Boys School**.
____/9	____/9	____/9	11. Post personal check from **Adrienne Cane**.
____/3	____/3	____/3	12. Add the proper endorsement for all checks received. Total the deposit and put them in an envelope with the bank slip.
______	______	______	Complete within specified time.
____/84	____/84	____/84	**Total points earned** (To obtain a percentage score, divide the total points earned by the number of points possible.)

Comments:

Evaluator's Signature: ______________________________ **Need to Repeat:** ____________

National Curriculum Competency: CAAHEP: Psychomotor: VI.P.2.a	ABHES: 8.h

JOB SKILL 15-5
Bookkeeping Day 1—Balance the Daysheet

Name ______________________________ Date ______________ Score ________

Performance Objective

Task: Total all columns on the daysheet, add previous page totals, and enter new figures in month-to-date areas.

Conditions: Daysheet (Day 1) used in Job Skills 15-3 and 15-4, calculator, and pencil. Refer to *textbook* Procedure 15-1 for step-by-step directions.

Standards: Complete all steps listed in this skill in _______ minutes with a minimum score of ________. (Time element and accuracy criteria may be given by instructor.)

Time: **Start:** ____________ **Completed:** ____________ **Total:** ____________ minutes

Scoring: One point for each step performed satisfactorily unless otherwise listed or weighted by instructor.

Directions with Performance Evaluation Checklist

1st Attempt	2nd Attempt	3rd Attempt	
_______	_______	_______	Gather materials (equipment and supplies) listed under "Conditions."

DAYSHEET TOTALS

_____/3	_____/3	_____/3	1. Total Column A, add "Previous Page" total, and enter the "Month-to-Date" figure.
_____/3	_____/3	_____/3	2. Total Column B-1, add "Previous Page" total, and enter the "Month-to-Date" figure.
_____/3	_____/3	_____/3	3. Total Column B-2, add "Previous Page" total, and enter the "Month-to-Date" figure.
_____/3	_____/3	_____/3	4. Total Column C, add "Previous Page" total, and enter the "Month-to-Date" figure.
_____/3	_____/3	_____/3	5. Total Column D, add "Previous Page" total, and enter the "Month-to-Date" figure.

PROOF OF POSTING

_____/5	_____/5	_____/5	6. Transfer today's daysheet totals as directed in the "Proof of Posting" section and add or subtract as instructed. If the total does not equal Column C, recalculate and look for errors.

ACCOUNTS RECEIVABLE CONTROL

_____/5	_____/5	_____/5	7. Enter figures from the "Proof of Posting" section to the "Accounts Receivable Control" section as indicated and add or subtract as instructed.

ACCOUNTS RECEIVABLE PROOF

_____/5	_____/5	_____/5	8. Enter "Month-to-Date" figures in the "Accounts Receivable Proof" section and add or subtract as instructed.

JOB SKILL 15-5 *(continued)*

BALANCE DAYSHEET

____/10 ____/10 ____/10 9. Compare the dollar amount in the "Total Accounts Receivable" from the "Accounts Receivable Control" section with the dollar amount in the "Total Accounts Receivable" from the "Accounts Receivable Proof" section; they should match. If not, follow instructions on common posting problems to locate the error.

RECORD DEPOSIT AND BALANCE CASH CONTROL

____/3 ____/3 ____/3 10. Add all cash received in the "Record of Deposits" section and enter the amount in the "Total Cash" area at the bottom.

____/6 ____/6 ____/6 11. Add all checks received in the "Record of Deposits" section and enter the amount in the "Total Checks" area at the bottom.

____/3 ____/3 ____/3 12. Add total cash received and total checks received to obtain the total deposit amount and enter it in the "Total Deposit" area at the bottom; this amount should equal the total of today's payments found in Column B-1.

____/5 ____/5 ____/5 13. Balance cash on hand by following the steps listed in "Cash Control."

____ ____ ____ Complete within specified time.

____/59 ____/59 ____/59 **Total points earned** (To obtain a percentage score, divide the total points earned by the number of points possible.)

Comments:

Evaluator's Signature: ____________________ **Need to Repeat:** ____________

National Curriculum Competency: CAAHEP: Cognitive: II.C.1, 2; Psychomotor: VI.P.2.a	ABHES: 8.k

JOB SKILL 15-6
Bookkeeping Day 2—Prepare the Daily Journal

Name ______________________________ Date ____________ Score ________

Performance Objective

Task: Set up the daily journal by inserting figures from the previous day's totals.

Conditions: Daily journal—Day 2 (Form 80) and pencil. You may want to enlarge this on a photocopy machine to legal size to ease handwritten entries. Refer to *textbook* Procedure 15-1 for step-by-step directions.

Standards: Complete all steps listed in this skill in _______ minutes with a minimum score of ________. (Time element and accuracy criteria may be given by instructor.)

Time: **Start:** ____________ **Completed:** ____________ **Total:** ____________ minutes

Scoring: One point for each step performed satisfactorily unless otherwise listed or weighted by instructor.

Directions with Performance Evaluation Checklist

1st Attempt	2nd Attempt	3rd Attempt	
_______	_______	_______	Gather materials (equipment and supplies) listed under "Conditions."
_____/2	_____/2	_____/2	1. It is June 29, current year. Enter this date on the top of the daysheet and in the "Record of Deposits" area and use it for all transactions that will occur today.
_____/2	_____/2	_____/2	2. All transactions for June 29, 20XX, will fit on one daysheet; label it page 1 of 1.
_____/2	_____/2	_____/2	3. Insert the "Previous Page" totals at the bottom of the daily journal (daysheet) by picking up the figures from June 28, 20XX, "Month-to-Date" totals for Columns A, B-1, B-2, C, and D.
_____/2	_____/2	_____/2	4. Insert the "Accounts Receivable Control" "Previous Day's Total" figure. This is the "Total Accounts Receivable" figure at the end of the previous day.
_____/2	_____/2	_____/2	5. Carry forward the "Accounts Receivable Proof " "First of Month" figure as indicated on the previous daysheet.
_____/2	_____/2	_____/2	6. Enter the "Beginning Cash On Hand" figure: $50.00.
_____/2	_____/2	_____/2	7. Insert your name at the bottom of the daysheet in the "Prepared by" area.
_______	_______	_______	Complete within specified time.
____/16	____/16	____/16	**Total points earned** (To obtain a percentage score, divide the total points earned by the number of points possible.)

JOB SKILL 15-6 *(continued)*

Comments:

Evaluator's Signature: ______________________________ **Need to Repeat:** ____________

National Curriculum Competency: CAAHEP: Psychomotor: VI.P.2.a	ABHES: 8.h

JOB SKILL 15-7

Bookkeeping Day 2—Post Charges, Payments, and Adjustments to Patient Ledger Cards and to the Daily Journal; Prepare Cash Receipts and the Bank Deposit

Name ______________________________ Date ______________ Score ________

Performance Objective

Task: Post charges and payments to patient ledger cards and calculate a running balance; prepare cash receipts. Duplicate posting entries on the daily journal (daysheet), record payments on the bank deposit slip, endorse checks, and prepare the bank deposit.

Conditions: Select ledger cards, which have been alphabetized, from Job Skill 15-1 and the daysheet prepared in Job Skill 15-6. Use three checks received by Practon Medical Group (Form 81), cash receipts (Form 78), number 10 envelope, calculator, and pencil. Refer to *textbook* Figure 15-2A for posting illustrations, Procedure 15-1 for step-by-step directions, and Figure 15-6 for a cash receipt example.

Standards: Complete all steps listed in this skill in _______ minutes with a minimum score of ________. (Time element and accuracy criteria may be given by instructor.)

Time: **Start:** _____________ **Completed:** _____________ **Total:** _____________ minutes

Scoring: One point for each step performed satisfactorily unless otherwise listed or weighted by instructor.

Directions with Performance Evaluation Checklist

It is June 29, current year. For this job skill, you will be posting to the patient's ledger card and then to the daily journal (daysheet); refer to specific instructions in Job Skill 15-4. Pull ledger cards for patients who are on today's schedule (they are highlighted in step-by-step instructions in **boldface**) and post entries as done in Job Skills 15-2 and 15-4. Post all charges (line by line) referring to the "Mock Fee Schedule" (Figure A-1 in Part III of this *Workbook*) to obtain fees; calculate a running balance for each line of posting. For all commercial (private) insurance programs, Medicaid, and TRICARE, use figures from the "Mock Fees" section. Cut checks apart and post all payments after charges have been posted, endorse checks, record on the deposit slip, total the bank deposit, and put into the envelope. Complete a receipt for all patients who paid cash; record all payments in the "Cash Control" section of the daily journal.

1st Attempt	2nd Attempt	3rd Attempt	
_______	_______	_______	Gather materials (equipment and supplies) listed under "Conditions."
____/11	____/11	____/11	1. Post charge on ledger for patient **Margaret Jenkins**. NP Office Consult Level IV (E/M Section) Post entry on daysheet.
____/21	____/21	____/21	2. Post charge on ledger for patient **Roger T. Simpson**. Est Pt OV Level IV (E/M Section) Post copayment received on ledger (see Form 81). Post entries on daysheet and record payment on bank deposit.
____/16	____/16	____/16	3. Post charges on ledger for patient **Joan Gomez**. ECG in office (Medicine Section) Admit to College Hospital; initial care—Level II (E/M Section) Post entries on daysheet.
____/11	____/11	____/11	4. Post charge on ledger for patient **Harold B. Mason**. Est Pt OV Level II (E/M Section) Post entry on daysheet.

JOB SKILL 15-7 *(continued)*

____/11 ____/11 ____/11 5. Post charge on ledger for patient **Maria Bargioni**.
Est Pt OV Level III (E/M Section)
Post entry on daysheet.

____/31 ____/31 ____/31 6. Post charges on ledger for patient **Jack J. Johnson**.
Est Pt OV Level I (E/M Section)
Tetanus inj (Medicine Section)
Immunization administration; IM (Medicine Section)
Post Medicaid copayment (check) on ledger (see Form 81).
Post entries on daysheet and record payment on bank deposit.

____/16 ____/16 ____/16 7. Post charges on ledger for patient **Lois A. Conrad**.
Est Pt OV Level III (E/M Section)
Pap smear collected and sent to laboratory. Note: The Pap smear is bundled into the office visit; however, there is a charge for the handling fee (Medicine Section—Special Services and Reports).
Post entries on daysheet.

____/21 ____/21 ____/21 8. Post charges on ledger for patient **Marylou Conrad**.
Est Pt OV Level II (E/M Section)
Poliovirus vaccine; oral immunization (Medicine Section)
Immunization administration (Medicine Section)
Post entries on daysheet.

____/16 ____/16 ____/16 9. Post charges on ledger for patient **Hannah F. Riley**.
Est Pt OV Level IV (E/M Section)
IUD insertion (Male/Female Genital System)
Post entries on daysheet.

____/30 ____/30 ____/30 10. Post charge on ledger for patient **Stephen B. Riley Jr**.
Office Consult Level IV (E/M Section)
Post cash payment on ledger; $25.
Complete cash receipt No. 149 (see Form 78).
Post entries on daysheet; record payment on bank deposit and cash control.

____/16 ____/16 ____/16 11. Post charges on ledger for patient **Rosa K. Okida**.
Est Pt OV Level I (E/M Section)
X-ray R hip, single view (Radiology Section)
Post entries on daysheet.

____/11 ____/11 ____/11 12. Post charge on ledger for patient **Howard S. Chan**.
Est Pt OV Level IV (E/M Section)
Post entries on daysheet.

____/11 ____/11 ____/11 13. Post charge on ledger for patient **Robert T. Jenner**.
HV (subsequent) Level I (E/M Section)
Post entry on daysheet.

INCOMING MAIL: The morning mail contained a check from Prudential Insurance Company for processing a life insurance examination report (Form 81).

____/6 ____/6 ____/6 14. Post the check and charge on the ledger from **Prudential Insurance Company**. Post charge and payment on the daysheet and record on the bank deposit.

____/3 ____/3 ____/3 15. Add the proper endorsement for all checks received. Total the deposit and put them in an envelope with the bank slip.

JOB SKILL 15-7 *(continued)*

_______	_______	_______	Complete within specified time.
___/233	___/233	___/233	**Total points earned** (To obtain a percentage score, divide the total points earned by the number of points possible.)

Comments:

Evaluator's Signature: ______________________________ **Need to Repeat:** ____________

National Curriculum Competency: CAAHEP: Psychomotor: VI.P.2.a	ABHES: 8.h

JOB SKILL 15-8
Bookkeeping Day 2—Balance the Daysheet

Name ______________________________ Date ______________ Score ________

Performance Objective

Task: Total all columns on the daysheet, add previous page totals, and enter new figures in month-to-date areas.

Conditions: Daysheet (Day 2) used in Job Skills 15-6 and 15-7, calculator, and pencil. Refer to *textbook* Procedure 15-1 for step-by-step directions.

Standards: Complete all steps listed in this skill in _______ minutes with a minimum score of ________. (Time element and accuracy criteria may be given by instructor.)

Time: **Start:** ____________ **Completed:** ____________ **Total:** ____________ minutes

Scoring: One point for each step performed satisfactorily unless otherwise listed or weighted by instructor.

Directions with Performance Evaluation Checklist

1st Attempt	2nd Attempt	3rd Attempt	
_______	_______	_______	Gather materials (equipment and supplies) listed under "Conditions."

DAYSHEET TOTALS

_____/3	_____/3	_____/3	1. Total Column A, add "Previous Page" total, and enter the "Month-to-Date" figure.
_____/3	_____/3	_____/3	2. Total Column B-1, add "Previous Page" total, and enter the "Month-to-Date" figure.
_____/3	_____/3	_____/3	3. Total Column B-2, add "Previous Page" total, and enter the "Month-to-Date" figure.
_____/3	_____/3	_____/3	4. Total Column C, add "Previous Page" total, and enter the "Month-to-Date" figure.
_____/3	_____/3	_____/3	5. Total Column D, add "Previous Page" total, and the enter "Month-to-Date" figure.

PROOF OF POSTING

_____/5	_____/5	_____/5	6. Transfer today's daysheet totals as directed in the "Proof of Posting" section and add or subtract as instructed. If the total does not equal Column C, recalculate and look for errors.

ACCOUNTS RECEIVABLE CONTROL

_____/5	_____/5	_____/5	7. Enter figures from the "Proof of Posting" section to the "Accounts Receivable Control" section as indicated and add or subtract as instructed.

ACCOUNTS RECEIVABLE PROOF

_____/5	_____/5	_____/5	8. Enter month-to-date figures in the "Accounts Receivable Proof" section and add or subtract as instructed.

JOB SKILL 15-8 *(continued)*

BALANCE DAYSHEET

____/10 ____/10 ____/10 9. Compare the dollar amount in the "Total Accounts Receivable" figure from the "Accounts Receivable Control" section with the dollar amount in the "Total Accounts Receivable" figure from the "Accounts Receivable Proof" section; they should match. If not, follow instructions on common posting problems to locate the error.

RECORD DEPOSIT AND BALANCE CASH CONTROL

____/3 ____/3 ____/3 10. Add all cash received in the "Record of Deposits" section and enter the amount in the "Total Cash" area at the bottom.

____/6 ____/6 ____/6 11. Add all checks received in the "Record of Deposits" section and enter the amount in the "Total Checks" area at the bottom.

____/3 ____/3 ____/3 12. Add total cash received and total checks received to obtain the total deposit amount and enter it in the "Total Deposit" area at the bottom; this amount should equal the total of today's payments found in Column B-1.

____/5 ____/5 ____/5 13. Balance cash on hand by following the steps listed in "Cash Control."

______ ______ ______ Complete within specified time.

____/59 ____/59 ____/59 **Total points earned** (To obtain a percentage score, divide the total points earned by the number of points possible.)

Comments:

Evaluator's Signature: ______________________________ **Need to Repeat:** ______________

National Curriculum Competency: CAAHEP: Cognitive: II.C.1, 2; Psychomotor: VI.P.2.a	ABHES: 8.h

JOB SKILL 15-9
Bookkeeping Day 3—Prepare the Daily Journal

Name ______________________________ Date ______________ Score ________

Performance Objective

Task: Set up the daily journal by inserting figures from the previous day's totals.

Conditions: Daily journal—Day 3 (Form 82) and pencil. You may want to use a photocopy machine to enlarge this to legal size to ease handwritten entries. Refer to *textbook* Procedure 15-1 for step-by-step directions.

Standards: Complete all steps listed in this skill in _______ minutes with a minimum score of ________. (Time element and accuracy criteria may be given by instructor.)

Time: **Start:** ____________ **Completed:** ____________ **Total:** ____________ minutes

Scoring: One point for each step performed satisfactorily unless otherwise listed or weighted by instructor.

Directions with Performance Evaluation Checklist

1st Attempt	2nd Attempt	3rd Attempt	
_____/2	_____/2	_____/2	Gather materials (equipment and supplies) listed under "Conditions."
_____/2	_____/2	_____/2	1. It is June 30, current year. Enter this date on the top of the daysheet and in the "Record of Deposits" area and use it for all transactions that will occur today.
_____/2	_____/2	_____/2	2. All transactions for June 30, 20XX, will fit on one daysheet; label it page number 1 of 1.
_____/2	_____/2	_____/2	3. Insert the "Previous Page" totals at the bottom of the daily journal (daysheet) by picking up the figures from June 29, 20XX, "Month-to-Date" totals for Columns A, B-1, B-2, C, and D.
_____/2	_____/2	_____/2	4. Insert the "Accounts Receivable Control" "Previous Day's Total" figure. This is the "Total Accounts Receivable" figure at the end of the previous day.
_____/2	_____/2	_____/2	5. Carry forward the "Accounts Receivable Proof" "First of Month" figure as indicated on the previous daysheet.
_____/2	_____/2	_____/2	6. Enter the "Beginning Cash On Hand" figure: $50.00.
_____/2	_____/2	_____/2	7. Insert your name at the bottom of the daysheet in the "Prepared by" area.
_______	_______	_______	Complete within specified time.
____/16	____/16	____/16	**Total points earned** (To obtain a percentage score, divide the total points earned by the number of points possible.)

JOB SKILL 15-9 *(continued)*

Comments:

Evaluator's Signature: ____ **Need to Repeat:** ________________

National Curriculum Competency: CAAHEP: Psychomotor: VI.P.2.a	ABHES: 8.h

JOB SKILL 15-10

Bookkeeping Day 3—Post Charges, Payments, and Adjustments to Patient Ledger Cards and to the Daily Journal; Prepare Cash Receipts and the Bank Deposit

Name ______________________________ Date ____________ Score ________

Performance Objective

Task: Post charges and payments to patient ledger cards and calculate a running balance; prepare cash receipts. Duplicate posting entries on the daily journal (daysheet), record payments on the bank deposit slip, endorse checks, and prepare the bank deposit.

Conditions: Select ledger cards, which have been alphabetized, from Job Skill 15-1 and the daysheet prepared in Job Skill 15-9. Use two checks received by Practon Medical Group (Form 83), cash receipts (Form 78), number 10 envelope, calculator, and pencil. Refer to *textbook* Figure 15-2A for posting illustrations, Procedure 15-1 for step-by-step directions, and Figure 15-6 for a cash receipt example.

Standards: Complete all steps listed in this skill in ________ minutes with a minimum score of ________. (Time element and accuracy criteria may be given by instructor.)

Time: **Start:** ____________ **Completed:** ____________ **Total:** ____________ minutes

Scoring: One point for each step performed satisfactorily unless otherwise listed or weighted by instructor.

Directions with Performance Evaluation Checklist

It is June 30, current year. For this job skill, you will be posting to the patient's ledger card and then to the daily journal (daysheet); refer to specific instructions in Job Skill 15-4. Pull ledger cards for patients who are on today's schedule (they are highlighted in step-by-step instructions in **boldface**) and post entries as done in Job Skills 15-2, 15-4, and 15-7. Post all charges (line by line), referring to the "Mock Fee Schedule" (Figure A-1 in Part III of this *Workbook*) to obtain fees; calculate a running balance for each line of posting. Doctors Fran and Gerald Practon are participating physicians in the Medicare program and bill using the "Medicare Participating" provider fee schedule. For all other insurance types, use figures from the "Mock Fees" column. Cut checks apart and post all payments after charges have been posted, endorse checks, record on the deposit slip, total the deposit, and put into an envelope. Complete a receipt for all patients who paid cash; record all payments in the "Cash Control" section of the daily journal.

1st Attempt	2nd Attempt	3rd Attempt	
______	______	______	Gather materials (equipment and supplies) listed under "Conditions."
____/11	____/11	____/11	1. Post charge on ledger for patient **J. B. Haupman**. Est Pt OV Level II (E/M Section) Post entry on daysheet.
____/21	____/21	____/21	2. Post charge on ledger for patient **Rachel T. O'Brien**. Est Pt OV Level II (E/M Section) Post copayment received (check) from managed care plan on ledger (see Form 83). Post entries on daysheet and record payment on bank deposit.
____/16	____/16	____/16	3. Post charges on ledger for patient **Martin P. Owens**. Est Pt OV Level II (E/M Section) Diathermy (Medicine Section—Physical Medicine) Post entries on daysheet.

JOB SKILL 15-10 *(continued)*

____/25 ____/25 ____/25 4. Post charges on ledger for patient **Joseph C. Smith**.
NP OV Level III (E/M Section)
Gastric motility with interpretation and report (Medical Section—Gastroenterology)
Post payment (check) on ledger (see Form 83).
Post entries on daysheet.

____/20 ____/20 ____/20 5. Post charge on ledger for patient **Kathryn L. Hope**.
Est Pt OV Level II (E/M Section)
Post HMO copayment on ledger; $10 cash.
Complete cash receipt No. 150 (see Form 78).
Post entries on daysheet.

____/11 ____/11 ____/11 6. Post charges on ledger for patient **Russell P. Smith**.
Est Pt OV Level II (E/M Section)
Post entry on daysheet.

____/21 ____/21 ____/21 7. Post charge on ledger for patient **Charlotte J. Brown.**
Est Pt OV Level III (E/M Section)
Post entry on daysheet.

____/11 ____/11 ____/11 8. Post charge on ledger for patient **Joan Gomez**.
HV (subsequent) Level I (E/M Section)
Post entry on daysheet.

____/11 ____/11 ____/11 9. Post charge on ledger for patient **Robert T. Jenner**.
Hospital discharge (E/M Section)
Post entry on daysheet.

TELEPHONE CALL: Mr. Howard S. Chan telephoned and said he was unable to pay his bill because he lost his job. You spoke with Dr. Practon and he told you to cancel the patient's debt.

____/12 ____/12 ____/12 10. Post an adjustment on the ledger for patient **Howard S. Chan**.
Reference Dr. G. Practon's name on the ledger.
Describe the adjustment as a "hardship."
Post entry on daysheet.

______ ______ ______ Complete within specified time.

___/161 ___/161 ___/161 **Total points earned** (To obtain a percentage score, divide the total points earned by the number of points possible.)

Comments:

Evaluator's Signature: ______________________________ **Need to Repeat:** ____________

National Curriculum Competency: CAAHEP: Psychomotor: VI.P.2.a	ABHES: 8.h

JOB SKILL 15-11
Bookkeeping Day 3—Balance the Daysheet

Name ______________________________ Date ______________ Score ________

Performance Objective

Task: Total all columns on the daysheet, add previous page totals, and enter new figures in month-to-date areas.

Conditions: Daysheet (Day 3) used in Job Skills 15-9 and 15-10, calculator, and pencil. Refer to *textbook* Procedure 15-1 for step-by-step directions.

Standards: Complete all steps listed in this skill in _______ minutes with a minimum score of ________. (Time element and accuracy criteria may be given by instructor.)

Time: **Start:** ____________ **Completed:** ____________ **Total:** ____________ minutes

Scoring: One point for each step performed satisfactorily unless otherwise listed or weighted by instructor.

Directions with Performance Evaluation Checklist

1st Attempt	2nd Attempt	3rd Attempt	
_______	_______	_______	Gather materials (equipment and supplies) listed under "Conditions."

DAYSHEET TOTALS

_____/3	_____/3	_____/3	1. Total Column A, add "Previous Page" total, and enter the "Month-to-Date" figure.
_____/3	_____/3	_____/3	2. Total Column B-1, add "Previous Page" total, and enter the "Month-to-Date" figure.
_____/3	_____/3	_____/3	3. Total Column B-2, add "Previous Page" total, and enter the "Month-to-Date" figure.
_____/3	_____/3	_____/3	4. Total Column C, add "Previous Page" total, and enter the "Month-to-Date" figure.
_____/3	_____/3	_____/3	5. Total Column D, add "Previous Page" total, and enter the "Month-to-Date" figure.

PROOF OF POSTING

_____/5	_____/5	_____/5	6. Transfer today's daysheet totals as directed in the "Proof of Posting" section and add or subtract as instructed. If the total does not equal Column C, recalculate and look for errors.

ACCOUNTS RECEIVABLE CONTROL

_____/5	_____/5	_____/5	7. Enter figures from the "Proof of Posting" section to the "Accounts Receivable Control" section as indicated and add or subtract as instructed.

ACCOUNTS RECEIVABLE PROOF

_____/5	_____/5	_____/5	8. Enter month-to-date figures in the "Accounts Receivable Proof" section and add or subtract as instructed.

JOB SKILL 15-11 *(continued)*

BALANCE DAYSHEET

____/10	____/10	____/10	9. Compare the dollar amount in the "Total Accounts Receivable" figure from the "Accounts Receivable Control" section with the dollar amount in the "Total Accounts Receivable" figure from the "Accounts Receivable Proof" section; they should match. If not, follow instructions on common posting problems to locate the error.

RECORD DEPOSIT AND BALANCE CASH CONTROL

____/3	____/3	____/3	10. Add all cash received in the "Record of Deposits" section and enter the amount in the "Total Cash" area at the bottom.
____/6	____/6	____/6	11. Add all checks received in the "Record of Deposits" section and enter the amount in the "Total Checks" area at the bottom.
____/3	____/3	____/3	12. Add total cash received and total checks received to obtain the total deposit amount and enter it in the "Total Deposit" area at the bottom; this amount should equal the total of today's payments found in Column B-1.
____/5	____/5	____/5	13. Balance cash on hand by following the steps listed in "Cash Control."
______	______	______	Complete within specified time.
____/59	____/59	____/59	**Total points earned** (To obtain a percentage score, divide the total points earned by the number of points possible.)

Comments:

Evaluator's Signature: ______________________________ **Need to Repeat:** ____________

National Curriculum Competency: CAAHEP: Cognitive: II.C.1.2; Psychomotor: VI.P.2.a	ABHES: 8.h

JOB SKILL 15-12
Bookkeeping Day 4—Set Up the Daysheet for a New Month

Name ______________________________ Date ______________ Score ________

Performance Objective

Task: Set up the daily journal for a new month by inserting figures from the previous month totals.

Conditions: Header and bottom section of daily journal (Form 84), daysheet from previous day/month (Day 3—Job Skill 15-11), and pencil.

Standards: Complete all steps listed in this skill in _______ minutes with a minimum score of ________. (Time element and accuracy criteria may be given by instructor.)

Time: **Start:** ____________ **Completed:** ____________ **Total:** ____________ minutes

Scoring: One point for each step performed satisfactorily unless otherwise listed or weighted by instructor.

Directions with Performance Evaluation Checklist

1st Attempt	2nd Attempt	3rd Attempt	
______	______	______	Gather materials (equipment and supplies) listed under "Conditions."
____/3	____/3	____/3	1. It is July 1, current year. Enter this date on the top of the daysheet and label it page 1 of 1.
____/5	____/5	____/5	2. Because it is the first of the month, there will be no "Previous Page" totals in Columns A, B-1, B-2, C, and D at the bottom of the daily journal; this area is used to calculate month-to-date figures. Enter zeros in the "Previous Page" columns.
____/2	____/2	____/2	3. Insert the "Accounts Receivable Control" "Previous Day's Total" at the bottom of the daysheet. This is the "Total Accounts Receivable" figure at the end of the previous day.
____/2	____/2	____/2	4. Insert the end-of-month total accounts receivable from June 30, 20XX, in the "Accounts Receivable Proof" "Accounts Receivable First of Month" area, found in the ending "Total Accounts Receivable" section. This will be the same total as the previous day's total (i.e., end-of-month total) entered into the "Accounts Receivable Control" section.
______	______	______	5. The daysheet is now setup to record the day's and month-to-date totals, along with the total accounts receivable to date. Insert your name at the bottom of the daysheet in the "Prepared by" area.
______	______	______	Complete within specified time.
____/15	____/15	____/15	**Total points earned** (To obtain a percentage score, divide the total points earned by the number of points possible.)

JOB SKILL 15-12 *(continued)*

Comments:

Evaluator's Signature: ____ **Need to Repeat:** ________________

National Curriculum Competency: CAAHEP: Psychomotor: VI.P.2.a	ABHES: 8.h

CHAPTER 16

Health Insurance Systems and Claim Submission

OBJECTIVES

After completing the exercises, the student will be able to:

1. Enhance knowledge of medical terminology, interpret abbreviations, and accurately spell medical words.
2. Complete a managed care authorization form (Job Skill 16-1).
3. Complete a health insurance claim form for a commercial case (Job Skill 16-2).
4. Complete a health insurance claim form for a Medicare case (Job Skill 16-3).
5. Complete a health insurance claim form for a TRICARE case (Job Skill 16-4).
6. Prepare ledger cards, post information, and calculate a running balance (Job Skills 16-2, 16-3, and 16-4).

FOCUS ON CERTIFICATION*

CMA Content Summary

- Third-party billing
- Capitated plans
- Commercial carriers
- Government plans (Medicare, Medicaid, TRICARE, CHAMPVA)
- Prepaid HMO, PPO, POS
- Workers' compensation
- Processing manual claims
- Processing electronic claims
- Tracing claims
- Sequence of filing claims
- Reconciling payments, rejections

*This *Workbook* and the accompanying *textbook* meet the entry-level administrative and general competencies for the CMA outlined by the AAMA Examination Content Outline and Occupational Analysis and for the RMA and CMAS outlined by the AMT Competencies, Construction Parameters, and Examination Specifications (see Competency Grid in Appendix B of the *textbook*).

- Inquiry and appeal process
- Applying managed care policies and procedures
- Referrals
- Precertification
- Methods of establishing fees
- Relative Value Studies
- Resource-based Relative Value Scale (RBRVS)
- Diagnosis Related Groups (DRGs)
- Contracted fees

RMA Content Summary

- Insurance terminology
- Insurance plans
- Identify and understand short-term and long-term disability
- Identify and understand workers' compensation (first and follow-up reports)
- Identify and understand Medicare (Advance Beneficiary Notice [ABN])
- Identify and understand Medicaid
- Identify and understand TRICARE and CHAMPVA
- Complete and file insurance claims
- File claims for paper and Electronic Data Interchange
- Understand and adhere to HIPAA Security and Uniformity Regulations
- Understand and evaluate explanation of benefits
- Evaluate claims rejection and utilize proper follow-up procedures
- Identify and comply with contractual requirements of insurance plans
- Track unpaid claims

CMAS Content Summary

- Understand private/commercial health care insurance plans
- Understand government health care insurance plans
- Process patient claims using appropriate forms and time frames
- Process workers' compensation/disability reports and forms
- Submit claims to third-party reimbursements including the use of electronic transmission methods
- Understand health care insurance terminology (deductible, copayment, preauthorization, capitation, coinsurance)
- Understand requirements for health care insurance plans
- Process insurance payments
- Track unpaid claims, and file and track appeals
- Understand fraud and abuse regulations

STOP AND THINK CASE SCENARIOS AND EXAM-STYLE REVIEW QUESTIONS

Refer to the end of Chapter 16 in the *textbook*.

Abbreviation and Spelling Review

Read the following patient's chart note and write the meanings for the abbreviations listed below the note. To decode any abbreviations you do not understand or that appear unfamiliar to you, refer to the list of abbreviations in Part IV of this *Workbook*. Step-by-step directions for this exercise are found in Procedure 1-1 of Chapter 1 in the *textbook*. Medical terms in the chart note are italicized; study them for spelling. Use your medical dictionary to look up their definitions. Your instructor may give a spelling and definition test that includes these words and abbreviations.

Brad Chieu

May 5, 20XX Pt came into the hosp c̄ a CC of *dyspnea* & pain in the RUQ. He was seen in the ED. Pt has had *diabetes* since childhood/*hypertension* for 3 years. Smoker. Increasing *malaise, nausea, anorexia* for past 5 days. *Polyuria, polydipsia.* The RN took his FH & vitals & recorded his TPR of 96.5°F & BP of 120/70 on the chart. After exam, the Dr. verified that the pt was suffering from COPD & scheduled him for an IPPB TX b.i.d. AP chest x-rays, a TB test and O2 therapy.

Gerald Practon, MD

Gerald Practon, MD

Pt	______________	BP	______________
c̄	______________	Dr.	______________
CC	______________	COPD	______________
RUQ	______________	IPPB	______________
ED	______________	TX	______________
RN	______________	b.i.d.	______________
FH	______________	AP	______________
TPR	______________	TB	______________
F	______________	O2	______________

Review Questions

Review the objectives, glossary, and chapter information before completing these review questions.

1. Match the terms in the left column with the definitions in the right column by writing letters in the blanks.

_______ copayment
_______ third-party payer
_______ indemnity
_______ deductible
_______ carrier
_______ adjuster
_______ fiscal intermediary
_______ elimination period
_______ assignment
_______ partial disability

a. employee of an insurance carrier with whom a case is assigned and who follows the case until it is settled
b. contractor that processes payments to providers on behalf of state or federal agencies or insurance companies
c. insurance carrier that intervenes to pay hospital or medical expenses on behalf of beneficiaries or recipients
d. benefits paid in a predetermined amount in the event of a covered loss
e. the transfer of one's right to collect an amount payable under an insurance contract
f. organization that offers protection against losses in exchange for a premium
g. form of cost sharing in which the insured pays a specific portion toward the amount of the professional services rendered
h. period of time after the beginning of a disability for which no benefits are payable
i. illness or injury preventing the insured from performing one or more functions of his or her occupation
j. amount the insured must pay in a fiscal year before an insurance company will begin the payment of benefits

2. Name and give a brief definition of three types of commercial (private) health insurance plans.

   a. ______________________________

   b. ______________________________

   c. ______________________________

3. The insured is also known as a/an ______________ or ______________.

4. The abbreviation for an insurance plan that has a high annual deductible is a/an:

   a. HSA

   b. HFSA

   c. HDHP

   d. UCR

   e. COB

5. An elimination period written in an insurance policy may also be known as a/an ______________ ______________ or ______________.

6. An attachment to a policy excluding certain illnesses or disabilities is called a/an ______________ ______________.

7. Managed care plans pay the physician by ______________.

8. Dr. Practon wants to know if Mrs. Snow's managed care plan covers a particular surgical procedure. This is a process known as ______________.

9. Dr. Practon completes a form for preauthorization of a diagnostic test to be ordered for Lee Cho. This process may also be called ______________ or ______________.

10. Before scheduling elective surgery on Phyllis Horton, Dr. Practon wants to know the maximum amount the insurance plan will pay. This is a process known as ______________ ______________.

11. Name five popular types of managed care health plans and list their abbreviations.

    a. ______________________________

    b. ______________________________

    c. ______________________________

    d. ______________________________

    e. ______________________________

12. Participating physicians receive ______________ percent of the allowable fee paid by Medicare.

13. Circle the correct answer. A [participating or nonparticipating] physician may not bill more than the Medicare limiting charge.

14. What is the time limit for submission of a Medicare claim? ______________ ______________

15. A document from the insurance company that arrives with a check for payment of an insurance claim is called a/an ____.

    In the Medicare program, this document is called a/an ______________________________,
    and the one sent to patients is called a/an ______________________________.

16. Circle the correct answer. Medicare Part D is [voluntary or involuntary] prescription drug coverage offered by [government or private] insurance carriers.

17. Circle the correct answer. When submitting a Medicare/Medicaid claim, the physician [should, should not, must always] accept assignment or payment will go to the patient.

18. A claim processed by Medicare and automatically processed by Medicaid is referred to as a/an ______________________________ claim.

19. The TRICARE fiscal year is from ____________________ to ____________________.

20. Define the following terms in relation to disability insurance.

    a. Temporary disability: ____

    b. Partial disability: ____

    c. Total disability: ____

21. After an initial workers' compensation report, insurance carriers want progress reports submitted on the injured worker each time the patient is seen, or on a/an ____________________ basis.

22. The paper insurance claim form that is accepted by most commercial (private) insurance companies, Medicare, Medicaid, and TRICARE is called the ______________________________.

23. If a patient signs an assignment of benefits statement, where is the insurance check sent? ____

24. The birthday rule:

    a. is honored in most states

    b. helps determine the primary insurance plan when a child is covered by both parents

    c. may not apply in divorce situations

    d. does not apply in Hawaii

    e. all are correct

25. The standard unique health identifier that all health care providers use when submitting claims is called the ____.

26. A service that receives insurance claims, edits and sorts them, and then electronically transmits them to insurance companies is called a/an ______________________________.

27. Indicate whether the following statements are true (T) or false (F).

    a. ________ Only an original CMS-1500 claim form may be optically scanned.

    b. ________ It is permissible to type data in lowercase for claims being optically scanned.

    c. ________ When entering data on a claim that is to be optically scanned, dates are keyed in using six digits.

    d. ________ Staples and paper clips may be used for attachments when sending insurance claims.

28. Which is the new version of the data element field that will need to be used for electronic billing starting January 1, 2012?

    a. 5010

    b. 1500

    c. 13

    d. 4010

    e. 640

29. If payment is not received after inquires have been made, a/an ______________ may need to be filed.

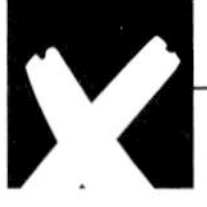

Critical Thinking Exercises

The following two scenarios are designed for students to role-play to gain experience interacting with insurance carriers and patients. Students should honor confidentiality, be courteous and demonstrate sensitivity, and display assertiveness and confidence while communicating with the provider and patient.

Divide students into groups of three—one can play a medical assistant, the second the insurance company employee, and the third can be the patient.

1. Dr. Gerald Practon has ordered a colonoscopy and has asked you to call the managed care company to see what policies and procedures are in place. The patient is waiting to see if the procedure can be scheduled immediately. Place a call to precertify benefits, predetermine the dollar amount allowed, and find out if preauthorization is needed; then notify the patient of your findings.

2. An insurance claim for a biopsy has evidently been lost. You think that it has been billed but cannot find a copy of the claim. A statement has been sent to the patient for the full charge, $383.34, and she is now in the office wanting an explanation. Call the insurance carrier to see if they received it and determine the status of the claim. Advise the patient of your findings.

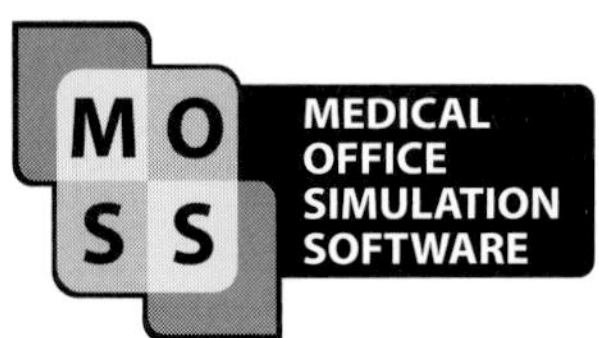

Computer Competency

Today's Date is Monday, 10/21/2013

Simulation: You are the medical biller for Douglasville Medicine Associates. At the end of each business day, the biller is responsible for submitting claims to insurance carriers for all office services provided to patients that day. *Note: You must complete the prior Computer Competency exercises in this Workbook prior to starting.*

1. Preparing Medical Claims

The medical biller will batch and submit medical claims for services provided on 10/21/2013 in the office. A Billing Worksheet Report and Claims Submitted Report will be printed for the office record.

A. Click on the *Insurance Billing* button on the *Main Menu*. The *Claims Preparation* screen will open.

B. Select the settings for the *Claims Preparation* screen as follows:

Field 1: Patient Name

Field 2: *Bill*
Provider: (All)
Service Dates: From 10/21/2013 Through 10/21/2013

Patient Name: (All)

Field 3: Paper

Field 4: Primary

Field 5: (All)

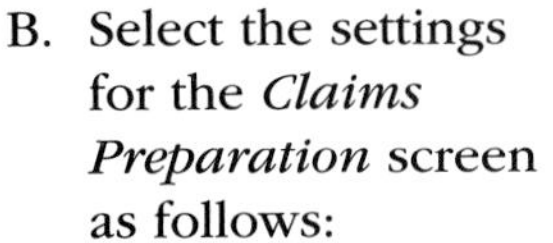

© Cengage Learning 2013

C. Click on the *Prebilling Worksheet* button to view claims in preparation for billing.

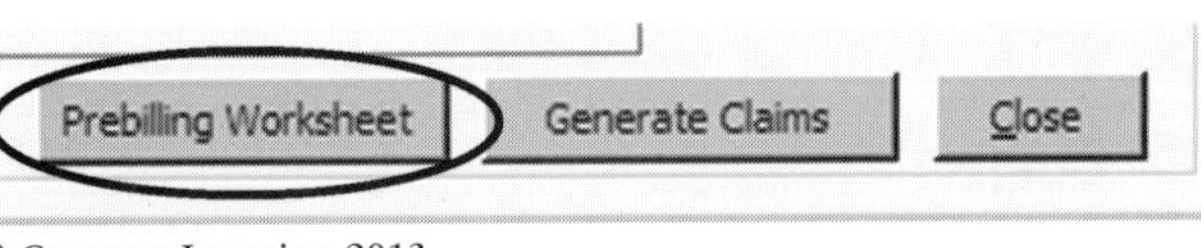

© Cengage Learning 2013

The generated worksheet should include five patients: Albertson, Merricks, Ybarra, Cartwright, and Ashby.

D. Print the *Insurance Prebilling Worksheet* and turn in the report to your instructor.

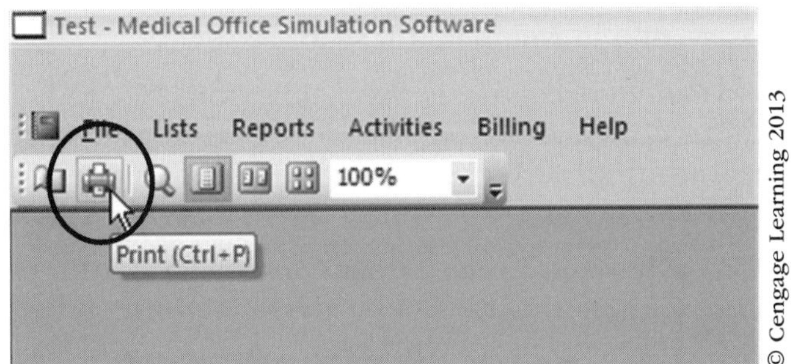

© Cengage Learning 2013

E. Close the *Insurance Prebilling Worksheet* window and return to the *Claims Preparation* screen.

Note: Be careful not to close MOSS when closing the *Insurance Prebilling Worksheet* (do not click on the close button on the upper right, but rather, the one below it).

F. On the *Claims Preparation* screen, click on the *Generate Claims* button. This will open the *Preview Claims* screen.

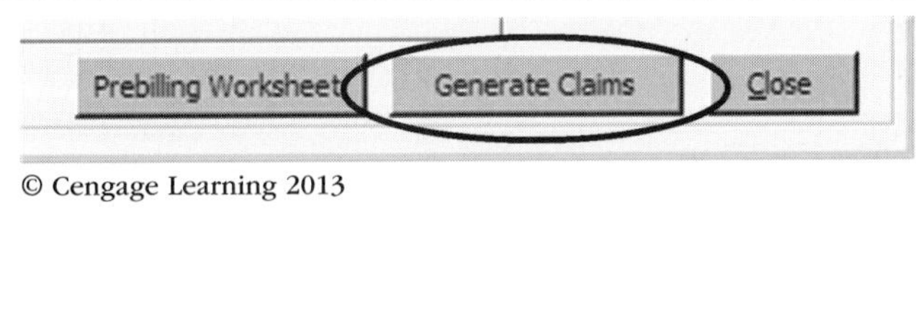

© Cengage Learning 2013

G. You may check the claims for accuracy against the *Insurance Prebilling Worksheet.* Use the record locator bar at the bottom to scroll through the five claim forms. When all of the claim forms have been reviewed, click on the *Print Forms* button.

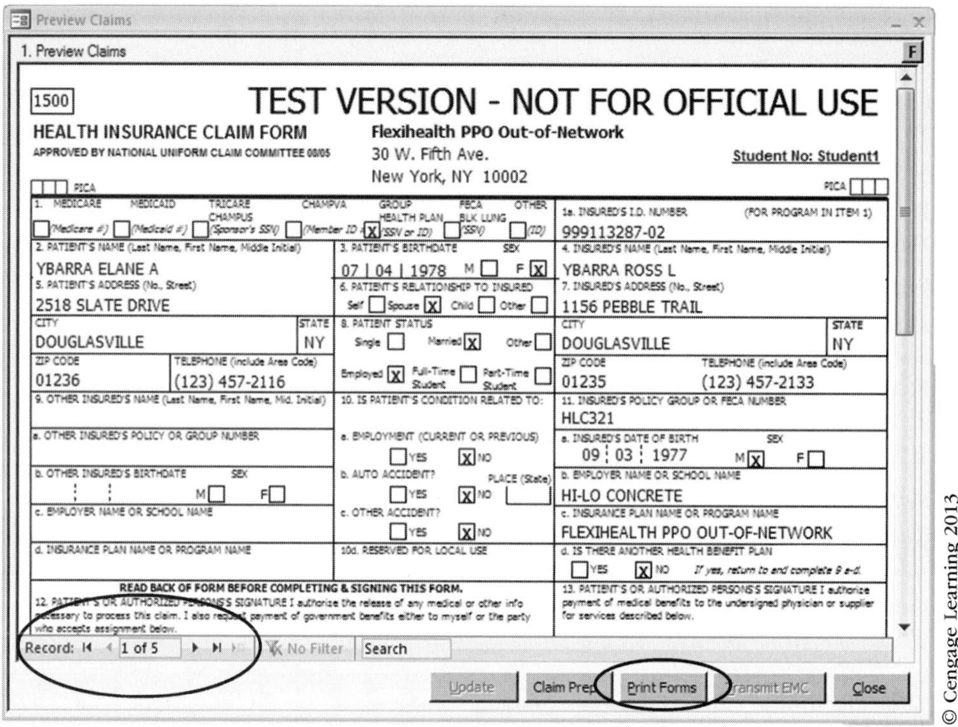

Preview Claims

1. Preview Claims

1500

TEST VERSION - NOT FOR OFFICIAL USE

HEALTH INSURANCE CLAIM FORM

APPROVED BY NATIONAL UNIFORM CLAIM COMMITTEE 08/05

Flexihealth PPO Out-of-Network
30 W. Fifth Ave.
New York, NY 10002

Student No: Student1

PICA

1. MEDICARE (Medicare #) MEDICAID (Medicaid #) TRICARE CHAMPUS (Sponsor's SSN) CHAMPVA (Member ID #) GROUP HEALTH PLAN [X] (SSN or ID) FECA BLK LUNG (SSN) OTHER (ID)

1a. INSURED'S I.D. NUMBER (FOR PROGRAM IN ITEM 1): 999113287-02

2. PATIENT'S NAME (Last Name, First Name, Middle Initial): YBARRA ELANE A

3. PATIENT'S BIRTHDATE: 07 | 04 | 1978 SEX: M [ ] F [X]

4. INSURED'S NAME (Last Name, First Name, Middle Initial): YBARRA ROSS L

5. PATIENT'S ADDRESS (No., Street): 2518 SLATE DRIVE

6. PATIENT'S RELATIONSHIP TO INSURED: Self [ ] Spouse [X] Child [ ] Other [ ]

7. INSURED'S ADDRESS (No., Street): 1156 PEBBLE TRAIL

CITY: DOUGLASVILLE STATE: NY

8. PATIENT STATUS: Single [ ] Married [X] Other [ ]

CITY: DOUGLASVILLE STATE: NY

ZIP CODE: 01236 TELEPHONE (include Area Code): (123) 457-2116

Employed [X] Full-Time Student [ ] Part-Time Student [ ]

ZIP CODE: 01235 TELEPHONE (include Area Code): (123) 457-2133

9. OTHER INSURED'S NAME (Last Name, First Name, Mid. Initial)

10. IS PATIENT'S CONDITION RELATED TO:

11. INSURED'S POLICY GROUP OR FECA NUMBER: HLC321

a. OTHER INSURED'S POLICY OR GROUP NUMBER

a. EMPLOYMENT (CURRENT OR PREVIOUS) [ ] YES [X] NO

a. INSURED'S DATE OF BIRTH: 09 | 03 | 1977 SEX: M [X] F [ ]

b. OTHER INSURED'S BIRTHDATE SEX M [ ] F [ ]

b. AUTO ACCIDENT? [ ] YES [X] NO PLACE (State)

b. EMPLOYER NAME OR SCHOOL NAME: HI-LO CONCRETE

c. EMPLOYER NAME OR SCHOOL NAME

c. OTHER ACCIDENT? [ ] YES [X] NO

c. INSURANCE PLAN NAME OR PROGRAM NAME: FLEXIHEALTH PPO OUT-OF-NETWORK

d. INSURANCE PLAN NAME OR PROGRAM NAME

10d. RESERVED FOR LOCAL USE

d. IS THERE ANOTHER HEALTH BENEFIT PLAN [ ] YES [X] NO If yes, return to and complete 9 a-d.

READ BACK OF FORM BEFORE COMPLETING & SIGNING THIS FORM.

12. PATIENT'S OR AUTHORIZED PERSON'S SIGNATURE I authorize the release of any medical or other info necessary to process this claim. I also request payment of government benefits either to myself or the party who accepts assignment below.

13. PATIENT'S OR AUTHORIZED PERSON'S SIGNATURE I authorize payment of medical benefits to the undersigned physician or supplier for services described below.

Record: 1 of 5 No Filter Search

Update Claim Prep Print Forms Transmit EMC Close

© Cengage Learning 2013

H. When the forms have printed, the program returns to the *Main Menu* in MOSS.

Today's Date is Friday, 11/15/2013

Simulation: You are the medical biller for Douglasville Medicine Associates. When payments are received from insurance carriers, the biller is responsible for posting payments, adjustments, and deductibles to patient accounts. **You will need to reference the MOSS source documents found below in the Source Documents: EOB and RA Forms section to complete these exercises.**

2. Posting Insurance Payments to Patient Accounts: Patient Albertson

The medical biller received a number of payments from insurance carriers when the mail was picked up today. Using the EOBs and RAs that came with each check, payments will be posted to each patient's account, including any applicable adjustments.

A. Refer to the EOB (Explanation of Benefits) received from ConsumerONE HRA **(Source Documents: EOB and RA Forms)**. Compare the details of the EOB with the information for Patient Albertson on the *Insurance Billing Worksheet* generated in Exercise 1.

B. Read the EOB from ConsumerONE, prepare the information before applying a payment to the patient's account. Use the guidelines below to read the EOB:

How much did the insurance allow?

$55.00

How much was disallowed?

$10.00

How much did the insurance pay?

$55.00

C. Click on the *Posting Payments* button on the *Main Menu*. *S*elect Patient Albertson, and then click on *Apply Payment.*

D. Click on the line item for 10/21/2013 in the *Procedure Charge History* area (Field 1), and then click on the *Select/ Edit* button. Make certain Field 13 shows the correct *Balance Due.*

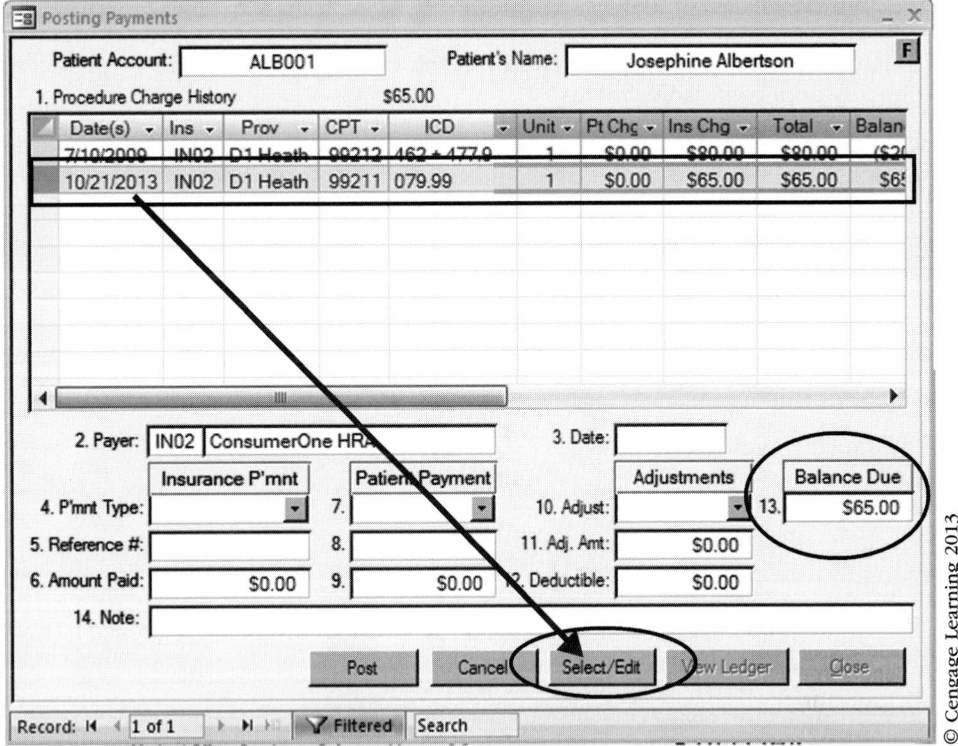

© Cengage Learning 2013

E. Input the date of posting (11/15/2013) and the insurance payment information as follows:

Payment by Insurance (Field 4)

Reference # 32155401 (Field 5)

Amount of payment $55.00 (Field 6)

Press *Enter* when finished to update the Balance Due (Field 13)

© Cengage Learning 2013

F. Input the disallowed amount as an insurance adjustment as follows:

Select *Insurance Adjustment* (ADJINS) (Field 10)

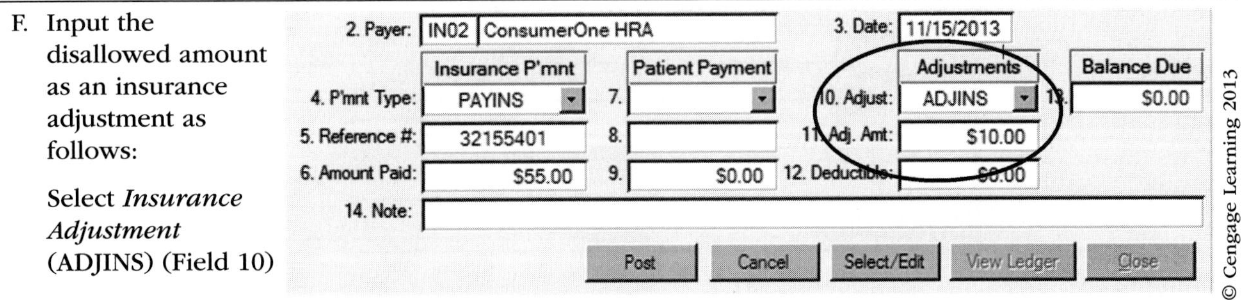

© Cengage Learning 2013

Enter $10.00 Adjustment Amount (Field 11)

Press *Enter* when finished to update the Balance Due (Field 13)

G. Click on the *Post* button to apply the payment and adjustment to the patient account.

H. Close all screens and return to the *Main Menu* in MOSS.

3. Posting Insurance Payments to Patient Accounts: Patient Merricks

The medical biller received a number of payments from insurance carriers when the mail was picked up today. Using the EOBs and RAs that came with each check, payments will be posted to each patient's account, including any applicable adjustments.

A. Refer to the EOB (Explanation of Benefits) received from FlexiHealth PPO **(Source Documents: EOB and RA Forms)**. There are two patients on one EOB (one in-network and the other out-of-network). Compare the details for each patient on the EOB with the information for Patient Merricks on the *Insurance Billing Worksheet.*

B. Read the FlexiHealth PPO EOB and prepare the information before applying a payment to the patient's account. Use the guidelines below to read the EOB for Patient Merricks only:

How much did the insurance allow?

$160.00

How much was disallowed?

$20.00

How much did the insurance pay?

$160.00

C. Click on the *Posting Payments* button on the *Main Menu.* Select Patient Merricks, and then click on *Apply Payment.*

D. Click on the line item for 10/21/2013 in the *Procedure Charge History* area (Field 1), and then click on the *Select/ Edit* button. Make certain Field 13 shows the correct *Balance Due.*

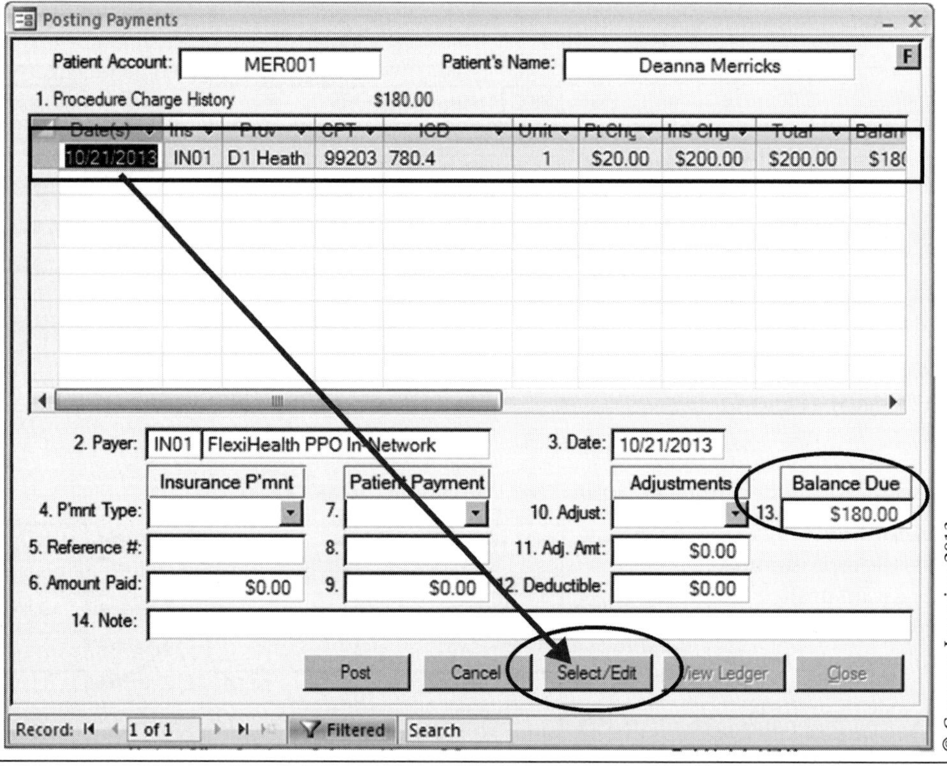

E. Input the date of posting (11/15/2013) and the insurance payment information as follows:

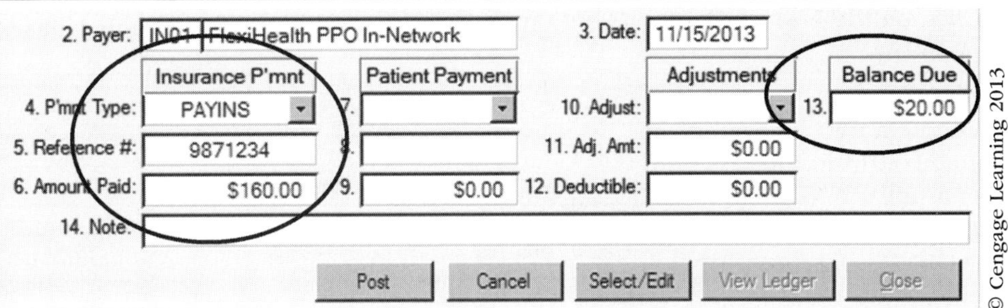

© Cengage Learning 2013

Payment by Insurance (Field 4)

Reference # 9871234 (Field 5)

Amount of payment $160.00 (Field 6)

Press *Enter* when finished to update the Balance Due (Field 13)

F. Input the noncovered amount as an insurance adjustment as follows:

2. Payer: IN01 FlexiHealth PPO In-Network
3. Date: 11/15/2013
Insurance P'mnt
Patient Payment
Adjustments
Balance Due
4. P'mnt Type: PAYINS
7.
10. Adjust: ADJINS
13. $0.00
5. Reference #: 9871234
8.
11. Adj. Amt: $20.00
6. Amount Paid: $160.00
9. $0.00
12. Deductible: $0.00
14. Note:
Post
Cancel
Select/Edit
View Ledger
Close

© Cengage Learning 2013

Select *Insurance Adjustment* (ADJINS) (Field 10)

Enter $20.00 Adjustment Amount (Field 11)

Press *Enter* when finished to update the Balance Due (Field 13)

G. Click on the *Post* button to apply the payment and adjustment to the patient account.

H. Close all screens and return to the *Main Menu* in MOSS.

4. Posting Insurance Payments to Patient Accounts: Patient Ybarra

The medical biller received a number of payments from insurance carriers when the mail was picked up today. Using the EOBs and RAs that came with each check, payments will be posted to each patient's account, including any applicable adjustments.

A. Refer to the EOB (Explanation of Benefits) received from FlexiHealth PPO **(Source Documents: EOB and RA Forms)**. Note that there are two patients on one EOB (one in-network and the other out-of-network). Compare the details for each patient on the EOB with the information for Patient Ybarra on the *Insurance Billing Worksheet*.

B. Read the FlexiHealth PPO EOB and prepare the information before applying a payment to the patient's account. Use the guidelines below to read the EOB for Patient Ybarra only:

How much did the insurance allow?

$153.00

How much was disallowed?

$27.00

How much did the insurance pay?

$122.40

C. Click on the *Posting Payments* button on the *Main Menu*. Select Patient Ybarra, and then click on *Apply Payment*.

D. Click on the line item for 10/21/2013 in the *Procedure Charge History* area (Field 1), and then click on the *Select/Edit* button. Make certain Field 13 shows the correct *Balance Due*.

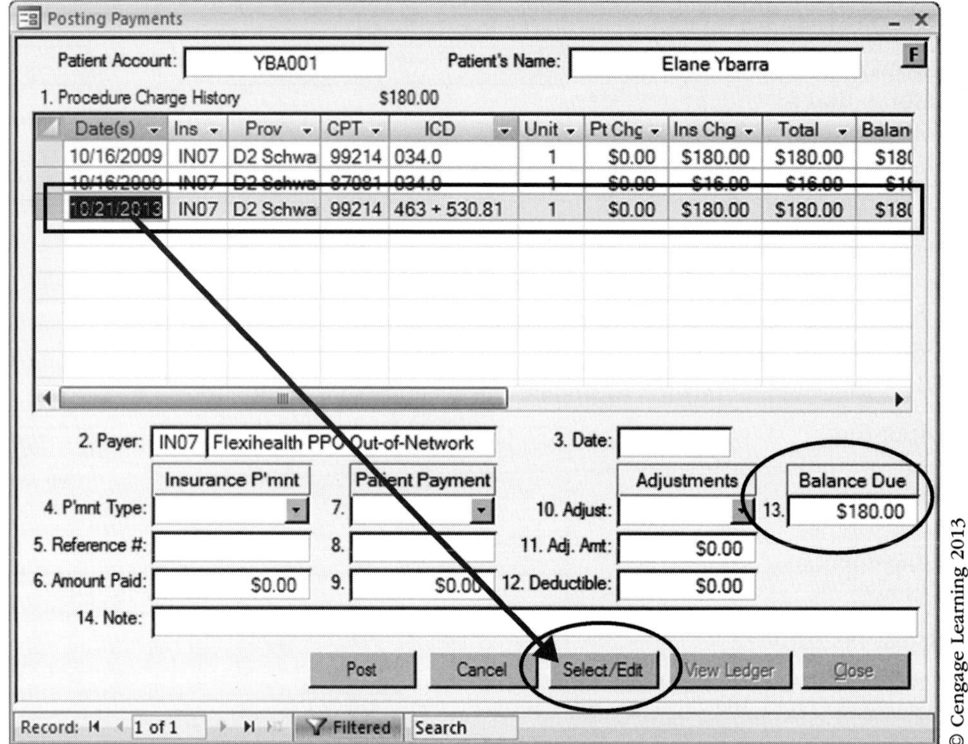

© Cengage Learning 2013

E. Input the date of posting (11/15/2013) and the insurance payment information as follows:

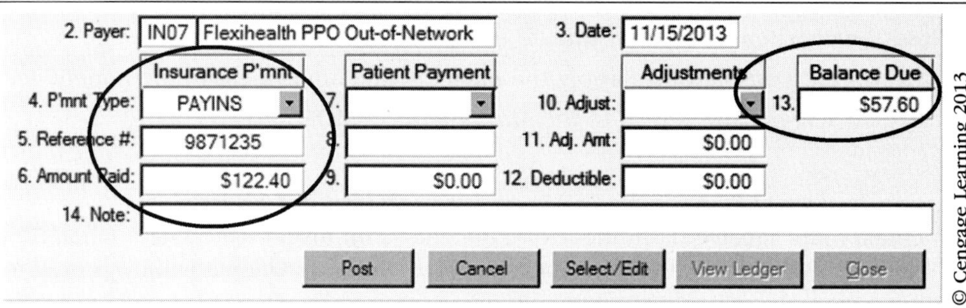

© Cengage Learning 2013

Payment by Insurance (Field 4)

Reference # 9871235 (Field 5)

Amount of payment $122.40 (Field 6)

Press *Enter* when finished to update the Balance Due (Field 13)

F. The noncovered amount will not be adjusted. As an out-of-network claim, the patient is responsible for the noncovered amount.

Notes on Benefit Determination:
A – Preferred provider discount. Patient is not required to pay this amount.
B – Patient is responsible for non-covered amounts for Out-of-Network providers.

© Cengage Learning 2013

The co-insurance of $30.60 and the noncovered amount will stay as a balance due on the patient's account (a total of $57.60).

G. Click on the *Post* button to apply the payment to the patient account.

H. Close all screens and return to the *Main Menu* in MOSS.

5. Posting Insurance Payments to Patient Accounts: Patient Cartwright

The medical biller received a number of payments from insurance carriers when the mail was picked up today. Using the EOBs and RAs that came with each check, payments will be posted to each patient's account, including any applicable adjustments.

A. Refer to the RA (Remittance Advice) received from Medicare **(Source Documents: EOB and RA Forms)**. Compare the details on the RA with the information for Patient Cartwright on the *Insurance Billing Worksheet.* Note that there are two separate procedures for which payment was made on this RA.

B. Read the Medicare RA and prepare the information before applying a payment to the patient's account. Use the guidelines below to read the RA for Patient Cartwright:

How much did Medicare allow for *CPT* 99203?*

$163.00

How much was disallowed?

$37.00

How much did Medicare pay?

$130.40

How much did Medicare allow for *CPT* 82465?

$14.00

How much was disallowed?

$0.00

How much did Medicare pay?

$14.00

C. Click on the *Posting Payments* button on the *Main Menu.* Select Patient Cartwright, and then click on *Apply Payment.*

D. Click on the line item for 10/21/2013, procedure 99203 in the *Procedure Charge History* area (Field 1), and then click on the *Select/Edit* button. Make certain Field 13 shows the correct *Balance Due.*

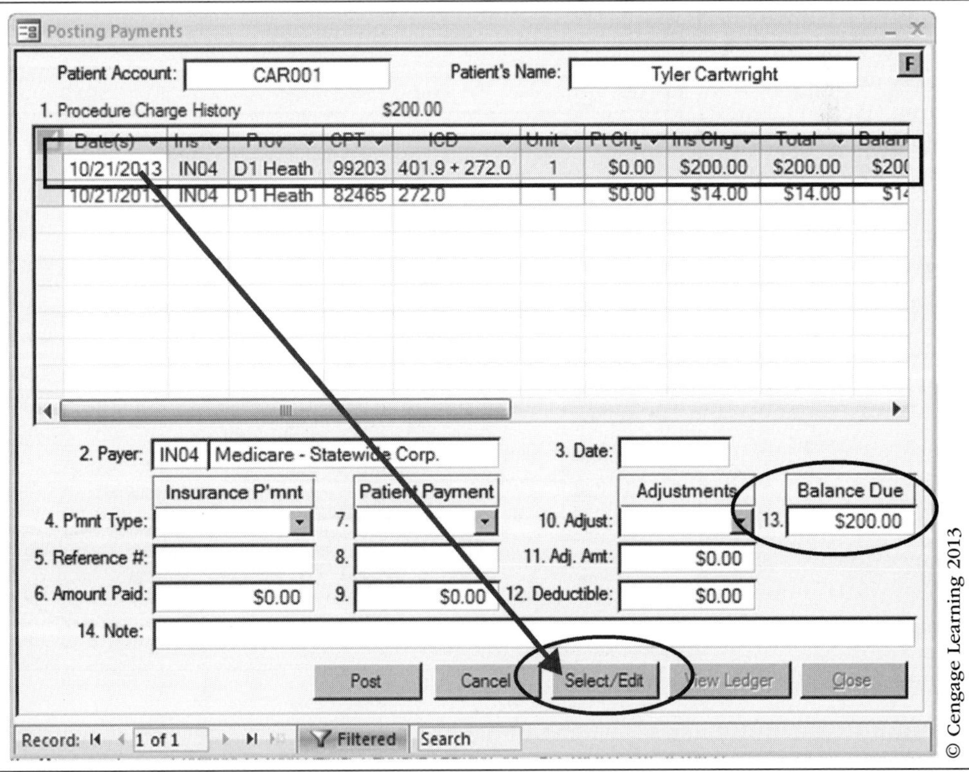

*2012 Current Procedural Terminology © *2011 American Medical Association.*

E. Input the date of posting (11/15/2013) and the insurance payment information as follows:

Payment by Insurance (Field 4)

Reference # 973333567 (Field 5)

Amount of payment $130.40 (Field 6)

Press *Enter* when finished to update the Balance Due (Field 13)

2. Payer: IN04 Medicare - Statewide Corp.
3. Date: 11/15/2013
Insurance P'mnt
Patient Payment
Adjustments
Balance Due
4. P'mnt Type: PAYINS
7.
10. Adjust:
13. $69.60
5. Reference #: 973333567
8.
11. Adj. Amt: $0.00
6. Amount Paid: $130.40
9. $0.00
12. Deductible: $0.00
14. Note:
Post
Cancel
Select/Edit
View Ledger
Close
© Cengage Learning 2013

F. Input the nonallowed amount as an insurance adjustment as follows:

Select *Insurance Adjustment* (ADJINS) (Field 10)

Enter $37.00 Adjustment Amount (Field 11)

Press *Enter* when finished to update the Balance Due (Field 13)

2. Payer: IN04 Medicare - Statewide Corp.
3. Date: 11/15/2013
Insurance P'mnt
Patient Payment
Adjustments
Balance Due
4. P'mnt Type: PAYINS
7.
10. Adjust: ADJINS
$32.60
5. Reference #: 973333567
8.
11. Adj. Amt: $37.00
6. Amount Paid: $130.40
9. $0.00
12. Deductible: $0.00
14. Note:
Post
Cancel
Select/Edit
View Ledger
Close
© Cengage Learning 2013

G. Click *Post* to apply the payment and adjustment to the patient account.

H. Now, click on the line item for 10/21/2013, procedure 82465 in the *Procedure Charge History* area (Field 1), and then click on the *Select/Edit* button. Make certain Field 13 shows the correct *Balance Due.*

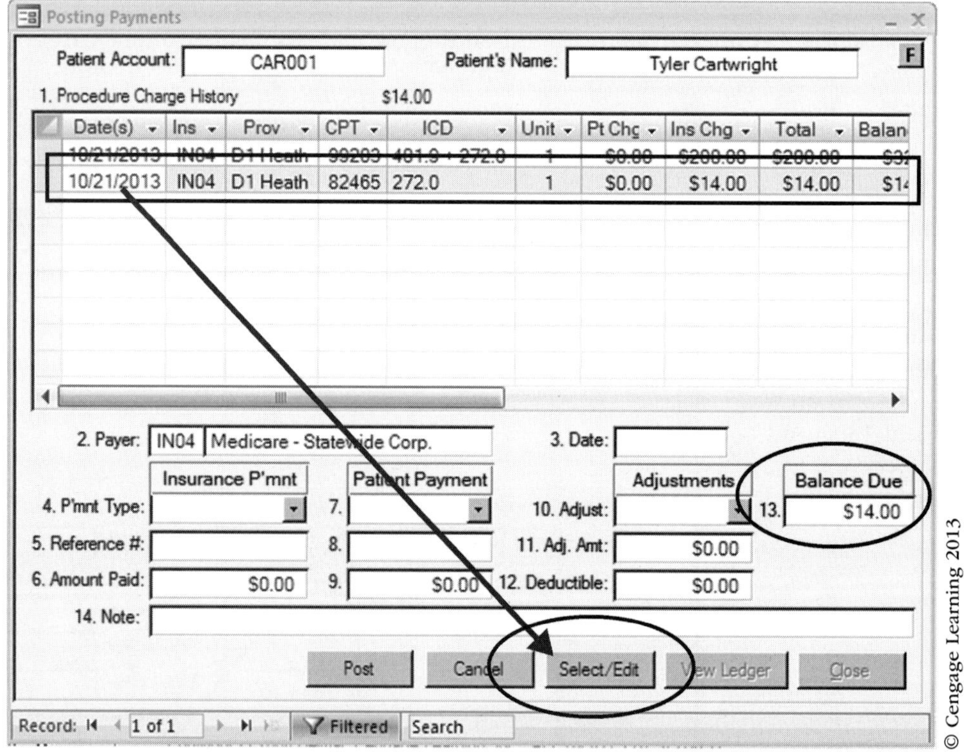

I. Input the date of posting (11/15/2013) and the insurance payment information as follows:

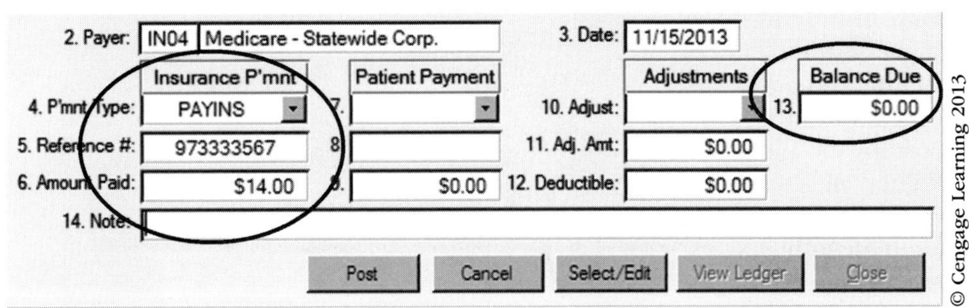

© Cengage Learning 2013

Payment by Insurance (Field 4)

Reference # 973333567 (Field 5)

Amount of payment $14.00 (Field 6)

Press *Enter* when finished to update the Balance Due (Field 13)

J. Click on the *Post* button to apply the payment to the patient account.

K. Close all screens and return to the *Main Menu* in MOSS.

6. Posting Insurance Payments to Patient Accounts: Patient Ashby

The medical biller received an electronic RA from Signal HMO. Using the electronic RA in MOSS, the payment will be posted to the patient's account, including any applicable adjustments.

A. Click on *Claims Tracking* from the *Main Menu*.

B. Input the selection into the prompts as follows:

Select Payer: Signal HMO

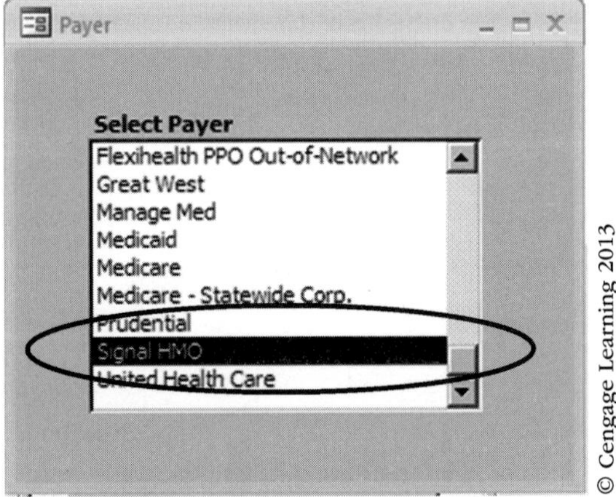

© Cengage Learning 2013

C. *Start Date:* 10/21/2013, then click *OK*

End Date: 10/21/2013, then click *OK*

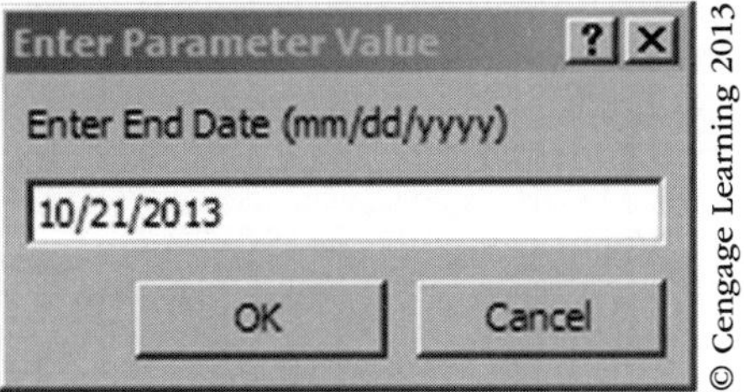

© Cengage Learning 2013

This will open the Signal HMO Remittance Advice (RA) for Patient Ashby

D. Print the electronic Signal HMO RA and refer to the hardcopy for posting. Close the RA and all screens and return to the *Main Menu* in MOSS.

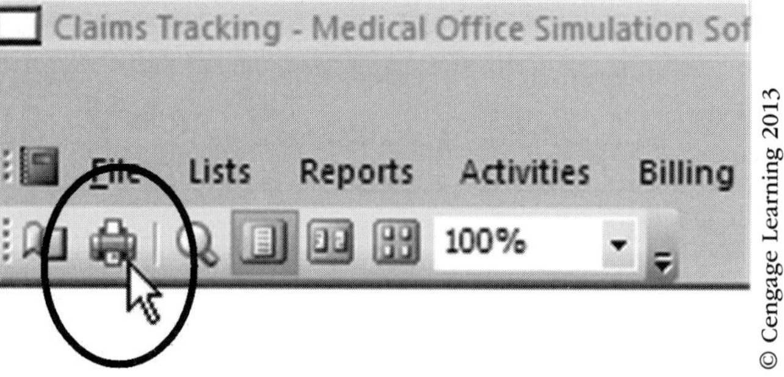

E. Click on the *Posting Payments* button on the *Main Menu*. Select Patient Ashby, and then click on *Apply Payment*.

F. Click on the line item for 10/21/2013, procedure 99212 in the *Procedure Charge History* area (Field 1), and then click on the *Select/Edit* button. Make certain Field 13 shows the correct *Balance Due*.

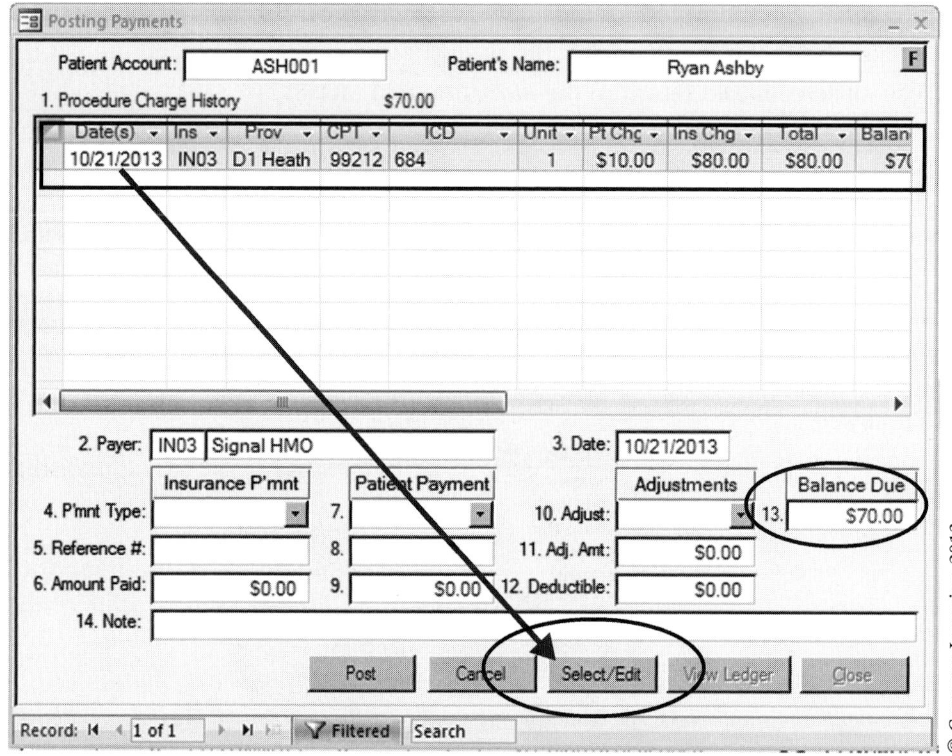

G. Input the date of posting (11/15/2013) and the insurance payment information as follows:

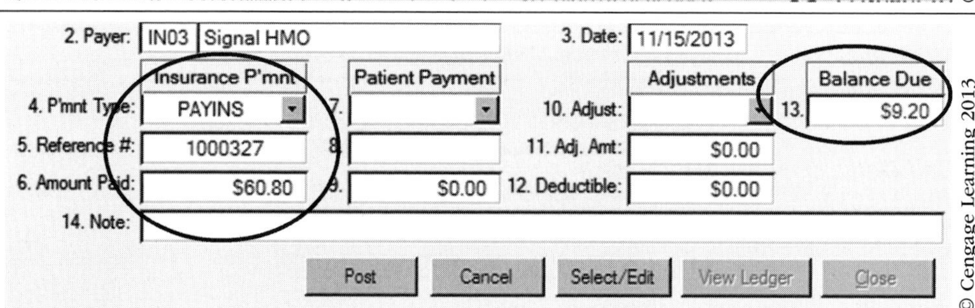

Payment by Insurance (Field 4)

Reference # 1000327 (Field 5)

Amount of payment $60.80 (Field 6)

Press *Enter* when finished to update the Balance Due (Field 13)

H. Input the nonallowed amount as an insurance adjustment as follows:

Select *Insurance Adjustment* (Field 10)

2. Payer:	IN03 Signal HMO			3. Date:	11/15/2013	
	Insurance P'mnt		Patient Payment		Adjustments	Balance Due
4. P'mnt Type:	PAYINS	7.		10. Adjust:	ADJINS	13. $0.00
5. Reference #:	1000327	8.		11. Adj. Amt:	$9.20	
6. Amount Paid:	$60.80	9.	$0.00	12. Deductible:	$0.00	
14. Note:						

Post | Cancel | Select/Edit | View Ledger | Close

Enter $9.20 Adjustment Amount (Field 11)

Press *Enter* when finished to update the Balance Due (Field 13)

I. Click on the *Post* button to apply the payment and adjustment to the patient account.

J. Close all screens and return to the *Main Menu* in MOSS.

Computer Competency Source Documents: EOB and RA Forms

Service Detail – ConsumerONE HRA
EXPLANATION OF BENEFITS

Date(s) of Service	Amount Charged	Amount Allowed	Amount Disallowed	Level One	Level Two	Level Three	Preventative Care	Patient Responsibility	Benefit Paid by HRA	*Remark Codes
Patient: Josephine Albertson		**Claim #: 32155401**			**Provider: HEATH**		**Douglasville Medicine Associates**			
102113	$65.00	$55.00	$10.00	$55.00	0.00	0.00	0.00	$0.00	$55.00	001
TOTALS	$65.00	$55.00	$10.00	$55.00	0.00	0.00	0.00	$0.00	$55.00	*

***Remark Codes:**

001 Level One EPA – Disallowed amount is an in-network provider write-off.

002 Level Two – Patient out-of-pocket responsibility up to $200.00; EPA exhausted

003 Level Three – In-Network 80/20 HRA reimbursement agreement.


```
Medicare Remittance Advice (MOSS Sample)

-----------------------------------------------------------------------------
 11-13-2013 MEDICARE CLAIMS SUBMITTED FOR L.D. Heath, MD  999501
-----------------------------------------------------------------------------
-----------------------------------------------------------------------------
CARTWRIGHT, TYLER           BILLED ALLOWED  DEDUCT   COINS PROV-PD  MC-ADJUSTMENT

  HIC 999316199A            ASG Y  ICN  973333567
  ACNT CAR001

1021  102113  11  99203    200.00 163.00   0         32.60 130.40    37.00
1021  102113  11  82465     14.00  14.00   0          0.00  14.00     0.00
           CLAIM TOTALS:   214.00 177.00   0         32.60 144.40    37.00

TOTAL PAID TO PROVIDER:  $144.40
```

Explanation of Medical Benefits **FlexiHealth PPO Plan**

Service Date	Type of Service	Charge(s) Submitted	Not Covered or Discount	Amount Covered	Patient Co-payment Co-insurance Deductible	Covered Balance	Plan Liability	See Note
Insured Name **MERRICKS, DEANNA**		Insured/Patient ID **999216812**			Patient Name **MERRICKS, DEANNA**			
Provider Name: L.D. Heath, MD – **In-Network Provider** Reference Number: 9871234								
10/21/2013	99203 Ext Prob Foc	$200.00	$ 20.00	$160.00	$20.00 co-pay	$160.00	$160.00	A
						Total Paid:	**$160.00**	
Insured Name **YBARRA, ROSS**		Insured/Patient ID **999113287**			Patient Name **YBARRA, ELANE**			
Provider Name: D.J. Schwartz MD – **Out-of-Network Provider** Reference Number: 9871235								
10/21/2013	99214 Est. Pat/Detail	$180.00	$27.00	$153.00	$30.60 co-ins	$122.40	$122.40	B
						Total Paid:	**$122.40**	

Notes on Benefit Determination:

A – Preferred provider discount. Patient is not required to pay this amount.

B – Patient is responsible for non-covered amounts for Out-of-Network providers.

JOB SKILL 16-1
Complete a Managed Care Authorization Form[1]

Name ______________________________ Date ______________ Score ________

Performance Objective

Task: Complete a managed care authorization form.

Conditions: Use Managed Care Plan Treatment Authorization Request (Form 85), computer or typewriter. Refer to *textbook* Figure 16-1 for a visual example.

Standards: Complete all steps listed in this skill in ________ minutes with a minimum score of ________. (Time element and accuracy criteria may be given by instructor.)

Time: **Start:** ____________ **Completed:** ____________ **Total:** ____________ minutes

Scoring: One point for each step performed satisfactorily unless otherwise listed or weighted by instructor.

Directions with Performance Evaluation Checklist

Read the following scenario and complete the Managed Care Authorization Form: On August 3, (current year), Antoyan Gagonian comes into Dr. Gerald Practon's office complaining of low back pain of 2 weeks' duration. He has difficulty walking, moving to a sitting position, and standing from a sitting position. Mr. Gagonian, born on October 10, 1963, lives at 2345 West Bath Street, Woodland Hills, XY 12345-0324; telephone number (555) 765-0720.

After taking a history and complete physical examination, Dr. Practon orders x-rays of the lower back and determines a working diagnosis of lumbago due to displacement of lumbar intervertebral disc. However, Mr. Gagonian's symptoms exceed typical criteria for this diagnosis. The patient is given a prescription for pain medication and muscle relaxant for muscle spasm. Dr. Practon recommends a magnetic resonance imaging (MRI) scan of the lumbar spine (without contrast) to investigate the problem further. The scan is to be done at College Hospital outpatient radiology.

Dr. Practon is the primary care physician for the managed care program, Health Net, of which Mr. Gagonian is a member. Dr. Practon's state license number is his member identification number with the insurance company. An authorization must be obtained for this study; the patient's insurance eligibility is verified today.

1st Attempt	2nd Attempt	3rd Attempt	
______	______	______	Gather materials (equipment and supplies) listed under "Conditions."
______	______	______	1. Complete the patient's demographic information on the authorization form.
____/5	____/5	____/5	2. Complete the information for the primary care physician, referring physician, and managed care plan.
____/8	____/8	____/8	3. List the description and code (M51.26[2]) for the diagnosis.
____/5	____/5	____/5	4. Indicate the treatment plan.
____/7	____/7	____/7	5. List the description and code (72148[3]) for the requested procedure.
____/3	____/3	____/3	6. Indicate the facility information.

[1] *International Classification of Diseases, 10th Revision, Clinical Modification* codes in this chapter are from the 2012 draft of *ICD-10-CM.*
[2] The 2012 *ICD-9-CM* code is 722.10.
[3] *Current Procedural Terminology* codes, descriptions, and two-digit numeric modifiers only are from *CPT 2012.* © 2011, American Medical Association. All rights reserved.

JOB SKILL 16-1 *(continued)*

_______	_______	_______	7. Obtain the physician's signature.
_____/4	_____/4	_____/4	8. Have Dr. Practon complete the primary care physician portion of the form.
_______	_______	_______	Complete within specified time.
____/41	____/41	____/41	**Total points earned** (To obtain a percentage score, divide the total points earned by the number of points possible.)

Comments:

Evaluator's Signature: ____ **Need to Repeat:** ________________

National Curriculum Competency: CAAHEP: Cognitive: VII.C.4; Psychomotor: VII.P.1, 5, 6	ABHES: 8.s

JOB SKILL 16-2
Complete a Health Insurance Claim Form for a Commercial Case

Name ______________________________ Date ______________ Score ________

Performance Objective

Task: Abstract information from a patient record and progress note to complete a health insurance claim form for a commercial case. Determine fees and post the information to the patient's ledger card.

Conditions:
1. Complete one health insurance claim form (Form 86).
2. Refer to Cathy B. Maywood's patient record and progress notes (*Workbook* Figure 16-1).
3. Locate physician information and charges in the fee schedule in Part III of this *Workbook*.
4. Refer to CMS-1500 field instructions for commercial insurance in Appendix A of this *textbook*.
5. View insurance template for a visual example of a completed commercial (private) insurance claim form (Figure A-1 in Appendix A of the *textbook*).
6. Complete a ledger card (Figure 16-2 in this *Workbook*).
7. Use a computer or typewriter and pen or pencil.

Standards: Complete all steps listed in this skill in ________ minutes with a minimum score of ________. (Time element and accuracy criteria may be given by instructor.)

Time: **Start:** _______ **Completed:** ________ **Total:** __________ minutes

Scoring: One point for each step performed satisfactorily unless otherwise listed or weighted by instructor.

Directions with Performance Evaluation Checklist

1st Attempt	2nd Attempt	3rd Attempt	
_______	_______	_______	Gather materials (equipment and supplies) listed under "Conditions."

CMS-1500 CLAIM FORM

1st Attempt	2nd Attempt	3rd Attempt	
_____/3	_____/3	_____/3	1. Address the claim form to the insurance carrier.
____/19	____/19	____/19	2. Obtain patient and insured information from the patient record, and complete the top portion of the claim form.
_____/3	_____/3	_____/3	3. On the initial date of service, obtain the patient's signature on the claim form indicating authorization to release medical information to the insurance carrier and assignment of benefits to the physician.
_______	_______	_______	4. Answer the question in Field 20 and mark the correct box.
_____/3	_____/3	_____/3	5. List the diagnostic codes in Fields 21.1 and 21.2 and reference them in Field 24 for each line of service.
_____/7	_____/7	_____/7	6. Insert the code for the office consult and complete the first line of service for June 2, 20XX.
_____/7	_____/7	_____/7	7. Insert the code for the handling of two specimens and complete the second line of service. Note: Multiply the charge by the number of units (2) and list the total in Field 24F. Indicate 2 units in Field 24G.
_____/7	_____/7	_____/7	8. Insert the code and complete the third line of service for the procedure on June 9, 20XX.

JOB SKILL 16-2 *(continued)*

____/7	____/7	____/7	9. Insert the code and complete the fourth line of service for the procedure on June 12, 20XX.
____/18	____/18	____/18	10. Total the claim and complete Fields 25 through 33 on the claim form; date the claim June 30, current year.

LEDGER CARD

____/4	____/4	____/4	11. List procedure codes in the Reference column on ledger card.
____/4	____/4	____/4	12. List charges in the Charge column on ledger card.
____/4	____/4	____/4	13. Calculate and record running balance for each charge posted.
____/4	____/4	____/4	14. Indicate when the insurance company has been billed.
____	____	____	Complete within specified time.
____/93	____/93	____/93	**Total points earned** (To obtain a percentage score, divide the total points earned by the number of points possible.)

Comments:

Evaluator's Signature: ________________________ **Need to Repeat:** ____________

National Curriculum Competency: CAAHEP: Cognitive: VII.C.4, 7, 8, 9; Psychomotor: VII.P.2, 3 ABHES: 8.r, u, v

FIGURE 16-1

No. 1612

PATIENT RECORD

LAST NAME	FIRST NAME	MIDDLE NAME	BIRTH DATE	SEX	HOME PHONE
Maywood	Cathy	B.	11-24-62	F	(555) 592-1841

ADDRESS	CITY	STATE	ZIP CODE
384 Gary Street	Woodland Hills	XY	12345

CELL PHONE	PAGER NO.	FAX NO.	E-MAIL ADDRESS
(555) 206-7788			Cmaywood@EM.com

PATIENT'S SOC. SEC. NO.	DRIVER'S LICENSE
XXX-XX-2601	CP22498X

PATIENT'S OCCUPATION	NAME OF COMPANY
public relations secretary	St. Joseph's Hospital

ADDRESS OF EMPLOYER	PHONE
4501 Main Street Woodland Hills, XY 1234	(555) 581-2600

SPOUSE OR PARENT	OCCUPATION
Robert M. Maywood	supervisor

EMPLOYER	ADDRESS	PHONE
United Parcel	261 Jeffers Street, Woodland Hills, XY 12345	(555) 521-8011

NAME OF INSURANCE	INSURED OR SUBSCRIBER
Colonial Health Ins. Co. 11 Royal St. Woodland Hills, 12345	self

POLICY/CERTIFICATE NO.	GROUP NO.
265012B	687SJ

REFERRED BY: Bert B. Evans, MD, NPI 00065411XX

DATE	PROGRESS
6/2/20XX	New patient was referred for consultation (comprehensive history and examination with moderate medical decision making – 99244**) with complaints of irregular vaginal bleeding after intercourse (N93.0*). Pelvic exam showed cervicitis (N72*) and cervical erosion. Pap smear and cervical mucosa smear taken and sent to outside laboratory (99000** X2). Patient to return in one week for possible cauterization of cervix. llf Fran Practon, MD
6/9/20XX	Lab results indicate Class IIB PAP. Patient has cryocauterization of cervix performed (57511**). Recommend endometrial biopsy. Pt. scheduled for outpatient surgery at College Hospital on June 12, 20XX. llf Fran Practon, MD
6/12/20XX	Pt reports to outpatient surgery at College Hospital at 5:30 a.m. Endometrial biopsy performed (58100**). Diagnosis: Postcoital bleeding. llf Fran Practon, MD

* The 2012 *ICD-9-CM* codes are 626.7 and 616.0.

** *Current Procedural Terminology* codes, descriptions, and two-digit numeric modifiers only are from *CPT 2012*, © 2011 American Medical Association. All rights reserved.

FIGURE 16-2

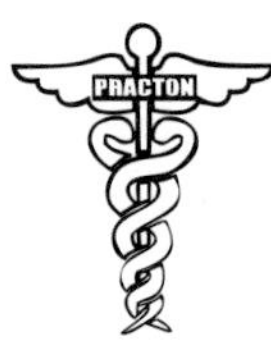

STATEMENT

PRACTON MEDICAL GROUP, INC.
4567 Broad Avenue
Woodland Hills, XY 12345-4700
Tel. 555-486-9002
Fax No. 555-488-7815

Cathy B. Maywood
384 Gary Street
Woodland Hills, XY 12345

Phone No.(H) 555-592-1841 (W) 555-581-2600 Birthdate 11-24-62
Insurance Co. Colonial Health Ins. Co. Policy No. 265012B / 687SJ

DATE	REFERENCE	DESCRIPTION	CHARGES	CREDITS Pymnts	CREDITS Adj	BALANCE
		BALANCE FORWARD				
6-2-XX		Consult NP				
6-2-XX		Handling of Specimens				
6-9-XX		Cauterization of Cervix				
6-12-XX		Endometrial Bx				

Pay last amount in balance column 

JOB SKILL 16-3

Complete a Health Insurance Claim Form for a Medicare Case

Name ______________________________ Date ____________ Score ________

Performance Objective

Task: Abstract information from a patient record and progress note and complete a health insurance claim form for a Medicare case. Determine fees and post the information to the patient's ledger card.

Conditions:
1. Complete one health insurance claim form (Form 87).
2. Refer to Michael T. Donlevy's patient record and progress notes (*Workbook* Figure 16-3).
3. Locate physician information and charges in the fee schedule in Part III of this *Workbook*.
4. Refer to CMS-1500 field instructions for the Medicare program in Appendix A of this *textbook*.
5. View insurance template for a visual example of a completed Medicare claim form in Figure 16-10 of the *textbook*.
6. Complete a ledger card (Figure 16-4 in this *Workbook*).
7. Use computer or typewriter and pen or pencil.

Standards: Complete all steps listed in this skill in ________ minutes with a minimum score of _________. (Time element and accuracy criteria may be given by instructor.)

Time: **Start:** _______ **Completed:** ________ **Total:** __________ minutes

Scoring: One point for each step performed satisfactorily unless otherwise listed or weighted by instructor.

Directions with Performance Evaluation Checklist

Dr. Gerald Practon is a participating physician with the Medicare program, so he accepts assignment; bill using the participating physician fees. After completing the claim form and ledger card, refer to the Mock Fee Schedule in Part III of this *Workbook* and answer the fee-related questions.

1st Attempt	2nd Attempt	3rd Attempt	
_______	_______	_______	Gather materials (equipment and supplies) listed under "Conditions."

CMS-1500 CLAIM FORM

1st Attempt	2nd Attempt	3rd Attempt	
_____/3	_____/3	_____/3	1. Address the claim form to the Medicare Administrative Contractor.
____/16	____/16	____/16	2. Obtain patient and insured information from the patient record and complete the top portion of the claim form.
_____/3	_____/3	_____/3	3. On the initial date of service, obtain the patient's signature on the claim form indicating authorization to release medical information to the insurance carrier and assignment of benefits to the physician.
_____/2	_____/2	_____/2	4. Fill in Field 14 and answer the question in Field 20; mark the correct box.
_____/3	_____/3	_____/3	5. List the diagnostic code in Field 21.1 and reference it in Field 24 for each line of service.
_____/7	_____/7	_____/7	6. Complete the first line of service for the emergency room visit on June 3, 20XX.
_____/7	_____/7	_____/7	7. Complete the second line of service for the procedure on June 3, 20XX.

JOB SKILL 16-3 (*continued*)

_______ _______ _______ 8. Determine whether or not you would bill for the follow-up office visit on 6/7/XX, and state the logic for your answer. ____________________________

____/17 ____/17 ____/17 9. Total the claim and complete Fields 25 through 33 on the claim form.

_______ _______ _______ 10. Date the claim June 30, current year.

LEDGER CARD

_____/2 _____/2 _____/2 11. List procedure codes in the Reference column on the ledger card.

_____/2 _____/2 _____/2 12. List charges in the Charge column on the ledger card.

_____/2 _____/2 _____/2 13. Calculate and record running balance for each charge posted.

_____/4 _____/4 _____/4 14. Indicate when the insurance company has been billed.

FEE SCHEDULE

When obtaining *precertification* you will need to verify benefits and make sure that the services and procedures performed are covered. When obtaining *predetermination* you will need to find out how much the insurance company pays for each service or procedure.

_____/2 _____/2 _____/2 15. If Dr. Practon is *participating* in the Medicare program, how much will he receive for the emergency room visit?

From Medicare: $ _____________

From the patient: $ _____________

_______ _______ _______ 16. If Dr. Practon is *not participating* in the Medicare program, how much will he receive for the emergency room visit from Medicare? $ _____________

_____/2 _____/2 _____/2 17. If Dr. Practon is *not participating* in the Medicare program and charges the maximum *limiting charge,* how much will he receive for the emergency room visit?

From Medicare: $ _____________

From the patient: $ _____________

_______ _______ _______ Complete within specified time.

____/77 ____/77 ____/77 **Total points earned** (To obtain a percentage score, divide the total points earned by the number of points possible.)

Comments:

Evaluator's Signature: ____ **Need to Repeat:** ________________

National Curriculum Competency: CAAHEP: Cognitive: VII.C.7, 9, 10; Psychomotor: VII.P.3, 4	ABHES: 8.r, u, v

FIGURE 16-3

No. 1613

PATIENT RECORD

Donlevy	Michael	T.	3/10/17	M	(555) 421-0015
LAST NAME	**FIRST NAME**	**MIDDLE NAME**	**BIRTH DATE**	**SEX**	**HOME PHONE**
282 Georgia Street		Woodland Hills	XY		12345
ADDRESS		**CITY**	**STATE**		**ZIP CODE**
CELL PHONE	**PAGER NO.**	**FAX NO.**	**E-MAIL ADDRESS**		
XXX-XX-9003			D033123X		
PATIENT'S SOC. SEC. NO.			**DRIVER'S LICENSE**		
Retired truck driver					
PATIENT'S OCCUPATION		**NAME OF COMPANY**			
ADDRESS OF EMPLOYER					**PHONE**

Patricia M. Donlevy	retired	
SPOUSE OR PARENT	**OCCUPATION**	
EMPLOYER	**ADDRESS**	**PHONE**
Medicare Administrator Contractor PO Box 123, Anytown, XY 12345	self	
NAME OF INSURANCE	**INSURED OR SUBSCRIBER**	
XXX-XX-9003A		
POLICY/CERTIFICATE NO.	**GROUP NO.**	

REFERRED BY: Harry Donlevy (brother)

DATE	PROGRESS
6/3/20XX	Called to ER at the request of patient who fell at home and cut his head (EPF HX & PX, LC MDM – 99282**). Sutured a 3.5 cm scalp wound – S01.1* (intermediate repair laceration – 12032**). RTO in 4 days for dressing change.
	llf Gerald Practon, MD
6/7/20XX	Dressing changed. Wound healing well, no signs of infection. Pt RTO next week for suture removal.
	llf M. Athins, CMA(AAMA)

* The 2012 *ICD-9-CM* code is 873.0.

** *Current Procedural Terminology* codes, descriptions, and two-digit numeric modifiers only are from *CPT 2012,* © 2011 American Medical Association. All rights reserved.

FIGURE 16-4

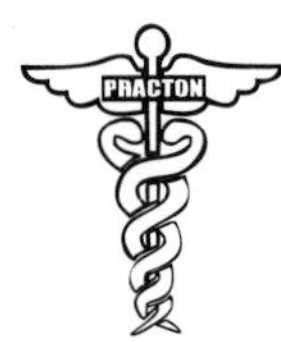

STATEMENT

PRACTON MEDICAL GROUP, INC.
4567 Broad Avenue
Woodland Hills, XY 12345-4700
Tel. 555-486-9002
Fax No. 555-488-7815

Michael T. Donlevy
282 Georgia Street
Woodland Hills, XY 12345

Phone No.(H) 555-421-0015 (W) ______ Birthdate 3/10/17
Insurance Co. Medicare Policy No. xxx-xx-9003A

DATE	REFERENCE	DESCRIPTION	CHARGES	CREDITS		BALANCE
				Pymnts	Adj	
		BALANCE FORWARD				
6-3-xx		ER Visit				
6-3-xx		Laceration repair				

Pay last amount in balance column 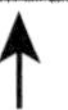

JOB SKILL 16-4

Complete a Health Insurance Claim Form for a TRICARE Case

Name ______________________________ Date ______________ Score ________

Performance Objective

Task: Abstract information from a patient record and progress note and complete a health insurance claim form for a TRICARE case. Determine fees and post the information to the patient's ledger card.

Conditions:
1. Complete one health insurance claim form (Form 88).
2. Refer to Frances O. Davidson's patient record and progress notes (*Workbook* Figure 16-5).
3. Locate physician information and charges in the fee schedule in Part III of this *Workbook.*
4. Refer to CMS-1500 field instructions for the TRICARE program in Appendix A of the *textbook.*
5. View insurance template for a visual example of a completed TRICARE claim form in Figure 16-13 of the *textbook.*
6. Complete a ledger card (Figure 16-6 in this *Workbook*).
7. Use typewriter, pen, or pencil.

Standards: Complete all steps listed in this skill in ________ minutes with a minimum score of ________. (Time element and accuracy criteria may be given by instructor.)

Time: **Start:** _______ **Completed:** ________ **Total:** ________ minutes

Scoring: One point for each step performed satisfactorily unless otherwise listed or weighted by instructor.

Directions with Performance Evaluation Checklist

Dr. Gerald Practon is a participating physician with the TRICARE program, so he accepts assignment; bill using the mock fees.

1st Attempt	2nd Attempt	3rd Attempt	
________	________	________	Gather materials (equipment and supplies) listed under "Conditions."

CMS-1500 CLAIM FORM

1st Attempt	2nd Attempt	3rd Attempt	
______/3	______/3	______/3	1. Address the claim form to TRICARE.
_____/26	_____/26	_____/26	2. Obtain patient and insured information from the patient record, and complete the top portion of the claim form.
______/3	______/3	______/3	3. On the initial date of service, obtain the patient's signature on the claim form indicating authorization to release medical information to the insurance carrier and assignment of benefits to the physician.
________	________	________	4. Answer the question in Field 20 and mark the correct box.
______/3	______/3	______/3	5. List the diagnostic code in Field 21.1 and reference it in Field 24 for each line of service.
______/7	______/7	______/7	6. Complete the first line of service for the office visit on June 4, 20XX.
______/7	______/7	______/7	7. Complete the second line of service for the electrocardiogram on June 4, 20XX.
______/7	______/7	______/7	8. Complete the third line of service for the spirometry on June 4, 20XX.

JOB SKILL 16-4 *(continued)*

_____/7 _____/7 _____/7 9. Complete the fourth line of service for the blood draw on June 4, 20XX.

_____/7 _____/7 _____/7 10. Complete the fifth line of service for the handling fee on June 4, 20XX.

_____/7 _____/7 _____/7 11. Complete the sixth line of service for the urinalysis on June 4, 20XX.

_____/18 _____/18 _____/18 12. Total the claim and complete Fields 25 through 33 on the claim form; date the claim June 30, current year .

LEDGER CARD

_____/6 _____/6 _____/6 13. List procedure codes in the Reference column on the ledger card.

_____/6 _____/6 _____/6 14. List charges in the Charge column on the ledger card.

_____/6 _____/6 _____/6 15. Calculate and record running balance for each charge posted.

_____/4 _____/4 _____/4 16. Indicate when the insurance company has been billed.

_____ _____ _____ Complete within specified time.

_____/120 _____/120 _____/120 **Total points earned** (To obtain a percentage score, divide the total points earned by the number of points possible.)

Comments:

Evaluator's Signature: ____________________ **Need to Repeat:** __________

National Curriculum Competency: CAAHEP: Cognitive: VII.C.4, 7, 8, 9, 10; Psychomotor: VII.P.2, 3 ABHES: 8.r, u, v

FIGURE 16-5

No. 1614

PATIENT RECORD

Davidson	Frances	O.	4/10/60	F	(555) 217-8105
LAST NAME	**FIRST NAME**	**MIDDLE NAME**	**BIRTH DATE**	**SEX**	**HOME PHONE**

128 Watson Street	Woodland Hills	XY	12345
ADDRESS	**CITY**	**STATE**	**ZIP CODE**

(555) 324-0088		(555) 217-8105	Fdavidson@EM.com
CELL PHONE	**PAGER NO.**	**FAX NO.**	**E-MAIL ADDRESS**

XXX-XX-1651	D034963X
PATIENT'S SOC. SEC. NO.	**DRIVER'S LICENSE**

tailor	Sampson Department Store
PATIENT'S OCCUPATION	**NAME OF COMPANY**

7841 Broadway St. Woodland Hills, XY 12345	(555) 289-7811
ADDRESS OF EMPLOYER	**PHONE**

Lieutenant William C. Davidson	U.S. Navy Lieutenant/Active Status NY	DOB 11/4/61
SPOUSE OR PARENT	**OCCUPATION**	

USN	PO Box 1878, APO New York, NY 09194	
EMPLOYER	**ADDRESS**	**PHONE**

TRICARE Standard, PO Box 444, Anytown, XY 12345	husband/sponsor
NAME OF INSURANCE	**INSURED OR SUBSCRIBER**

Social Security no. XXX-XX-2601	
POLICY/CERTIFICATE NO.	**GROUP NO.**

REFERRED BY: Martha B. Emory (friend)

DATE	PROGRESS
6/4/20XX	New patient comes in with CC of chest pain (moderate to severe), difficulty breathing, weakness, fatigue, & dizziness (Level 4 E/M – 99204**). Performed ECG (93000**); normal sinus rhythm. Performed spirometry (94010**) total and timed capacity; reduced lung capacity. Took blood specimen (36415**) and sent to outside lab (99000**) for CBC and basic metabolic panel. UA (non-automated with microscopy – 81000** neg. Edema throughout lower extremities. Dx: congestive heart failure I50.9*. Start patient on diuretic; may need hospitalization. RTO tomorrow. llf Gerald Practon, MD

* The 2012 *ICD-9-CM* code is 428.0.

** *Current Procedural Terminology* codes, descriptions, and two-digit numeric modifiers only are from *CPT 2012,* © 2011 American Medical Association. All rights reserved.

FIGURE 16-6

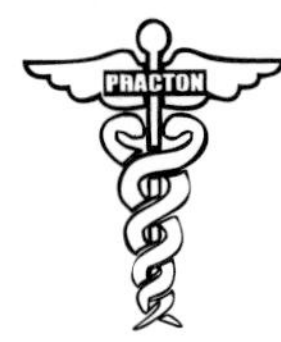

STATEMENT

PRACTON MEDICAL GROUP, INC.
4567 Broad Avenue
Woodland Hills, XY 12345-4700
Tel. 555-486-9002
Fax No. 555-488-7815

Frances O. Davidson
128 Watson Street
Woodland Hills, XY 12345

Phone No.(H) 555-217-8105 (W) 555-289-7811 Birthdate 4/10/50
Insurance Co. TRICARE Standard Policy No. XXX-XX-2601

DATE	REFERENCE	DESCRIPTION	CHARGES	CREDITS Pymnts	CREDITS Adj	BALANCE
	BALANCE FORWARD					
6-4-XX		OV NP				
6-4-XX		ECG				
6-4-XX		Spirometry				
6-4-XX		Venipuncture				
6-4-XX		Handling Spec				
6-4-XX		UA				

Pay last amount in balance column ↑

CHAPTER 17

Procedural and Diagnostic Coding

OBJECTIVES

After completing the exercises, the student will be able to:

1. Enhance knowledge of coding terminology, interpret abbreviations, and accurately spell medical words.
2. Review *Current Procedural Terminology* codebook sections (Job Skill 17-1).
3. Code evaluation and management services (Job Skill 17-2).
4. Code surgical services and procedures (Job Skill 17-3).
5. Code radiology and laboratory services and procedures (Job Skill 17-4).
6. Code procedures and services in the Medicine section (Job Skill 17-5).
7. Code clinical examples (Job Skill 17-6).
8. Code diagnoses from Chapters 1, 2, 3, 4 and 5 in *ICD-10-CM* (Job Skill 17-7).
9. Code diagnoses from Chapters 6, 7, 8, 9, and 10 in *ICD-10-CM* (Job Skill 17-8).
10. Code diagnoses from Chapters 11, 12, 13, 14, and 15 in *ICD-10-CM* (Job Skill 17-9).
11. Code diagnoses from Chapters 16, 17, 18, 19, and 20 in *ICD-10-CM* (Job Skill 17-10).
12. Code diagnoses from Chapter 21 and the Table of Drugs and Chemicals in *ICD-10-CM* (Job Skill 17-11).

FOCUS ON CERTIFICATION*

CMA Content Summary

- *Current Procedural Terminology (CPT)* coding system
- *International Classification of Diseases, 10th Revision, Clinical Modifications (ICD-10-CM)* coding system
- *Healthcare Financing Common Procedural Coding System (HCPCS Level II)*
- Relationship between procedure and diagnostic codes

RMA Content Summary

- Identify HIPAA-mandated coding systems and references
- *ICD-10-CM*
- *CPT*
- *HCPCS*
- Properly apply diagnosis and procedure codes to insurance claims

CMAS Content Summary

- Understand procedure and diagnoses codes
- Employ *Current Procedural Terminology (CPT)* and Evaluation and Management codes appropriately
- Employ *International Classification of Diseases (ICD-10-CM)* codes appropriately
- Employ *Healthcare Financing Administration Common Procedure Coding System (HCPCS)* codes appropriately

STOP AND THINK CASE SCENARIOS AND EXAM-STYLE REVIEW QUESTIONS

Refer to the end of Chapter 17 in the *textbook*.

Abbreviation and Spelling Review

Read the following patient's chart note and write the meanings for the abbreviations listed following the note. To decode any abbreviations you do not understand or that appear unfamiliar to you, refer to the list of abbreviations in Part IV of this *Workbook*. Step-by-step directions for this exercise are found in Procedure 1-1 of Chapter 1 in the *textbook*. Medical terms in the chart note are italicized; study them for spelling. Use your medical dictionary to look up their definitions. Your instructor may give a spelling and definition test that includes these words and abbreviations.

> Julie Odegard
>
> March 31, 20XX Wendy Smith, CMA (AAMA) accompanied me to 679 Chapel Street, Woodland Hills, XY this afternoon for a HC on pregnant pt Julie Odegard; G III, Para I. She has been at bed rest for 3 wks due to HBP. She is in her third *trimester*; LMP 7/1/XX, approx EDC 4/7/XX. Pt lying on L side, BP 170/92. Pt seems to be in good spirits. Collected sample for a UA, FHS strong. Perf. a PE, C/O abd discomfort, has not started to *dilate*. Will come into ofc in 3 days for a *non-stress test*. Adv to call if any concerns arise.

*This *Workbook* and the accompanying *textbook* meet the entry-level administrative and general competencies for the CMA outlined by the AAMA Examination Content Outline and Occupational Analysis and for the RMA and CMAS outlined by the AMT Competencies, Construction Parameters, and Examination Specifications (see Competency Grid in Appendix B of the *textbook*).

CMA (AAMA)	____________	L	____________
HC	____________	BP	____________
pt	____________	UA	____________
G III	____________	FHS	____________
Para I	____________	perf.	____________
wks	____________	PE	____________
HBP	____________	C/O	____________
LMP	____________	abd	____________
approx	____________	ofc	____________
EDC	____________	adv	____________

Review Questions

Review the objectives, glossary, and chapter information before completing these review questions.

1. When coding insurance claims, the ____________ code will determine whether the physician gets paid, and the ____________ code will determine how much the practice receives.
2. When completing health insurance claims electronically, list the types of codes required on the claim according to the Standard Code Set.
   a. ____________
   b. ____________
   c. ____________
3. An automated system that can assign codes to clinical procedures and services is called ____________
4. What is the commonly used code system called for coding workers' compensation claims? ____________
5. What is the codebook called used for complementary and alternative medicine? ____________
6. For coding purposes, the definition of *new patient* is ____________.
7. True or False. Critical care must always be provided in some type of critical care unit.
8. Explain the difference between a consult and a patient referral.
   a. Consult: ____________
   b. Referral: ____________

9. Write the definition of these three symbols that appear in the *Current Procedural Terminology** codebook.

   a. + ____________________

   b. • ____________________

   c. ▲ ____________________

10. Write the definition of a "bundled code." ____________________

    ____

    ____

11. Procedure codes consist of __________ -digit number(s) with __________ -digit modifiers.

12. In what section of *CPT* are office visits and hospital visits found? ____________________

13. To code from the Evaluation and Management section of *CPT*, what three things must be determined?

    a. ____________________

    b. ____________________

    c. ____________________

14. Which section of *CPT* has the most subsections? ____________________

15. Surgical package rules are established by ____________________, and global package rules are established by ____________________.

16. Repairs of lacerations are coded according to:

    a. ____________________

    b. ____________________

    c. ____________________

17. When coding fractures, name two things that need to be determined.

    a. ____________________

    b. ____________________

18. Endoscopes should always reflect the __________ area of visualization.

19. What is the less invasive surgical approach called when coding abdominal procedures? __________

    ____

20. True or False. When coding lesion removals on male or female genitalia, always select codes from the Integumentary subsection of the Surgery section in *CPT*.

21. The documentation required in a patient's medical record when an injection is given includes:

    a. ____________________

    b. ____________________

    c. ____________________

22. Diagnostic codes using *ICD-10-CM* can vary from __________ to __________ digits.

23. The first Classification of Causes of Death was introduced by the French physician Jacques Bertillon in the year __________.

**Current Procedural Terminology* codes, descriptions, and two-digit numeric modifiers only are from *CPT 2012*. ©2011, American Medical Association. All rights reserved.

24. What is the compliance implementation date for using *ICD-10-CM* codes? ______________________

25. To code diagnoses, start in Volume ______________ and verify the code in Volume ______________.

26. Explain a "qualified diagnosis," and state what descriptions (terms) to code instead.

____

____

____

____

____

27. In your own words, describe what the following terms mean.

    a. NEC: ____

    b. NOS: ____

28. When coding an underlying cause of a disease, along with the disease that resulted, name the rule to follow and state which is coded first and second.

    a. Rule: ____

    b. Code first: ____

    c. Code second: ____

29. When coding neoplasms, name the five titles that codes are listed under and give a brief definition of each term.

    a. ____

    b. ____

    c. ____

    d. ____

    e. ____

30. When coding burns, name the three elements in which burns are classified and give a brief description of each term.

    a. ____

    b. ____

    c. ____

31. Codes for external causes of morbidity start with the letters ____, ____, ____, and ____. Codes for factors that influence health status and contact with health services start with the letter ____.

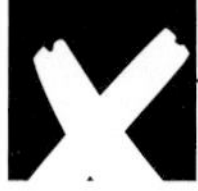

Critical Thinking Exercises

1. Underline the "main term" in the following diagnostic statements. When determining the main term, do not forget to ask, "What is wrong with the patient?"

    a. The patient received an insect bite on the index finger of her right hand.

    b. The newborn baby is experiencing spasmodic colic.

    c. The patient is suffering from gastrointestinal anthrax.

    d. The patient experienced lung edema due to flying at a high altitude.

e. After having a vaginal hysterectomy, the patient developed a vaginoperineal fistula.
f. The patient has all the symptoms of Bright's disease.
g. The patient had an infection during labor.
h. The baby has jaundice due to preterm delivery.
i. The patient has bilateral glaucoma with increased episcleral venous pressure.
j. The patient is a drug addict and has drug-induced Korsakoff's with an amnesic disorder.
k. The patient has lymphoid leukemia but is in remission.
l. The patient is experiencing an acute post-traumatic headache.
m. The patient is suffering from acute purulent otitis media in the right ear.
n. The patient was hospitalized with acute alcohol-induced hemorrhagic pancreatitis.
o. The baby was born with facial neuritis.
p. The patient has myocarditis due to streptococcus.
q. After childbirth, the patient developed an incomplete rectocele with uterine prolapse.
r. The patient has gangrenous quinsy.
s. The patient is seen today for gonococcal urethritis with a periurethral abscess.
t. The patient has postmenopausal atrophic vaginitis.
u. After a bone scan, the patient was diagnosed with hereditary bone xanthoma.
v. The patient has rhinocerebral zygomycosis.
w. The patient was hospitalized with thrombosis due to a breast implant.
x. The patient is experiencing psychogenic yawning.
y. The patient was hospitalized with a penetrating wound in the abdominal cavity.
z. The patient returned from Palm Springs, where it was 110 degrees, and is still experiencing lower limb swelling in both legs.

2. You desire to communicate to the physician the importance of the relationship between correct coding and reimbursement. Role-play a meeting in which you emphasize various aspects of accurate procedure and diagnostic coding.

JOB SKILL 17-1
Review *Current Procedural Terminology* Codebook Sections

Name ______________________________ Date ______________ Score ________

Performance Objective

Task: Locate procedure codes in various sections of the *Current Procedural Terminology* (*CPT*)* codebook.

Conditions: *Current Procedural Terminology* codebook and pen or pencil.

Standards: Complete all steps listed in this skill in _______ minutes with a minimum score of ________. (Time element and accuracy criteria may be given by instructor.)

Time: **Start:** ____________ **Completed:** ____________ **Total:** ____________ minutes

Scoring: One point for each step performed satisfactorily unless otherwise listed or weighted by instructor.

Directions with Performance Evaluation Checklist

Insert the section of *CPT* where each of the following codes are located.

1st Attempt	2nd Attempt	3rd Attempt	
_______	_______	_______	Gather materials (equipment and supplies) listed under "Conditions."
_______	_______	_______	1. 99202 ______________________
_______	_______	_______	2. 27500 ______________________
_______	_______	_______	3. 73500 ______________________
_______	_______	_______	4. 00500 ______________________
_______	_______	_______	5. 80055 ______________________
_______	_______	_______	6. 90713 ______________________
_______	_______	_______	7. 75970 ______________________
_______	_______	_______	8. 41872 ______________________
_______	_______	_______	9. 86805 ______________________
_______	_______	_______	10. 95004 ______________________
_______	_______	_______	11. 99281 ______________________
_______	_______	_______	12. 01810 ______________________
_______	_______	_______	Complete within specified time.
____/14	____/14	____/14	**Total points earned** (To obtain a percentage score, divide the total points earned by the number of points possible.)

**Current Procedural Terminology* codes, descriptions, and two-digit numeric modifiers only are from *CPT 2012*. ©2011, American Medical Association. All rights reserved.

JOB SKILL 17-1 *(continued)*

Comments:

Evaluator's Signature: ______________________ **Need to Repeat:** __________

National Curriculum Competency: CAAHEP: Cognitive: VIII.C.1

JOB SKILL 17-2
Code Evaluation and Management Services

Name ______________________________ Date ______________ Score ________

Performance Objective

Task: Locate evaluation and management codes in various subsections of the E/M section of *CPT.*

Conditions: *Current Procedural Terminology* codebook, "Evaluation and Management Services Guidelines" found at the beginning of the E/M section, and *CPT* notes that appear prior to the subsections and within categories of the E/M section. Refer to the section "Coding for Professional Services" in the *textbook* and Procedure 17-1 for step-by-step directions.

Standards: Complete all steps listed in this skill in ________ minutes with a minimum score of _________. (Time element and accuracy criteria may be given by instructor.)

Time: **Start:** ____________ **Completed:** ____________ **Total:** ____________ minutes

Scoring: One point for each step performed satisfactorily unless otherwise listed or weighted by instructor.

Directions with Performance Evaluation Checklist

The following divisions in this job skill are designed to acquaint you with various subsections in the Evaluation and Management (E/M) section of *CPT.* The problems become more difficult as you progress.

E/M codes are used by physicians to report a significant portion of their services. Some physicians rank E/M codes on a scale of 1 to 5, with 5 as the highest, most complex level, and 1 as the lowest, least-complex level. This terminology appears on multipurpose billing forms. The levels are determined by the last digit and are broken down as follows:

	OFFICE VISITS		CONSULTATIONS	
	New	**Established**	**Office**	**Hospital**
Level 1	99201	99211	99241	99251
Level 2	99202	99212	99242	99252
Level 3	99203	99213	99243	99253
Level 4	99204	99214	99244	99254
Level 5	99205	99215	99245	99255

Remember, it is the physician's responsibility to assign E/M codes, and this job skill is for familiarization purposes. The problems will acquaint you with terminology for this section of the *CPT* codebook.

1st Attempt	2nd Attempt	3rd Attempt	
______	______	______	Gather materials (equipment and supplies) listed under "Conditions."

NEW PATIENT OFFICE VISIT CODES: Select by level of service and key components.

______ ______ ______ 1. This is a level 2 case:
Expanded problem-focused history ____________
Expanded problem-focused examination
Straightforward medical decision making

______ ______ ______ 2. This is a level 4 case:
Comprehensive examination ____________
Comprehensive history
Moderate complexity medical decision making

JOB SKILL 17-2 (*continued*)

______ ______ ______ 3. This is a level 1 case: ____________
Problem-focused history
Problem-focused examination
Straightforward decision making

ESTABLISHED PATIENT OFFICE VISIT CODES: Select by level of service and key components, taking into consideration the rule that states you need "two out of three" key components to assign a code for an established patient.

______ ______ ______ 4. This is a level 2 case: ____________
Problem-focused history
Problem-focused examination
Straightforward medical decision making

______ ______ ______ 5. This is a level 4 case: ____________
Detailed history
Detailed examination
Moderate-complexity medical decision making

______ ______ ______ 6. This is a level 5 case: ____________
Comprehensive history
Comprehensive examination
High-complexity decision making

CODE RANGE 99201 TO 99238—Services provided in physician's office, hospital inpatient/outpatient, or other ambulatory facility. Select codes according to key components.

_____/3 _____/3 _____/3 7. Office visit for a 4-year-old male, established patient, with an expanded problem-focused history and physical examination for earache and dyshidrosis of feet and low-complexity medical decision making. ____________

_____/3 _____/3 _____/3 8. Office visit for a 35-year-old male, established patient, with a detailed history and examination for a new-onset RLQ pain. Medical decision making is of moderate complexity. ____________

_____/3 _____/3 _____/3 9. Initial hospital visit for a 15-year-old male with a detailed history and examination for infectious mononucleosis and dehydration. Medical decision making is of low complexity. ____________

_____/3 _____/3 _____/3 10. Subsequent hospital visit for a 9-year-old female admitted for lobar pneumonia with vomiting and dehydration. A problem-focused interval history is taken because she is becoming afebrile but tolerates oral fluids. An expanded problem-focused examination is done, with straightforward decision making. ____________

_____/3 _____/3 _____/3 11. Office visit for a 9-year-old male, established patient, who has been taking swimming lessons and now presents with a two-day history of left ear pain with purulent drainage. This visit requires a problem-focused history and examination, with straightforward decision making. ____________

CODE RANGE 99241 TO 99255—Consultation services provided in the physician's office, hospital inpatient/outpatient, or other ambulatory facility. Select codes according to key components.

_____/3 _____/3 _____/3 12. Office consultation for a 67-year-old male with chronic low back pain radiating to the left leg requiring a detailed history and examination and low-complexity decision making. ____________

JOB SKILL 17-2 *(continued)*

____/3 ____/3 ____/3 13. Initial office consultation for a 21-year-old female with acute upper respiratory tract symptoms that require an expanded problem-focused history and examination with straightforward decision making. ____________

____/3 ____/3 ____/3 14. Office consult for 30-year-old female with chronic pelvic inflammatory disease who now has left lower quadrant pain with a palpable pelvic mass. This visit requires a comprehensive history and examination and moderate-complexity decision making. ____________

____/3 ____/3 ____/3 15. Initial office consultation for a 60-year-old carpenter with olecranon bursitis requiring a problem-focused history and examination. Medical decision making is straightforward. ____________

____/3 ____/3 ____/3 16. Hospital consultation for a highly functional 70-year-old male to review laboratory studies. A problem-focused history and examination is performed. Medical decision making is straightforward. ____________

CODE RANGE 99281 TO 99499—Services provided in a hospital emergency or critical care department, nursing facility, rest home or custodial care facility, and patient's home as well as prolonged physician standby, case management, care plan, and preventive medicine services. Select codes according to key components or time.

____/3 ____/3 ____/3 17. First hour of critical care of a 16-year-old male with acute respiratory failure from asthma. ____________

____/3 ____/3 ____/3 18. A child is seen in the emergency department with a rash on both legs after exposure to poison ivy. This visit requires an expanded problem-focused history and examination but low-complexity medical decision making. ____________

____/3 ____/3 ____/3 19. Initial nursing facility visit to evaluate a 70-year-old male found confused and wandering, admitted by Adult Protective Services without a qualifying stay or inpatient diagnostic workup. Patient lives alone and has no relatives in the area. A comprehensive history and examination is performed. Medical decision making is of moderate complexity. ____________

____/3 ____/3 ____/3 20. Subsequent visit in a skilled nursing facility to a female with controlled dementia, hypertension, and diabetes. During the visit, she seems to exhibit flu symptoms. An expanded problem-focused interval history and examination is performed. Medical decision making is straightforward. ____________

____/3 ____/3 ____/3 21. Emergency department visit for a female who received an abrasion and needs a tetanus toxoid immunization. A problem-focused history and examination is performed, and medical decision making is straightforward. ____________

____/3 ____/3 ____/3 22. A 16-year-old patient presents for her yearly physical examination. ____________

JOB SKILL 17-2 *(continued)*

____/3 ____/3 ____/3 23. Rest home visit for the evaluation and management of a new 86-year-old patient with a detailed history and examination and moderate-complexity medical decision making. ____________

____/3 ____/3 ____/3 24. Complex interval history and examination done during a home visit for an established patient; high-complexity medical decision making. ____________

____/3 ____/3 ____/3 25. A 26-year-old new patient presents for an initial comprehensive preventive medicine visit. The physician performs a history and examination, then counsels the patient regarding birth control. ____________

______ ______ ______ Complete within specified time.

____/65 ____/65 ____/65 **Total points earned** (To obtain a percentage score, divide the total points earned by the number of points possible.)

Comments:

Evaluator's Signature: ______________________________ **Need to Repeat:** ____________

National Curriculum Competency: CAAHEP: Psychomotor: VIII.P.1	ABHES: 8.t

JOB SKILL 17-3
Code Surgical Procedures and Services

Name ______________________________ Date ______________ Score ________

Performance Objective

Task: Locate the correct procedure code within the Surgery section of *CPT* for each description listed.

Conditions: *Current Procedural Terminology* codebook, "Surgery Guidelines" found at the beginning of the Surgery section, *CPT* notes that appear prior to and within the subsections and categories of the Surgery section, and pen or pencil. Refer to "How to Code from the Surgery Section" and the section "Coding for Professional Services" in the *textbook* as well as Procedure 17-1 for step-by-step directions.

Standards: Complete all steps listed in this skill in _______ minutes with a minimum score of ________. (Time element and accuracy criteria may be given by instructor.)

Time: **Start:** ____________ **Completed:** ____________ **Total:** ____________ minutes

Scoring: One point for each step performed satisfactorily unless otherwise listed or weighted by instructor.

Directions with Performance Evaluation Checklist

Surgery codes 10021 to 69990 are divided according to body systems, then anatomic parts of the body. Use the *CPT* codebook to obtain the correct code number for each descriptor given. Critical thinking enters this job skill as you use your judgment to determine the correct code, since some cases do not contain full details. Read each case and code description carefully.

1st Attempt	2nd Attempt	3rd Attempt		
_____	_____	_____	Gather materials (equipment and supplies) listed under "Conditions."	
INTEGUMENTARY SYSTEM 10021–19499				
____/5	____/5	____/5	1. Excision, benign lesion, face, 0.5 cm	________
____/5	____/5	____/5	2. Repair layered closure of lt leg 2.7 cm laceration	________
MUSCULOSKELETAL SYSTEM 20005–29999				
____/5	____/5	____/5	3. Closed reduction of rt humeral shaft fracture, no manipulation	________
____/5	____/5	____/5	4. Subsequent application of long leg cast (walker)	________
RESPIRATORY SYSTEM 30000–32999				
____/5	____/5	____/5	5. Remove fried potato from left nostril of child	________
____/5	____/5	____/5	6. Simple excision of small nasal polyp	________
CARDIOVASCULAR SYSTEM 33010–37799				
____/5	____/5	____/5	7. Introduction of catheter into superior vena cava	________
____/5	____/5	____/5	8. Coronary artery bypass using single arterial graft	________
HEMIC/LYMPHATIC & MEDIASTINUM/DIAPHRAGM 38100–39599				
____/5	____/5	____/5	9. Biopsy of cervical lymph nodes; open, deep	________
____/5	____/5	____/5	10. Open excision for removal of total spleen	________

JOB SKILL 17-3 *(continued)*

DIGESTIVE SYSTEM 40490–49999

____/5 ____/5 ____/5 11. Liver biopsy; needle; percutaneous ____________

____/5 ____/5 ____/5 12. Open excision to remove gallbladder (cholecystectomy) ____________

URINARY SYSTEM 50010–53899

____/5 ____/5 ____/5 13. Drainage of deep periurethral abscess ____________

____/5 ____/5 ____/5 14. Aspiration of bladder by needle ____________

MALE GENITAL/INTERSEX/FEMALE GENITAL/MATERNITY CARE AND DELIVERY 54000–59899

____/5 ____/5 ____/5 15. Removal of IUD ____________

____/5 ____/5 ____/5 16. Cesarean delivery including obstetric/ antepartum/postpartum care ____________

ENDOCRINE/NERVOUS SYSTEMS 60000–64999

____/5 ____/5 ____/5 17. Complete thyroidectomy ____________

____/5 ____/5 ____/5 18. Cervical laminoplasty with decompression of spinal cord; two segments ____________

EYE AND OCULAR ADNEXA/AUDITORY/OPERATING MICROSCOPE 65091–69990

____/5 ____/5 ____/5 19. Subconjunctival injection ____________

____/5 ____/5 ____/5 20. Removal of temporal bone tumor ____________

______ ______ ______ Complete within specified time. ____________

___/102 ___/102 ___/102 **Total points earned** (To obtain a percentage score, divide the total points earned by the number of points possible.)

Comments:

Evaluator's Signature: ______________________________ **Need to Repeat:** ____________

National Curriculum Competency: CAAHEP: Psychomotor: VIII.P.1	ABHES: 8.t

JOB SKILL 17-4
Code Radiology and Laboratory Procedures and Services

Name ______________________________ Date ____________ Score ________

Performance Objective

Task: Locate the correct procedure code in the Radiology and Pathology/Laboratory section of *CPT* for each description.

Conditions: *Current Procedural Terminology* codebook, "Radiology" and "Pathology/Laboratory" Guidelines found at the beginning of each section of *CPT*, *CPT* notes that appear prior to and within the subsections and categories of each section, and pen or pencil. Refer to the section "Coding for Professional Services" in the *textbook* and Procedure 17-1 for step-by-step directions.

Standards: Complete all steps listed in this skill in _______ minutes with a minimum score of ________. (Time element and accuracy criteria may be given by instructor.)

Time: **Start:** ____________ **Completed:** ____________ **Total:** ____________ minutes

Scoring: One point for each step performed satisfactorily unless otherwise listed or weighted by instructor.

Directions with Performance Evaluation Checklist

1st Attempt	2nd Attempt	3rd Attempt		
_______	_______	_______	Gather materials (equipment and supplies) listed under "Conditions."	

RADIOLOGY 70010–79999 AND PATHOLOGY/LABORATORY 80048–89398

1st Attempt	2nd Attempt	3rd Attempt		
____/5	____/5	____/5	1. X-rays of hand, four views	____________
____/5	____/5	____/5	2. Internal mammary angiography; radiological supervision and interpretation	____________
____/5	____/5	____/5	3. Computed tomography of the abdomen with contrast material	____________
____/5	____/5	____/5	4. Retrograde urethrocystography with supervision and interpretation	____________
____/5	____/5	____/5	5. Lipid panel	____________
____/5	____/5	____/5	6. Bacterial culture quantitative, urine	____________
____/5	____/5	____/5	7. Bone marrow (blood cells) tissue culture for neoplastic disorders	____________
____/5	____/5	____/5	8. Surgical pathology examination of the gallbladder	____________
_______	_______	_______	Complete within specified time.	
____/42	____/42	____/42	**Total points earned** (To obtain a percentage score, divide the total points earned by the number of points possible.)	

JOB SKILL 17-4 *(continued)*

Comments:

Evaluator's Signature: ________________________ **Need to Repeat:** ____________

National Curriculum Competency: CAAHEP: Psychomotor: VIII.P.1	ABHES: 8.t

JOB SKILL 17-5
Code Procedures and Services in the Medicine Section

Name ______________________________ Date ______________ Score ________

Performance Objective

Task: Locate the correct procedure code from the Medicine section of *CPT* for each scenario.

Conditions: *Current Procedural Terminology* codebook, "Medicine Guidelines" found at the beginning of the Medicine section, *CPT* notes that appear prior to and within the subsections and categories of the Medicine section, and pen or pencil. Refer to the section "Coding for Professional Services" in the *textbook* and Procedure 17-1 for step-by-step directions.

Standards: Complete all steps listed in this skill in _______ minutes with a minimum score of ________. (Time element and accuracy criteria may be given by instructor.)

Time: **Start:** ____________ **Completed:** ____________ **Total:** ____________ minutes

Scoring: One point for each step performed satisfactorily unless otherwise listed or weighted by instructor.

Directions with Performance Evaluation Checklist

1st Attempt	2nd Attempt	3rd Attempt		
_____	_____	_____	Gather materials (equipment and supplies) listed under "Conditions."	
____/10	____/10	____/10	1. Immune globulin injection, botulism, intravenous push	
			Product:	__________
			Administration:	__________
____/10	____/10	____/10	2. Influenza virus vaccine (split virus) intramuscular injection (IM), to a 62-year-old patient	
			Product:	__________
			Administration:	__________
____/5	____/5	____/5	3. Replacement of contact lens	__________
____/5	____/5	____/5	4. Cardiovascular stress test (treadmill) with continuous electrocardiographic monitoring with physician supervision, interpretation, and report	__________
____/5	____/5	____/5	5. Handling of specimen for transfer from the physician's office to a laboratory	__________
_____	_____	_____	Complete within specified time.	
____/37	____/37	____/37	**Total points earned** (To obtain a percentage score, divide the total points earned by the number of points possible.)	

JOB SKILL 17-5 *(continued)*

Comments:

Evaluator's Signature: ______________________ **Need to Repeat:** __________

National Curriculum Competency: CAAHEP: Psychomotor: VIII.P.1	ABHES: 8.t

JOB SKILL 17-6
Code Clinical Examples

Name ______________________________ Date ______________ Score ________

Performance Objective

Task: Read each scenario; select the correct *CPT* or *HCPCS Level II* procedure code.

Conditions: Use *Current Procedural Terminology* codebook or Tables 17-2 and 17-3 in the *textbook*, Mock Fee Schedule and *HCPCS Level II* codes found in Part III of the *Workbook,* and pen or pencil.

Standards: Complete all steps listed in this skill in _______ minutes with a minimum score of ________. (Time element and accuracy criteria may be given by instructor.)

Time: **Start:** ____________ **Completed:** ____________ **Total:** ____________ minutes

Scoring: One point for each step performed satisfactorily unless otherwise listed or weighted by instructor.

Directions with Performance Evaluation Checklist

This job skill will familiarize you with the parts of the CMS-1500 claim form, coding from SOAP chart notes, and *HCPCS Level II* codes. All sections of *CPT* will be used. Answer the questions and insert data in Field 24 of the CMS-1500 claim form.

1st Attempt	2nd Attempt	3rd Attempt	
______	______	______	Gather materials (equipment and supplies) listed under "Conditions."

CMS-1500 CLAIM FORM—SCENARIO A: On February 3, current year, a private insurance patient is taken to an ambulatory surgery center with effusion of fluid (hydrarthrosis) of the right knee. The physician does an arthrocentesis and aspirates. A dressing is applied and patient is to return to office in one week.

____/7 ____/7 ____/7 1. What is the date of the service or procedure? Indicate the eight-digit date in the unshaded area of Field 24A (left portion only).

____/7 ____/7 ____/7 2. What is the correct procedure code? Insert this in the unshaded area of Field 24D (*CPT/HCPCS*).

____/7 ____/7 ____/7 3. What is the mock fee for this service? Insert this in the unshaded area of Field 24F.

____/7 ____/7 ____/7 4. How many times was this procedure performed? Indicate this in the unshaded area of Field 24G (DAYS OR UNITS).

24. A. DATE(S) OF SERVICE From MM DD YY To MM DD YY	B. PLACE OF SERVICE	C. EMG	D. PROCEDURES, SERVICES, OR SUPPLIES (Explain Unusual Circumstances) CPT/HCPCS | MODIFIER	E. DIAGNOSIS POINTER	F. $ CHARGES	G. DAYS OR UNITS	H. EPSDT Family Plan	I. ID. QUAL.	J. RENDERING PROVIDER ID. #
								NPI	

Courtesy of the Centers for Medicare and Medicaid Services

CMS-1500 CLAIM FORM—SCENARIO B: On May 6, a new patient is seen in the office of an otologist after referral by a family physician to evaluate and treat diminished hearing in the right ear. The physician performs an expanded problem-focused history and examination. A comprehensive audiometry threshold evaluation and speech recognition test is performed, revealing a conductive right ear low-frequency loss of hearing. Patient is referred to an audiologist for hearing aid examination and selection. Decision making is straightforward. Patient is asked to return in one month.

JOB SKILL 17-6 *(continued)*

_____/7 _____/7 _____/7 5. What is the date of the service for each procedure? Indicate the eight-digit date in the unshaded area of Field 24A (left portion only).

_____/7 _____/7 _____/7 6. What are the correct procedure codes? Insert these in the unshaded area of Field 24D (*CPT/HCPCS*).

_____/7 _____/7 _____/7 7. What are the mock fees for these services? Insert these in the unshaded area of Field 24F.

_____/7 _____/7 _____/7 8. How many times were these procedures performed? Indicate this in the unshaded area of Field 24G (DAYS OR UNITS).

24. A. DATE(S) OF SERVICE From MM	DD	YY	To MM	DD	YY	B. PLACE OF SERVICE	C. EMG	D. PROCEDURES, SERVICES, OR SUPPLIES (Explain Unusual Circumstances) CPT/HCPCS	MODIFIER	E. DIAGNOSIS POINTER	F. $ CHARGES	G. DAYS OR UNITS	H. EPSDT Family Plan	I. ID. QUAL.	J. RENDERING PROVIDER ID. #
														NPI	
														NPI	

Courtesy of the Centers for Medicare and Medicaid Services

SOAP CHART NOTE A:

4/15/XX Maria Gomez

S: A 35-year-old female established patient is seen for a new complaint of left lower quadrant pain; 1 wk. duration. Symptoms: mild fever, decreased appetite, and mild constipation for 1 wk. Pt denies abdominal injury, change in urination, or abnormal menstruation. LMP: 3/12/XX.

O: Temp: 100.2°F; BP 130/80, HR 80; RR 18.

Lungs: Clear.

Abdomen: Both sides mildly hyperactive, flat, mild guarding LLQ, rebound neg; fullness LLQ; no discrete masses; no HSM.

Rectal: Normal tone; no masses; guaiac positive.

Pelvic: Cervix closed, uterus and ovaries normal, fullness lt lat adnexa c̄ tenderness.

Lab: CBC, elevated. WBC c̄ mild lt shift; UA, normal; HCG, pregnancy test negative.

A: Probable diverticulitis of sigmoid colon based on clinical picture.

P: Obtain barium enema to R/O diverticulitis. Begin antibiotics and dietary restriction during acute phase and follow up in three days.

_____/5 _____/5 _____/5 9. Read the SOAP note and select the correct E/M code. _____________

CHART NOTE B:

A physician does a history and examination on an established patient for 5 minutes, performs acne surgery (code 10040), and counsels the patient on skin care and diet for 10 minutes.

_____/5 _____/5 _____/5 10. Read the chart note and select the correct E/M code. _____________

HCPCS LEVEL II CODES

_____/3 _____/3 _____/3 11. Select the correct *HCPCS* Level II code for one sterile eye pad. _____________

_____/3 _____/3 _____/3 12. Select the correct *HCPCS* Level II code for metal underarm crutches. _____________

JOB SKILL 17-6 *(continued)*

____/3	____/3	____/3	13. Select the correct *HCPCS* Level II code for 1 cc gamma globulin inj IM.	________
____/3	____/3	____/3	14. Select the correct *HCPCS* Level II code for the physician interpretation of a screening Pap smear.	________
____	____	____	Complete within specified time.	
____/80	____/80	____/80	**Total points earned** (To obtain a percentage score, divide the total points earned by the number of points possible.)	

Comments:

Evaluator's Signature: ____________________ **Need to Repeat:** ________

National Curriculum Competency: CAAHEP: Psychomotor: VIII.P.1	ABHES: 8.t

JOB SKILL 17-7
Code Diagnoses from Chapters 1, 2, 3, 4, and 5 in *ICD-10-CM*

Name ______________________ Date __________ Score ______

PERFORMANCE OBJECTIVE

Task: Code diagnoses from the first five chapters of *ICD-10-CM,* Volumes 1 and 2.

Conditions: Use *International Classification of Diseases, 10th Revision, Clinical Modification**, Volumes 1 and 2; and pen or pencil. Refer to Procedure 17-2 in the *textbook* for step-by-step directions.

Standards: Complete all steps listed in this job skill in ______ minutes with a minimum score of ______.
(Time element and accuracy criteria may be given by instructor.)

Time: **Start:** __________ **Completed:** __________ **Total:** __________ minutes

Scoring: One point for each step performed satisfactorily unless otherwise listed or weighted by instructor.

DIRECTIONS WITH PERFORMANCE EVALUATION CHECKLIST

Read the following statements, look up main terms in Volume 2, the Alphabetic Index of the diagnostic codebook, and then confirm the code selection in Volume 1, the Tabular List.

1st Attempt	2nd Attempt	3rd Attempt		
______	______	______	Gather materials (equipment and supplies) listed under "Conditions."	
____/5	____/5	____/5	1. Code human immunodeficiency virus.	__________
____/5	____/5	____/5	2. Code blackwater fever malaria.	__________
____/5	____/5	____/5	3. Code malignant melanoma in situ of the shoulder and left upper arm.	__________
____/5	____/5	____/5	4. Code benign neoplasm of the right testes.	__________
____/5	____/5	____/5	5. Code hereditary hemolytic anemia.	__________
____/5	____/5	____/5	6. Code primary thrombocytopenia.	__________
____/5	____/5	____/5	7. Code type 2 diabetes mellitus without complications.	__________
____/5	____/5	____/5	8. Code active rickets.	__________
____/5	____/5	____/5	9. Code anxiety.	__________
____/5	____/5	____/5	10. Code mild mental retardation.	__________
______	______	______	Complete within specified time.	
____/52	____/52	____/52	**Total points earned** (To obtain a percentage score, divide the total points earned by the number of points possible.)	

International Classification of Diseases, 10th Revision, Clinical Modification codes in this chapter are from the 2012 draft of *ICD-10-CM.*

JOB SKILL 17-7 *(continued)*

Comments:

Evaluator's Signature: ________________________ **Need to Repeat:** __________

National Curriculum Competency: CAAHEP: Psychomotor: VIII.P.2	ABHES: 8.t

JOB SKILL 17-8
Code Diagnoses from Chapters 6, 7, 8, 9, and 10 in *ICD-10-CM*

Name ________________________________ Date ______________ Score ________

PERFORMANCE OBJECTIVE

Task: Code diagnoses from Chapters 6 through 10 of *ICD-10-CM,* Volumes 1 and 2.

Conditions: Use *International Classification of Diseases, 10th Revision, Clinical Modification,* Volumes 1 and 2; and pen or pencil. Refer to Procedure 17-2 in the *textbook* for step-by-step directions.

Standards: Complete all steps listed in this job skill in _______ minutes with a minimum score of _______. (Time element and accuracy criteria may be given by instructor.)

Time: **Start:** ____________ **Completed:** ____________ **Total:** ____________ minutes

Scoring: One point for each step performed satisfactorily unless otherwise listed or weighted by instructor.

DIRECTIONS WITH PERFORMANCE EVALUATION CHECKLIST

Read the following statements, look up main terms in Volume 2, the Alphabetic Index of the diagnostic codebook, and then confirm the code selection in Volume 1, the Tabular List.

1st Attempt	2nd Attempt	3rd Attempt		
_____	_____	_____	Gather materials (equipment and supplies) listed under "Conditions."	
____/5	____/5	____/5	1. Code epileptic seizure.	__________
____/5	____/5	____/5	2. Code pneumococcal meningitis.	__________
____/5	____/5	____/5	3. Code borderline glaucoma.	__________
____/5	____/5	____/5	4. Code right, lower eyelid cyst.	__________
____/5	____/5	____/5	5. Code bilateral otorrhea.	__________
____/5	____/5	____/5	6. Code acute eustachian salpingitis of the right ear.	__________
____/5	____/5	____/5	7. Code malignant hypertension.	__________
____/5	____/5	____/5	8. Code nontraumatic cerebral hemorrhage; brain stem.	__________
____/5	____/5	____/5	9. Code viral pneumonia.	__________
____/5	____/5	____/5	10. Code chronic bronchitis.	__________
_____	_____	_____	Complete within specified time.	
___/52	___/52	___/52	**Total points earned** (To obtain a percentage score, divide the total points earned by the number of points possible.)	

JOB SKILL 17-8 *(continued)*

Comments:

Evaluator's Signature: ______________________ **Need to Repeat:** ______________

National Curriculum Competency: CAAHEP: Psychomotor: VIII.P.2	ABHES: 8.t

JOB SKILL 17-9

Code Diagnoses from Chapters 11, 12, 13, 14, and 15 in *ICD-10-CM*

Name ______________________________ Date ______________ Score ________

PERFORMANCE OBJECTIVE

Task: Code diagnoses from Chapters 11 through 15 of *ICD-10-CM,* Volumes 1 and 2.

Conditions: Use *International Classification of Diseases, 10th Revision, Clinical Modification,* Volumes 1 and 2; and pen or pencil. Refer to Procedure 17-2 in the *textbook* for step-by-step directions.

Standards: Complete all steps listed in this job skill in ________ minutes with a minimum score of ________. (Time element and accuracy criteria may be given by instructor.)

Time: **Start:** ____________ **Completed:** ____________ **Total:** ____________ minutes

Scoring: One point for each step performed satisfactorily unless otherwise listed or weighted by instructor.

DIRECTIONS WITH PERFORMANCE EVALUATION CHECKLIST

Read the following statements, look up main terms in Volume 2, the Alphabetic Index of the diagnostic codebook, and then confirm the code selection in Volume 1, the Tabular List.

1st Attempt	2nd Attempt	3rd Attempt		
______	______	______	Gather materials (equipment and supplies) listed under "Conditions."	
____/5	____/5	____/5	1. Code ulcerative stomatitis.	__________
____/5	____/5	____/5	2. Code acute peptic ulcer with hemorrhage.	__________
____/5	____/5	____/5	3. Code impetigo.	__________
____/5	____/5	____/5	4. Code dermatitis due to cold weather.	__________
____/5	____/5	____/5	5. Code Kaschin-Beck disease affecting multiple sites.	__________
____/5	____/5	____/5	6. Code spondylosis of the lumbar spine without myelopathy or radiculopathy.	__________
____/5	____/5	____/5	7. Code stage II chronic renal disease.	__________
____/5	____/5	____/5	8. Code fibroadenosis of the left breast.	__________
____/5	____/5	____/5	9. Code excessive vomiting in early pregnancy causing dehydration.	__________
____/5	____/5	____/5	10. Code postpartum condition of retained placenta without hemorrhage.	__________
______	______	______	Complete within specified time.	
____/52	____/52	____/52	**Total points earned** (To obtain a percentage score, divide the total points earned by the number of points possible.)	

JOB SKILL 17-9 (*continued*)

Comments:

Evaluator's Signature: ______________________________ **Need to Repeat:** ______________

National Curriculum Competency: CAAHEP: Psychomotor: VIII.P.2	ABHES: 8.t

JOB SKILL 17-10

Code Diagnoses from Chapters 16, 17, 18, 19, and 20 in *ICD-10-CM*

Name ______________________________ Date ______________ Score ________

PERFORMANCE OBJECTIVE

Task: Code diagnoses from Chapters 16 through 20 of *ICD-10-CM,* Volumes 1 and 2.

Conditions: Use *International Classification of Diseases, 10th Revision, Clinical Modification,* Volumes 1 and 2; and pen or pencil. Refer to Procedure 17-2 in the *textbook* for step-by-step directions.

Standards: Complete all steps listed in this job skill in _______ minutes with a minimum score of _______. (Time element and accuracy criteria may be given by instructor.)

Time: **Start:** ____________ **Completed:** ____________ **Total:** ____________ minutes

Scoring: One point for each step performed satisfactorily unless otherwise listed or weighted by instructor.

DIRECTIONS WITH PERFORMANCE EVALUATION CHECKLIST

Read the following statements, look up main terms in Volume 2, the Alphabetic Index of the diagnostic codebook, and then confirm the code selection in Volume 1, the Tabular List.

1st Attempt	2nd Attempt	3rd Attempt		
______	______	______	Gather materials (equipment and supplies) listed under "Conditions."	
____/5	____/5	____/5	1. Code bradycardia in a neonate.	____________
____/5	____/5	____/5	2. Code neonatal diabetes mellitus.	____________
____/5	____/5	____/5	3. Code bilateral cleft lip and palate (hard and soft).	____________
____/5	____/5	____/5	4. Code accessory toe on right foot.	____________
____/5	____/5	____/5	5. Code frequent urination.	____________
____/5	____/5	____/5	6. Code microcalcification found on mammogram.	____________
____/5	____/5	____/5	7. Code fracture of two ribs, right side.	____________
____/5	____/5	____/5	8. Code left ankle sprain.	____________
____/5	____/5	____/5	9. Code drowning due to an overturned sailboat.	____________
____/5	____/5	____/5	10. Code an initial encounter for exposure to excessive natural heat.	____________
______	______	______	Complete within specified time.	
____/52	____/52	____/52	**Total points earned** (To obtain a percentage score, divide the total points earned by the number of points possible.)	

JOB SKILL 17-10 (*continued*)

Comments:

Evaluator's Signature: ______________________ **Need to Repeat:** __________

National Curriculum Competency: CAAHEP: Psychomotor: VIII.P.2	ABHES: 8.t

JOB SKILL 17-11
Code Diagnoses from Chapter 21 and the Table of Drugs and Chemicals in *ICD-10-CM*

Name ______________________________ Date ____________ Score ________

PERFORMANCE OBJECTIVE

Task: Code diagnoses from Chapter 21 and the Table of Drugs and Chemicals of *ICD-10-CM,* Volumes 1 and 2.

Conditions: Use *International Classification of Diseases, 10th Revision, Clinical Modification,* Volumes 1 and 2; and pen or pencil. Refer to Procedure 17-2 in the textbook for step-by-step directions.

Standards: Complete all steps listed in this job skill in ________ minutes with a minimum score of ________. (Time element and accuracy criteria may be given by instructor.)

Time: **Start:** ____________ **Completed:** ____________ **Total:** ____________ minutes

Scoring: One point for each step performed satisfactorily unless otherwise listed or weighted by instructor.

DIRECTIONS WITH PERFORMANCE EVALUATION CHECKLIST

Read the following statements, look up main terms in Volume 2, the Alphabetic Index of the diagnostic codebook, and then confirm the code selection in Volume 1, the Tabular List. Use the Table of Drugs and Chemicals, found at the end of Volume 2 when selecting "X" codes.

1st Attempt	2nd Attempt	3rd Attempt		
______	______	______	Gather materials (equipment and supplies) listed under "Conditions."	
____/5	____/5	____/5	1. Code supervision of first normal pregnancy.	__________
____/5	____/5	____/5	2. Code personal history of blood disease.	__________
____/5	____/5	____/5	3. Code encounter for influenza vaccination.	__________
____/5	____/5	____/5	4. Code encounter for patient with positive HIV test result with no symptoms.	__________
____/5	____/5	____/5	5. Code rattlesnake bite reaction.	__________
____/5	____/5	____/5	6. Code accidental poisoning using tranquilizers.	__________
______	______	______	Complete within specified time.	
____/32	____/32	____/32	**Total points earned** (To obtain a percentage score, divide the total points earned by the number of points possible.)	

JOB SKILL 17-11 *(continued)*

Comments:

Evaluator's Signature: ______________________________ **Need to Repeat:** ____________

National Curriculum Competency: CAAHEP: Psychomotor: VIII.P.2	ABHES: 8.t

CHAPTER 18

Office Managerial Responsibilities

OBJECTIVES

After completing the exercises, the student will be able to:

1. Enhance knowledge of medical terminology, interpret abbreviations, and accurately spell medical words.
2. Document patient complaints and determine actions to resolve problems (Job Skill 18-1).
3. Write an agenda for an office meeting (Job Skill 18-2).
4. Prepare material for an office procedures manual (Job Skill 18-3).
5. Perform inventory control and keep an equipment maintenance log (Job Skill 18-4).
6. Abstract data from a catalog and key an order form (Job Skill 18-5).
7. Complete an order form for office supplies (Job Skill 18-6).
8. Perform mathematic calculations of an office manager (Job Skill 18-7).
9. Prepare two order forms (Job Skill 18-8).
10. Prepare a travel expense report (Job Skill 18-9).

FOCUS ON CERTIFICATION*

CMA Content Summary

- Americans with Disabilities Act
- Employment laws
- Personnel records
- Performance evaluation
- Maintenance and repairs
- Inventory control
- Purchasing
- Personnel manual
- Policy and procedures manual
- Job readiness and seeking employment

RMA Content Summary

- Maintain inventory of medical/office supplies and equipment
- Coordinate maintenance and repair of office equipment
- Maintain office sanitation and comfort
- Employ appropriate interpersonal skills with employer, coworkers, vendors, and business associates
- Understand and utilize proper documentation of instruction

CMAS Content Summary

- Know basic laws pertaining to the medical practice
- Observe and maintain confidentiality of records
- Facilitate staff meetings and in-service, and ensure communication of essential information to staff
- Manage medical office business functions
- Manage outside vendors and supplies
- Comply with licensure and accreditation requirements
- Manage/supervise medical office staff
- Conduct performance reviews and disciplinary action
- Maintain office policy manual
- Manage staff recruiting in compliance with state and federal laws
- Orient and train new staff
- Manage medical and office supply inventories and order supplies
- Maintain office equipment and arrange for equipment maintenance and repair
- Maintain office facilities environment

STOP AND THINK CASE SCENARIOS AND EXAM-STYLE REVIEW QUESTIONS

Refer to the end of Chapter 18 in the *textbook*.

Abbreviation and Spelling Review

Read the following patient's chart note and write the meanings for the abbreviations listed below the note. To decode any abbreviations you do not understand or that appear unfamiliar to you, refer to the list of abbreviations in Part IV of this *Workbook*. Step-by-step directions for this exercise are found in Procedure 1-1 of Chapter 1 in the *textbook*. Medical terms in the chart note are italicized; study them for spelling. Use your medical dictionary to look up their definitions. Your instructor may give a spelling and definition test that includes these words and abbreviations.

*This *Workbook* and the accompanying *textbook* meet the entry-level administrative and general competencies for the CMA outlined by the AAMA Examination Content Outline and Occupational Analysis and for the RMA and CMAS outlined by the AMT Competencies, Construction Parameters, and Examination Specifications (see Competency Grid in Appendix B of the *textbook*).

DATE	PROGRESS
12-14-20XX	Helen P. Craig CC: Back pain originating in the *flank* + radiating across the *abdomen*. Pt complains of *abdominal distention* & difficulty *urinating*. Exam reveals increased *sensitivity* in lumbar & *groin* areas. Considerable discomfort c̄ marked *urethral stenosis*. U/A: 5-10 RBC, occ wbc, sp gr 1.012; X: KUB & IVP revealed small *calculus* in R UPJ dilat to 24F c̄ Brev. Inc fluid intake, low *calcium* diet. RX *Aluminum hydroxide* gel 60 ml q.i.d. RTC 1 wk for FU + decision on whether to operate.
	G Practon, MD G Practon, MD

CC __________

Pt __________

c̄ __________

U/A __________

RBC __________

occ __________

wbc __________

sp gr __________

X __________

KUB __________

IVP __________

R __________

UPJ __________

dilat __________

F __________

Brev __________

inc __________

RX __________

ml __________

q.i.d. __________

RTC __________

wk __________

FU __________

Review Questions

Review the objectives, glossary, and chapter information before completing the following review questions.

1. Why is it important for the office manager to be a mentor and coach? __________

2. What two mechanisms can be put into place in a medical office to help patient relations, promote patient satisfaction, and learn what policies and procedures need improvement? __________

3. To boost job performance, what three things should be emphasized during a staff meeting?

   a. __________

   b. __________

   c. __________

4. As a new employee, where would you look to find your job description? ______________________

____

5. List one federal agency that administers statutes and regulations that employers must adhere to, and name a resource it publishes that can be used to determine which statutes apply to your office.

____

____

6. What is the name of the act that covers most benefit plans in the private sector? ______________

____

____

7. What laws prohibit job discrimination based on race, color, religion, sex, or national origin? ________

____

8. How would you know if the Family and Medical Leave Act applies to your job in a medical office?

____

____

9. As an office manager, what two questions will you be expected to answer if a case of sexual harassment goes to court? ____

____

____

10. What is the purpose of an office policies and procedures manual? ____________________

____

____

11. When hiring a new employee, what are four responsibilities of an office manager? What would you do first, second, third, and fourth? ____

____

12. After an employee has been hired and before he or she is expected to perform all tasks, what are two responsibilities of the office manager? ______________________________________

13. What observations should be included when an office manager evaluates a new employee? ________

____

____

14. Before selecting a housecleaning service, what must be done? ______________________

____

15. When selecting a new piece of equipment for the medical office, what are some things to consider?

    a. ______

    b. ______

    c. ______

    d. ______

    e. ______

    f. ______

    g. ______

16. What are three important points to consider when selecting a vendor from which to order office or medical supplies?

    a. ______

    b. ______

    c. ______

17. State four reasons why it may be unsatisfactory to order supplies in bulk.

    a. ______

    b. ______

    c. ______

    d. ______

18. When an order for merchandise arrives, what steps should be taken after the package is opened? ______

19. Name three items that must appear on a running-inventory card.

    a. ______

    b. ______

    c. ______

20. If the physician is planning to attend a medical convention, at what point should the office manager start making the arrangements? ______

Critical Thinking Exercises

1. As an office manager, what strategy would you use to correct an employee who is a gossip and spreads a harmful rumor about another employee? ______

2. List some methods that an office manager might implement to promote open and honest communication.

____

____

____

____

____

____

3. As an office manager, describe how you would make a new employee feel more relaxed during his or her first week at work. ____

____

____

____

____

____

JOB SKILL 18-1

Document Patient Complaints and Determine Actions to Resolve Problems

Name ______________________ Date ____________ Score ________

Performance Objective

Task: Document two patient complaints then determine the action to take to resolve each problem.

Conditions: Scenarios, Patient Complaint Documents (Forms 89 and 90), and pen or pencil. Refer to *textbook* Figure 18-1 for a visual example and Procedure 18-1 for step-by-step directions.

Standards: Complete all steps listed in this job skill in ________ minutes with a minimum score of ________. (Time element and accuracy criteria may be given by instructor.)

Time: **Start:** ____________ **Completed:** ____________ **Total:** ____________ minutes

Scoring: One point for each step performed satisfactorily unless otherwise listed or weighted by instructor.

Directions with Performance Evaluation Checklist

Scenario A: You are working as the receptionist and patient Margaret Williams walks in and is very upset. She requested and received a copy of her medical records last week and while reading them discovered several errors. She wants to cancel her appointment later today and is thinking of changing doctors. Mrs. Williams' account number is 987-23A and her account balance is $132.28.

1st Attempt	2nd Attempt	3rd Attempt	
______	______	______	Gather materials (equipment and supplies) listed under "Conditions."
______	______	______	1. Use Form 89 and fill in the current date.
______	______	______	2. Record the patient's account number.
______	______	______	3. Record the patient's name.
______	______	______	4. List the account balance.
____/5	____/5	____/5	5. Document the patient's complaint, using quotation marks when writing her exact words; demonstrate empathy and use active listening skills.
____10	____/10	____/10	6. Determine what action you would take and document the plan.

Scenario B. It is 4:00 p.m. and patient Susan Robles (account 689-41A, balance $250.00) calls and starts complaining to you about how she is never able to get through to Dr. Practon when she needs him. She says, "The telephone lines are always busy, busy, busy!" You ask how many times she has called and she indicates her telephone has been on automatic dialing on and off for 2 hours.

1st Attempt	2nd Attempt	3rd Attempt	
______	______	______	7. Use Form 90 and fill in the current date.
______	______	______	8. Record the patient's account number.
______	______	______	9. Record the patient's name.
______	______	______	10. List the account balance.
____/5	____/5	____/5	11. Document the patient's complaint, using quotation marks when writing her exact words; demonstrate empathy and use active listening skills.
____/10	____/10	____/10	12. Determine what action you would take and document the plan.
______	______	______	Complete within specified time.
____/40	____/40	____/40	**Total points earned** (To obtain a percentage score, divide the total points earned by the number of points possible.)

JOB SKILL 18-1 *(continued)*

Comments:

Evaluator's Signature: ______________________________ **Need to Repeat:** ____________

National Curriculum Competency: CAAHEP: Psychomotor: IV.P.2, 4; Affective: IV.A.1, 2	ABHES: 8.d, aa, bb, dd

JOB SKILL 18-2
Write an Agenda for an Office Meeting

Name ______________________________ Date ______________ Score ________

Performance Objective

Task: Assemble information and key or type an outline for an office meeting agenda.

Conditions: One sheet of white paper, computer or typewriter, example of an agenda outlining items covered in the previous staff meeting (see *textbook* Figure 18-4), agenda suggestions posted on a bulletin board (see *Workbook* Figure 18-1), and step-by-step directions found in Procedure 18-3 in the *textbook*.

Standards: Complete all steps listed in this skill in _______ minutes with a minimum score of _______. (Time element and accuracy criteria may be given by instructor.)

Time: **Start:** ____________ **Completed:** ____________ **Total:** ____________ minutes

Scoring: One point for each step performed satisfactorily unless otherwise listed or weighted by instructor.

Directions with Performance Evaluation Checklist

Refer to *textbook* Figure 18-4 to learn what occurred at the previous meeting and to determine unfinished business. Study the notes in *Workbook* Figure 18-1, gathered from members of the staff, indicating actions they wish to introduce at the meeting and when the meeting is scheduled. List all subject matter for the agenda in rough draft outline form.

1st Attempt	2nd Attempt	3rd Attempt	
______	______	______	Gather materials (equipment and supplies) listed under "Conditions."
____/2	____/2	____/2	1. Key a heading for the staff meeting agenda.
____/3	____/3	____/3	2. Indicate when the meeting will take place.
______	______	______	3. Indicate that the office manager, Jane Paulsen, will act as the chairperson and will call the meeting to order.
______	______	______	4. Indicate that the minutes from the previous meeting will be read.
______	______	______	5. Indicate who will be present (all staff members).
____/5	____/5	____/5	6. Under Committee Reports, indicate that staff members Amy Fluor (transcription) and Mike O'Shea (bookkeeping) will be reporting as committee chairpersons.
____/5	____/5	____/5	7. Indicate that Jane Paulsen and Dr. Fran Practon will be reposting unfinished business.
____/5	____/5	____/5	8. Indicate that Dr. Gerald Practon and Carla Haskins will be reporting new business.
______	______	______	9. Note that the next meeting is scheduled at 8:30 a.m. on March 20, 20XX.
______	______	______	10. Indicate that the meeting is adjourned.
______	______	______	Complete within specified time.
____/27	____/27	____/27	**Total points earned** (To obtain a percentage score, divide the total points earned by the number of points possible.)

JOB SKILL 18-2 (*continued*)

FIGURE 18-1

Mon.
I want to discuss possibility of moving transcription station to Rm. A, which is away from reception room interruptions.
Amy Fluor

from the desk of Gerald Practon...
I will present summer vacation schedule for sign-ups.
G.P.

staff Meeting scheduled for 2/25/XX in conference room at 12 noon. Lunch will be provided. Please make plans to attend.
Jane Paulsen-OM

I PLAN TO INTRODUCE GARY KLEIN, FROM MEDICAL ARTS PRESS, WHO WILL PRESENT THE ADVANTAGES OF ALPH/COLOR FILING SYSTEM. (I THINK HIS REPORT SHOULD BE SCHEDULED LAST ON THE AGENDA.)
CARLA HASKINS

F.P. and G.P.
At our last meeting I was asked to investigate cleaning services. I'm going to recommend we hire Todd's Cleaning to begin on March 15, and I'll make a motion to this effect.
Also, someone needs to notify Martha's Maids soon that we are terminating their services. Would you like me to do this?
Jane Paulsen-OM

I am going to suggest hiring an accting firm to audit the books yearly on Jan. 1.
Mike O'Shea
bookkeeper

From the desk of Fran Practon...
I will suggest that since flex-time is to be initiated in May, a committee should be named to spell out scheduling, compensation, and benefits for the staff and incorporate it into the office procedures manual; also there should be a discussion of circumstances under which an alternative work schedule will be used.

Comments:

Evaluator's Signature: ______________________ **Need to Repeat:** __________

National Curriculum Competency: CAAHEP: Psychomotor: IV.P.2	ABHES: 8.hh

JOB SKILL 18-3
Prepare Material for an Office Procedures Manual

Name ______________________ Date ____________ Score ________

Performance Objective

Task: Assemble information on office appointments for Practon Medical Group, Inc., and key or type a sample reference sheet for an office procedures manual.

Conditions: One or two sheets of white paper; computer or typewriter. Refer to Procedure 18-6 in the *textbook* for step-by-step directions. Refer to the *Appointment* section of *Office Policies* listed in Part III of the *Workbook* to obtain specific appointment information. Refer to Chapter 7 for general appointment guidelines and *textbook* Figure 18-6 to help you plan a well-organized reference sheet.

Standards: Complete all steps listed in this skill in _______ minutes with a minimum score of _______. (Time element and accuracy criteria may be given by instructor.)

Time: **Start:** ____________ **Completed:** ____________ **Total:** ____________ minutes

Scoring: One point for each step performed satisfactorily unless otherwise listed or weighted by instructor.

Directions with Performance Evaluation Checklist

Doctors Gerald and Fran Practon have asked you to prepare a reference sheet for the office procedures manual detailing appointment procedures. Create a page listing information regarding appointments that is easy for all employees to follow.

1st Attempt	2nd Attempt	3rd Attempt	
______	______	______	Gather materials (equipment and supplies) listed under "Conditions."
______	______	______	1. Key a heading for the reference sheet.
______	______	______	2. Key a heading for "Appointment Office Hours."
____/5	____/5	____/5	3. List appointment days and times as well as office policy for routine appointments.
____/5	____/5	____/5	4. List appointment days and times as well as office policy for emergency appointments, work-ins, callbacks, and dictation.
____/5	____/5	____/5	5. List hospital surgery days and times for doctors Gerald and Fran Practon.
____/2	____/2	____/2	6. List the appropriate times for house calls.
____/7	____/7	____/7	7. Create a heading for time allotment for office visits and procedures and state office scheduling policy.
______	______	______	8. List the time allotment for initial office visits.
______	______	______	9. List the time allotment for consultations.
______	______	______	10. List the time allotment for follow-up office visits.
____/6	____/6	____/6	11. List the time allotment for brief office visits for such things as suture removal; name various procedures that fit into this category.
______	______	______	12. List the time allotment for office procedures.
______	______	______	13. List the office policy for house calls.
______	______	______	14. Create a heading for questions to be asked when an appointment is made over the telephone.

JOB SKILL 18-3 (*continued*)

____/5 ____/5 ____/5 15. List five basic questions to ask when an appointment is made over the telephone.

a. ________________________________

b. ________________________________

c. ________________________________

d. ________________________________

e. ________________________________

_____ _____ _____ Complete within specified time.

____/45 ____/45 ____/45 **Total points earned** (To obtain a percentage score, divide the total points earned by the number of points possible.)

Comments:

Evaluator's Signature: ____________________ **Need to Repeat:** __________

National Curriculum Competency: CAAHEP: Psychomotor: IV.P.4	ABHES: 8.d

JOB SKILL 18-4
Perform Inventory Control and Keep an Equipment Maintenance Log

Name ______________________________ Date ______________ Score ________

Performance Objective

Task: List office equipment on an inventory control sheet and track the maintenance of each piece of equipment.

Conditions: List of office equipment with manufacturer, model number, length of warranty, date of purchase, and purchase price; Inventory Control Sheet/Maintenance Log (Form 91); pen or pencil.

Standards: Complete all steps listed in this job skill in ________minutes with a minimum score of ________. (Time element and accuracy criteria may be given by instructor.)

Time: **Start:** ____________ **Completed:** ____________ **Total:** ____________ minutes

Scoring: One point for each step performed satisfactorily unless otherwise listed or weighted by instructor.

Directions with Performance Evaluation Checklist

Scenario: You have just been promoted to office manager and Dr. Practon has asked you to look in your file cabinet and locate the warranties for each piece of office equipment. He presents you with an inventory control sheet with a maintenance log and asks you to record the file information so that you can make sure the equipment undergoes routine maintenance; it has been neglected in the past. You have located files for the equipment; their contents are listed in steps 2 through 7. Read the information about each piece of equipment, then abstract and record the pertinent data.

1st Attempt	2nd Attempt	3rd Attempt	
______	______	______	Gather materials (equipment and supplies) listed under "Conditions."
______	______	______	1. Using the Inventory Control Sheet/Maintenance Log (Form 91), record information for the equipment listed below; list each in alphabetical order by name (e.g., fax machine), recording data in each section of the form.
____/7	____/7	____/7	2. Macintosh iMac computer (3.2 GHz) with a 27-inch screen, bought October 3, 2011, for $1,699. There is a warranty for 3 years and it went through a routine service on October 12, 2012. You cannot find the serial number so you look it up on the computer (W88000XZX00) and record it on the warranty.
____/6	____/6	____/6	3. There is a file for the office stereo with two speakers. It has a CD player with FM/AM radio. The brand is "Denon," Model M37. It has a 2-year warranty and was purchased December 2, 2008, for $369.
____/12	____/12	____/12	4. You locate a file under "Philips" that includes a couple of items. A Desktop Dictaphone Cassette Transcriber/Recorder machine and a Dictaphone SpeechMike III. They were both purchased on June 20, 2008, and each has a 5-year warranty; it does not look like either has been serviced. The machine (model 3742) cost $440.98 and the handheld "mike" (model LFH3215) cost $70.

JOB SKILL 18-4 *(continued)*

____/13	____/13	____/13	5. There is a big file for the Sharp copy machine but that is not the one in the office; it is a Xerox machine. After sifting through all the papers you locate the sales receipt—it was purchased on February 11, 2005, and cost $4,299. You have to look at the machine to find the model number (5225); it is called a "Xerox WorkCentre." You locate paperwork that says it has a 3-year warranty so it has run out. There is a service book that lists service calls on the following dates: 2/15/06, 3/1/07, 3/12/08, 3/14/09, 2/25/10, 3/3/11, and 1/15/12.
____/6	____/6	____/6	6. The Panasonic fax machine (model UF-4000) was purchased on February 12, 2012, for $517. It has a 1-year warranty.
____/7	____/7	____/7	7. You cannot find a record for the Hewlett Packard LaserJet printer, model P2035, so you look in the check register and find that it was purchased on September 14, 2010, for $1,476. You call Hewlett Packard and give them the serial number and find out it has a 3-year warranty. Dr. Practon says it was serviced around the middle of March 2012.
______	______	______	8. You cannot find any more paperwork for the other equipment in the office so you will have to go to each piece of equipment and record the pertinent data.
______	______	______	Complete within specified time.
____/55	____/55	____/55	**Total points earned** (To obtain a percentage score, divide the total points earned by the number of points possible)

Comments:

Evaluator's Signature: ______________________________ **Need to Repeat:** ____________

National Curriculum Competency: CAAHEP: Psychomotor: V.P.9, 10	ABHES: 8.y, z

JOB SKILL 18-5
Abstract Data from a Catalog and Key an Order Form

Name ______________________ Date ____________ Score ________

Performance Objective

Task: Abstract information from catalog data sheets, determine charges, accurately key or type an order form, calculate discounts and sales tax, and compute a total.

Conditions: Order form (Form 92), catalog sheets (*Workbook* Figure 18-2 and Figure 18-3), calculator, and pen or pencil. Refer in the *textbook* to Procedure 18-10 for step-by-step directions, Figure 18-8 for an illustration, and Example 18-3 for an example of calculating sales tax.

Standards: Complete all steps listed in this skill in ________ minutes with a minimum score of ________. (Time element and accuracy criteria may be given by instructor.)

Time: **Start:** ____________ **Completed:** ____________ **Total:** ____________ minutes

Scoring: One point for each step performed satisfactorily unless otherwise listed or weighted by instructor.

Directions with Performance Evaluation Checklist

Doctors Fran and Gerald Practon want to order some printed letterhead, second sheets, and envelopes from Medical Arts Press. Study and abstract the correct information from the catalog sheets, noting the discount offered for second sheets. Then, complete the order form using the name, address, and so forth of Practon Medical Group, Inc. Determine the cost for each item, calculate discounts, and insert this information on the order form.

1st Attempt	2nd Attempt	3rd Attempt	
______	______	______	Gather materials (equipment and supplies) listed under "Conditions."
____/6	____/6	____/6	1. Complete the "Bill to" information on the order form.
______	______	______	2. Fill in the e-mail address for Practon Medical Group, Inc. (PMGI@aol.com).
______	______	______	3. Indicate "SAME" in the "Ship to" location on the order form.
____/2	____/2	____/2	4. Fill in the customer order number (0001002345) and the source code (BTGF) from the catalog.
____/2	____/2	____/2	5. List your name as the person to call for questions and the office telephone number; you are at extension 12.
______	______	______	6. List the practice specialty and number of doctors.
______	______	______	7. Indicate the method of shipping as UPS 2nd Day.
____/7	____/7	____/7	8. List the first item ordered: 2,000 raised-printed 25% rag content bond paper (8½″ by 11″); black ink, type style NR, product color ivory, order number PNB-530.
____/5	____/5	____/5	9. List the second item ordered: 1,000 Hammermill bond unprinted second sheets (8½″ by 11″), color ivory. See pricing under "Hammermill Bond Stock-Raised Printed" and apply the discount.
____/7	____/7	____/7	10. List the third item ordered: 1,000 raised-printed 25% rag content bond envelopes (number 10); black ink, type style NR, color ivory.
______	______	______	11. Total the merchandise order and insert figure.

JOB SKILL 18-5 *(continued)*

_______ _______ _______ 12. Calculate 7% sales tax and insert figure.

_______ _______ _______ 13. Add the sales tax to the total of the order and insert figure.

_______ _______ _______ Complete within specified time.

____/38 ____/38 ____/38 **Total points earned** (To obtain a percentage score, divide the total points earned by the number of points possible.)

Comments:

Evaluator's Signature: ______________________________ **Need to Repeat:** ____________

National Curriculum Competency: ABHES: 8.z

JOB SKILL 18-5 *(continued)*

FIGURE 18-2

letterheads

Distinctive. Dignified. Four popular sizes in your choice of paper stocks with flat or raised printing. Select either Hammermill Bond, an extremely popular paper noted for its bright white, smooth surface or 25% Rag Content Bond with Its cockle surface and crisp finish. We take an Intense pride In these papers and the craftsmanship of the printing. All copy in black ink.

SECOND SHEETS
Unprinted. Available at 60% of the Hammermill Bond price. Choice of onlonskin or Hammermill.

555 896 1114
RAYMOND S. STRONG, M.D.
SUITE 315 PROFESSIONAL BUILDING
1616 SHERIDAN WAY LAKESIDE CITY XY 12345-0000

Raymond S. Strong, M.D.
1616 Sheridan Way
Suite 315, Professional Building
Lakeside City, XY 12345-0000
(555) 896-1114

Raymond S Strong MD
1616 Sheridan Way
Suite 315 Professional Building
Lakeside City XY 12345-0000
555-896-1114

555/896-1114 Suite 315 Professional Bldg
Raymond S. Strong
1616 Sheridan Way
Lakeside City XY 12345-0000

5½ 8½ inches **6¼ 9¼ inches** **7¼ 10½ inches** **8½ 11 inches**

HAMMERMILL BOND STOCK

	Quantity	5½×8½ HB-407	6¼×9¼ HB-690	7¼×10½ HB-403	8½×11 HB-401
FLAT-PRINTED	500	$9.85	$12.25	$13.55	$15.95
	1000	13.95	18.35	20.70	23.10
	2000	24.95	30.65	34.95	39.60
	5000	58.15	70.60	80.10	83.65
	Quantity	5½×8½ PE-144	6¼×9¼ PE-695	7¼×10½ PE-146	8½×11 PE-140
RAISED-PRINTED	500	$11.70	$14.50	$16.00	$17.65
	1000	16.45	20.45	22.75	25.25
	2000	28.35	35.40	40.65	45.15
	5000	56.30	75.15	86.90	99.65

25% RAG CONTENT BOND

Quantity	5½×8½ NB-675	6¼×9¼ NB-69	7¼×10½ NB-70	8½×11 NB-81
500	$11.35	$13.55	$16.40	$18.65
1000	16.25	22.00	24.55	26.80
2000	27.25	37.55	42.10	48.60
5000	59.55	82.15	93.25	113.50
Quantity	5½×8½ PNB-560	6¼×9¼ PNB-695	7¼×10½ PNB-540	8½×11 PNB-530
500	$13.15	$16.00	$17.60	$21.50
1000	18.70	22.15	26.15	29.65
2000	32.80	40.75	45.50	51.15
5000	71.90	92.50	104.65	114.40

JOB SKILL 18-5 *(continued)*

FIGURE 18-3

envelopes

RAYMOND S. STRONG, M.D.
SUITE 315 PROFESSIONAL BUILDING
1616 SHERIDAN WAY
LAKESIDE CITY XY 12345-0000

SIZE 10 ENVELOPES: 4½×9½ inches. For 8½×11-inch letterheads.

SIZE 7½ ENVELOPES: 3½×7½ inches. For 7¼×10½-inch letterheads.

Raymond S. Strong, M.D.
1616 Sheridan Way Suite 315
Lakeside City, XY 12345-0000

Raymond S Strong MD
1616 Sheridan Way Ste 315
Lakeside City XY 12345-0000

SIZE 6¼ ENVELOPES: 3½×6½ inches. For 6¼×9¼-inch letterheads.

Unless specified, we print your copy in ther upper left-hand corner on the front of the envelope, Flat-printed envelopes can be Imprinted on the back flap as shown.

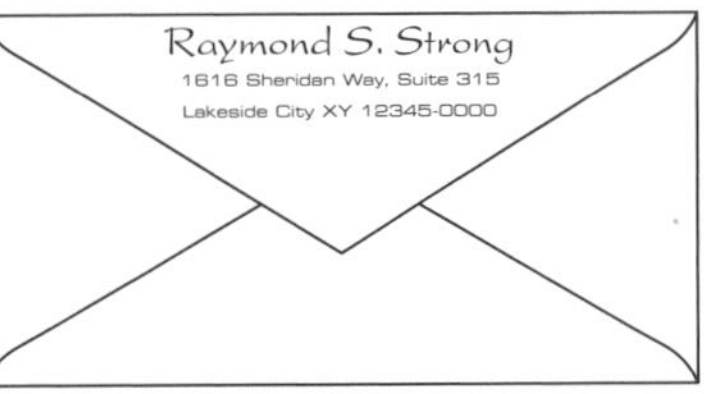

Envelopes are produced on the same fine stocks as our letterheads. Hammermill Bond is a bright white, smooth-surfaced paper. 25% Rag Content Bond is a crisp paper with a cockle finish - a most distinctive stationery. Both available in either flat or raised printing with your copy in 3 or 4 lines in the upper left-hand corner or on ther back flap (flat-printed only). All printing in black ink.

HAMMERMILL BOND
FLAT-PRINTED

Quantity	Size 6¾ L-500	Size 7½ L-510	Size 10 L-502
500	$13.50	$17.25	$18.50
1000	24.25	28.80	34.55
2000	45.15	50.15	59.30
5000	98.25	110.85	132.75

HAMMERMILL BOND
RAISED-PRINTED

Quantity	Size 6¾ PE-220	Size 7½ PE-192	Size 10 PE-190
500	$16.00	$20.50	$21.25
1000	26.30	28.90	34.75
2000	45.40	53.35	59.60
5000	99.00	124.25	133.45

25% RAG CONTENT BOND
FLAT-PRINTED

Quantity	Size 6¾ NB-800	Size 7½ NB-600	Size 10 NB-700
500	$18.90	$24.55	$25.20
1000	33.40	34.95	44.60
2000	57.80	67.75	76.95
5000	126.50	149.95	171.90

25% RAG CONTENT BOND
RAISED-PRINTED

Quantity	Size 6¾ PNB-520	Size 7½ PNB-510	Size 10 PNB-500
500	$21.60	$27.25	$27.90
1000	33.40	39.55	44.70
2000	58.15	70.95	77.20
5000	127.15	152.55	172.60

JOB SKILL 18-6
Complete an Order Form for Office Supplies

Name ______________________________ Date ______________ Score ________

Performance Objective

Task: Complete an order form for office supplies, filling in designated spaces and computing total amount ordered.

Conditions: Order form (Form 93) and pen or pencil. Refer to Procedure 18-10 in the *textbook* for step-by-step directions.

Standards: Complete all steps listed in this skill in ________ minutes with a minimum score of ________. (Time element and accuracy criteria may be given by instructor.)

Time: **Start:** ____________ **Completed:** ____________ **Total:** ____________ minutes

Scoring: One point for each step performed satisfactorily unless otherwise listed or weighted by instructor.

Directions with Performance Evaluation Checklist

Doctors Fran and Gerald Practon have asked you to order some office supplies. Neatly and accurately complete the order form.

1st Attempt	2nd Attempt	3rd Attempt	
______	______	______	Gather materials (equipment and supplies) listed under "Conditions."
______	______	______	1. Fill in the customer number (667-32-7118-4006).
____/5	____/5	____/5	2. Complete the customer contact information.
____/7	____/7	____/7	3. Order four 1,000 single-sheet cartons of CMS-1500 laser-printed insurance claim forms (8½″ by 11″), $29.95/carton, Cat. No. RED-25104, page 53.
____/7	____/7	____/7	4. Order four boxes of end-tab file folders with two fasteners (blue, letter size), ¾″ expansions, $40.90/box, Cat No. GLW-FF113, page 32.
____/7	____/7	____/7	5. Order six daily group practice wire-bound appointment books with 15-minute appointments, four columns per page, appointments from 8 a.m. to 7:45 p.m. (11″ by 7 7/8″), $29.15 each (price break: for each five ordered, one is free), Cat. No. GLW-AB402, page 65.
____/7	____/7	____/7	6. Order five packages of large envelopes (9″ by 12″) with clasp, 28-lb heavyweight Kraft, 25/pkg., $3.75 pkg., Cat No. 42SH-11, page 61.
____/7	____/7	____/7	7. Order two packages of double-prong clasp envelopes (9″ by 12″), reinforced eyelet, gummed flaps, $4.25/pkg., Cat. No. 387-ACJ, page 62.
____/7	____/7	____/7	8. Order two dozen packages of Post-it flags, Style No. 680-1 (1″ by 1.7″), one dozen red, one dozen yellow, $1.49 pkg., Cat. No. 49WEX-52, page 50.
______	______	______	9. Total order and insert figure.
______	______	______	10. Calculate and insert sales tax at 6%.
______	______	______	11. Determine the two-day shipping and handling fee, which is 5% of the total order. This is waived for orders over $400; and a flat fee of $15.00 is charged.
______	______	______	12. Add the sales tax and shipping and handling fee to determine the total amount for the order; insert this figure on the order form.

JOB SKILL 18-6 *(continued)*

_____/4 _____/4 _____/4 13. You will be paying for the order with the company credit card, which is a Visa card, number 2222-3333-4444-0000, expiration date August 2017. You have signature authority on the card; complete this section.

_______ _______ _______ Complete within specified time.

____/58 ____/58 ____/58 **Total points earned** (To obtain a percentage score, divide the total points earned by the number of points possible.)

Comments:

Evaluator's Signature: ______________________________ **Need to Repeat:** ____________

National Curriculum Competency: ABHES: 8.z

JOB SKILL 18-7
Perform Mathematic Calculations of an Office Manager

Name ______________________ Date ____________ Score ______

Performance Objective

Task: Perform basic mathematic calculations when ordering supplies to determine the cost, taking advantage of special discounts, and applying sales tax.

Conditions: Calculator, paper, and pencil.

Standards: Complete all steps listed in this skill in ______ minutes with a minimum score of ______. (Time element and accuracy criteria may be given by instructor.)

Time: **Start:** __________ **Completed:** __________ **Total:** __________ minutes

Scoring: One point for each step performed satisfactorily unless otherwise listed or weighted by instructor.

Directions with Performance Evaluation Checklist

The office manager may be responsible for ordering supplies, and he or she should be able to perform basic mathematics to calculate discounts and sales tax amounts. Wise purchasing and correct math procedures can save the office added expense. Solve the following problems, assuming that you pay all bills within the discount period stated. Discounts are subtracted before sales tax is added.

1st Attempt	2nd Attempt	3rd Attempt		
______	______	______	Gather materials (equipment and supplies) listed under "Conditions."	
____/2	____/2	____/2	1. The laundry bill is $33.80. If paid within 10 days, the company allows a 2.5% discount. Calculate the amount of the bill.	$ __________
____/5	____/5	____/5	2. Mr. Carl McFadden had five office visits at $25 each, three injections at $8.50 each, an x-ray at $26.60, and a home visit at $40.00. He has a $4.60 credit on his account. What will be the amount of his next bill?	$ __________
____/2	____/2	____/2	3. Mr. Bill Nelson is scheduled to have corrective surgery, which will be $385. He is asked to make a down payment of $50 before the operation, and then his payments will be divided into six equal installments. What will be the amount of each installment?	$ __________
____/10	____/10	____/10	4. The following items are on an invoice that arrived today. You are required to check to see that the bill is correct and that the supplies received are the ones ordered. The physician will receive a 3% discount, and sales tax is 6%. The total shown on the invoice is $26.14. Calculate and verify that the amount is correct. 4 bottles rubbing alcohol @ $2.25 each 3 thermometers @ $1.95 each 6 boxes cotton @ $.29 each 6 bottles mouthwash @ $.89 each 11 cartons cotton swabs @ $.39 each 3 hypodermic needles @ $.39 each The correct amount for which the check would be written is	$ __________

JOB SKILL 18-7 *(continued)*

____/5 ____/5 ____/5 5. Paper towels are sold at the rate of $6.50 per dozen rolls. Figure the cost of 10 dozen rolls of towels with a 3.5% discount and a 6% sales tax. $ __________

____/6 ____/6 ____/6 6. Dr. Fran Practon needs 500 needles priced at $2.60 per hundred. If she pays within 10 days, she receives a 2% discount; sales tax is 5.5%. What amount would you pay with the discount? $ __________

____/6 ____/6 ____/6 7. An advertisement states that eight thermometers cost $12.42 minus a 3% discount. Dr. Practon wants to order a dozen to take advantage of the savings; sales tax is 5%. What would the cost be? $ __________

____/3 ____/3 ____/3 8. Robert Mason's account of $98.50 has been delinquent for 3 months. According to the office procedures manual, after 90 days a 2% service charge, compounded monthly, is added to future bills. What will be the amount owed after 9 months? $ __________

____/2 ____/2 ____/2 9. Steri-Strips cost $4.95 per box; there are 100 in a box.

a. How much would 300 Steri-Strips cost? $ __________

b. How much would 700 Steri-Strips cost? $ __________

____/12 ____/12 ____/12 10. If the Steri-Strips are purchased in large lots of 1,000 or more, the manufacturer allows a discount of 15%.

a. How much would 3,000 Steri-Strips cost? $ __________

b. How much would 14,000 Steri-Strips cost? $ __________

c. If an orthopedic surgical group uses 200 Steri-Strips a month, how much would be saved in a year by making a single purchase for a year's supply rather than 12 monthly purchases? $ __________

______ ______ ______ Complete within specified time.

____/55 ____/55 ____/55 **Total points earned** (To obtain a percentage score, divide the total points earned by the number of points possible.)

Comments:

Evaluator's Signature: ____________________ **Need to Repeat:** __________

National Curriculum Competency: CAAHEP: Cognitive: II.C.1

JOB SKILL 18-8
Prepare Two Order Forms

Name ______________________________ Date ______________ Score ________

Performance Objective

Task: Key or type two order forms for medical supplies using the given information and determine the total amount owed after taking advantage of all discounts.

Conditions: Order forms (Forms 94 and 95) and computer or typewriter. Refer to Procedure 18-10 in the *textbook* for step-by-step directions and Figure 18-8 in the *textbook* for a visual example.

Standards: Complete all steps listed in this skill in ________ minutes with a minimum score of ________. (Time element and accuracy criteria may be given by instructor.)

Time: **Start:** ____________ **Completed:** ____________ **Total:** ____________ minutes

Scoring: One point for each step performed satisfactorily unless otherwise listed or weighted by instructor.

Directions with Performance Evaluation Checklist

Use the following information to order office and medical supplies. Determine the total for all merchandise, subtract the physician's discount, and then add the sales tax. The supplies are to be shipped to Practon Medical Group, Inc. Note: Photocopies would be made before sending off the order; all prices are fictitious.

1st Attempt	2nd Attempt	3rd Attempt	
______	______	______	Gather materials (equipment and supplies) listed under "Conditions."
____/10	____/10	____/10	1. Complete the "Bill to" information on both order forms.
____/2	____/2	____/2	2. Fill in the e-mail address for Practon Medical Group, Inc. (PMGI@aol.com), on both forms.
____/2	____/2	____/2	3. Indicate "SAME" in the "Ship to" location on both order forms.
____/4	____/4	____/4	4. Fill in the customer order number (0001002345) and the source code (BTGF) from the catalog.
____/4	____/4	____/4	5. List your name as the person to call for questions and the office telephone number; you are at extension 12.
____/2	____/2	____/2	6. List the practice specialty and number of doctors.
____/2	____/2	____/2	7. Indicate the method of shipping as UPS 2nd Day.

ORDER NO. 1

____/6	____/6	____/6	8. Order four reams of white 8½″ by 11″ bond paper, 20# weight, catalog number P20, unit price $12.95.
____/5	____/5	____/5	9. Order five boxes security-lined envelopes, 500/box, No. 6¾ , catalog number E60, unit price 19.99.
____/5	____/5	____/5	10. Order 1,500 large No. 10 envelopes, catalog number E10, unit price $5.50M.*
____/5	____/5	____/5	11. Order six boxes red fine-line ballpoint pens, catalog number B23, unit price $3.95.
______	______	______	12. Subtotal the merchandise order and insert figure.

*M is the Roman numeral that means one thousand.

JOB SKILL 18-8 *(continued)*

_______ _______ _______ 13. Calculate 2% discount and insert figure.

_______ _______ _______ 14. Subtract discount from subtotal.

_______ _______ _______ 15. Insert total on order form.

_______ _______ _______ 16. Calculate 5.5% sales tax and insert figure.

_______ _______ _______ 17. Add the sales tax and insert total for order.

ORDER NO. 2

_____/4 _____/4 _____/4 18. Order three surgeon's blade handles (Model No. B872C), catalog number BH3, unit price $2.95.

_____/4 _____/4 _____/4 19. Order two dozen scalpel blades (No. F112), 12 to a box, catalog number SB2, unit price $1.39.

_____/4 _____/4 _____/4 20. Order four Oval Duplex thermometers, rectal, catalog number T66, unit price $2.95.

_____/4 _____/4 _____/4 21. Order 3M* tongue blades, catalog number RB2, unit price $2.50M.

_____/8 _____/8 _____/8 22. Order 5,000 laser (8.5″ by 11″), OCR-scannable red ink insurance claim forms (single sheets) for Dr. Fran Practon. Catalog number CMS29, unit prices: $43.99/1,000; $77.99/2,000; $144.99/5,000; $239.99/10,000; $389.99/20,000.

_______ _______ _______ 23. Subtotal the merchandise order and insert this figure on line 6 of the order form (e.g., Sub total 123.45).

_______ _______ _______ 24. Calculate a 3% discount and subtract it from the subtotal. Write this figure on line 7 of the order form (e.g., Less 3% discount 1.23).

_______ _______ _______ 25. List the merchandise total.

_______ _______ _______ 26. Calculate 4% sales tax and insert figure.

_______ _______ _______ 27. Add the sales tax to the total of the order and insert figure.

_______ _______ _______ Complete within specified time.

____/84 ____/84 ____/84 **Total points earned** (To obtain a percentage score, divide the total points earned by the number of points possible.)

Comments:

Evaluator's Signature: ________________________________ **Need to Repeat:** ______________

National Curriculum Competency: ABHES: 8a

*M is the Roman numeral that means one thousand.

JOB SKILL 18-9
Prepare a Travel Expense Report

Name ______________________________ Date ______________ Score ________

Performance Objective

Task: Complete a travel expense report for the accountant.

Conditions: Travel Expense Report (Form 96) and pen or pencil. Refer to *textbook* Procedure 18-13 for step-by-step directions and *textbook* Figure 18-14 for a visual example.

Standards: Complete all steps listed in this skill in ________ minutes with a minimum score of ________. (Time element and accuracy criteria may be given by instructor.)

Time: **Start:** ____________ **Completed:** ____________ **Total:** ____________ minutes

Scoring: One point for each step performed satisfactorily unless otherwise listed or weighted by instructor.

Directions with Performance Evaluation Checklist

Dr. Gerald Practon presented a research paper at a medical convention in Boston, Massachusetts. He kept a detailed record of all expenses for the week of May 9 (Sat.) through May 16 (Sat.). Set up a travel expense report, transferring the figures that follow by placing them in the proper columns. Calculate totals.

1st Attempt	2nd Attempt	3rd Attempt	
______	______	______	Gather materials (equipment and supplies) listed under "Conditions."
____/2	____/2	____/2	1. Enter beginning and ending dates of trip.
____/8	____/8	____/8	2. Record dates for column headings that will be used on the travel report.
______	______	______	3. Record parking fees for Monday: $5.20.
______	______	______	4. Record parkway toll fees for Monday: $4.00.
____/5	____/5	____/5	5. Record tips for the week: $2 on Saturday, $3 on Sunday, $6 on Wednesday, $5.50 on Friday, and $6.25 on Saturday.
____/7	____/7	____/7	6. Record the discounted Hertz car rental, which was $25 per day for seven days.
____/2	____/2	____/2	7. Record gasoline expenses, which were $30.90 on Monday and $44.20 on Saturday.
____/7	____/7	____/7	8. Record the hotel expenses: Conroy Hotel was $150 per night for the first four nights, Commonwealth Hotel was $135 per night for the next two nights, and Shoreham Hotel was $165 per night for the last night.
______	______	______	9. Record one telephone call ($1.91) on Sunday, May 10, which was made to confirm the time for the speaking engagement.
____/16	____/16	____/16	10. Record all meal expenses.

Day	Breakfast	Lunch	Dinner
Sunday	$8.90	$15.40	$36.20
Monday	5.10	—	26.14
Tuesday	3.40	10.90	31.50
Wednesday	—	13.98	48.14
Thursday	9.15	10.00	20.02
Friday	10.82	22.08	36.33

JOB SKILL 18-9 *(continued)*

____/7	____/7	____/7	11. Calculate and record total for Lodging.
____/5	____/5	____/5	12. Calculate and record total for Breakfasts.
____/5	____/5	____/5	13. Calculate and record total for Lunches.
____/6	____/6	____/6	14. Calculate and record total for Dinners.
______	______	______	15. Calculate and record total for Local Fares.
____/7	____/7	____/7	16. Calculate and record total for Auto Expenses.
______	______	______	17. Calculate and record total for Parking Fees.
______	______	______	18. Calculate and record total for Phone and E-mail.
______	______	______	19. Calculate and record total for Entertainment.
____/5	____/5	____/5	20. Calculate and record total for Tips.
______	______	______	21. Calculate and record total for Toll Charges.
____/2	____/2	____/2	22. Calculate and record total for Other/Miscellaneous.
____/3	____/3	____/3	23. Calculate and record total for May 9.
____/7	____/7	____/7	24. Calculate and record total for May 10.
____/7	____/7	____/7	25. Calculate and record total for May 11.
____/5	____/5	____/5	26. Calculate and record total for May 12.
____/5	____/5	____/5	27. Calculate and record total for May 13.
____/5	____/5	____/5	28. Calculate and record total for May 14.
____/6	____/6	____/6	29. Calculate and record total for May 15.
____/2	____/2	____/2	30. Calculate and record total for May 16.
____/10	____/10	____/10	31. Add and record all totals in the right column.
____/8	____/8	____/8	32. Add and record all totals listed for each day and verify against the figure obtained in step 31; they should be the same. If not, recalculate and compare again.
____/2	____/2	____/2	33. Write a brief description for the purpose of the trip and enter on report.
______	______	______	Complete within specified time.
____/154	____/154	____/154	**Total points earned** (To obtain a percentage score, divide the total points earned by the number of points possible.)

Comments:

Evaluator's Signature: ______________________________ **Need to Repeat:** ____________

National Curriculum Competency: ABHES: 4.a; 8.a

CHAPTER 19

Financial Management of the Medical Practice

OBJECTIVES

After completing the exercises, the student will be able to:

1. Enhance knowledge of medical terminology, interpret abbreviations, and accurately spell medical words.
2. Perform accounts payable functions: write checks and record disbursements (Job Skill 19-1).
3. Pay bills and record expenditures (Job Skill 19-2).
4. Replenish and balance the petty cash fund (Job Skill 19-3).
5. Balance a check register (Job Skill 19-4).
6. Reconcile a bank statement (Job Skill 19-5).
7. Prepare payroll (Job Skill 19-6).
8. Complete a payroll register (Job Skill 19-7).
9. Complete an employee earning record (Job Skill 19-8).
10. Complete an employee's withholding allowance certificate (Job Skill 19-9).
11. Complete an employee benefit form (Job Skill 19-10).

FOCUS ON CERTIFICATION*

CMA Content Summary

- Document reporting to the Internal Revenue Service (IRS)
- Accounts payable
- Employee payroll
- Calculating payroll and payroll forms
- Practice management software
- Report generation
- Applying managed care policies and procedures

RMA Content Summary

- Identify and apply plan policies and regulations for HMO, PPO, EPO, indemnity, and open programs
- Generate aging reports
- Employ appropriate accounting procedures
- Understand and manage petty cash
- Maintain checking accounts
- Process payables and practice obligations
- Understand and maintain disbursement accounts
- Prepare employee payroll
- Understand hourly and salary payroll procedures
- Understand and maintain payroll records
- Prepare and maintain payroll tax deduction/withholding records
- Prepare employee tax forms
- Prepare quarterly tax forms
- Understand terminology pertaining to payroll and payroll tax
- Understand and perform appropriate calculations related to patient and practice accounts

CMAS Content Summary

- Understand basic principles of accounting
- Perform bookkeeping procedures including balancing accounts
- Perform financial computations
- Manage accounts payable
- Prepare monthly trial balance reports
- Understand basic audit controls
- Manage other financial aspects of office management
- Understand banking services and procedures
- Manage petty cash
- Prepare employee payroll and reports
- Maintain payroll tax deduction procedures and records
- Possess fundamental knowledge of computing in the medical office
- Manage staff payroll and scheduling
- Manage employee benefits

STOP AND THINK CASE SCENARIOS AND EXAM-STYLE REVIEW QUESTIONS

Refer to the end of Chapter 19 in the *textbook*.

Abbreviation and Spelling Review

Read the following patients' chart notes and write the meanings for the abbreviations listed below each note. To decode any abbreviations you do not understand or that appear unfamiliar to you, refer to the list of abbreviations in Part IV of this *Workbook*. Step-by-step directions for this exercise are found in Procedure 1-1 of Chapter 1 in the *textbook*. Medical terms in the chart note are italicized; study them for spelling. Use your medical dictionary to look up their definitions. Your instructor may give a spelling and definition test that includes these words and abbreviations.

*This *Workbook* and the accompanying *textbook* meet the entry-level administrative and general competencies for the CMA outlined by the AAMA Examination Content Outline and Occupational Analysis and for the RMA and CMAS outlined by the AMT Competencies, Construction Parameters, and Examination Specifications (see Competency Grid in Appendix B of the *textbook*).

Bernice Saxon

April 10, 20XX Pt had closed reduction of *telescoping* nasal *ethmoidal fracture* with sutures and application of an *external nasal* splint. When pt ret'nd from surg, she was given 100 mg of *Demerol* q. 3h. IM. Her vital signs were taken q.i.d. for the first 2 days & then b.i.d. p̄ that. Sleeping medication was given h.s. She will be seen in the office in 4 days for follow-up.

Gerald Practon, MD
Gerald Practon, MD

Pt	______	IM	______
ret'nd	______	q.i.d.	______
surg	______	b.i.d.	______
mg	______	p̄	______
q. 3h.	______	h.s.	______

Lucy Corsentino

July 7, 20XX Pt, a 3-year-old, has had temp 100.1° for 2 days. Exam reveals strep throat. DX: Acute *streptococcal pharyngitis*. Plan: *Penicillin* V *potassium* 250 mg/tsp to be taken in a dose of 1 tsp q.i.d. x 10 days, *Tylenol* up to 1 gm q. 4h. for pain & fever. Mother advised not to give ASA.

Fran Practon, MD
Fran Practon, MD

Pt	______	1 gm	______
DX	______	q. 4h.	______
mg/tsp	______	ASA	______
q.i.d. x 10 days	______		

Review Questions

Review the objectives, glossary, and chapter information before completing the following review questions.

1. List several ways a computerized financial management system benefits a medical practice.
   a. ______
   b. ______
   c. ______
   d. ______
   e. ______
2. What projection does the office manager look at to determine how much actual cash should be available each month? ______

3. Income received and expenses paid are presented in a report called a ______________________________
______________________________.

4. What important report is used to begin a financial analysis of a medical practice? ____________
____

5. Explain an insurance aging report and list ways it can be broken down for analysis. ____________
____
____
____
____

6. What are some of the things that are looked at and learned when an office manager analyzes a medical practice's productivity?
   a. ______________________________
   b. ______________________________
   c. ______________________________
   d. ______________________________

7. An office manager calculates the accounts receivable ratio in order to determine how well which person is performing his or her job?
____
____
____

8. To track the accounts payable, expenditures are recorded in a ______________________________.

9. Name some responsibilities of the office manager or medical assistant when he or she is in complete charge of the payroll.
   a. ______________________________
   b. ______________________________
   c. ______________________________
   d. ______________________________
   e. ______________________________
   f. ______________________________

10. What law covers minimum wage and overtime standards? ______________________________

11. The office manager must post notices in the medical office according to the ____________________.

12. Explain how to obtain a tax identification number for a physician-employer.
____
____

13. Why do you have an employee complete an Employee's Withholding Allowance Certificate, Form W-4?
____

14. Under FICA, both the ______________ and ______________ contribute at a rate specified by law.

15. Name three programs financed under Social Security (FICA) from one payroll tax, and list what they provide.

    a. Program 1: ______________________________

       Provides: ______________________________

    b. Program 2: ______________________________

       Provides: ______________________________

    c. Program 3: ______________________________

       Provides: ______________________________

16. List three names used for state disability insurance deductions.

    a. ______________________________

    b. ______________________________

    c. ______________________________

17. You may have difficulty remembering whether *biweekly* means "twice a week" or "every two weeks"; it can mean both. However, *semiweekly* is usually used for "twice a week," and in accounting *biweekly* is used for "every two weeks." In the following list, check the correct definitions.

biyearly	________	a. twice a year	semiannually	________	a. every six months
	________	b. once a year		________	b. every two years
	________	c. every two years		________	c. once a year
biweekly	________	a. twice a week	semimonthly	________	a. every half month
	________	b. every two weeks		________	b. twice a month
	________	c. semiweekly		________	c. every other month
quarterly	________	a. twice a year	weekly	________	a. every day
	________	b. every four weeks		________	b. once a week
	________	c. four times a year		________	c. every week

18. List several optional payroll deductions; also called ______________________________.

    a. ______________________________

    b. ______________________________

    c. ______________________________

    d. ______________________________

    e. ______________________________

    f. ______________________________

    g. ______________________________

19. How often must employers report payments by using Form 940?

    ____

20. In what publication does the Department of the Treasury, Internal Revenue Service, publish submission guidelines and requirements for quarterly reports, federal tax deposits, and unemployment tax payments?

    ____

21. The employer's quarterly federal tax return must be filed by an employer on or before ______________, ______________, ______________, and ______________ on Form ______________.

22. Spell out the following payroll abbreviations.

    FICA ______________________________

    FUTA ______________________________

    UCD ______________________________

23. Agnes Baker terminated her employment with Dr. Jeffries on August 31. What document must be given to her by the employer and what is the time limit?

    ____

    ____

Critical Thinking Exercises

1. Why is it a federal requirement that the Wage and Tax Statement (W-2) tax form be sent by the employer to both the IRS and to each employee? ______________________________

    ____

2. State the deductions from a payroll check required in your state.

    a. ______________________________

    b. ______________________________

    c. ______________________________

    d. ______________________________

    e. ______________________________

3. Looking ahead to when you are employed as an administrative medical assistant, list what kind of fringe benefits you would prefer and why.

    ____

    ____

JOB SKILL 19-1
Perform Accounts Payable Functions: Write Checks and Record Disbursements

Name ______________________________ Date ______________ Score ________

Performance Objective

Task: Write checks for disbursement, enter transactions on the check register, and post deposits.

Conditions: Check register (Forms 97, 98, and 99), twelve checks (4 sheets: Forms 100 through 103), calculator, and pencil. Refer to Procedure 19-1 in the *textbook* for step-by-step directions. Note: Job Skills 19-1, 19-2, 19-3, and 19-4 will use the same information and check register.

Standards: Complete all steps listed in this skill in _______ minutes with a minimum score of ________. (Time element and accuracy criteria may be given by instructor.)

Time: **Start:** ____________ **Completed:** ____________ **Total:** ____________ minutes

Scoring: One point for each step performed satisfactorily unless otherwise listed or weighted by instructor.

Directions with Performance Evaluation Checklist

Read the entire job skill before beginning. You may want to enlarge Forms 97, 98, and 99 onto legal size paper to make it easier to handwrite entries. Blank forms can also be downloaded from the Premium Website to accompany this *textbook* (access at www.CengageBrain.com) and complete electronically. Another option would be to complete the job skill on the computer using an Excel spreadsheet.

Check Stub: List date and record deposit(s), and then add to the balance forward; list the check amount and a brief description subtracting the amount to determine the checkbook balance; *always carry the balance forward to the next check.*

Check Entries: Write out the amount of the check and enter the numerical figure in the "Check Amount." Record the company name and address to which the check is written; use the date indicated.

Check Register: Study the column headings to familiarize yourself with the various categories. Write the amount of the check in the "Gross" column and in the "Amount of Check" column (page 1); indicate the check number. Then, post each check amount on the appropriate line in the correct disbursement column on page 2 or 3 of the check register.

1st Attempt	2nd Attempt	3rd Attempt	
_____	_____	_____	Gather materials (equipment and supplies) listed under "Conditions."
____/5	____/5	____/5	1. Prepare pages 1, 2, and 3 of the check register (Forms 97, 98, and 99) for checks drawn on "The First National Bank" for the month of June 20XX.
____/2	____/2	____/2	2. Record the beginning checkbook balance of $9,745.45 on the first check stub (No. 479) and on page 2 of the check register bank deposit slip.
____/2	____/2	____/2	3. Record a deposit of $130 on June 1, 20XX, on the first check stub (No. 479) and on the bank deposit slip.
____/8	____/8	____/8	4. Make out check No. 479 on June 1, 20XX, for rent to Security Pacific Company, 2091 Mission Street, Woodland Hills, XY 12345, in the amount of $1,900.00, and make the appropriate calculations on the check stub.
____/6	____/6	____/6	5. Record check No. 479 on the check register.
____/2	____/2	____/2	6. Record a deposit of $95 on June 3, 20XX, on check stub No. 480 and on the bank deposit slip.

JOB SKILL 19-1 *(continued)*

____/8 ____/8 ____/8 7. Make out check No. 480 on June 3, 20XX, for medical supplies to Central Laboratories, 351 Robin Avenue, Woodland Hills, XY 12345, in the amount of $74.50, and make the appropriate calculations on the check stub.

____/6 ____/6 ____/6 8. Record check No. 480 on the check register.

____/8 ____/8 ____/8 9. Make out check No. 481 on June 3, 20XX, for parking fees to Broadway Garage, 4560 Broad Avenue, Woodland Hills, XY 12345, in the amount of $300.00, and make the appropriate calculations on the check stub.

____/6 ____/6 ____/6 10. Record check No. 481 on the check register.

____/2 ____/2 ____/2 11. Record a deposit of $195 on June 4, 20XX, on check stub No. 482 and on the bank deposit slip.

____/8 ____/8 ____/8 12. Make out check No. 482 on June 4, 20XX, for diesel fuel to Union Oil Company, PO Box 232, Woodland Hills, XY 12345, in the amount of $87.75, and make the appropriate calculations on the check stub.

____/6 ____/6 ____/6 13. Record check No. 482 on the check register.

____/2 ____/2 ____/2 14. Record a deposit of $80 on June 15, 20XX, on check stub No. 483 and on the bank deposit slip.

____/8 ____/8 ____/8 15. Make out check No. 483 on June 15, 20XX, for quarterly city tax to Woodland Hills Tax Commission, 2200 James Street, Woodland Hills, XY 12345, in the amount of $162.00, and make the appropriate calculations on the check stub.

____/6 ____/6 ____/6 16. Record check No. 483 on the check register.

____/8 ____/8 ____/8 17. Make out check No. 484 on June 15, 20XX, for medications to Eli Lilly and Company, Lilly Corporate Center, Indianapolis, IN 46285, in the amount of $226.00, and make the appropriate calculations on the check stub.

____/6 ____/6 ____/6 18. Record check No. 484 on the check register.

____/2 ____/2 ____/2 19. Record a deposit of $160 on June 20, 20XX, on check stub No. 485 and on the bank deposit slip.

____/8 ____/8 ____/8 20. Make out check No. 485 on June 20, 20XX, for utilities to Woodland Hills Gas Company, 50 South M Street, Woodland Hills, XY 12345, in the amount of $87.80, and make the appropriate calculations on the check stub.

____/6 ____/6 ____/6 21. Record check No. 485 on the check register.

____/8 ____/8 ____/8 22. Make out check No. 486 on June 20, 20XX, for drugs and medical supplies to Sargents Pharmacy, 711 Wheeler Road, Woodland Hills, XY 12345, in the amount of $38.75, and make the appropriate calculations on the check stub.

____/6 ____/6 ____/6 23. Record check No. 486 on the check register.

____/8 ____/8 ____/8 24. Make out check No. 487 on June 20, 20XX, for a donation to United Fund, PO Box 400, New York, NY 10015, in the amount of $200.00, and make the appropriate calculations on the check stub.

____/6 ____/6 ____/6 25. Record check No. 487 on the check register.

____/2 ____/2 ____/2 26. Record a deposit of $105 on June 25, 20XX, on check stub No. 488 and on the bank deposit slip.

JOB SKILL 19-1 *(continued)*

_____/8 _____/8 _____/8 27. Make out check No. 488 on June 25, 20XX, for utilities to Woodland Hills Telephone Company, 505 Peppermint Street, Woodland Hills, XY 12345, in the amount of $79.60, and make the appropriate calculations on the check stub.

_____/6 _____/6 _____/6 28. Record check No. 488 on the check register.

_____/8 _____/8 _____/8 29. Make out check No. 489 on June 25, 20XX, for utilities to Woodland Hills Electric Company, 320 Banyon Avenue, Woodland Hills, XY 12345, in the amount of $85.78, and make the appropriate calculations on the check stub.

_____/6 _____/6 _____/6 30. Record check No. 489 on the check register.

_____/8 _____/8 _____/8 31. Make out check No. 490 on June 25, 20XX, for office linens to Rite-Way Laundry, 2500 Torrance Way, Woodland Hills, XY 12345, in the amount of $45.00, and make the appropriate calculations on the check stub.

_____/6 _____/6 _____/6 32. Record check No. 490 on the check register.

_____ _____ _____ Complete within specified time.

___/189 ___/189 ___/189 **Total points earned** (To obtain a percentage score, divide the total points earned by the number of points possible.)

Comments:

Evaluator's Signature: ______________________________ **Need to Repeat:** ____________

National Curriculum Competency: CAAHEP: Cognitive: II.C.1; VI.C.1, 6	ABHES: 8.g, j

JOB SKILL 19-2
Pay Bills and Record Expenditures

Name ______________________________ Date ______________ Score ________

Performance Objective

Task: Write checks for invoices received, complete the check register, and enter the deposit.

Conditions: Four invoices (*Workbook* Figure 19-1), check register used in Job Skill 19-1 (Forms 97, 98, and 99), four checks (Forms 104 and 105), calculator, and pencil. Refer to Procedure 19-1 in the *textbook* for step-by-step directions.

Standards: Complete all steps listed in this skill in ________ minutes with a minimum score of ________. (Time element and accuracy criteria may be given by instructor.)

Time: **Start:** ____________ **Completed:** ____________ **Total:** ____________ minutes

Scoring: One point for each step performed satisfactorily unless otherwise listed or weighted by instructor.

Directions with Performance Evaluation Checklist

Read the entire job skill before beginning. Use the date June 30, 20XX.

1st Attempt	2nd Attempt	3rd Attempt	
______	______	______	Gather materials (equipment and supplies) listed under "Conditions."
______	______	______	1. Carry the checkbook balance forward from the previous job skill to check No. 491.
____/6	____/6	____/6	2. You have deposited money on the following dates for the amounts listed: 6/28 \$410.99, 6/29 \$70, 6/30 \$95. Include these deposits on the first check stub that you will be using (No. 491) and on page 2 of the check register bank deposit slip.
____/3	____/3	____/3	3. If possible, copy the invoices in Figure 19-1 on the following page and cut them apart.
____/56	____/56	____/56	4. Write checks for the invoices shown in Figure 19-1 and record the information on the check register as in Job Skill 19-1.
____/12	____/12	____/12	5. Indicate the following on each invoice: date paid, check number, and check amount.
______	______	______	Complete within specified time.
____/80	____/80	____/80	**Total points earned** (To obtain a percentage score, divide the total points earned by the number of points possible.)

Comments:

JOB SKILL 19-2 *(continued)*

FIGURE 19-1

Central Medical Supply Company
859 East Santa Clara Drive
Woodland Hills, XY 12345-0012

STATEMENT

20XX

6-15	Ophthalmoscope	$350.00
	tax	24.50
	Shipping & handling	10.00
	BALANCE DUE	$384.50

Thrifty Drug Store
540 West Main Street
Woodland Hills, XY 12345-6785

STATEMENT

20XX

6-20	1 roll bandages	$6.50
	2 boxes tissues	3.00
	1 box cotton swabs	4.50
	tax	.98
	TOTAL	$14.98

Prudential Life Insurance
2603 Underpass Street
Woodland Hills, XY 12345-9822

INVOICE

20XX

6-30 Gerald Practon
Life Insurance
6 months premium

PLEASE PAY $1969.42

ABC MOTORS
610 Main Street
Woodland Hills, XY 12345-2389

INVOICE

20XX

6-15	Lube and oil	
	1998 Toyota	$65.00
	5 qts oil	10.00
	filter	5.00
	TOTAL BALANCE DUE	$80.00

Evaluator's Signature: ______________________ **Need to Repeat:** ____________

National Curriculum Competency: CAAHEP: Cognitive: II.C.1, VI.C.1; Psychomotor: VI.P.1 ABHES: 8.g, j

JOB SKILL 19-3
Replenish and Balance the Petty Cash Fund

Name ______________________________ Date ______________ Score ________

Performance Objective

Task: Record entries on a petty cash envelope, calculate totals, balance the cash drawer, and write a check to replenish the petty cash fund.

Conditions: Check register used in Job Skills 19-1 and 19-2 (Forms 97, 98, and 99), one check No. 495 (Form 106), petty cash envelope (Form 107), calculator, and pencil. Refer to Procedure 19-1 in the *textbook* for step-by-step instructions.

Standards: Complete all steps listed in this job skill in _______ minutes with a minimum score of _______. (Time element and accuracy criteria may be given by instructor.)

Time: **Start:** ____________ **Completed:** ____________ **Total:** ____________ minutes

Scoring: One point for each step performed satisfactorily unless otherwise listed or weighted by instructor.

Directions with Performance Evaluation Checklist

1st Attempt	2nd Attempt	3rd Attempt	
_____	_____	_____	Gather materials (equipment and supplies) listed under "Conditions."
____/2	____/2	____/2	1. Indicate on the petty cash receipt envelope (Form 107) the beginning petty cash amount of $100 for June 1, 20XX.
____/30	____/30	____/30	2. Enter the following expenses that occurred during the month of June on the petty cash receipt envelope listing the date paid, voucher number, to whom it was paid, a brief description of the item, under which account heading it would be listed (i.e., office supplies, postage, medical supplies, miscellaneous), and the amount.

Date	Voucher	Vendor	Item	Amount
6/3/XX	103	Crown Stationers	stationery supplies	$2.70
6/7/XX	104	U.S. Postal Service	postage due	.95
6/15/XX	105	Thrifty Drug Store	medical supplies	10.32
6/20/XX	106	TG & Y Store	miscellaneous (office plant)	3.40
6/22/XX	107	U.S. Postal Service	postage	45.00
6/27/XX	108	Thrifty Drug Store	medical supplies	2.62

1st Attempt	2nd Attempt	3rd Attempt	
____/6	____/6	____/6	3. Total the amount of all items and record on the last line.
____/4	____/4	____/4	4. List the following headings in the "Distribution of Petty Cash": Office Supplies, Postage, Medical Supplies, Miscellaneous.
____/6	____/6	____/6	5. Itemize each of the expenditures under the correct heading.
____/4	____/4	____/4	6. Total each column under "Distribution of Petty Cash" and list the total on the last line.
____/4	____/4	____/4	7. Add all totals listed and record on the last line under "Totals." This number should be the same as the total in step 3.
_____	_____	_____	8. List the amount of all vouchers paid under "Receipts Paid."
_____	_____	_____	9. Count the cash in the cash drawer and list under "Cash on Hand."

JOB SKILL 19-3 *(continued)*

____/2	____/2	____/2	10. Add the receipts paid and the cash on hand; it should equal the beginning amount in the office fund account.
______	______	______	11. List this amount in "Total Receipts and Cash."
____/2	____/2	____/2	12. Subtract the "Total Receipts and Cash" from the "Office Fund Amount" and list the amount of money that is over or short.
____/6	____/6	____/6	13. Write check No. 495, made out to "Petty Cash," for the amount necessary to replenish the petty cash.
___/11	___/11	___/11	14. List petty cash amounts on the check register. Note: Add together items in the same category; office supplies and postage will be combined and listed under "Office Supplies."
______	______	______	15. Indicate this transaction on the "Petty Cash Receipt Envelope."
______	______	______	Complete within specified time.
___/83	___/83	___/83	**Total points earned** (To obtain a percentage score, divide the total points earned by the number of points possible.)

Comments:

Evaluator's Signature: ________________________________ **Need to Repeat:** ______________

National Curriculum Competency: CAAHEP: Cognitive: II.C.1	ABHES: 8.j, l

JOB SKILL 19-4
Balance a Check Register

Name ______________________________ Date ______________ Score ________

Performance Objective

Task: Total all columns (pages 1, 2, and 3) and balance the check register.

Conditions: Check register with figures entered that were used in Job Skills 19-1, 19-2, and 19-3, calculator and pencil. Refer to Procedure 19-1 in the *textbook* for step-by-step directions.

Standards: Complete all steps listed in this job skill in _______ minutes with a minimum score of _______. (Time element and accuracy criteria may be given by instructor.)

Time: **Start:** ____________ **Completed:** ____________ **Total:** ____________ minutes

Scoring: One point for each step performed satisfactorily unless otherwise listed or weighted by instructor.

Directions with Performance Evaluation Checklist

1st Attempt	2nd Attempt	3rd Attempt	
_______	_______	_______	Gather materials (equipment and supplies) listed under "Conditions."
____/20	____/20	____/20	1. Total both columns on page 1 of the check register and record at the bottom of the form; they should equal.
____/8	____/8	____/8	2. Total the bank deposit and all columns on page 2 of the check register and record at the bottom of the form.
____/6	____/6	____/6	3. Total all columns on page 3 of the check register and record at the bottom of the form.
____/14	____/14	____/14	4. Balance the check register by adding all disbursement column totals on pages 2 and 3; they should equal Total C listed on page 1.
_______	_______	_______	Complete within specified time.
____/50	____/50	____/50	**Total points earned** (To obtain a percentage score, divide the total points earned by the number of points possible.)

Comments:

Evaluator's Signature: ______________________________ **Need to Repeat:** ____________

National Curriculum Competency: CAAHEP: Cognitive: II.C.1	ABHES: 8.g, j

JOB SKILL 19-5
Reconcile a Bank Statement

Name ______________________________ Date ______________ Score ________

Performance Objective

Task: Reconcile a bank statement.

Conditions: One bank account reconciliation form (Form 108); checkbook stubs completed in Job Skills 19-1, 19-2, and 19-3; bank statement (*Workbook* Figure 19-2); calculator; and pen or pencil. Refer to Job Skill 14-7 in Chapter 14 to review the steps for reconciling a bank statement.

Standards: Complete all steps listed in this skill in _______ minutes with a minimum score of _______. (Time element and accuracy criteria may be given by instructor.)

Time: **Start:** ____________ **Completed:** ____________ **Total:** ____________ minutes

Scoring: One point for each step performed satisfactorily unless otherwise listed or weighted by instructor.

Directions with Performance Evaluation Checklist

You have received the bank statement from The First National Bank for June 20XX. Use the checks written for the month of June 20XX (No. 479 through 495) and the bank statement shown in *Workbook* Figure 19-2 to reconcile the bank statement.

1st Attempt	2nd Attempt	3rd Attempt	
______	______	______	Gather materials (equipment and supplies) listed under "Conditions."
____/9	____/9	____/9	1. Mark off all checks made out during the month of June that have been returned by the bank and appear on the bank statement.
____/16	____/16	____/16	2. List all checks that have not been returned on the reconciliation form under "Outstanding Checks or Other Withdrawals."
____/8	____/8	____/8	3. Add all outstanding checks and record the total on the reconciliation form.
____/6	____/6	____/6	4. Check off all deposits that have been made during the month of June that appear on the bank statement.
____/6	____/6	____/6	5. List all deposits that do not appear on the statement on the reconciliation form under "Deposits Not Credited."
____/3	____/3	____/3	6. Add all deposits not credited to the account and record the total on the reconciliation form.
____/4	____/4	____/4	7. Balance the checking account using the steps indicated on the reconciliation form under "Balance Your Account."
____/2	____/2	____/2	8. Compare this figure with the ending figure in the checkbook (see check No. 495); they should match.
______	______	______	Complete within specified time.
____/56	____/56	____/56	**Total points earned** (To obtain a percentage score, divide the total points earned by the number of points possible.)

JOB SKILL 19-5 *(continued)*

FIGURE 19-2

Account Statement — THE FIRST NATIONAL BANK

CHECKING ACCOUNT #00012345 WOODLAND HILLS 140

0020
100

PRACTON MEDICAL GROUP, INC 140
4567 BROAD AVENUE
WOODLAND HILLS XY 12345

CHECKING ACCOUNT SUMMARY AS OF 06-27-20XX 3

BEGINNING BALANCE	TOTAL DEPOSITS	TOTAL WITHDRAWALS	SERVICE CHARGES	ENDING BALANCE
9,745 45	765 00	3076 80	00	7,433 65

-CHECKING ACCOUNT TRANSACTIONS-

DEPOSITS	DATE	AMOUNT
BRANCH DEPOSIT	06-01	130.00
BRANCH DEPOSIT	06-03	95.00
BRANCH DEPOSIT	06-04	195.00
BRANCH DEPOSIT	06-15	80.00
BRANCH DEPOSIT	06-20	160.00
BRANCH DEPOSIT	06-25	105.00

CHECKS ITEM	DATE	AMOUNT	CHECKS ITEM	DATE	AMOUNT	BALANCES DATE	BALANCES
479	06-01	1,900.00	484	06-15	226.00	06-01	7,975.45
480	06-03	74.50	485	06-20	87.80	06-03	7,695.95
481	06-03	300.00	486	06-20	38.75	06-04	7,803.20
482	06-04	87.75	487	06-20	200.00	06-15	7,495.20
483	06-15	162.00				06-20	7,328.65
						06-25	7,433.65

Comments:

Evaluator's Signature: ______________________ **Need to Repeat:** ____________

National Curriculum Competency: CAAHEP: Cognitive: II.C.1, 2	ABHES: 8.g

JOB SKILL 19-6
Prepare Payroll

Name ______________________________ Date ______________ Score ________

Performance Objective

Task: Prepare payroll for seven employees; calculate gross pay and all deductions to determine net pay.

Conditions: Income tax tables (*Workbook* Figure 19-3 through Figure 19-11), calculator, and pen or pencil. Refer to Procedure 19-2 in the *textbook* for step-by-step directions and *textbook* Figure 19-14 and Figure 19-15 for examples of a completed employee earning record and monthly payroll register.

Standards: Complete all steps listed in this skill in _______ minutes with a minimum score of ________. (Time element and accuracy criteria may be given by instructor.)

Time: **Start:** ____________ **Completed:** ____________ **Total:** ____________ minutes

Scoring: One point for each step performed satisfactorily unless otherwise listed or weighted by instructor.

Directions with Performance Evaluation Checklist

It is May 28, 20XX, and you will be preparing the payroll for seven employees. Following are payroll guidelines:

1. Hourly employees are paid once each month, on the first.
2. Salaried employees are paid semimonthly.
3. A few employees have elected to pay 2% of their gross pay into the Practon Medical Group, Inc., insurance plan.
4. If you reside in California, Hawaii, New Jersey, New York, Puerto Rico, or Rhode Island, assume state disability insurance (SDI) is 1% of gross pay; in all other states, disregard this deduction.
5. Determine the employee's status and refer to the tax tables that follow this exercise to determine federal and state deductions. If the amount of income is shown on two lines (e.g., at least $540 but less than $560 and at least $560 but less than $580), use the higher deduction.
6. Calculate FICA deductions at 6.2% of gross earnings.
7. Calculate Medicare deductions at 1.45% of gross earnings.
8. Divorced persons are considered "single" on federal tax tables and "head of household" on state tax tables that appear in this exercise.
9. Single persons with a dependent parent are considered "unmarried head of household" with the state.
10. Read the following scenarios and refer to these directions while using the worksheet provided to indicate whether the person is single (S), married (M), or divorced (D); the number of exemptions claimed; whether the employee is on salary or hourly and number of hours worked, if hourly; and frequency of pay (e.g., semimonthly, monthly). Then calculate and record the gross pay, all necessary deductions, and net pay.

1st Attempt	2nd Attempt	3rd Attempt	
______	______	______	Gather materials (equipment and supplies) listed under "Conditions."
____/13	____/13	____/13	1. Prepare payroll for Hillary Sheehan who is the physician's bookkeeper. She is married and claims herself as an exemption. She earns $13 an hour and worked 168 hours this month with no overtime.

JOB SKILL 19-6 *(continued)*

Status	Exemptions	Salary/Hrs Worked	Frequency of Pay
S M D	0 1 2 3	______________	Monthly/Semimonthly

Gross Pay	FICA	Fed. Inc. Tax	State Inc. Tax	SDI	Medicare	Other	Total Deduc.	Net Pay

___/13 ___/13 ___/13 2. Prepare payroll for Roger Young, who works part-time as a custodian on weekends. He is single and claims himself and a dependent mother. He is paid $7.50 per hour. He worked 18 hours this month.

Status	Exemptions	Salary/Hrs Worked	Frequency of Pay
S M D	0 1 2 3	______________	Monthly/Semimonthly

Gross Pay	FICA	Fed. Inc. Tax	State Inc. Tax	SDI	Medicare	Other	Total Deduc.	Net Pay

___/13 ___/13 ___/13 3. Prepare payroll for Kelley Jones, who is the office receptionist. She is single and claims herself only. She is paid $1,650 per month, and she elected not to enroll in the hospital insurance plan.

Status	Exemptions	Salary/Hrs Worked	Frequency of Pay
S M D	0 1 2 3	______________	Monthly/Semimonthly

Gross Pay	FICA	Fed. Inc. Tax	State Inc. Tax	SDI	Medicare	Other	Total Deduc.	Net Pay

___/13 ___/13 ___/13 4. Prepare payroll for Maryjane Moran, who works part-time doing insurance. She is paid hourly and earns $12.50 per hour. She is married and claims no dependents because her husband claims her. She worked 80 hours this month.

Status	Exemptions	Salary/Hrs Worked	Frequency of Pay
S M D	0 1 2 3	______________	Monthly/Semimonthly

Gross Pay	FICA	Fed. Inc. Tax	State Inc. Tax	SDI	Medicare	Other	Total Deduc.	Net Pay

___/13 ___/13 ___/13 5. Prepare payroll for Carla O'Hare, who is the administrative medical assistant. She is divorced and has three children. She claims herself and her children. She is paid $1,675 a month, and she is a member of the hospital insurance plan.

Status	Exemptions	Salary/Hrs Worked	Frequency of Pay
S M D	0 1 2 3	______________	Monthly/Semimonthly

Gross Pay	FICA	Fed. Inc. Tax	State Inc. Tax	SDI	Medicare	Other	Total Deduc.	Net Pay

JOB SKILL 19-6 *(continued)*

___/13 ___/13 ___/13 6. Prepare payroll for Amy Seaforth, who is a part-time laboratory technician. She is married; her husband does not claim her, and she does not wish to claim herself either. She joined the hospital insurance plan. She is paid a salary of $145 per week plus car expense figured at $0.34 per mile. She drove 36 miles this pay period. Amy is a new employee hired on May 1, 20XX. You will be completing an employee earning record card for her in a future job skill. Her address is 29926 West Ridgeway Avenue, Woodland Hills, XY 12345; telephone 555-692-4408; Social Security number XXX-XX-1945; birth date 08-04-50.

Status	Exemptions	Salary/Hrs Worked	Frequency of Pay
S M D	0 1 2 3	__________	Monthly/Semimonthly

Gross Pay	FICA	Fed. Inc. Tax	State Inc. Tax	SDI	Medicare	Other	Total Deduc.	Net Pay

___/13 ___/13 ___/13 7. Prepare payroll for Lisa Adams, who is the clinical medical assistant. She is married and has one child, whom she claims along with herself as deductions. She is paid $1,750 per month, and she joined the hospital insurance plan.

Status	Exemptions	Salary/Hrs Worked	Frequency of Pay
S M D	0 1 2 3	__________	Monthly/Semimonthly

Gross Pay	FICA	Fed. Inc. Tax	State Inc. Tax	SDI	Medicare	Other	Total Deduc.	Net Pay

_____ _____ _____ Complete within specified time.

___/93 ___/93 ___/93 **Total points earned** (To obtain a percentage score, divide the total points earned by the number of points possible.)

Comments:

Evaluator's Signature: ____________________ **Need to Repeat:** __________

National Curriculum Competency: CAAHEP: Cognitive: II.C.1	ABHES: 8.j

FIGURE 19-3

SINGLE Persons—**SEMIMONTHLY** Payroll Period (For Wages Paid through December 2011)												**FEDERAL**
And the wages are–		And the number of withholding allowances claimed is—										
At least	But less than	0	1	2	3	4	5	6	7	8	9	10
		The amount of income tax to be withheld is —										
$ 800	$ 820	$ 91	$ 68	$ 44	$ 26	$ 11	$ 0	$ 0	$ 0	$ 0	$ 0	$ 0
820	840	94	71	47	28	13	0	0	0	0	0	0
840	860	97	74	50	30	15	0	0	0	0	0	0
860	880	100	77	53	32	17	1	0	0	0	0	0
880	900	103	80	56	34	19	3	0	0	0	0	0
900	920	106	83	59	36	21	5	0	0	0	0	0
920	940	109	86	62	39	23	7	0	0	0	0	0
940	960	112	89	65	42	25	9	0	0	0	0	0
960	980	115	92	68	45	27	11	0	0	0	0	0
980	1,000	118	95	71	48	29	12	0	0	0	0	0
1,000	1,020	121	98	74	51	31	15	0	0	0	0	0
1,020	1,040	124	101	77	54	33	17	2	0	0	0	0
1,040	1,060	127	104	80	57	35	19	4	0	0	0	0
1,060	1,080	130	107	83	60	37	21	6	0	0	0	0
1,080	1,100	133	110	86	63	40	23	8	0	0	0	0
1,100	1,120	136	113	89	66	43	25	10	0	0	0	0
1,120	1,140	139	116	92	69	46	27	12	0	0	0	0
1,140	1,160	142	119	95	72	49	29	14	0	0	0	0
1,160	1,180	145	122	98	75	52	31	16	0	0	0	0
1,180	1,200	148	125	101	78	55	33	18	2	0	0	0
1,200	1,220	151	128	104	81	58	35	20	4	0	0	0
1,220	1,240	154	131	107	84	61	38	22	6	0	0	0
1,240	1,260	157	134	110	87	64	41	24	8	0	0	0
1,260	1,280	160	137	113	90	67	44	26	10	0	0	0
1,280	1,300	163	140	116	93	70	47	28	12	0	0	0
1,300	1,320	166	143	119	96	73	50	30	14	0	0	0
1,320	1,340	169	146	122	99	76	53	32	16	1	0	0
1,340	1,360	172	149	125	102	79	56	34	18	3	0	0
1,360	1,380	175	152	128	105	82	59	36	20	5	0	0
1,380	1,400	178	155	131	108	85	62	39	22	7	0	0
1,400	1,420	181	158	134	111	88	65	42	24	9	0	0
1,420	1,440	184	161	137	114	91	68	45	26	11	0	0
1,440	1,460	184	164	140	117	94	71	48	28	13	0	0
1,460	1,480	190	167	143	120	97	74	51	30	15	0	0
1,480	1,500	193	170	146	123	100	77	54	32	17	2	0
1,500	1,520	196	173	149	126	103	80	57	34	19	4	0
1,520	1,540	199	176	152	129	106	83	60	37	21	6	0
1.540	1,560	204	179	155	132	109	86	63	40	23	8	0
1,560	1,580	209	182	158	135	112	89	66	43	25	10	0
1,580	1,600	214	185	161	138	115	92	69	46	27	12	0
1,600	1,620	219	188	164	141	118	95	72	49	29	14	0
1,620	1,640	224	191	167	144	121	98	75	52	31	16	0
1,640	1,660	229	194	170	147	124	101	78	55	33	18	2
1,660	1,680	234	197	173	150	127	104	81	58	35	20	4
1,680	1,700	239	201	176	153	130	107	84	61	38	22	6
1,700	1,720	244	206	179	156	133	110	87	64	41	24	8
1,720	1,740	249	211	182	159	136	113	90	67	44	26	10
1,740	1,760	254	216	185	162	139	116	93	70	47	28	12
1,760	1,780	259	221	188	165	142	119	96	73	50	30	14
1,780	1,800	264	226	191	168	145	122	99	76	53	32	16
1,800	1,820	269	231	194	171	148	125	102	79	56	34	18
1,820	1,840	274	236	197	174	151	128	105	82	59	36	20
1,840	1,860	279	241	202	177	154	131	108	85	62	39	22
1,860	1,880	284	246	207	180	157	134	111	88	65	42	24
1,880	1,900	289	251	212	183	160	137	114	91	68	45	26
1,900	1,920	294	256	217	186	163	140	117	94	71	48	28
1,920	1,940	299	261	222	189	166	143	120	97	74	51	30
1,940	1,960	304	266	227	192	169	146	123	100	77	54	32
1,960	1,980	309	271	232	195	172	149	126	103	80	57	34
1,980	2,000	314	276	237	199	175	152	129	106	83	60	36
2,000	2,020	319	281	242	204	178	155	132	109	86	63	39
2,020	2,040	324	286	247	209	181	158	135	112	89	66	42
2,040	2,060	329	291	252	214	184	161	138	115	92	69	45
2,060	2,080	334	296	257	219	187	164	141	118	95	72	48
2,080	2,100	339	301	262	224	190	167	144	121	98	75	51
2,100	2,120	344	306	267	229	198	170	147	124	101	78	54
2,120	2,140	349	311	272	234	196	173	150	127	104	81	57

Internal Revenue Service, www.irs.gov.

FIGURE 19-4

SINGLE Persons—**MONTHLY** Payroll Period **FEDERAL**
(For Wages Paid through December 2011)

And the wages are–		And the number of withholding allowances claimed is—										
At least	But less than	0	1	2	3	4	5	6	7	8	9	10
		The amount of income tax to be withheld is —										
$ 0	$ 220	$ 0	$ 0	$ 0	$ 0	$ 0	$ 0	$ 0	$0	$0	$0	$0
220	230	5	0	0	0	0	0	0	0	0	0	0
230	240	6	0	0	0	0	0	0	0	0	0	0
240	250	7	0	0	0	0	0	0	0	0	0	0
250	260	8	0	0	0	0	0	0	0	0	0	0
260	270	9	0	0	0	0	0	0	0	0	0	0
270	280	10	0	0	0	0	0	0	0	0	0	0
280	290	11	0	0	0	0	0	0	0	0	0	0
290	300	12	0	0	0	0	0	0	0	0	0	0
300	320	14	0	0	0	0	0	0	0	0	0	0
320	340	16	0	0	0	0	0	0	0	0	0	0
340	360	18	0	0	0	0	0	0	0	0	0	0
360	380	20	0	0	0	0	0	0	0	0	0	0
380	400	22	0	0	0	0	0	0	0	0	0	0
400	420	24	0	0	0	0	0	0	0	0	0	0
420	440	26	0	0	0	0	0	0	0	0	0	0
440	460	28	0	0	0	0	0	0	0	0	0	0
460	480	30	0	0	0	0	0	0	0	0	0	0
480	500	32	1	0	0	0	0	0	0	0	0	0
500	520	34	3	0	0	0	0	0	0	0	0	0
520	540	36	5	0	0	0	0	0	0	0	0	0
540	560	38	7	0	0	0	0	0	0	0	0	0
560	580	40	9	0	0	0	0	0	0	0	0	0
580	600	42	11	0	0	0	0	0	0	0	0	0
600	640	45	14	0	0	0	0	0	0	0	0	0
640	680	49	18	0	0	0	0	0	0	0	0	0
680	720	53	22	0	0	0	0	0	0	0	0	0
720	760	57	26	0	0	0	0	0	0	0	0	0
760	800	61	30	0	0	0	0	0	0	0	0	0
800	840	65	34	3	0	0	0	0	0	0	0	0
840	880	69	38	7	0	0	0	0	0	0	0	0
880	920	73	42	11	0	0	0	0	0	0	0	0
920	960	79	46	15	0	0	0	0	0	0	0	0
960	1,000	85	50	19	0	0	0	0	0	0	0	0
1,000	1,040	91	54	23	0	0	0	0	0	0	0	0
1,040	1,080	97	58	27	0	0	0	0	0	0	0	0
1,080	1,120	103	62	31	0	0	0	0	0	0	0	0
1,120	1,160	109	66	35	4	0	0	0	0	0	0	0
1,160	1,200	115	70	39	8	0	0	0	0	0	0	0
1,200	1,240	121	75	43	12	0	0	0	0	0	0	0
1,240	1,280	127	81	47	16	0	0	0	0	0	0	0
1,280	1,320	133	87	51	20	0	0	0	0	0	0	0
1,320	1,360	139	93	55	24	0	0	0	0	0	0	0
1,360	1,400	145	99	59	28	0	0	0	0	0	0	0
1,400	1,440	151	105	63	32	1	0	0	0	0	0	0
1,440	1,480	157	111	67	36	5	0	0	0	0	0	0
1,480	1,520	163	117	71	40	9	0	0	0	0	0	0
1,520	1,560	169	123	77	44	13	0	0	0	0	0	0
1,560	1,600	175	129	83	48	17	0	0	0	0	0	0
1,600	1,640	181	135	89	52	21	0	0	0	0	0	0
1,640	1,680	187	141	95	56	25	0	0	0	0	0	0
1,680	1,720	193	147	101	60	29	0	0	0	0	0	0
1,720	1,760	199	153	107	64	33	2	0	0	0	0	0
1,760	1,800	205	159	113	68	37	6	0	0	0	0	0
1,800	1,840	211	165	119	73	41	10	0	0	0	0	0
1,840	1,880	217	171	125	79	45	14	0	0	0	0	0
1,880	1,920	223	177	131	85	49	18	0	0	0	0	0
1,920	1,960	229	183	137	91	53	22	0	0	0	0	0
1,960	2,000	235	189	143	97	57	26	0	0	0	0	0
2,000	2,040	241	195	149	103	61	30	0	0	0	0	0
2,040	2,080	247	201	155	109	65	34	4	0	0	0	0
2,080	2,120	253	207	161	115	69	38	8	0	0	0	0
2,120	2,160	259	213	167	121	74	42	12	0	0	0	0
2,160	2,200	265	219	173	127	80	46	16	0	0	0	0
2,200	2,240	271	225	179	133	86	50	20	0	0	0	0
2,240	2,280	277	231	185	139	92	54	24	0	0	0	0
2,280	2,320	283	237	191	145	98	58	28	0	0	0	0
2,320	2,360	289	243	197	151	104	62	32	1	0	0	0
2,360	2,400	295	249	203	157	110	66	36	5	0	0	0

Internal Revenue Service, www.irs.gov.

FIGURE 19-5

MARRIED Persons—**MONTHLY** Payroll Period **FEDERAL**

(For Wages Paid through December 2011)

And the wages are–		And the number of withholding allowances claimed is—										
At least	But less than	0	1	2	3	4	5	6	7	8	9	10
		The amount of income tax to be withheld is —										
$ 0	$ 680	$ 0	$ 0	$ 0	$ 0	$ 0	$ 0	$ 0	$ 0	$ 0	$ 0	$ 0
680	720	4	0	0	0	0	0	0	0	0	0	0
720	760	8	0	0	0	0	0	0	0	0	0	0
760	800	12	0	0	0	0	0	0	0	0	0	0
800	840	16	0	0	0	0	0	0	0	0	0	0
840	880	20	0	0	0	0	0	0	0	0	0	0
880	920	24	0	0	0	0	0	0	0	0	0	0
920	960	28	0	0	0	0	0	0	0	0	0	0
960	1,000	32	1	0	0	0	0	0	0	0	0	0
1,000	1,040	36	5	0	0	0	0	0	0	0	0	0
1,040	1,080	40	9	0	0	0	0	0	0	0	0	0
1,080	1,120	44	13	0	0	0	0	0	0	0	0	0
1,120	1,160	48	17	0	0	0	0	0	0	0	0	0
1,160	1,200	52	21	0	0	0	0	0	0	0	0	0
1,200	1,240	56	25	0	0	0	0	0	0	0	0	0
1,240	1,280	60	29	0	0	0	0	0	0	0	0	0
1,280	1,320	64	33	3	0	0	0	0	0	0	0	0
1,320	1360	68	37	7	0	0	0	0	0	0	0	0
1360	1,400	72	41	11	0	0	0	0	0	0	0	0
1,400	1,440	76	45	15	0	0	0	0	0	0	0	0
1,440	1,480	80	49	19	0	0	0	0	0	0	0	0
1,480	1,520	84	53	23	0	0	0	0	0	0	0	0
1,520	1,560	88	57	27	0	0	0	0	0	0	0	0
1,560	1,600	92	61	31	0	0	0	0	0	0	0	0
1,600	1,640	96	65	35	4	0	0	0	0	0	0	0
1,640	1,680	100	69	39	8	0	0	0	0	0	0	0
1,680	1,720	104	73	43	12	0	0	0	0	0	0	0
1,720	1,760	108	77	47	16	0	0	0	0	0	0	0
1,760	1,800	112	81	51	20	0	0	0	0	0	0	0
1,800	1,840	116	85	55	24	0	0	0	0	0	0	0
1,840	1,880	120	89	59	28	0	0	0	0	0	0	0
1,880	1,920	124	93	63	32	1	0	0	0	0	0	0
1,920	1,960	128	97	67	36	5	0	0	0	0	0	0
1,960	2,000	132	101	71	40	9	0	0	0	0	0	0
2,000	2,040	136	105	75	44	13	0	0	0	0	0	0
2,040	2,080	140	109	79	48	17	0	0	0	0	0	0
2,080	2,120	145	113	83	52	21	0	0	0	0	0	0
2,120	2,160	151	117	87	56	25	0	0	0	0	0	0
2,160	2,200	157	121	91	60	29	0	0	0	0	0	0
2,200	2,240	163	125	95	64	33	2	0	0	0	0	0
2,240	2,280	169	129	99	68	37	6	0	0	0	0	0
2,280	2,320	175	133	103	72	41	10	0	0	0	0	0
2,320	2,360	181	137	107	76	45	14	0	0	0	0	0
2,360	2,400	187	141	111	80	49	18	0	0	0	0	0
2,400	2,440	193	147	115	84	53	22	0	0	0	0	0
2,440	2,480	199	153	119	88	57	26	0	0	0	0	0
2,480	2,520	205	159	123	92	61	30	0	0	0	0	0
2,520	2,560	211	165	127	96	65	34	3	0	0	0	0
2,560	2,600	217	171	131	100	69	38	7	0	0	0	0
2,600	2,640	223	177	135	104	73	42	11	0	0	0	0
2,640	2,680	229	183	139	108	77	46	15	0	0	0	0
2,680	2,720	235	189	143	112	81	50	19	0	0	0	0
2,720	2,760	241	195	149	116	85	54	23	0	0	0	0
2,760	2,800	247	201	155	120	89	58	27	0	0	0	0
2,800	2,840	253	207	161	124	93	62	31	0	0	0	0
2,840	2,880	259	213	167	128	97	66	35	4	0	0	0
2,880	2,920	265	219	173	132	101	70	39	8	0	0	0
2,920	2,960	271	225	179	136	105	74	43	12	0	0	0
2,960	3,000	277	231	185	140	109	78	47	16	0	0	0
3,000	3,040	283	237	191	145	113	82	51	20	0	0	0
3,040	3,080	289	243	197	151	117	86	55	24	0	0	0
3,080	3,120	295	249	203	157	121	90	59	28	0	0	0
3,120	3,160	301	255	209	163	125	94	63	32	2	0	0
3,160	3,200	307	261	215	169	129	98	67	36	6	0	0
3,200	3,240	313	267	221	175	133	102	71	40	10	0	0
3,240	3,280	319	273	227	181	137	106	75	44	14	0	0
3,280	3,320	325	279	233	187	141	110	79	48	18	0	0
3,320	3,360	331	285	239	193	146	114	83	52	22	0	0
3,360	3,400	337	291	245	199	152	118	87	56	26	0	0

Internal Revenue Service, www.irs.gov.

JOB SKILL 19-6 *(continued)*

FIGURE 19-6

MARRIED Persons—**MONTHLY** Payroll Period (For Wages Paid through December 2011)												**FEDERAL**
And the wages are–		And the number of withholding allowances claimed is—										
At least	But less than	0	1	2	3	4	5	6	7	8	9	10
		The amount of income tax to be withheld is —										
$ 0	$ 330	$ 0	$ 0	$ 0	$ 0	$ 0	$ 0	$ 0	$0	$ 0	$0	$0
330	340	1	0	0	0	0	0	0	0	0	0	0
340	350	2	0	0	0	0	0	0	0	0	0	0
350	360	3	0	0	0	0	0	0	0	0	0	0
360	370	4	0	0	0	0	0	0	0	0	0	0
370	380	5	0	0	0	0	0	0	0	0	0	0
380	390	6	0	0	0	0	0	0	0	0	0	0
390	400	7	0	0	0	0	0	0	0	0	0	0
400	410	8	0	0	0	0	0	0	0	0	0	0
410	420	9	0	0	0	0	0	0	0	0	0	0
420	430	10	0	0	0	0	0	0	0	0	0	0
430	440	11	0	0	0	0	0	0	0	0	0	0
440	450	12	0	0	0	0	0	0	0	0	0	0
450	460	13	0	0	0	0	0	0	0	0	0	0
460	470	14	0	0	0	0	0	0	0	0	0	0
470	480	15	0	0	0	0	0	0	0	0	0	0
480	490	16	0	0	0	0	0	0	0	0	0	0
490	500	17	1	0	0	0	0	0	0	0	0	0
500	520	18	3	0	0	0	0	0	0	0	0	0
520	540	20	5	0	0	0	0	0	0	0	0	0
540	560	22	7	0	0	0	0	0	0	0	0	0
560	580	24	9	0	0	0	0	0	0	0	0	0
580	600	26	11	0	0	0	0	0	0	0	0	0
600	620	28	13	0	0	0	0	0	0	0	0	0
620	640	30	15	0	0	0	0	0	0	0	0	0
640	660	32	17	1	0	0	0	0	0	0	0	0
660	680	34	19	3	0	0	0	0	0	0	0	0
680	700	36	21	5	0	0	0	0	0	0	0	0
700	720	38	23	7	0	0	0	0	0	0	0	0
720	740	40	25	9	0	0	0	0	0	0	0	0
740	760	42	27	11	0	0	0	0	0	0	0	0
760	780	44	29	13	0	0	0	0	0	0	0	0
780	800	46	31	15	0	0	0	0	0	0	0	0
800	820	48	33	17	2	0	0	0	0	0	0	0
820	840	50	35	19	4	0	0	0	0	0	0	0
840	860	52	37	21	6	0	0	0	0	0	0	0
860	880	54	39	23	8	0	0	0	0	0	0	0
880	900	56	41	25	10	0	0	0	0	0	0	0
900	920	58	43	27	12	0	0	0	0	0	0	0
920	940	60	45	29	14	0	0	0	0	0	0	0
940	960	62	47	31	16	0	0	0	0	0	0	0
960	980	64	49	33	18	2	0	0	0	0	0	0
980	1,000	66	51	35	20	4	0	0	0	0	0	0
1,000	1,020	68	53	37	22	6	0	0	0	0	0	0
1,020	1,040	70	55	39	24	8	0	0	0	0	0	0
1,040	1,060	73	57	41	26	10	0	0	0	0	0	0
1,060	1,080	76	59	43	28	12	0	0	0	0	0	0
1,080	1,100	79	61	45	30	14	0	0	0	0	0	0
1,100	1,120	82	63	47	32	16	1	0	0	0	0	0
1,120	1,140	85	65	49	34	18	3	0	0	0	0	0
1,140	1,160	88	67	51	36	20	5	0	0	0	0	0
1,160	1,180	91	69	53	38	22	7	0	0	0	0	0
1,180	1,200	94	71	55	40	24	9	0	0	0	0	0
1,200	1,220	97	74	57	42	26	11	0	0	0	0	0
1,220	1,240	100	77	59	44	28	13	0	0	0	0	0
1,240	1,260	103	80	61	46	30	15	0	0	0	0	0
1,260	1,280	106	83	63	48	32	17	2	0	0	0	0
1,280	1,300	109	86	65	50	34	19	4	0	0	0	0
1,300	1,320	112	89	67	52	36	21	6	0	0	0	0
1,320	1,340	115	92	69	54	38	23	8	0	0	0	0
1,340	1,360	118	95	71	56	40	25	10	0	0	0	0
1,360	1,380	121	98	74	58	42	27	12	0	0	0	0
1,380	1,400	124	101	77	60	44	29	14	0	0	0	0
1,400	1,420	127	104	80	62	46	31	16	0	0	0	0
1,420	1,440	130	107	83	64	48	33	18	2	0	0	0
1,440	1,460	133	110	86	66	50	35	20	4	0	0	0
1,460	1,480	136	113	89	68	52	37	22	6	0	0	0
1,480	1,500	139	116	92	70	54	39	24	8	0	0	0

Internal Revenue Service, www.irs.gov.

JOB SKILL 19-6 *(continued)*

FIGURE 19-7

SINGLE PERSONS, DUAL INCOME MARRIED
OR MARRIED WITH MULTIPLE EMPLOYERS----SEMI-MONTHLY PAYROLL PERIOD

IF WAGES ARE... AND THE NUMBER OF WITHHOLDING ALLOWANCES CLAIMED IS... **STATE**

AT LEAST	BUT LESS THAN	0	1	2	3	4	5	6	7	8	9	10 OR MORE
		...THE AMOUNT OF INCOME TAX TO BE WITHHELD SHALL BE...										
$1	$300											
300	320	1.74										
320	340	1.94										
340	360	2.14										
360	380	2.34										
380	400	2.54										
400	420	2.86										
420	440	3.26										
440	460	3.66	0.03									
460	480	4.06	0.43									
480	500	4.46	0.83									
500	540	5.06	1.43									
540	580	5.86	2.23									
580	620	6.66	3.03									
620	660	7.46	3.83	0.20								
660	700	8.26	4.63	1.00								
700	740	9.06	5.43	1.80								
740	780	9.87	6.24	2.61								
780	820	11.47	7.84	4.21	0.58							
820	860	13.07	9.44	5.81	2.18							
860	900	14.67	11.04	7.41	3.78	0.15						
900	940	16.27	12.64	9.01	5.38	1.75						
940	980	17.87	14.24	10.61	6.98	3.35						
980	1020	19.47	15.84	12.21	8.58	4.95	1.32					
1020	1060	21.07	17.44	13.81	10.18	6.55	2.92					
1060	1100	22.67	19.04	15.41	11.78	8.15	4.52	0.89				
1100	1140	24.27	20.64	17.01	13.38	9.75	6.12	2.49				
1140	1180	26.66	23.03	19.40	15.77	12.14	8.51	4.88	1.25			
1180	1220	29.06	25.43	21.80	18.17	14.54	10.91	7.28	3.65	0.02		
1220	1260	31.46	27.83	24.20	20.57	16.94	13.31	9.68	6.05	2.42		
1260	1300	33.86	30.23	26.60	22.97	19.34	15.71	12.08	8.45	4.82	1.19	
1300	1340	36.26	32.63	29.00	25.37	21.74	18.11	14.48	10.85	7.22	3.59	
1340	1380	38.66	35.03	31.40	27.77	24.14	20.51	16.88	13.25	9.62	5.99	2.36
1380	1420	41.06	37.43	33.80	30.17	26.54	22.91	19.28	15.65	12.02	8.39	4.76
1420	1460	43.46	39.83	36.20	32.57	28.94	25.31	21.68	18.05	14.42	10.79	7.16
1460	1500	45.86	42.23	38.60	34.97	31.34	27.71	24.08	20.45	16.82	13.19	9.56
1500	1540	48.60	44.97	41.34	37.71	34.08	30.45	26.82	23.19	19.56	15.93	12.30
1540	1580	51.80	48.17	44.54	40.91	37.28	33.65	30.02	26.39	22.76	19.13	15.50
1580	1620	55.00	51.37	47.74	44.11	40.48	36.85	33.22	29.59	25.96	22.33	18.70
1620	1660	58.20	54.57	50.94	47.31	43.68	40.05	36.42	32.79	29.16	25.53	21.90
1660	1700	61.40	57.77	54.14	50.51	46.88	43.25	39.62	35.99	32.36	28.73	25.10
1700	1750	65.00	61.37	57.74	54.11	50.48	46.85	43.22	39.59	35.96	32.33	28.70
1750	1800	69.00	65.37	61.74	58.11	54.48	50.85	47.22	43.59	39.96	36.33	32.70
1800	1850	73.00	69.37	65.74	62.11	58.48	54.85	51.22	47.59	43.96	40.33	36.70
1850	1900	77.15	73.52	69.89	66.26	62.63	59.00	55.37	51.74	48.11	44.48	40.85
1900	1950	81.80	78.17	74.54	70.91	67.28	63.65	60.02	56.39	52.76	49.13	45.50
1950	2000	86.45	82.82	79.19	75.56	71.93	68.30	64.67	61.04	57.41	53.78	50.15
2000	2100	93.43	89.80	86.17	82.54	78.91	75.28	71.65	68.02	64.39	60.76	57.13
2100	2200	102.73	99.10	95.47	91.84	88.21	84.58	80.95	77.32	73.69	70.06	66.43
2200	2300	112.03	108.40	104.77	101.14	97.51	93.88	90.25	86.62	82.99	79.36	75.73
2300	2400	121.33	117.70	114.07	110.44	106.81	103.18	99.55	95.92	92.29	88.66	85.03
2400 and over		(Table Amount PLUS 9.3 Percent of the Amount Over 2350)										

Internal Revenue Service, www.irs.gov.

JOB SKILL 19-6 (*continued*)

FIGURE 19-8

MARRIED PERSONS----SEMI-MONTHLY PAYROLL PERIOD

IF WAGES ARE... AND THE NUMBER OF WITHHOLDING ALLOWANCES CLAIMED IS... **STATE**

AT LEAST	BUT LESS THAN	0	1	2	3	4	5	6	7	8	9	10 OR MORE
		...THE AMOUNT OF INCOME TAX TO BE WITHHELD SHALL BE...										
$1	$300											
300	320	1.74										
320	340	1.94										
340	360	2.14										
360	380	2.34										
380	400	2.54										
400	420	2.74										
420	440	2.94										
440	460	3.14										
460	480	3.34										
480	500	3.54										
500	520	3.74	0.11									
520	540	3.94	0.31									
540	560	4.14	0.51									
560	580	4.34	0.71									
580	600	4.54	0.91									
600	620	4.74	1.11									
620	640	4.94	1.31									
640	660	5.14	1.51									
660	680	5.43	1.80									
680	700	5.83	2.20									
700	720	6.23	2.60									
720	740	6.63	3.00									
740	760	7.03	3.40									
760	780	7.43	3.80									
780	800	7.83	4.20									
800	820	8.23	4.60									
820	840	8.63	5.00									
840	860	9.03	5.40									
860	880	9.43	5.80									
880	900	9.83	6.20									
900	920	10.23	6.60	0.26								
920	940	10.63	7.00	0.66								
940	960	11.03	7.40	1.06								
960	980	11.43	7.80	1.46								
980	1000	11.83	8.20	1.86								
1000	1040	12.43	8.80	2.46								
1040	1080	13.23	9.60	3.26								
1080	1120	14.03	10.40	4.06	0.43							
1120	1160	14.83	11.20	4.86	1.23							
1160	1200	15.63	12.00	5.66	2.03							
1200	1240	16.43	12.80	6.46	2.83							
1240	1280	17.23	13.60	7.26	3.63							
1280	1320	18.03	14.40	8.06	4.43	0.80						
1320	1360	18.83	15.20	8.86	5.23	1.60						
1360	1400	19.63	16.00	9.66	6.03	2.40						
1400	1440	21.16	17.53	10.46	6.83	3.20						
1440	1480	22.76	19.13	11.26	7.63	4.00	0.37					
1480	1520	24.36	20.73	12.06	8.43	4.80	1.17					
1520	1560	25.96	22.33	13.27	9.64	6.01	2.38					
1560	1600	27.56	23.93	14.87	11.24	7.61	3.98	0.35				

Internal Revenue Service, www.irs.gov.

JOB SKILL 19-6 *(continued)*

FIGURE 19-9

UNMARRIED HEAD OF HOUSEHOLD----SEMI-MONTHLY PAYROLL PERIOD

IF WAGES ARE... AND THE NUMBER OF WITHHOLDING ALLOWANCES CLAIMED IS... **STATE**

AT LEAST	BUT LESS THAN	0	1	2	3	4	5	6	7	8	9	10 OR MORE
		...THE AMOUNT OF INCOME TAX TO BE WITHHELD SHALL BE...										
$1	$600											
600	620	3.39										
620	640	3.59										
640	660	3.79	0.16									
660	680	3.99	0.36									
680	700	4.19	0.56									
700	720	4.39	0.76									
720	740	4.59	0.96									
740	760	4.79	1.16									
760	780	4.99	1.36									
780	800	5.19	1.56									
800	820	5.51	1.88									
820	840	5.91	2.28									
840	860	6.31	2.68									
860	880	6.71	3.08									
880	900	7.11	3.48									
900	920	7.51	3.88	0.25								
920	940	7.91	4.28	0.65								
940	960	8.31	4.68	1.05								
960	980	8.71	5.08	1.45								
980	1000	9.11	5.48	1.85								
1000	1025	9.56	5.93	2.30								
1025	1050	10.06	6.43	2.80								
1050	1075	10.56	6.93	3.30								
1075	1100	11.06	7.43	3.80	0.17							
1100	1125	11.56	7.93	4.30	0.67							
1125	1150	12.06	8.43	4.80	1.17							
1150	1175	12.56	8.93	5.30	1.67							
1175	1200	13.06	9.43	5.80	2.17							
1200	1225	13.56	9.93	6.30	2.67							
1225	1250	14.06	10.43	6.80	3.17							
1250	1275	14.56	10.93	7.30	3.67	0.04						
1275	1300	15.06	11.43	7.80	4.17	0.54						
1300	1325	15.56	11.93	8.30	4.67	1.04						
1325	1350	16.06	12.43	8.80	5.17	1.54						
1350	1375	16.56	12.93	9.30	5.67	2.04						
1375	1400	17.06	13.43	9.80	6.17	2.54						
1400	1450	17.81	14.18	10.55	6.92	3.29						
1450	1500	18.81	15.18	11.55	7.92	4.29	0.66					
1500	1550	19.92	16.29	12.66	9.03	5.40	1.77					
1550	1600	21.92	18.29	14.66	11.03	7.40	3.77	0.14				
1600	1650	23.92	20.29	16.66	13.03	9.40	5.77	2.14				
1650	1700	25.92	22.29	18.66	15.03	11.40	7.77	4.14	0.51			
1700	1750	27.92	24.29	20.66	17.03	13.40	9.77	6.14	2.51			
1750	1800	29.92	26.29	22.66	19.03	15.40	11.77	8.14	4.51	0.88		
1800	1850	31.92	28.29	24.66	21.03	17.40	13.77	10.14	6.51	2.88		
1850	1900	33.92	30.29	26.66	23.03	19.40	15.77	12.14	8.51	4.88	1.25	
1900	2000	38.32	34.69	31.06	27.43	23.80	20.17	16.54	12.91	9.28	5.65	2.02
2000	2100	44.32	40.69	37.06	33.43	29.80	26.17	22.54	18.91	15.28	11.65	8.02
2100	2200	50.32	46.69	43.06	39.43	35.80	32.17	28.54	24.91	21.28	17.65	14.02
2200	2300	56.32	52.69	49.06	45.43	41.80	38.17	34.54	30.91	27.28	23.65	20.02
2300 and over		(Table Amount PLUS 9.3 Percent of the Amount Over 2250)										

Internal Revenue Service, www.irs.gov.

JOB SKILL 19-6 *(continued)*

FIGURE 19-10

MARRIED PERSONS----MONTHLY PAYROLL PERIOD

IF WAGES ARE... AND THE NUMBER OF WITHHOLDING ALLOWANCES CLAIMED IS... **STATE**

AT LEAST	BUT LESS THAN	0	1	2	3	4	5	6	7	8	9	10 OR MORE
		...THE AMOUNT OF INCOME TAX TO BE WITHHELD SHALL BE...										
$1	$600											
600	640	3.49										
640	680	3.89										
680	720	4.29										
720	760	4.69										
760	800	5.09										
800	840	5.49										
840	880	5.89										
880	920	6.29										
920	960	6.69										
960	1000	7.09										
1000	1040	7.49	0.23									
1040	1080	7.89	0.63									
1080	1120	8.29	1.03									
1120	1160	8.69	1.43									
1160	1200	9.09	1.83									
1200	1240	9.49	2.23									
1240	1280	9.89	2.63									
1280	1320	10.29	3.03									
1320	1360	10.86	3.60									
1360	1400	11.66	4.40									
1400	1440	12.46	5.20									
1440	1480	13.26	6.00									
1480	1520	14.06	6.80									
1520	1560	14.86	7.60									
1560	1600	15.66	8.40									
1600	1640	16.46	9.20									
1640	1680	17.26	10.00									
1680	1720	18.06	10.80									
1720	1760	18.86	11.60									
1760	1800	19.66	12.40									
1800	1840	20.46	13.20	0.51								
1840	1880	21.26	14.00	1.31								
1880	1920	22.06	14.80	2.11								
1920	1960	22.86	15.60	2.91								
1960	2000	23.66	16.40	3.71								
2000	2040	24.46	17.20	4.51								
2040	2080	25.26	18.00	5.31								
2080	2140	26.26	19.00	6.31								
2140	2200	27.46	20.20	7.51	0.25							
2200	2260	28.66	21.40	8.71	1.45							
2260	2320	29.86	22.60	9.91	2.65							
2320	2380	31.06	23.80	11.11	3.85							
2380	2440	32.26	25.00	12.31	5.05							
2440	2500	33.46	26.20	13.51	6.25							
2500	2560	34.66	27.40	14.71	7.45	0.19						
2560	2620	35.86	28.60	15.91	8.65	1.39						
2620	2680	37.06	29.80	17.11	9.85	2.59						
2680	2740	38.26	31.00	18.31	11.05	3.79						
2740	2800	39.51	32.25	19.51	12.25	4.99						
2800	2860	41.91	34.65	20.71	13.45	6.19						

Internal Revenue Service, www.irs.gov.

JOB SKILL 19-6 *(continued)*

FIGURE 19-11

UNMARRIED HEAD OF HOUSEHOLD----MONTHLY PAYROLL PERIOD

IF WAGES ARE... AND THE NUMBER OF WITHHOLDING ALLOWANCES CLAIMED IS... **STATE**

AT LEAST	BUT LESS THAN	0	1	2	3	4	5	6	7	8	9	10 OR MORE
		...THE AMOUNT OF INCOME TAX TO BE WITHHELD SHALL BE...										
$1	1400											
1400	1420	8.68	1.42									
1420	1440	8.88	1.62									
1440	1460	9.08	1.82									
1460	1480	9.28	2.02									
1480	1500	9.48	2.22									
1500	1520	9.68	2.42									
1520	1540	9.88	2.62									
1540	1560	10.08	2.82									
1560	1580	10.28	3.02									
1580	1600	10.48	3.22									
1600	1620	10.81	3.55									
1620	1640	11.21	3.95									
1640	1660	11.61	4.35									
1660	1680	12.01	4.75									
1680	1720	12.61	5.35									
1720	1760	13.41	6.15									
1760	1800	14.21	6.95									
1800	1840	15.01	7.75	0.49								
1840	1880	15.81	8.55	1.29								
1880	1920	16.61	9.35	2.09								
1920	1960	17.41	10.15	2.89								
1960	2000	18.21	10.95	3.69								
2000	2040	19.01	11.75	4.49								
2040	2080	19.81	12.55	5.29								
2080	2120	20.61	13.35	6.09								
2120	2160	21.41	14.15	6.89								
2160	2200	22.21	14.95	7.69	0.43							
2200	2250	23.11	15.85	8.59	1.33							
2250	2300	24.11	16.85	9.59	2.33							
2300	2350	25.11	17.85	10.59	3.33							
2350	2400	26.11	18.85	11.59	4.33							
2400	2450	27.11	19.85	12.59	5.33							
2450	2500	28.11	20.85	13.59	6.33							
2500	2550	29.11	21.85	14.59	7.33	0.07						
2550	2600	30.11	22.85	15.59	8.33	1.07						
2600	2650	31.11	23.85	16.59	9.33	2.07						
2650	2700	32.11	24.85	17.59	10.33	3.07						
2700	2800	33.61	26.35	19.09	11.83	4.57						
2800	2900	35.61	28.35	21.09	13.83	6.57						
2900	3000	37.61	30.35	23.09	15.83	8.57	1.31					
3000	3100	39.85	32.59	25.33	18.07	10.81	3.55					
3100	3200	43.85	36.59	29.33	22.07	14.81	7.55	0.29				
3200	3300	47.85	40.59	33.33	26.07	18.81	11.55	4.29				
3300	3400	51.85	44.59	37.33	30.07	22.81	15.55	8.29	1.03			
3400	3500	55.85	48.59	41.33	34.07	26.81	19.55	12.29	5.03			
3500	3600	59.85	52.59	45.33	38.07	30.81	23.55	16.29	9.03	1.77		
3600	3800	65.85	58.59	51.33	44.07	36.81	29.55	22.29	15.03	7.77	0.51	
3800	4000	76.64	69.38	62.12	54.86	47.60	40.34	33.08	25.82	18.56	11.30	4.04
4000	4200	88.64	81.38	74.12	66.86	59.60	52.34	45.08	37.82	30.56	23.30	16.04
4200	4400	100.64	93.38	86.12	78.86	71.60	64.34	57.08	49.82	42.56	35.30	28.04
4400 and over		(Table Amount PLUS 9.3 Percent of the Amount Over 4300)										

Internal Revenue Service, www.irs.gov.

JOB SKILL 19-7
Complete a Payroll Register

Name ______________________________ Date ______________ Score ________

Performance Objective

Task: Insert employee payroll data to complete a payroll register.

Conditions: Use the payroll information obtained for seven employees from Job Skill 19-6, one payroll register (Form 109), and pen or pencil. Refer to Procedure 19-2 in the *textbook* for step-by-step directions and *textbook* Figure 19-15 for a visual example.

Standards: Complete all steps listed in this skill in _______ minutes with a minimum score of _______. (Time element and accuracy criteria may be given by instructor.)

Time: **Start:** ____________ **Completed:** ____________ **Total:** ____________ minutes

Scoring: One point for each step performed satisfactorily unless otherwise listed or weighted by instructor.

Directions with Performance Evaluation Checklist

Refer to the employees in Job Skill 19-6. Alphabetize their names (last name first), and record the information in the payroll register.

1st Attempt	2nd Attempt	3rd Attempt	
______	______	______	Gather materials (equipment and supplies) listed under "Conditions."
___/14	___/14	___/14	1. Complete payroll register information for employee Lisa Adams.
___/13	___/13	___/13	2. Complete payroll register information for employee Kelley Jones.
___/13	___/13	___/13	3. Complete payroll register information for employee Maryjane Moran.
___/13	___/13	___/13	4. Complete payroll register information for employee Carla O'Hare.
___/14	___/14	___/14	5. Complete payroll register information for employee Amy Seaforth.
___/13	___/13	___/13	6. Complete payroll register information for employee Hillary Sheehan.
___/11	___/11	___/11	7. Complete payroll register information for employee Roger Young.
______	______	______	Complete within specified time.
___/93	___/93	___/93	**Total points earned** (To obtain a percentage score, divide the total points earned by the number of points possible.)

Comments:

Evaluator's Signature: ______________________________ **Need to Repeat:** ______________

National Curriculum Competency: CAAHEP: Cognitive: II.C.1	ABHES: 8.j

JOB SKILL 19-8
Complete an Employee Earning Record

Name ______________________________ Date ______________ Score ________

Performance Objective

Task: Complete an employee earning record.

Conditions: Use information from Job Skill 19-6, one employee earning record (Form 110), and pen or pencil.

Standards: Complete all steps listed in this skill in _______ minutes with a minimum score of ________. (Time element and accuracy criteria may be given by instructor.)

Time: **Start:** ____________ **Completed:** ____________ **Total:** ____________ minutes

Scoring: One point for each step performed satisfactorily unless otherwise listed or weighted by instructor.

Directions with Performance Evaluation Checklist

Refer to Amy Seaforth's employment information in Job Skill 19-6 and complete an employee earning record; she is a new employee.

1st Attempt	2nd Attempt	3rd Attempt	
______	______	______	Gather materials (equipment and supplies) listed under "Conditions."
____/5	____/5	____/5	1. Fill in the employee's name, address, telephone number, and Social Security number.
____/8	____/8	____/8	2. Fill in the employee's date of hire, birth date, position, number of exemptions, and rate of pay indicating (with a circle) whether she is part-time or full-time; single or married; and paid hourly, weekly, or monthly.
____/12	____/12	____/12	3. Complete all line items in the earning record that are applicable to Amy Seaforth for May 28, 20XX.
______	______	______	Complete within specified time.
____/27	____/27	____/27	**Total points earned** (To obtain a percentage score, divide the total points earned by the number of points possible.)

Comments:

Evaluator's Signature: ______________________________ **Need to Repeat:** ____________

National Curriculum Competency: CAAHEP: Cognitive: II.C.1	ABHES: 8.j

JOB SKILL 19-9
Complete an Employee's Withholding Allowance Certificate

Name ______________________________ Date ______________ Score ________

Performance Objective

Task: Complete an employee's withholding allowance certificate.

Conditions: One Employee's Withholding Allowance Certificate (Form 111), and typewriter, pen, or pencil. Refer to *textbook* Figure 19-9 for an illustration of a completed W-4 form and Part III of the *Workbook* for physician information.

Standards: Complete all steps listed in this skill in _______ minutes with a minimum score of ________. (Time element and accuracy criteria may be given by instructor.)

Time: **Start:** ____________ **Completed:** ____________ **Total:** ____________ minutes

Scoring: One point for each step performed satisfactorily unless otherwise listed or weighted by instructor.

Directions with Performance Evaluation Checklist

Complete an Employee's Withholding Allowance Certificate for yourself as if you were being hired by Drs. Gerald and Fran Practon.

1st Attempt	2nd Attempt	3rd Attempt	
_____	_____	_____	Gather materials (equipment and supplies) listed under "Conditions."
____/5	____/5	____/5	1. Read through Items A through G, and mark which allowances you would like to claim.
_____	_____	_____	2. Total all deductions and enter in Line H.
____/4	____/4	____/4	3. Fill in your last name, first name, and address.
_____	_____	_____	4. Fill in your Social Security number. You may use a mock SSN or the last 4 digits for confidentiality.
_____	_____	_____	5. Indicate whether you are single, married, or married and withholding at a higher single rate.
_____	_____	_____	6. Verify your last name with that appearing on your Social Security card and indicate if it is different.
_____	_____	_____	7. Indicate the number of allowances in Item 5.
_____	_____	_____	8. Read Items 6 and 7 and mark if applicable.
____/2	____/2	____/2	9. Sign and date the form.
____/3	____/3	____/3	10. Complete the employer's name and address in Item 8.
_____	_____	_____	11. Fill in the Tax Identification Number for Practon Medical Group, Inc.
_____	_____	_____	Complete within specified time.
____/23	____/23	____/23	**Total points earned** (To obtain a percentage score, divide the total points earned by the number of points possible.)

JOB SKILL 19-9 *(continued)*

Comments:

Evaluator's Signature: ______________________________ **Need to Repeat:** ____________

National Curriculum Competency: ABHES: 8.a

JOB SKILL 19-10
Complete an Employee Benefit Form

Name ______________________________ Date ______________ Score ________

Performance Objective

Task: Extract information from the case scenario, calculate employee benefits, and complete an employee benefit form.

Conditions: Employee benefit form (Form 112); calculator; and computer, typewriter, pen, or pencil. Refer to *textbook* Figure 19-11 for an illustration of a completed benefit form.

Standards: Complete all steps listed in this skill in ________ minutes with a minimum score of ________. (Time element and accuracy criteria may be given by instructor.)

Time: **Start:** ____________ **Completed:** ____________ **Total:** ____________ minutes

Scoring: One point for each step performed satisfactorily unless otherwise listed or weighted by instructor.

Directions with Performance Evaluation Checklist

Extract information for the following case scenario and complete an employee benefit form.

Scenario: You have just been hired by Drs. Gerald and Fran Practon as a full-time administrative medical assistant, and they have agreed to pay you $1,760 per month, which amounts to approximately $10 per hour. You receive six paid holidays per year and one week (5 days) paid vacation after the first year. You have 10 sick days per year and $150 yearly uniform allowance. There are no retirement benefits; there may be an incentive bonus if the practice does well. The practice pays for your medical insurance, which costs $60 per month, and you elect to get life insurance at your own expense, at $12 per month for $100,000 coverage. You also elect to get accident insurance at an additional $4.60 per month for $200,000 coverage. Drs. Practon pay $15.35 per month for your workers' compensation insurance and an additional $17.60 per month for your disability insurance. They pay for your dues to the American Association of Medical Assistants, which are $90 per year.

1st Attempt	2nd Attempt	3rd Attempt	
______	______	______	Gather materials (equipment and supplies) listed under "Conditions."
______	______	______	1. Calculate the employer/employee benefits for medical insurance.
______	______	______	2. Calculate the employer/employee benefits for life insurance.
______	______	______	3. Calculate the employer/employee benefits for accident insurance.
______	______	______	4. Calculate the employer/employee benefits for disability insurance.
______	______	______	5. Calculate the employer/employee benefits for workers' compensation.
______	______	______	6. Calculate the employer/employee benefits for holidays.
______	______	______	7. Calculate the employer/employee benefits for vacation.
______	______	______	8. Calculate the employer/employee benefits for sick leave.
______	______	______	9. Complete the employer/employee benefits for personal leave.
______	______	______	10. Complete the employer/employee benefits for education.
______	______	______	11. Complete the employer/employee benefits for incentive bonus.
______	______	______	12. Complete the employer/employee benefits for retirement.
______	______	______	13. Complete the employer/employee benefits for uniforms.
______	______	______	14. Complete other employer/employee benefits.

JOB SKILL 19-10 (*continued*)

______	______	______	15. Total all employer-paid benefits.
______	______	______	16. Total all employee-paid benefits.
______	______	______	17. Fill in the wage of the employee.
______	______	______	18. Calculate the gross wage for the year.
____/5	____/5	____/5	19. Calculate the amount for the total employee package paid by the employer.
____/5	____/5	____/5	Complete within specified time.
___/30	___/30	___/30	**Total points earned** (To obtain a percentage score, divide the total points earned by the number of points possible.)

Comments:

Evaluator's Signature: ______________________________ **Need to Repeat:** ____________

National Curriculum Competency: ABHES: 8.a

CHAPTER 20

Seeking a Position as an Administrative Medical Assistant

ACCESS THIS CHAPTER EXCLUSIVELY ON THE PREMIUM WEBSITE AT WWW.CENGAGEBRAIN.COM

Directions for accessing can be found in the preface of this book or on your Printed Access Card.

OBJECTIVES

After completing the exercises, the student will be able to:

1. Enhance knowledge of medical terminology, interpret abbreviations, and accurately spell medical words.
2. Complete a job application form (Job Skill 20-1).
3. Compose a letter of introduction (Job Skill 20-2).
4. Key a résumé (Job Skill 20-3).
5. Prepare a follow-up thank-you letter (Job Skill 20-4).

PART II

Blank Forms

To fill out forms electronically, and e-mail them to the instructor or print them, go to the Premium Website that accompanies this text at www.CengageBrain.com. At the CengageBrain.com home page, search for the ISBN of the *text* (from the back cover of your book) using the search box at the top of the page. This will take you to the product page where the Premium Website can be accessed. The forms are included in a downloadable file in the Book Resources section of the Premium Website.

LIST OF FORMS

Number	Name
1	Authorization for Release of Information
2	Patient Registration Information Form
3	Disabled Person Parking Placard Application
4	Telephone Message Forms
5	Telephone Message Forms
6	Telephone Message Forms
7	Telephone Message Forms
8	Telephone Message Forms
9	Telephone Message Forms
10	Appointment Record
11	Appointment Record
12	Appointment Record
13	Appointment Cards
14	Hospital/Surgery Scheduling Form
15	Surgical Form Letter
16	Laboratory Requisition Form
17	X-Ray Request Form
18	File Labels
19	File Labels
20	File Labels
21	Patient Record
22	Patient Record
23	Medical Record Abstract Form
24	Patient Record
25	Flow Sheet
26	Prescription Labels
27	Prescription Form
28	Medication Schedule
29	Letterhead
30	Letterhead
31	Letterhead
32	Letterhead
33	Letterhead
34	Interoffice Memo
35	Interoffice Memo
36	Letterhead

Number	Name
37	Letterhead
38	Number 6 Envelope
39	Number 6 Envelope
40	U.S. Postal Service Stamps by Mail Order Form
41	Letterhead
42	Number 10 Envelope
43	U.S. Postal Service Certified Mail Receipt Form
44	Fax Transmittal Sheet
45	Letterhead
46	Number 6 Envelope
47	U.S. Postal Service Certified Mail Receipt
48	Letterhead
49	Number 10 Envelope
50	U.S. Postal Service Certified Mail Receipt
51	Ledger/Statement (with dates and figures inserted)
52	Ledger/Statement
53	Cash Receipt Forms
54	Letterhead
55	Number 10 Envelope
56	Ledger/Statement
57	Authorization to Charge Credit Card Form
58	Financial Agreement Form
59	Deposit Slip
60	Invoices and Blank Checks
61	Bank Statement Reconciliation
62	Ledger Card
63	Ledger Card
64	Ledger Card
65	Ledger Card
66	Ledger Card
67	Ledger Card
68	Ledger Card
69	Ledger Card
70	Ledger Card

Number	Name
71	Ledger Card
72	Ledger Card
73	Ledger Card
74	Ledger Card
75	Ledger Card
76	Checks
77	Checks
78	Cash Receipts
79	Daily Journal—Day 1
80	Daily Journal—Day 2
81	Checks
82	Daily Journal—Day 3
83	Checks
84	Daily Journal Heading and Bottom Section
85	Managed Care Plan Treatment Authorization Request
86	CMS-1500 Health Insurance Claim Form
87	CMS-1500 Health Insurance Claim Form
88	CMS-1500 Health Insurance Claim Form
89	Patient Complaint Document
90	Patient Complaint Document
91	Inventory Control/Maintenance Log
92	Order Form
93	Order Form

Number	Name
94	Order Form
95	Order Form
96	Travel Expense Report
97	Check Register Form
98	Check Register Form
99	Check Register Form
100	Checks
101	Checks
102	Checks
103	Checks
104	Checks
105	Checks
106	Checks
107	Petty Cash Receipt Envelope
108	Bank Account Reconciliation Form
109	Payroll Register
110	Employee Earning Record
111	Employee's Withholding Allowance Certificate
112	Employee Benefit Form
113	Employment Application Form
114	Preemployment Worksheet
115	Number 10 Envelope
116	Number 6 Envelope

AUTHORIZATION FOR RELEASE OF INFORMATION

Section A: Must be completed for all authorizations.

I hereby authorize the use or disclosure of my individually identifiable health information as described below.
I understand that this authorization is voluntary. I understand that if the organization authorized to receive the information is not a health plan or health care provider, the released information may no longer be protected by federal privacy regulations.

Patient name: ______________________ **ID Number:** ______________________

Persons/organizations providing information: **Persons/organizations receiving information:**

______________________ ______________________
______________________ ______________________
______________________ ______________________

Specific description of information [including from and to date(s)]:
____

Section B: Must be completed only if a health plan or a heath care provider has requested the authorization.

1. The health plan or health care provider must complete the following:
   a. What is the purpose of the use or disclosure?______________________
   ____
   b. Will the health plan or health care provider requesting the authorization receive financial or in-kind compensation in exchange for using or disclosing the health information described above? Yes__ No__

2. The patient or the patient's representative must read and initial the following statements:
   a. I understand that my health care and the payment for my health care will not be affected if I do not sign this form.
   Initials: ______________
   b. I understand that I may see and copy the information described on this form if I ask for it, and that I get a copy of this form after I sign it.
   Initials: ______________

Section C: Must be completed for all authorizations.

The patient or the patient's representative must read and initial the following statements:

1. I understand that this authorization will expire on____/____/______(DD/MM/YR).
   Initials: ______________
2. I understand that I may revoke this authorization at any time by notifying the providing organization in writing, but if I do not it will not have any effect on any actions they took before they received the revocation.
   Initials: ______________
3. I understand that any disclosure of information carries with it the potential for an unauthorized redisclosure and the information may not be protected by federal confidentiality rules.
   Initials: ______________

______________________ ______________________
Signature of patient or patient's representative **Date**
(Form MUST be completed before signing)

Printed name of patient's representative:______________________

Relationship to the patient:______________________

YOU MAY REFUSE TO SIGN THIS AUTHORIZATION
You may not use this form to release information for treatment or payment except when the information to be released is psychotherapy notes or certain research information.

Form 1

Insurance cards copied ❑
Date: ___________

Patient Registration Information

Account # : ___________
Insurance # : ___________
Co-Payment: $ ___________

Please PRINT AND complete ALL sections below!

Is your condition a result of a work injury? YES NO An auto accident? YES NO Date of injury: ___________

PATIENT'S PERSONAL INFORMATION Marital Status: ❑ Single ❑ Married ❑ Divorced ❑ Widowed Sex: ❑ Male ❑ Female

Name: ___________ (last name) ___________ (first name) ___________ (initial)

Street address: ___________ (Apt # ___) City: ___________ State: ______ Zip: ______

Home phone: (___) ___________ Work phone: (___) ___________ Social Security # ______ - ______ - ______

Date of Birth: ______ (month) / ______ (day) / ______ (year) Driver's License: (State & Number) ___________

Employer / Name of School ___________ ❑ Full Time ❑ Part Time

Spouse's Name: ___________ (last name) ___________ (first name) ______ (initial) Spouse's Work phone: (___) ___________

How do you wish to be addressed? ___________ Social Security # ______ - ______ - ______

PATIENT'S / RESPONSIBLE PARTY INFORMATION

Responsible party: ___________ Date of Birth: ___________

Relationship to Patient: ❑ Self ❑ Spouse ❑ Other ___________ Social Security # ______ - ______ - ______

Responsible party's home phone: (____) ___________ Work phone: (____) ___________

Address: ___________ (Apt # ____) City: ___________ State: ______ Zip: ______

Employer's name: ___________ Phone number: (____) ___________

Address: ___________ City: ___________ State: ______ Zip: ______

Your occupation: ___________

Spouse's Employer's name: ___________ Spouse's Work phone: (___) ___________

Address: ___________ City: ___________ State: ______ Zip: ______

PATIENT'S INSURANCE INFORMATION Please present insurance cards to receptionist.

PRIMARY insurance company's name: ___________

Insurance address: ___________ City: ___________ State: ______ Zip: ______

Name of insured: ___________ Date of Birth: ______ Relationship to insured: ☐ Self ☐ Spouse ☐ Other ☐ Child

Insurance ID number: ___________ Group number: ___________

SECONDARY insurance company's name: ___________

Insurance address: ___________ City: ___________ State: ______ Zip: ______

Name of insured: ___________ Date of Birth: ______ Relationship to insured: ☐ Self ☐ Spouse ☐ Other ☐ Child

Insurance ID number: ___________ Group number: ___________

Check if appropriate: ❑ Medigap policy ❑ Retiree coverage

PATIENT'S REFERRAL INFORMATION (please circle one)

Referred by: ___________ If referred by a friend, may we thank her or him? YES NO

Name(s) of other physician(s) who care for you: ___________

EMERGENCY CONTACT

Name of person not living with you: ___________ Relationship: ___________

Address: ___________ City: ___________ State: ______ Zip: ______

Phone number (home): (_____) ___________ Phone number (work): (_____) ___________

Assignment of Benefits • Financial Agreement

I hereby give lifetime authorization for payment of insurance benefits to be made directly to ___________, and any assisting physicians, for services rendered. I understand that I am financially responsible for all charges whether or not they are covered by insurance. In the event of default, I agree to pay all costs of collection, and reasonable attorney's fees. I hereby authorize this healthcare provider to release all information necessary to secure the payment of benefits.

I further agree that a photocopy of this agreement shall be as valid as the original.

Date: ___________ Your Signature: ___________

Method of Payment: ❑ Cash ❑ Check ❑ Credit Card

FORM # 58-8424 • BIBBERO SYSTEMS, INC. • PETALUMA, CA. • TO ORDER CALL TOLL FREE : 800-BIBBERO (800-242-2376) • FAX (800) 242-9330 © 7/94

PATIENT REGISTRATION

Courtesy of Bibbero Systems, Inc., Petaluma, CA. Phone: 800-242-2376; Fax: 800-242-9330; Web site: http://www.bibbero.com

Form 2

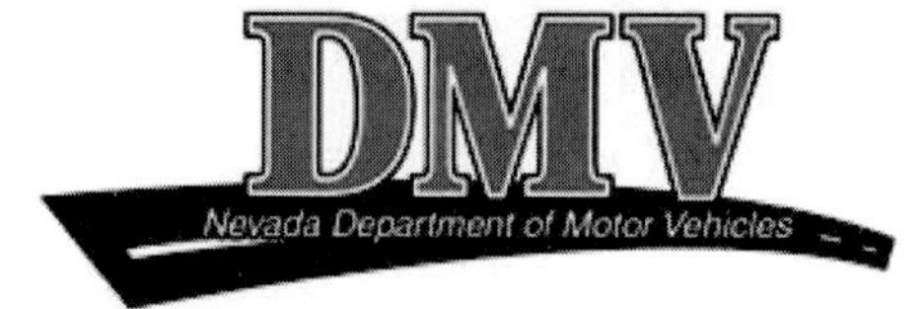

555 Wright Way
Carson City, NV 89711
Reno/Sparks/Carson City (775) 684-4DMV (4368)
Las Vegas area (702) 486-4DMV (4368)
Rural Nevada or Out of State (877) 368-7828
www.dmvnv.com

APPLICATION FOR DISABLED PERSONS LICENSE PLATES AND/OR PLACARDS

NRS 482.384

☐ Disabled Plates *(permanent disability only)* Disabled Placard(s) ☐ One ☐ Two

You may select either plates and one (1) placard, or two (2) placards.

Disabled Motorcycle Sticker ☐ One ☐ Other ____________

First time applications for a Disabled Persons license plate or motorcycle sticker must be made in person.

In order to apply for disabled persons license plates or disabled motorcycle stickers(s) your name must appear on the vehicle registration certificate. If your vehicle is currently registered, you have the option of maintaining your current vehicle registration expiration date, or renewing for a full twelve (12) month period. Credit for any unused portion of your current registration is transferable to your disabled license plate registration. In applicable counties, if you are renewing for a full 12-month period, and your previous evidence of compliance with emissions standards was obtained more than 90 days ago, the vehicle must be re-inspected prior to registration. **You must have a permanent disability to qualify for Disabled Persons license plates *(see description below)*.**

Please Print or Type

Applicant's Name ______________________________ ____/____/____
(Disabled Person) First Middle Last Date of Birth

Address ______________________________
Address City State Zip Code

County of Residence ____________ Nevada DL or ID No. ____________ Daytime Telephone No. (____)____________

Signature of Applicant ______________________________ Date ____________

A LICENSED PHYSICIAN MUST COMPLETE THIS PORTION*

As a Physician for the above-named patient, I hereby certify that the applicant:

1. ________ Cannot walk two hundred feet without stopping to rest.
2. ________ Cannot walk without the use of a brace, cane, crutch, wheelchair, or other device or another person.
3. ________ Has a cardiac condition to the extent that functional limitations are classified as a Class III or Class IV according to standards adopted by the American Heart Association.
4. ________ Is restricted by a lung disease.
5. ________ Is severely limited in his/her ability to walk because of an arthritic, neurological, or orthopedic condition.
6. ________ Is visually handicapped.
7. ________ Uses portable oxygen.

I further certify that my patient's condition is a:

☐ **Temporary Disability** (6 months or less) Must indicate length of time not to exceed 6 months *beginning* ____________ *ending* ____________

☐ **Moderate Disability** (reversible but disabled longer than 6 months)
Must indicate length of time not to exceed 2 years *beginning* ____________ *ending* ____________

☐ **Permanent Disability** (irreversible, permanently disabled in his/her ability to walk, certification is valid indefinitely)

Please Print or Type

Physician's Name ______________________________

Mailing Address ______________________________
Address City State Zip Code

Physician's License Number ____________ Telephone No. (________)____________

Physician's Signature ______________________________ Date ____________

*** Physicians Assistant Certified (PA-C) or Advanced Practice Nurse (APN) are not authorized to complete this document.**

SP27 (Rev 4/2007)

Nevada Department of Motor Vehicles

Form 3

72623

PRIORITY ☐	
PATIENT	AGE
CALLER	
TELEPHONE	
REFERRED TO	
CHART #	
CHART ATTACHED ☐ YES ☐ NO	
DATE / /	TIME / REC'D BY

Copyright © 1978 Bibbero Systems, Inc.
Printed in the U.S.A.

TELEPHONE RECORD

MESSAGE			
		TEMP	ALLERGIES
RESPONSE			
PHY/RN INITIALS	DATE / /	TIME	HANDLED BY

PRIORITY ☐	
PATIENT	AGE
CALLER	
TELEPHONE	
REFERRED TO	
CHART #	
CHART ATTACHED ☐ YES ☐ NO	
DATE / /	TIME / REC'D BY

Copyright © 1978 Bibbero Systems, Inc.
Printed in the U.S.A.

TELEPHONE RECORD

MESSAGE			
		TEMP	ALLERGIES
RESPONSE			
PHY/RN INITIALS	DATE / /	TIME	HANDLED BY

PRIORITY ☐	
PATIENT	AGE
CALLER	
TELEPHONE	
REFERRED TO	
CHART #	
CHART ATTACHED ☐ YES ☐ NO	
DATE / /	TIME / REC'D BY

Copyright © 1978 Bibbero Systems, Inc.
Printed in the U.S.A.

TELEPHONE RECORD

MESSAGE			
		TEMP	ALLERGIES
RESPONSE			
PHY/RN INITIALS	DATE / /	TIME	HANDLED BY

PRIORITY ☐	
PATIENT	AGE
CALLER	
TELEPHONE	
REFERRED TO	
CHART #	
CHART ATTACHED ☐ YES ☐ NO	
DATE / /	TIME / REC'D BY

Copyright © 1978 Bibbero Systems, Inc.
Printed in the U.S.A.

TELEPHONE RECORD

MESSAGE			
		TEMP	ALLERGIES
RESPONSE			
PHY/RN INITIALS	DATE / /	TIME	HANDLED BY

Courtesy of Bibbero Systems, Inc., Petaluma, CA. Phone: 800-242-2376; Fax: 800-242-9330; Web site: http://www.bibbero.com

Form 4

72623

PRIORITY ☐	
PATIENT	AGE
CALLER	
TELEPHONE	
REFERRED TO	
CHART #	
CHART ATTACHED ☐ YES ☐ NO	
DATE / /	TIME	REC'D BY
Copyright © 1978 Bibbero Systems, Inc. Printed in the U.S.A.	

TELEPHONE RECORD			
MESSAGE			
		TEMP	ALLERGIES
RESPONSE			
PHY/RN INITIALS	DATE / /	TIME	HANDLED BY

PRIORITY ☐	
PATIENT	AGE
CALLER	
TELEPHONE	
REFERRED TO	
CHART #	
CHART ATTACHED ☐ YES ☐ NO	
DATE / /	TIME	REC'D BY
Copyright © 1978 Bibbero Systems, Inc. Printed in the U.S.A.	

TELEPHONE RECORD			
MESSAGE			
		TEMP	ALLERGIES
RESPONSE			
PHY/RN INITIALS	DATE / /	TIME	HANDLED BY

PRIORITY ☐	
PATIENT	AGE
CALLER	
TELEPHONE	
REFERRED TO	
CHART #	
CHART ATTACHED ☐ YES ☐ NO	
DATE / /	TIME	REC'D BY
Copyright © 1978 Bibbero Systems, Inc. Printed in the U.S.A.	

TELEPHONE RECORD			
MESSAGE			
		TEMP	ALLERGIES
RESPONSE			
PHY/RN INITIALS	DATE / /	TIME	HANDLED BY

PRIORITY ☐	
PATIENT	AGE
CALLER	
TELEPHONE	
REFERRED TO	
CHART #	
CHART ATTACHED ☐ YES ☐ NO	
DATE / /	TIME	REC'D BY
Copyright © 1978 Bibbero Systems, Inc. Printed in the U.S.A.	

TELEPHONE RECORD			
MESSAGE			
		TEMP	ALLERGIES
RESPONSE			
PHY/RN INITIALS	DATE / /	TIME	HANDLED BY

Courtesy of Bibbero Systems, Inc., Petaluma, CA. Phone: 800-242-2376; Fax: 800-242-9330; Web site: http://www.bibbero.com

Form 5

72623

PRIORITY ☐		
PATIENT	AGE	
CALLER		
TELEPHONE		
REFERRED TO		
CHART #		
CHART ATTACHED ☐ YES ☐ NO		
DATE / /	TIME	REC'D BY
Copyright © 1978 Bibbero Systems, Inc. Printed in the U.S.A.		

TELEPHONE RECORD			
MESSAGE			
	TEMP	ALLERGIES	
RESPONSE			
PHY/RN INITIALS	DATE / /	TIME	HANDLED BY

PRIORITY ☐		
PATIENT	AGE	
CALLER		
TELEPHONE		
REFERRED TO		
CHART #		
CHART ATTACHED ☐ YES ☐ NO		
DATE / /	TIME	REC'D BY
Copyright © 1978 Bibbero Systems, Inc. Printed in the U.S.A.		

TELEPHONE RECORD			
MESSAGE			
	TEMP	ALLERGIES	
RESPONSE			
PHY/RN INITIALS	DATE / /	TIME	HANDLED BY

PRIORITY ☐		
PATIENT	AGE	
CALLER		
TELEPHONE		
REFERRED TO		
CHART #		
CHART ATTACHED ☐ YES ☐ NO		
DATE / /	TIME	REC'D BY
Copyright © 1978 Bibbero Systems, Inc. Printed in the U.S.A.		

TELEPHONE RECORD			
MESSAGE			
	TEMP	ALLERGIES	
RESPONSE			
PHY/RN INITIALS	DATE / /	TIME	HANDLED BY

PRIORITY ☐		
PATIENT	AGE	
CALLER		
TELEPHONE		
REFERRED TO		
CHART #		
CHART ATTACHED ☐ YES ☐ NO		
DATE / /	TIME	REC'D BY
Copyright © 1978 Bibbero Systems, Inc. Printed in the U.S.A.		

TELEPHONE RECORD			
MESSAGE			
	TEMP	ALLERGIES	
RESPONSE			
PHY/RN INITIALS	DATE / /	TIME	HANDLED BY

Courtesy of Bibbero Systems, Inc., Petaluma, CA. Phone: 800-242-2376; Fax: 800-242-9330; Web site: http://www.bibbero.com

Form 6

72623

PRIORITY ☐	TELEPHONE RECORD
PATIENT AGE	MESSAGE
CALLER	
TELEPHONE	
REFERRED TO	TEMP / ALLERGIES
CHART #	RESPONSE
CHART ATTACHED ☐ YES ☐ NO	
DATE / / · TIME · REC'D BY	
Copyright © 1978 Bibbero Systems, Inc. Printed in the U.S.A.	PHY/RN INITIALS · DATE / / · TIME · HANDLED BY

PRIORITY ☐	TELEPHONE RECORD
PATIENT AGE	MESSAGE
CALLER	
TELEPHONE	
REFERRED TO	TEMP / ALLERGIES
CHART #	RESPONSE
CHART ATTACHED ☐ YES ☐ NO	
DATE / / · TIME · REC'D BY	
Copyright © 1978 Bibbero Systems, Inc. Printed in the U.S.A.	PHY/RN INITIALS · DATE / / · TIME · HANDLED BY

PRIORITY ☐	TELEPHONE RECORD
PATIENT AGE	MESSAGE
CALLER	
TELEPHONE	
REFERRED TO	TEMP / ALLERGIES
CHART #	RESPONSE
CHART ATTACHED ☐ YES ☐ NO	
DATE / / · TIME · REC'D BY	
Copyright © 1978 Bibbero Systems, Inc. Printed in the U.S.A.	PHY/RN INITIALS · DATE / / · TIME · HANDLED BY

PRIORITY ☐	TELEPHONE RECORD
PATIENT AGE	MESSAGE
CALLER	
TELEPHONE	
REFERRED TO	TEMP / ALLERGIES
CHART #	RESPONSE
CHART ATTACHED ☐ YES ☐ NO	
DATE / / · TIME · REC'D BY	
Copyright © 1978 Bibbero Systems, Inc. Printed in the U.S.A.	PHY/RN INITIALS · DATE / / · TIME · HANDLED BY

Courtesy of Bibbero Systems, Inc., Petaluma, CA. Phone: 800-242-2376; Fax: 800-242-9330; Web site: http://www.bibbero.com

Form 7

MESSAGE FROM

For Dr.	Name of Caller	Rel. to Pt.	Patient	Pt. Age	Pt. Temp.	Message Date / /	Message Time AM PM	Urgent ☐ Yes ☐ No

Message:	Allergies

Respond to Phone #	Best Time to Call AM PM	Pharmacy Name / #	Patient's Chart Attached ☐ Yes ☐ No	Patient's Chart #	Initials

DOCTOR - STAFF RESPONSE

Doctor's / Staff Orders / Follow-Up Action

	Call Back ☐ Yes ☐ No	Chart Mess. ☐ Yes ☐ No	Follow-Up Date / /	Follow-Up Completed-Date/Time / / AM PM	Response by

Product #78-9156 Pkg., #78-9157 Pads, Bibbero Systems, Inc., Petaluma, CA. To order, call toll free 800-Bibbero (800-242-2376) or Fax 800-242-9330.

Courtesy of Bibbero Systems, Inc., Petaluma, CA. Phone: 800-242-2376; Fax: 800-242-9330; Web site: http://www.bibbero.com

Form 8

MESSAGE FROM

For Dr.	Name of Caller	Rel. to Pt.	Patient	Pt. Age	Pt. Temp.	Message Date	Message Time	Urgent
						/ /	AM PM	❑ Yes ❑ No

Message:	Allergies

Respond to Phone #	Best Time to Call	Pharmacy Name / #	Patient's Chart Attached	Patient's Chart #	Initials
	AM PM		❑ Yes ❑ No		

DOCTOR - STAFF RESPONSE

Doctor's / Staff Orders / Follow-Up Action

	Call Back	Chart Mess.	Follow-Up Date	Follow-Up Completed-Date/Time	Response by
	❑ Yes ❑ No	❑ Yes ❑ No	/ /	/ / AM PM	

Product #78-9156 Pkg., #78-9157 Pads, Bibbero Systems, Inc., Petaluma, CA. To order, call toll free 800-Bibbero (800-242-2376) or Fax 800-242-9330.

Courtesy of Bibbero Systems, Inc., Petaluma, CA. Phone: 800-242-2376; Fax: 800-242-9330; Web site: http://www.bibbero.com

Form 9

APPOINTMENT RECORD

		DOCTOR			
		DATE			
		DAY			
		AM	00		
		8	15		
			30		
			45		
		9	00		
			15		
			30		
			45		
		10	00		
			15		
			30		
			45		
		11	00		
			15		
			30		
			45		
		12	00		
			15		
			30		
			45		
		PM	00		
		1	15		
			30		
			45		
		2	00		
			15		
			30		
			45		
		3	00		
			15		
			30		
			45		
		4	00		
			15		
			30		
			45		
		5	00		
			15		
			30		
			45		

Form 10

APPOINTMENT RECORD

		DOCTOR			
		DATE			
		DAY			
		AM	00		
		8	15		
			30		
			45		
		9	00		
			15		
			30		
			45		
		10	00		
			15		
			30		
			45		
		11	00		
			15		
			30		
			45		
		12	00		
			15		
			30		
			45		
		PM	00		
		1	15		
			30		
			45		
		2	00		
			15		
			30		
			45		
		3	00		
			15		
			30		
			45		
		4	00		
			15		
			30		
			45		
		5	00		
			15		
			30		
			45		

Form 11

APPOINTMENT RECORD

		DOCTOR			
		DATE			
		DAY			
		AM	00		
		8	15		
			30		
			45		
		9	00		
			15		
			30		
			45		
		10	00		
			15		
			30		
			45		
		11	00		
			15		
			30		
			45		
		12	00		
			15		
			30		
			45		
		PM	00		
		1	15		
			30		
			45		
		2	00		
			15		
			30		
			45		
		3	00		
			15		
			30		
			45		
		4	00		
			15		
			30		
			45		
		5	00		
			15		
			30		
			45		

Form 12

M______________________________

has an appointment with:
☐ Fran Practon MD ☐ Gerald Practon MD
PRACTON MEDICAL GROUP, INC.
4567 Broad Avenue
Woodland Hills, XY 12345
Tel. 555/486-9002

for

Mon. _______________ at________

Tues. _______________ at________

Wed. _______________ at________

Thurs. _______________ at________

Fri. _______________ at________

Sat. _______________ at________

If unable to keep this appointment kindly give 24 hours notice.

M______________________________

has an appointment with:
☐ Fran Practon MD ☐ Gerald Practon MD
PRACTON MEDICAL GROUP, INC.
4567 Broad Avenue
Woodland Hills, XY 12345
Tel. 555/486-9002

for

Mon. _______________ at________

Tues. _______________ at________

Wed. _______________ at________

Thurs. _______________ at________

Fri. _______________ at________

Sat. _______________ at________

If unable to keep this appointment kindly give 24 hours notice.

M______________________________

has an appointment with:
☐ Fran Practon MD ☐ Gerald Practon MD
PRACTON MEDICAL GROUP, INC.
4567 Broad Avenue
Woodland Hills, XY 12345
Tel. 555/486-9002

for

Mon. _______________ at________

Tues. _______________ at________

Wed. _______________ at________

Thurs. _______________ at________

Fri. _______________ at________

Sat. _______________ at________

If unable to keep this appointment kindly give 24 hours notice.

M______________________________

has an appointment with:
☐ Fran Practon MD ☐ Gerald Practon MD
PRACTON MEDICAL GROUP, INC.
4567 Broad Avenue
Woodland Hills, XY 12345
Tel. 555/486-9002

for

Mon. _______________ at________

Tues. _______________ at________

Wed. _______________ at________

Thurs. _______________ at________

Fri. _______________ at________

Sat. _______________ at________

If unable to keep this appointment kindly give 24 hours notice.

Form 13

HOSPITAL/SURGERY SCHEDULING FORM

Section 1 **Completed by physician**

1. _____ Patient's name____
2. _____ Procedure____
3. _____ Emergency: Urgent_____ Elective_____
4. _____ Diagnoses 1. ____
   2. ____
5. _____ Hospital/Facility name____
6. _____ Inpatient_____ Outpatient___________ Day Surgery________
7. _____ Surgical assistant required? Yes_____ No_____
   Who preferred?____
8. _____ Anesthesia required? Yes_____ No_____ General_____ Local_______
   Who preferred?____
9. _____ Referring physician____

Section 2 **Completed by patient**

10. _____ Age of patient_____ Date of birth __________ Smoker_____Nonsmoker_____
11. _____ Room accommodations: Private_____ Semi-private_____ Ward_____
12. _____ Telephone numbers: Home (_____)____________ Work (_____)__________
13. _____ Insurance company______________________ Policy number_________
    Secondary insurance______________________ Policy number_________
14. _____ Second surgical opinion needed for insurance? Yes_____ No_____
15. _____ Name of nearest relative____
    Address______________________________Phone number________
16. _____ Admitted to this facility previous? Yes_____ No_____
    Date_________________ Type of procedure______________________
17. _____ Patient has had preadmission testing of CBC_____, EKG_____,
    Chest x-ray_______within ______ weeks.
18. _____ Admission and procedures reported to patient on Date:_______________
19. _____ Preadmission and operation instructions given to me? Yes_____ No_____
20. _____ Insurance and financial arrangements discussed with me? Yes_____ No_____

Section 3 **Completed by medical assistant**

21. _____ Operation room reserved for surgery on this date____________and time________
22. _____ Name of hospital employee who scheduled surgery______________________
23. _____ Name of surgical assistant scheduled and called______________________
24. _____ Name of anesthesiologist scheduled and called______________________
25. _____ Reported to referring physician's office and talked to______________________
26. _____ Hospital/Facility admission confirmed/preadmission test scheduled
27. _____ Prior authorizations/second opinions obtained
    Authorization/precertification #____________________Date provided__________
    Who provided number?____
28. _____ Admitting date and surgical procedure entered in appointment book
29. _____ Arrangements confirmed with patient
30. _____ History and physical report ready
    Name of office employee who scheduled surgery______________Date__________

Form 14

PRACTON MEDICAL GROUP, INC.
4567 BROAD AVENUE • WOODLAND HILLS, XY 12345-4700
OFFICE: (555) 486-9002 • FAX: (555) 488-7815

____

____
____
____
____

The following arrangements have been made for your hospitalization under the care of ______________________. You are to enter ____________ on ____________, ______________________ at ________________________________.

Your procedure, ____________________, is scheduled for __________, __________ at ______ (subject to change in time). A _____ room has been reserved for you as requested. You should take robe, slippers, and personal grooming articles with you. Please leave valuables at home. If it should become necessary for you to cancel these arrangements, please notify me immediately.

Sincerely,

____________________, Medical Assistant

Surgeon: ____________________

Assistant Surgeon: ____________________

Anesthetist: ____________________

SPECIAL NOTE to patients covered by Medicare. Medicare will only pay for a semiprivate room; therefore, patients requesting private rooms will be required to pay the difference in cost.

Form 15

LABORATORY REQUISITION

I.D.#	PATIENT LAST NAME	FIRST	M.I.	REFERRING PHYSICIAN

REFERRED BY

SS #: ___ ___ ___ - ___ ___ - ___ ___ ___ ___

BILL: ☐ PHYSICIAN ☐ MEDI-CAL ☐ HMO ☐ CHDP ☐ MEDICARE ☐ INSURANCE ☐ PATIENT
PLEASE COMPLETE BILLING INFORMATION AT BOTTOM

D.O.B.	AGE	SEX

ADDRESS	PHONE NUMBER ( )	DATE COLLECTED	TIME COLLECTED

CITY	STATE	ZIP CODE	FASTING YES | NO	STAT	CALL RESULT

MEDICARE #	MEDICAL #	INFO. BELOW WILL APPEAR ON REPORT

CUSTOM PROFILES & ADDITIONAL TESTS

173 [ ] CHEMISTRY PANEL, COMPLETE BLOOD COUNT (ZPP), LIPID PROFILE, T4
05050 [ ] CHOL, TRIG, HDL CHOL, VLDL CHOL, LDL CHOL, RISK FACTOR

PROFILES

Code		Profile	Tube	Code		Profile	Tube
00011	☐	SPECIAL COMPREHENSIVE	2 SS,L	03536	☐	HYPERTHYROID PROFILE	SS
00001	☐	COMPREHENSIVE HEALTH SURVEY	SS,L	05037	☐	HYPOTHYROID PROFILE	SS
00002	☐	GENERAL SURVEY	SS,L	05051	☐	LIPID PROFILE	SS
00003	☐	CHEMISTRY PANEL	SS	05021	☐	LIVER PROFILE	SS
CH7	☐	CHEM 7 PANEL	SS	03350	☐	LUPUS PROFILE	SS
03280	☐	ANEMIA PROFILE	SS,L	03959	☐	MENOPAUSAL PROFILE SS / 03960 ☐ POST MENOPAUSAL	SS
05016	☐	ARTHRITIS PROFILE	SS,L	02280	☐	OVARIAN FUNCTION PROFILE SS / 02281 ☐ TESTICULAR FUNC. PROF.	SS
05726	☐	COMPREHENSIVE THYROID SURVEY	SS	02808	☐	PRENATAL PROFILE	L,R
02691	☐	EPSTEIN BARR PROFILE	SS	05006	☐	THYROID PROFILE	SS
05010	☐	ELECTROLYTES	SS	03191	☐	TORCH PANEL	SS
06826	☐	HEPATITIS PROFILE	SS	5756	☐	URINE DRUG SCREEN U / ☐ VENIPUNCTURE	

TESTS

Code		Test	Tube	Code		Test	Tube	Code		Test	Tube	Code		Test	Tube
0361	☐	ABO & Rh TYPE	R, L	0141	☐	C-REACTIVE PROTEIN	SS	0673	☐	HEPATITIS B SURFACE ANTIGEN	SS	0237	☐	PTT	B
0302	☐	ALKALINE PHOSPHATASE	SS	1341	☐	DHEA-S	SS	0245	☐	HEPATITIS C ANTIBODY	SS	0317	☐	RA FACTOR	SS
0109	☐	AMYLASE	SS	0119	☐	DIGOXIN	SS	0257	☐	IRON	SS	0321	☐	RUBELLA	SS
0613	☐	ANA	SS	0224	☐	DILANTIN	SS	LDL-A	☐	LDL CHOLESTEROL	SS	0381	☐	RPR	SS
0366	☐	ANTIBODY SCREEN	R	0835	☐	ESTRADIOL	SS	0283	☐	LEAD BLOOD	RB	0335	☐	SEMEN ANALYSIS	SEMEN
0110	☐	ASO (STREPTOZYME)	SS	0833	☐	FERRITIN	SS	0281	☐	LIPASE	SS	0328	☐	SEDIMENTATION RATE (ESR)	L
0126	☐	BILIRUBIN TOTAL	SS	0003	☐	FOLIC ACID & VITAMIN B12	SS	8225	☐	LH	SS	0349	☐	SGOT (AST)	SS
0132	☐	BUN	SS	0651	☐	FSH	SS	0247	☐	MONONUCLEOSIS	SS	0348	☐	SGPT (ALT)	SS
8728	☐	CA125	SS	0140	☐	FTA-ABS	SS	0778	☐	PHENOBARBITAL	SS	0330	☐	SICKLE CELL SCREEN	L
0142	☐	CALCIUM	SS	0210	☐	GGTP	SS	0307	☐	POTASSIUM	SS	0354	☐	T4 (THYROXINE)	SS
0130	☐	CBC	L	0536	☐	GLUCOSE, FASTING	GY	0557	☐	PREGNANCY (SERUM)	SS	1358	☐	T4 FREE	SS
0388	☐	CEA-ROCHE	SS		☐	GLUCOSE, ______ HR PP	GY	0308	☐	PREGNANCY (URINE)	U	8456	☐	TESTOSTERONE	SS
0152	☐	CHOLESTEROL	SS	0771	☐	GLYCOHEMOGLOBIN	L	0859	☐	PROGESTERONE	SS	0824	☐	THEOPHYLLINE	SS
0786	☐	CORTISOL	SS	0534	☐	H. PYLORI	SS	8041	☐	PROLACTIN	SS	0360	☐	TRIGLYCERIDE	SS
0162	☐	CPK	SS	0823	☐	HCG QUANTITATIVE	SS	0103	☐	PROTEIN, TOTAL	SS	0672	☐	TSH	SS
0445	☐	CKMB ISOENZYME	SS	1856	☐	HIV (ANTIBODY)	SS	2000	☐	PROSTATE SPECIFIC ANTIGEN (PSA)	SS	0373	☐	URIC ACID	SS
0161	☐	CREATININE	SS	0558	☐	HDL CHOLESTEROL	SS	0310	☐	PT (PROTHROMBIN TIME)	B	0219	☐	URINALYSIS	U

CYTOPATHOLOGY

☐ PREGNANT ☐ ABORTION ☐ POST-PARTUM ☐ POST-MENOPAUSE
HISTORY ______

PREV. ABNORMAL CYTOL FINDINGS ______
DATE ______

☐ CONTRACEPTIVES ☐ HORMONES ☐ IUD
☐ HYSTERECTOMY ☐ TOTAL ☐ SUPRA CX
☐ OOPHORECTOMY DATE ______
☐ RADIATION Rx ☐ HORMONES Rx ☐ CHEMO Rx
☐ OTHER

LMP: ______ DATE COLLECTED: ______
SOURCE ☐ CERVIX ☐ ENDOCERVIX ☐ VAGINA
☐ CYTOBRUSH ☐ OTHER SITE ______

LAB USE ONLY (DO NOT WRITE BELOW THIS SPACE)

DATE RECEIVED	DATE REPORTED

STATEMENT OF SPECIMEN ADEQUACY

GENERAL CATEGORIZATION

DESCRIPTIVE DIAGNOSIS

HORMONAL EVALUATION MI

ADDITIONAL COMMENT

CYTOTECHNOLOGIST	PATHOLOGIST

MICROBIOLOGY

THCUL	☐	THROAT	URTHC	☐	URETHRAL	9391	☐	CHLAMYDIA DNA
EACUL	☐	EAR	VACUL	☐	VAGINAL	9390	☐	GONORRHEA DNA
EYCUL	☐	EYE	WOCUL	☐	WOUND	OBR	☐	OCCULT BLOOD
GOCUL	☐	GC	ROCUL	☐	CULTURE (Routine)	0293	☐	OVA & PARASITE
SPCUL	☐	SPUTUM	URCUL	☐	URINE	WTM	☐	WET MOUNT
STCUL	☐	STOOL	GSP	☐	GRAM STAIN			

SOURCE ______ OTHER ______

DIAGNOSIS OR COMMENTS

BILLING INFORMATION

PRIMARY INSURED	INSURANCE COMPANY
ADDRESS	
POLICY NO. & I.D. NO.	ICD-10 CODE

LEGEND

SS	Serum Separator	GY	Grey	B	Blue	U	Urine
R	Red	L	Lavender	RB	Royal Blue	G	Green

Form 16

DATE ORDERED ______ AGE ______ **X-RAY REQUEST** DATE PERFORMED ______

PATIENT ______ X-RAY # ______

CHART # [| | | | | | |] DOB ______ REFERRING PHYSICIAN: ______

BILL TO: ______ CALL REPORT EXT: ______

STREET ______

CITY ______ TYPE

✔ NEW ADDRESS ☐ ASAP ☐ TODAY

Examination ______

Chief Complaint ______

Clinical Findings ______

✔	SC	Description	CPT	Mod	Fee	✔	SC	Description	CPT	Mod	Fee	✔	SC	Description	CPT	Mod	Fee
		CHEST						**UPPER EXTREMITY**						**HEAD**			
	5085	P.A. & Lat Chest	71020				5158	Shoulder Complete	73030				5042	Facial Bones	70150		
	5083	P.A. Chest	71010				5155	Clavicle	73000				5043	Nose	70160		
	5088	Chest Fluoro	71023				5156	Scapula	73010				5048	Sinuses	70220		
	5098	Ribs Unilateral	71101				5160	A-C Joints	73050				5047	Sinuses, Ltd.	70210		
	5100	Ribs Bilateral	71111				5102	S-C Joints	71130				5051	Skull, Complete	70260		
	5101	Sternum	71120				5161	Humerus	73060				5050	Skull, Ltd.	70250		
	5352	Mammo, Diag	77056				5163	Elbow, Complete	73080				5039	Mastoids	70130		
	5351	Mammo, Unilat	77055				5162	Elbow, 2 views	73070				5046	Orbits	70200		
	5353	Mammo, Screen	77057				5165	Forearm	73090				5037	Mandible	70110		
							5168	Wrist Complete	73110				5056	T.M. Joints	70330		
		ABDOMEN					5167	Wrist, 2 views	73100								
	5204	A.P.	74000				5171	Hand, Complete	73130					**SPINE-PELVIS**			
	5207	Acute Series	74022				5170	Hand, 2 views	73120				5110	C-Spine, Comp	72050		
							5172	Finger(s)	73140				5108	C-Spine, Ltd.	72020		
		GASTROINTESTINAL					5341	Bone Age	77072				5113	T-Spine	72070		
	5212	Swallowing - Eso	74210										5119	L-Spine, Comp	72110		
	5213	Esophagram	74220					**LOWER EXTREMITY**					5118	L-Spine, Ltd.	72100		
	5217	UGI Series	74241				5179	Hip	73510				5140	Pelvis	72170		
	5218	UGI & Sm Bowel	74245				5180	Bilateral Hips	73520				5147	Sacro-Iliac Joints	72202		
	5224	BA Enema	74270				5183	Infant Hips	73540				5148	Sacrum/Coccyx	72220		
	5225	BA Air Contrast	74280				5184	Femur (Thigh)	73550				5112	Scoliosis Study	72069		
	5227	GB Oral	74290				5187	Knee, Complete	73564								
	5228	GB Repeat	74291				5185	Knee, 2 views	73560					**MISCELLANEOUS**			
	5222	Small Bowel	74250				5186	Patella	73562				5337	Fluoroscopy	76000		
	5231	T-Tube Cholangio	74305				5190	Leg (Tibia)	73590				5344	Bone Survey	77076		
	5348	Sinogram	76080				5193	Ankle, Complete	73610				5362	Outside Films	76140		
	5061	Soft Tissue Neck	70360				5192	Ankle, 2 views	73600				5354	Foreign Body	76010		
							5196	Foot, Complete	73630				5356	Specimen Film	76098		
		GENITOURINARY					5195	Foot, 2 views	73620				5159	Shoulder Arthro	73040		
	5242	I.VP.	74400				5197	Os Calcis	73650								
	5258	Salpingogram	74740				5198	Toe(s)	73660					**SUPPLIES**			
	5248	Cystogram	74430				5342	Bone Length Scan	77073								

5-10

Form 17

1. Walter Louis McDougall
2. Marilyn Marvel
3. Ms. Margaret McKinney
4. Roberta Nelson
   6428 Lorraine Rd., Sherman Oaks, XY
5. Rev. Jack Rowe
   462 Twelve Oaks Dr., Encino, XY
6. Renee T. Moore (Mrs. C. H.)
7. Marilyn P. Marvel (Mrs. Paul P.)
8. Roger C. Camp
9. Mrs. John M. White (Jane B.)
10. Anna F. Rolf
11. Mrs. Roger G. Camp (Jane)
12. Raymond E. Stokes Jr.
13. Nancy Jeffers
14. Mrs. Alfred Hall (Martha)
15. Ms. Carla St. John
16. Wm. L. MacPherson
17. Benjamin Thomas
18. L. William McPherson
19. A. Buckley
20. Vincent DeLuca

Form 18

21. John Lee-Barry

31. Paul P. Marvel

22. Alice Buckley

32. Carl Saintelley

23. Tufo Skroff

33. Professor Carl Procter

24. Mrs. Andrew Hall (Mary Jones)

34. Frank Albert

25. Mrs. Winifred LaSalle (Robert L.)

35. Mr. C. H. Moore

26. Alice-Ruth Buckely

36. Larry J. Riley

27. Dr. Jack Rowe
409 23 St., Encino, XY

37. Karen Ruth-Ann Klein

28. Robert Nelson III
321 April Ave., Woodland Hills, XY

38. Robert Nelson III
421 April Ave., Woodland Hills, XY

29. Professor Carl Starr

39. Mr. C. Howard Moore

30. Margo Hawkins, RN

40. Mary Faye Jeffers

Form 19

41. Edward R. Mackey

42. M. Robert DeAriolla

43. Marvin N. Riley

44. Hannah R. Sentry (Mrs. Randolph E.)

45. Rock C. Stetson

46. Senator Griffith

47. Mr. Donald Morris, III
771 So. Main St., Long Beach, XY

48. Dr. John S. Richards

49. Robert LaVelle

50. John C. Richards, MD

51. Edward S. Mackey

52. Raymond E. Stokes

53. Walter L. McDougall

54. Mary MacKay

55. Donald Morris, Mr., II
26 Avocado Place, Logan, XY

56. Chas. R. Bennett

57. C. Richard Bennett

58. Donald Morris
14 Meridian St., Logan, XY

X

X

Form 20

PATIENT RECORD

LAST NAME	FIRST NAME	MIDDLE NAME	BIRTH DATE	SEX	HOME PHONE
ADDRESS		CITY	STATE		ZIP CODE
CELL PHONE	PAGER NO.	FAX NO.	E-MAIL ADDRESS		
PATIENT'S SOC. SEC. NO.			DRIVER'S LICENSE		
PATIENT'S OCCUPATION		NAME OF COMPANY			
ADDRESS OF EMPLOYER					PHONE
SPOUSE OR PARENT		OCCUPATION			
EMPLOYER		ADDRESS			PHONE
NAME OF INSURANCE		INSURED OR SUBSCRIBER			
POLICY/CERTIFICATE NO.		GROUP NO.		REFERRED BY:	

DATE	PROGRESS

Form 21

PATIENT RECORD

LAST NAME	FIRST NAME	MIDDLE NAME	BIRTH DATE	SEX	HOME PHONE
ADDRESS		CITY	STATE		ZIP CODE
CELL PHONE	PAGER NO.	FAX NO.	E-MAIL ADDRESS		
PATIENT'S SOC. SEC. NO.			DRIVER'S LICENSE		
PATIENT'S OCCUPATION		NAME OF COMPANY			
ADDRESS OF EMPLOYER					PHONE
SPOUSE OR PARENT		OCCUPATION			
EMPLOYER		ADDRESS			PHONE
NAME OF INSURANCE		INSURED OR SUBSCRIBER			
POLICY/CERTIFICATE NO.		GROUP NO.		REFERRED BY:	

DATE	PROGRESS

Form 22

MEDICAL RECORD ABSTRACT FORM

Patient's Name: ______________________________

Date(s) of treatment: ______________________________

Patient's physician: ______________________________

Was patient hospitalized? _____ If so, where? ______________________________

____

Did patient have surgery? _____ If so, what was done? ______________________________

What is the patient's chief complaint? ______________________________

____

What is the diagnosis? ______________________________

Was any medication prescribed? _____ If, so, what is the name of the

medication and dosage? ______________________________

Does the patient have any drug or food allergies? _____ If so, list them: __

____

Was any laboratory work performed? _____ If so, list all tests and results:_

____

What is the prognosis of this case? ______________________________

Form 23

PATIENT RECORD

LAST NAME	FIRST NAME	MIDDLE NAME	BIRTH DATE	SEX	HOME PHONE
ADDRESS		CITY	STATE		ZIP CODE
CELL PHONE	PAGER NO.	FAX NO.	E-MAIL ADDRESS		
PATIENT'S SOC. SEC. NO.			DRIVER'S LICENSE		
PATIENT'S OCCUPATION		NAME OF COMPANY			
ADDRESS OF EMPLOYER					PHONE
SPOUSE OR PARENT		OCCUPATION			
EMPLOYER		ADDRESS			PHONE
NAME OF INSURANCE		INSURED OR SUBSCRIBER			
POLICY/CERTIFICATE NO.		GROUP NO.		REFERRED BY:	

DATE	PROGRESS

Form 24

Freeman, Richard		FLOW SHEET				Acct No. 08051944RF
DATE	TRIGLYCERIDES	TOTAL CHOLESTEROL	HDL	LDL	CHOL/HDLC RATIO	GLUCOSE (fasting)
6/15/10	114	204	59	116	3.5	120
7/01/11	158	232	61	160	3.8	136
6/24/12	190	170	49	92	3.5	147

Form 25

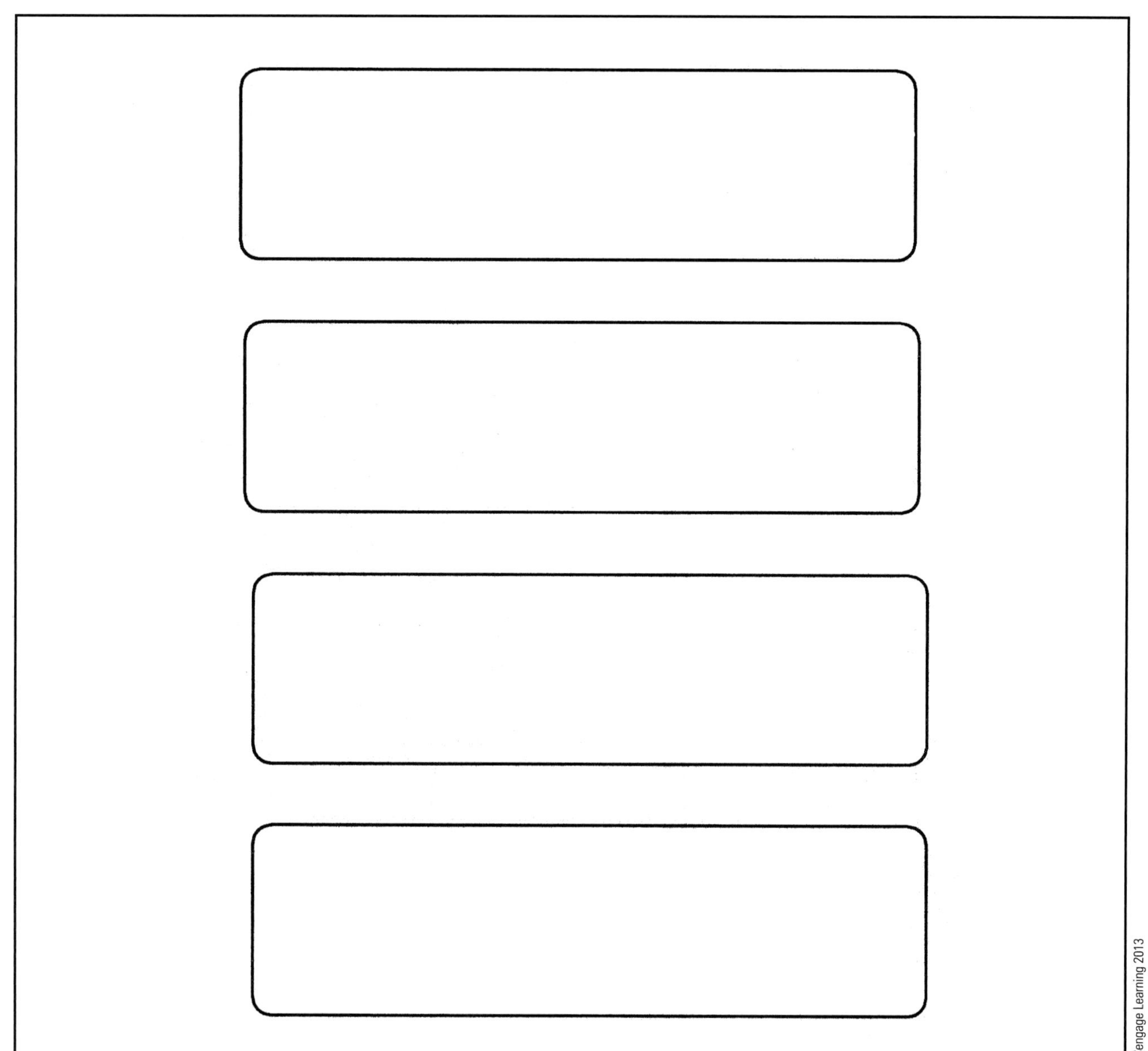

Form 26

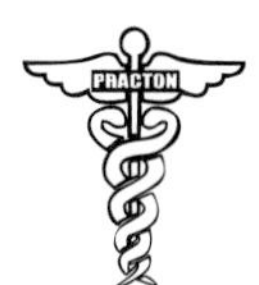

PRACTON MEDICAL GROUP, INC.
4567 BROAD AVENUE
WOODLAND HILLS, XY 12345-4700

Phone: (555) 486-9002 Fax: (555) 488-7815

NAME ______________________________ DATE __________
ADDRESS ______________________ CITY ______________ STATE ____

Rx

N.E. REP. __________ ____________________ MD
REP. ________ TIMES Gerald M. Practon, M.D. C 14021
BNDD NO. H 835190X Fran T. Practon, M.D. C 15038

Form 27

PRACTON MEDICAL GROUP, INC.
4567 Broad Avenue
Woodland Hills, XY 12345-4700
Tel. 555/486-9002

Patient's name:

____

Please bring this card with you for each appointment.

Your primary physician is:

____

With so many potent medicines available today, the possibility of undesirable effects of single drugs, or adverse interactions of multiple drugs, is always present. If there is any question of side effects of drugs, or their potential toxicity, feel free to call and discuss this with your physician.

It is vital that you, and all health care professionals involved in your care, know exactly the names and dosages of ALL medicines you are currently taking. Please keep this card with you and show it to your doctor or dentist, during office visits, and to your pharmacist when prescriptions and/or over-the-counter preparations are purchased.

MEDICATION SCHEDULE

Name of Medication	Strength	Times to be Taken						

If you have any questions or problems with medications, please call 486-9002

Form 28

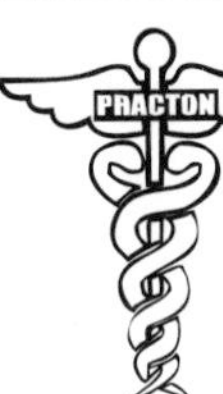

PRACTON MEDICAL GROUP, INC.

4567 BROAD AVENUE • WOODLAND HILLS, XY 12345-4700
OFFICE: (555) 486-9002 • FAX: (555) 488-7815

Fran Practon, M.D.
Gerald Practon, M.D.

Form 29

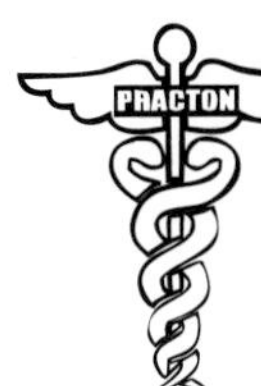

PRACTON MEDICAL GROUP, INC.

4567 BROAD AVENUE • WOODLAND HILLS, XY 12345-4700
OFFICE: (555) 486-9002 • FAX: (555) 488-7815

Fran Practon, M.D.
Gerald Practon, M.D.

Form 30

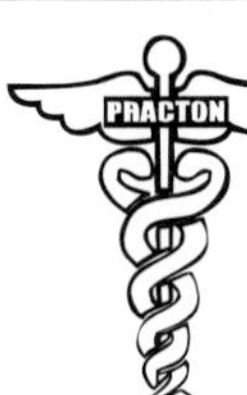

PRACTON MEDICAL GROUP, INC.

4567 BROAD AVENUE • WOODLAND HILLS, XY 12345-4700
OFFICE: (555) 486-9002 • FAX: (555) 488-7815

Fran Practon, M.D.
Gerald Practon, M.D.

Form 31

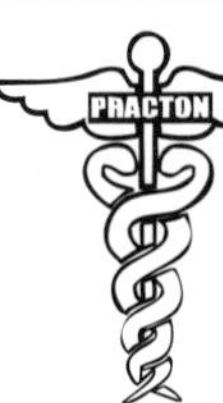

PRACTON MEDICAL GROUP, INC.

4567 BROAD AVENUE • WOODLAND HILLS, XY 12345-4700
OFFICE: (555) 486-9002 • FAX: (555) 488-7815

Fran Practon, M.D.
Gerald Practon, M.D.

Form 32

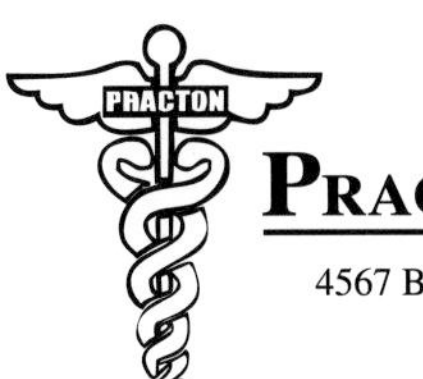

PRACTON MEDICAL GROUP, INC.

4567 BROAD AVENUE • WOODLAND HILLS, XY 12345-4700
OFFICE: (555) 486-9002 • FAX: (555) 488-7815

Fran Practon, M.D.
Gerald Practon, M.D.

Form 33

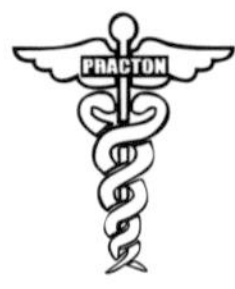

PRACTON MEDICAL GROUP, INC.

4567 BROAD AVENUE
WOODLAND HILLS, XY 12345-4700
TEL: (555) 486-9002
FAX NO. (555) 488-7815

INTEROFFICE MEMO

DATE:
TO:
FROM:
RE:

Form 34

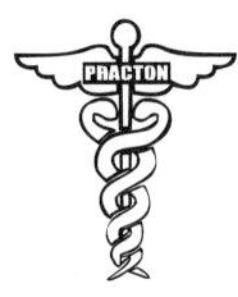

PRACTON MEDICAL GROUP, INC.

4567 BROAD AVENUE
WOODLAND HILLS, XY 12345-4700
TEL: (555) 486-9002
FAX NO. (555) 488-7815

INTEROFFICE MEMO

TO:	DATE:
FROM:	RE:

Form 35

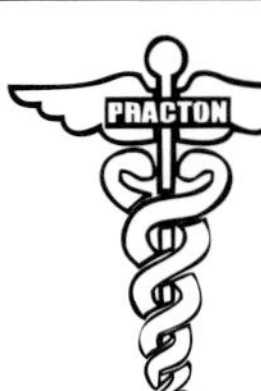

PRACTON MEDICAL GROUP, INC.

4567 BROAD AVENUE • WOODLAND HILLS, XY 12345-4700
OFFICE: (555) 486-9002 • FAX: (555) 488-7815

Fran Practon, M.D.
Gerald Practon, M.D.

Form 36

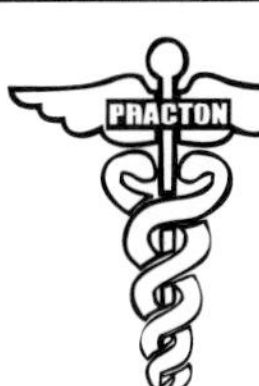

PRACTON MEDICAL GROUP, INC.

4567 BROAD AVENUE • WOODLAND HILLS, XY 12345-4700
OFFICE: (555) 486-9002 • FAX: (555) 488-7815

Fran Practon, M.D.
Gerald Practon, M.D.

Form 37

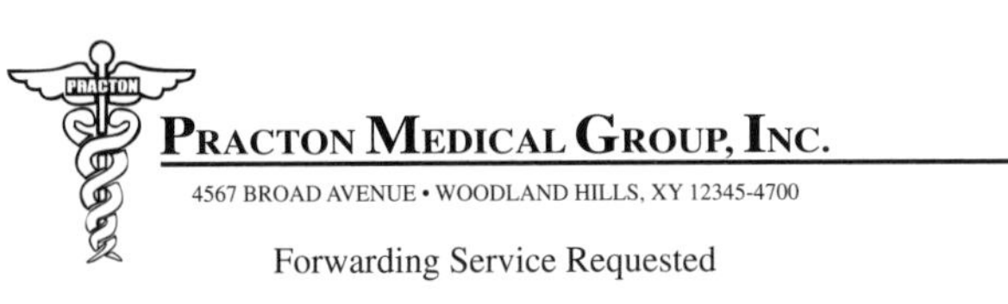

Forwarding Service Requested

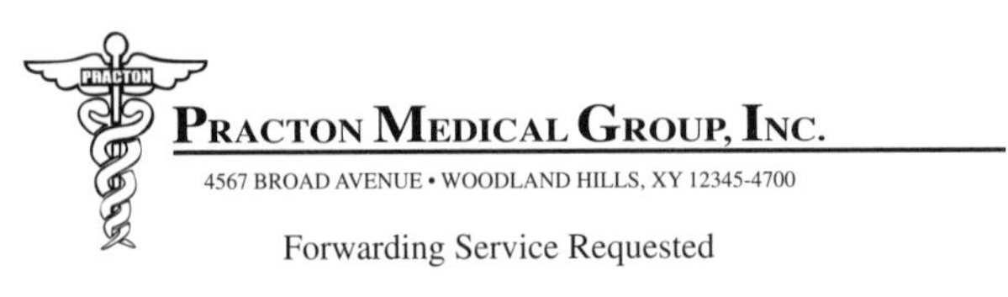

Forwarding Service Requested

Form 38

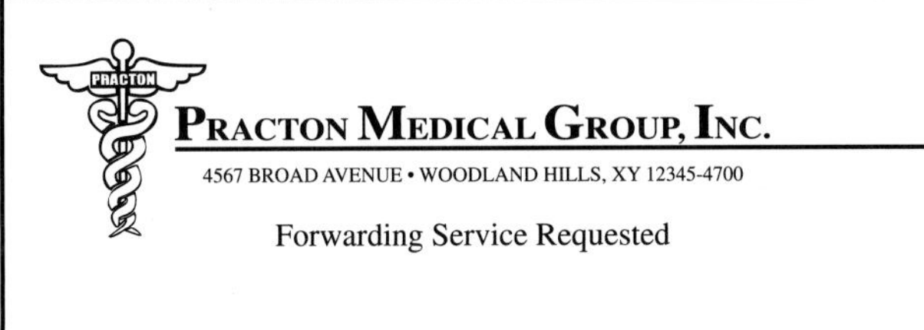

PRACTON MEDICAL GROUP, INC.
4567 BROAD AVENUE • WOODLAND HILLS, XY 12345-4700

Forwarding Service Requested

Form 39

U.S. POSTAL SERVICE®
STAMPS BY MAIL® ORDER FORM

Please fill out clearly and completely.

AREA CODE | DAYTIME PHONE NUMBER

0311
03/11

First Name Middle Initial Last Name

Company Name (if applicable)

Mailing Address/PO Box Apt./Suite

City State ZIP+4®

ITEM	DESCRIPTION	PRICE	QTY.	COST
1	**U.S. Flag** 45 cents – First-Class Roll(s) – 100 stamps per roll	$45.00		
2	**Forever Stamp** 45 cents – First-Class Booklet(s) – 20 stamps per booklet	$9.00		
3	**Navajo Jewelry*** 2 cents – 20 stamps	$.40		
4	**George Washington**** 20 cents – 20 stamps	$4.00		
5	**Tiffany Lamp*** 1 cent – 20 stamps	$.20		

*May be combined to equal the $.44 First-Class Mail price.
**Additional ounce for First-Class price for Letter and Flat-Size Mail.z

Total Cost of Order $ ____________

moving somewhere?

Don't leave your mail behind. Just visit usps.com® and click "Change your address." Then follow the five simple steps to complete the form and we'll e-mail you a confirmation of the change.

Privacy Act Statement: Your information will be used to fulfill your request. Collection is authorized by 39 U.S.C. 401, 403 & 404.

Providing the information is voluntary, but if not provided, we may not process your transaction. We do not disclose your information to third parties without your consent, except to facilitate the transaction, to act on your behalf or request, or as legally required. This includes the following limited circumstances: to a congressional office on your behalf; to financial entities regarding financial transaction issues; to a U.S. Postal Service auditor; to entities, including law enforcement, as required by law or in legal proceedings; and to contractors and other entities aiding us to fulfill the service (service providers). For more information regarding our privacy policy, visit us at usps.com/privacypolicy.

PS Form 3227-A – March 2011

United States Postal Service

Form 40

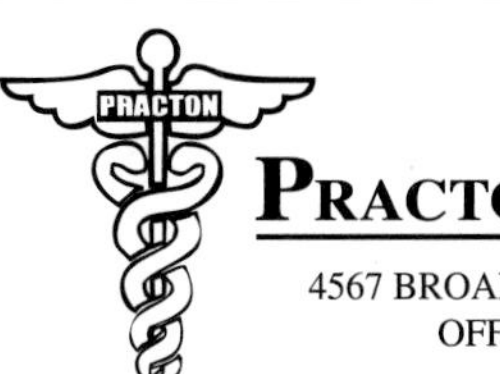

PRACTON MEDICAL GROUP, INC.

4567 BROAD AVENUE • WOODLAND HILLS, XY 12345-4700
OFFICE: (555) 486-9002 • FAX: (555) 488-7815

Fran Practon, M.D.
Gerald Practon, M.D.

Form 41

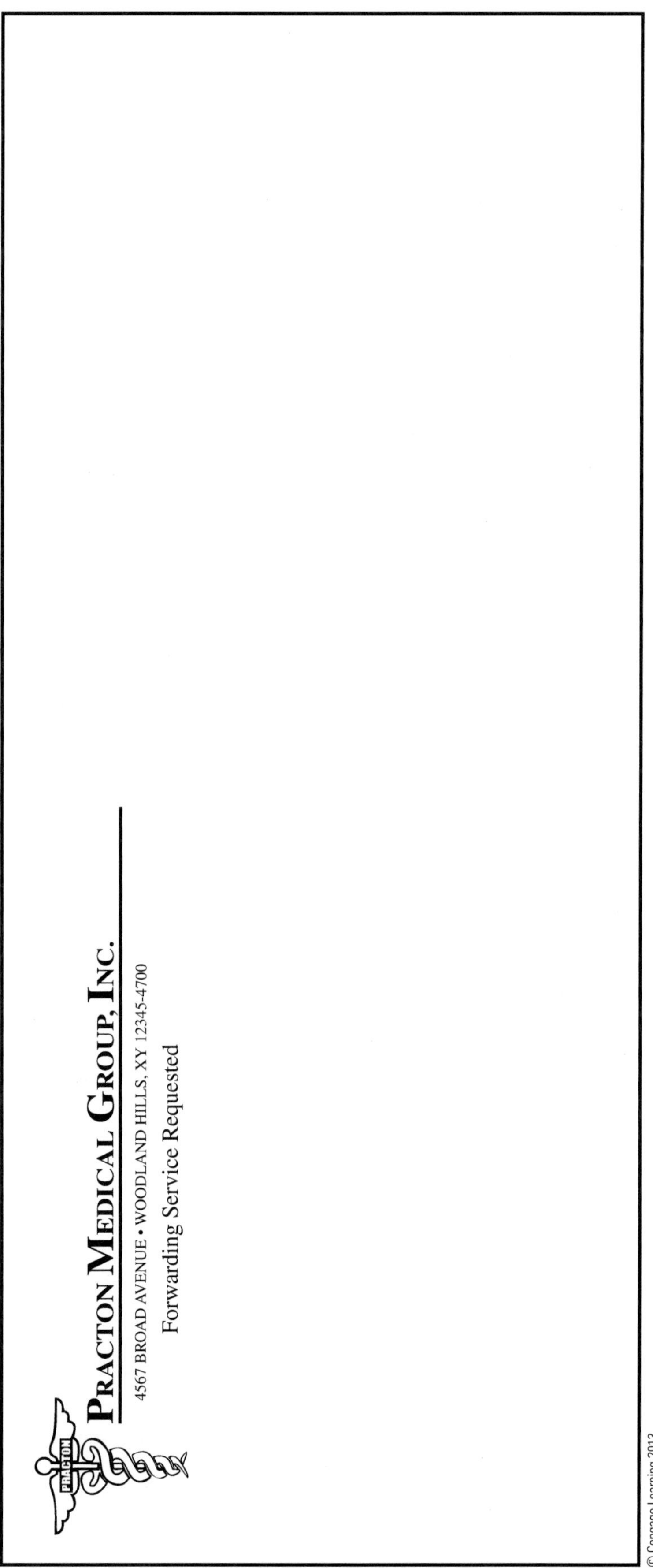
PRACTON MEDICAL GROUP, INC.
4567 BROAD AVENUE • WOODLAND HILLS, XY 12345-4700
Forwarding Service Requested

Form 42

UNITED STATES POSTAL SERVICE

First-Class Mail
Postage & Fees Paid
USPS
Permit No. G-10

• Print your name, address, and ZIP Code in this box •

SENDER: *COMPLETE THIS SECTION*

- Complete items 1,2, and 3. Also complete item 4 if Restricted Delivery is desired.
- Print your name and address on the reverse so that we can return the card to you.
- Attach this card to the back of the mailpiece, or on the front if space permits.

1. Article Addressed to:

2. Article Number
(Transfer from service label)

COMPLETE THIS SECTION ON DELIVERY

A. Signature
X ☐ Agent ☐ Addressee

B. Received by *(Printed Name)*

C. Date of Delivery

D. Is delivery address different from item 1? ☐ Yes
If YES, enter delivery address below: ☐ No

3. Service Type
☐ Certified Mail ☐ Express Mail
☐ Registered ☐ Return Receipt for Merchandise
☐ Insured Mail ☐ C.O.D

4. Restricted Delivery? *(Extra Fee)* ☐ Yes

PS Form 3811, February 2004 Domestic Return Receipt 102595-02-M-1540

7007 0710 0004 3603 0444

PLACE STICKER AT TOP OF ENVELOPE TO THE RIGHT OF THE RETURN ADDRESS, FOLD AT DOTTED LINE

CERTIFIED MAIL™

7007 0710 0004 3603 0444

7007 0710 0004 3603 0444

U.S. Postal Service™
CERTIFIED MAIL™ RECEIPT
(Domestic Mail Only; No Insurance Coverage Provided)

For delivery information visit our website at www.usps.com®

OFFICIAL USE

Postage	$
Certified Fee	
Return Receipt Fee (Endorsement Required)	
Restricted Delivery Fee (Endorsement Required)	
Total Postage & Fees	$

Postmark Here

Sent To

Street, Apt. No.; or PO Box No.

City, State, ZIP+4

PS Form 3800, August 2006 See Reverse for Instructions

United State Postal Service

Form 43

FAX TRANSMITTAL SHEET

To: ______________________________ Date: ______________

Fax Number: ______________________________ Time: ______________

Telephone No.: ______________________________

Number of Pages (including this one): ______________________________

From: ______________________________ Telephone No. ______________

Note: This transmittal is intended only for the use of the individual or entity to which it is addressed and may contain information that is privileged, confidential, and exempt from disclosure under applicable law. If you are not the intended recipient, any dissemination, distribution, or photocopying of this communication is strictly prohibited. If you have received this communication in error, please notify this office immediately by telephone and return the original fax to us at the address below by U.S. Postal Service. Thank you.

Remarks: ____

____

____

If you cannot read this fax or if pages are missing, please contact:

PRACTON

PRACTON MEDICAL GROUP, INC.

4567 BROAD AVENUE • WOODLAND HILLS, XY 12345-4700
OFFICE: (555) 486-9002 • FAX: (555) 488-7815

INSTRUCTIONS TO THE AUTHORIZED RECEIVER: PLEASE COMPLETE THIS STATEMENT OF RECEIPT AND RETURN TO SENDER VIA THE ABOVE FAX NUMBER.

I, ______________, verify that I have received ______________
(no. of pages including cover sheet)
from ______________________________.
(sending facility's name)

Form 44

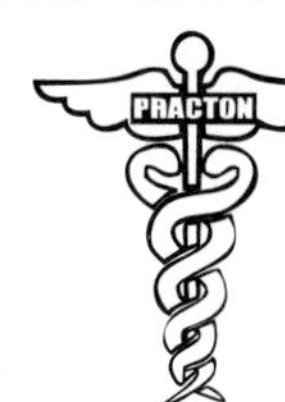

Practon Medical Group, Inc.

4567 BROAD AVENUE • WOODLAND HILLS, XY 12345-4700
OFFICE: (555) 486-9002 • FAX: (555) 488-7815

Fran Practon, M.D.
Gerald Practon, M.D.

Form 45

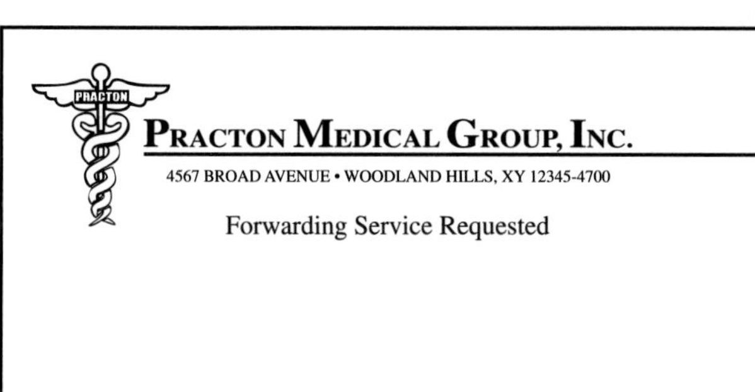
PRACTON
PRACTON MEDICAL GROUP, INC.
4567 BROAD AVENUE • WOODLAND HILLS, XY 12345-4700
Forwarding Service Requested

Form 46

UNITED STATES POSTAL SERVICE

First-Class Mail
Postage & Fees Paid
USPS
Permit No. G-10

• Print your name, address, and ZIP Code in this box •

SENDER: *COMPLETE THIS SECTION*

- Complete items 1,2, and 3. Also complete item 4 if Restricted Delivery is desired.
- Print your name and address on the reverse so that we can return the card to you.
- Attach this card to the back of the mailpiece, or on the front if space permits.

1. Article Addressed to:

COMPLETE THIS SECTION ON DELIVERY

A. Signature
X ☐ Agent ☐ Addressee

B. Received by *(Printed Name)* | C. Date of Delivery

D. Is delivery address different from item 1? ☐ Yes
If YES, enter delivery address below: ☐ No

3. Service Type
☐ Certified Mail ☐ Express Mail
☐ Registered ☐ Return Receipt for Merchandise
☐ Insured Mail ☐ C.O.D

4. Restricted Delivery? *(Extra Fee)* ☐ Yes

2. Article Number
(Transfer from service label)

PS Form 3811, February 2004 Domestic Return Receipt 102595-02-M-1540

7007 0710 0004 3603 0451

PLACE STICKER AT TOP OF ENVELOPE TO THE RIGHT OF THE RETURN ADDRESS, FOLD AT DOTTED LINE

CERTIFIED MAIL™

7007 0710 0004 3603 0451

7007 0710 0004 3603 0451

U.S. Postal Service™
CERTIFIED MAIL™ RECEIPT
(Domestic Mail Only; No Insurance Coverage Provided)

For delivery information visit our website at www.usps.com®

OFFICIAL USE

Postage	$	Postmark Here
Certified Fee		
Return Receipt Fee (Endorsement Required)		
Restricted Delivery Fee (Endorsement Required)		
Total Postage & Fees	$	

Sent To

Street, Apt. No.; or PO Box No.

City, State, ZIP+4

PS Form 3800, August 2006 See Reverse for Instructions

United States Postal Service

Form 47

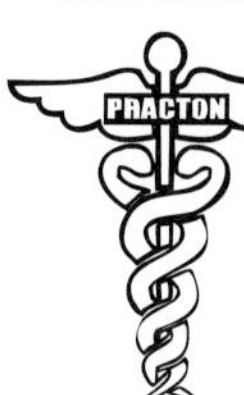

PRACTON MEDICAL GROUP, INC.

4567 BROAD AVENUE • WOODLAND HILLS, XY 12345-4700
OFFICE: (555) 486-9002 • FAX: (555) 488-7815

Fran Practon, M.D.
Gerald Practon, M.D.

Form 48

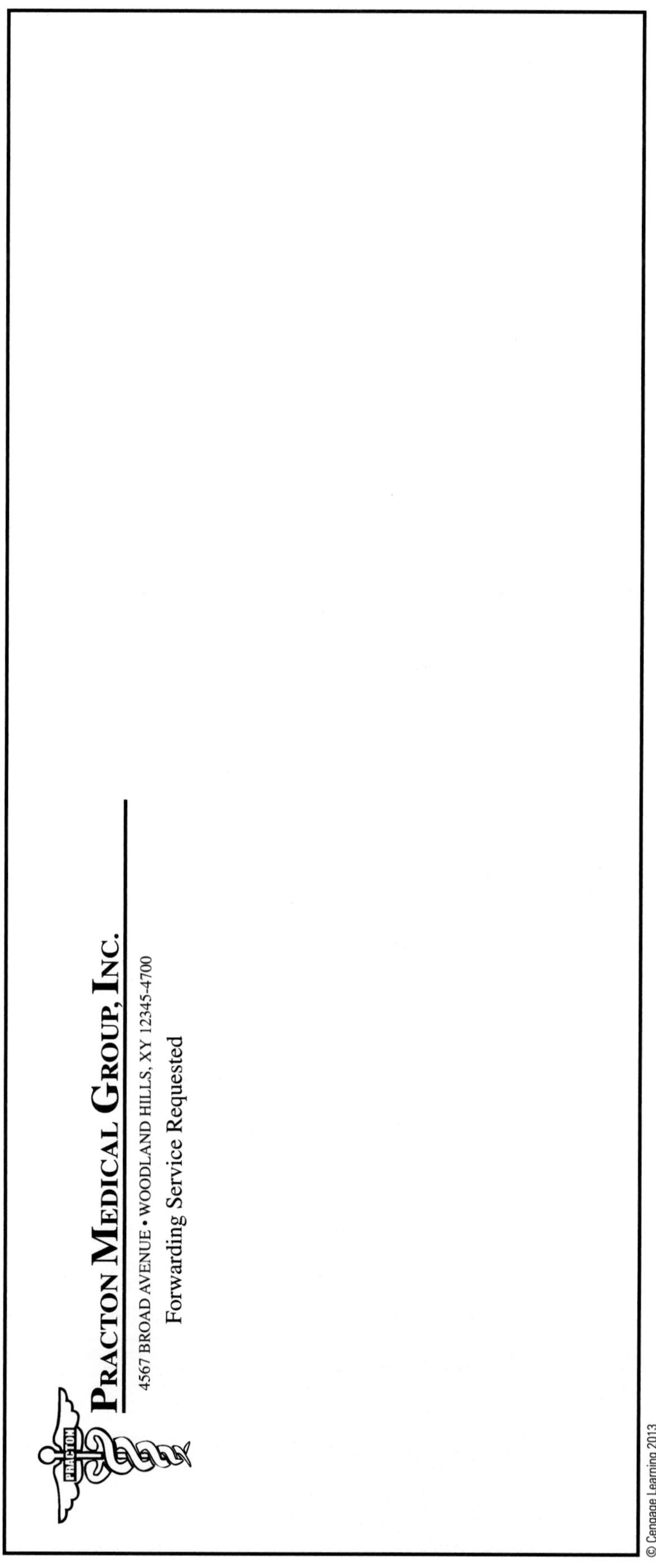
PRACTON MEDICAL GROUP, INC.
4567 BROAD AVENUE • WOODLAND HILLS, XY 12345-4700
Forwarding Service Requested

Form 49

UNITED STATES POSTAL SERVICE

First-Class Mail
Postage & Fees Paid
USPS
Permit No. G-10

• Print your name, address, and ZIP Code in this box •

SENDER: *COMPLETE THIS SECTION*

- Complete items 1,2, and 3. Also complete item 4 if Restricted Delivery is desired.
- Print your name and address on the reverse so that we can return the card to you.
- Attach this card to the back of the mailpiece, or on the front if space permits.

1. Article Addressed to:

COMPLETE THIS SECTION ON DELIVERY

A. Signature
X ☐ Agent ☐ Addressee

B. Received by *(Printed Name)* | C. Date of Delivery

D. Is delivery address different from item 1? ☐ Yes
If YES, enter delivery address below: ☐ No

3. Service Type
☐ Certified Mail ☐ Express Mail
☐ Registered ☐ Return Receipt for Merchandise
☐ Insured Mail ☐ C.O.D

4. Restricted Delivery? *(Extra Fee)* ☐ Yes

2. Article Number
(Transfer from service label)

PS Form 3811, February 2004 Domestic Return Receipt 102595-02-M-1540

7007 0710 0004 3603 0468

PLACE STICKER AT TOP OF ENVELOPE TO THE RIGHT OF THE RETURN ADDRESS, FOLD AT DOTTED LINE

CERTIFIED MAIL™

7007 0710 0004 3603 0468

7007 0710 0004 3603 0468

U.S. Postal Service™
CERTIFIED MAIL™ RECEIPT
(Domestic Mail Only; No Insurance Coverage Provided)

For delivery information visit our website at www.usps.com®

OFFICIAL USE

Postage	$	Postmark Here
Certified Fee		
Return Receipt Fee (Endorsement Required)		
Restricted Delivery Fee (Endorsement Required)		
Total Postage & Fees	$	

Sent To

Street, Apt. No.; or PO Box No.

City, State, ZIP+4

PS Form 3800, August 2006 See Reverse for Instructions

United States Postal Service

Form 50

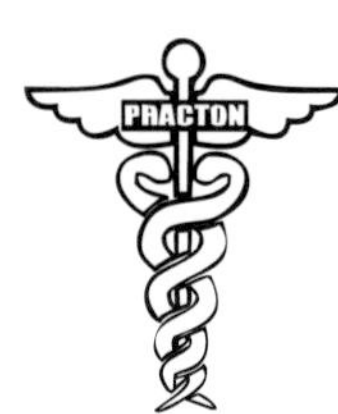

STATEMENT

PRACTON MEDICAL GROUP, INC.
4567 Broad Avenue
Woodland Hills, XY 12345-4700
Tel. 555-486-9002
Fax No. 555-488-7815

Phone No.(H)__________(W)__________ Birthdate__________
Insurance Co.____________________Policy No.__________

	DATE	REFERENCE	DESCRIPTION	CHARGES		CREDITS PYMNTS.		CREDITS ADJ.		BALANCE	
			BALANCE FORWARD →							25	00
1.	1/25/XX	99213	OV level III	40	20						
2.	1/25/XX	93000	ECG	34	26						
3.	1/25/XX	94010	Spirometry	38	57						
4.	1/25/XX	99000	Handling spec.	5	00						
5.	1/25/XX	81000	Ua Non-auto.& micr.	8	00						
6.	1/26/XX	1/25/XX	Billed Aetna Ins.								
7.	2/12/XX	99212	OV level II	28	55						
8.	2/12/XX	99000	ECG	34	26						
9.	2/12/XX	CK #1692	ROA pt			25	00				
10.	3/2/XX	CK #5093	ROA Aetna CK.			90	74				
11.	3/2/XX	1/25/XX	Aetna adj.					12	60		
12.	3/2/XX	2/12/XX	Billed Aetna								
13.	3/17/XX	CK #1701	ROA pt			22	69				
14.	4/11/XX	CK #7948	ROA Aetna			45	22				
15.	4/11/XX	2/12/XX	Aetna adj.					6	28		

RB40BC-2-96

PLEASE PAY LAST AMOUNT IN BALANCE COLUMN ↑

THIS IS A COPY OF YOUR ACCOUNT AS IT APPEARS ON OUR RECORDS

Form 51

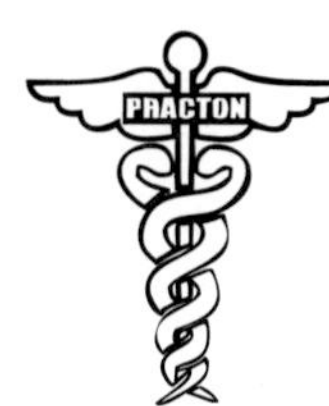

STATEMENT

PRACTON MEDICAL GROUP, INC.
4567 Broad Avenue
Woodland Hills, XY 12345-4700
Tel. 555-486-9002
Fax No. 555-488-7815

Phone No.(H)____________(W)______________ Birthdate______________
Insurance Co.______________________________Policy No.____________

DATE	REFERENCE	DESCRIPTION	CHARGES		CREDITS				BALANCE	
					PYMNTS.		ADJ.			
	BALANCE FORWARD →									

RB40BC-2-96

PLEASE PAY LAST AMOUNT IN BALANCE COLUMN →

THIS IS A COPY OF YOUR ACCOUNT AS IT APPEARS ON OUR RECORDS

Form 52

DATE	REFERENCE	DESCRIPTION	CHARGES	CREDITS PYMNTS.	CREDITS ADJ.	BALANCE	PREVIOUS BALANCE	NAME

This is your RECEIPT for this amount
This is a STATEMENT of your account to date

Please present this slip to receptionist before leaving office.

PRACTON MEDICAL GROUP, INC.
4567 Broad Avenue
Woodland Hills, XY 12345-4700
Tel.555-486-9002
Fax. No.555-488-7815

Thank You!

ROA – Received on Account

OT – Other ______________________

NEXT APPOINTMENT ______________

RB40BC-3-96

143

DATE	REFERENCE	DESCRIPTION	CHARGES	CREDITS PYMNTS.	CREDITS ADJ.	BALANCE	PREVIOUS BALANCE	NAME

This is your RECEIPT for this amount
This is a STATEMENT of your account to date

Please present this slip to receptionist before leaving office.

PRACTON MEDICAL GROUP, INC.
4567 Broad Avenue
Woodland Hills, XY 12345-4700
Tel.555-486-9002
Fax. No.555-488-7815

Thank You!

ROA – Received on Account

OT – Other ______________________

NEXT APPOINTMENT ______________

RB40BC-3-96

144

DATE	REFERENCE	DESCRIPTION	CHARGES	CREDITS PYMNTS.	CREDITS ADJ.	BALANCE	PREVIOUS BALANCE	NAME

This is your RECEIPT for this amount
This is a STATEMENT of your account to date

Please present this slip to receptionist before leaving office.

PRACTON MEDICAL GROUP, INC.
4567 Broad Avenue
Woodland Hills, XY 12345-4700
Tel.555-486-9002
Fax. No.555-488-7815

Thank You!

ROA – Received on Account

OT – Other ______________________

NEXT APPOINTMENT ______________

RB40BC-3-96

145

DATE	REFERENCE	DESCRIPTION	CHARGES	CREDITS PYMNTS.	CREDITS ADJ.	BALANCE	PREVIOUS BALANCE	NAME

This is your RECEIPT for this amount
This is a STATEMENT of your account to date

Please present this slip to receptionist before leaving office.

PRACTON MEDICAL GROUP, INC.
4567 Broad Avenue
Woodland Hills, XY 12345-4700
Tel.555-486-9002
Fax. No.555-488-7815

Thank You!

ROA – Received on Account

OT – Other ______________________

NEXT APPOINTMENT ______________

RB40BC-3-96

146

Form 53

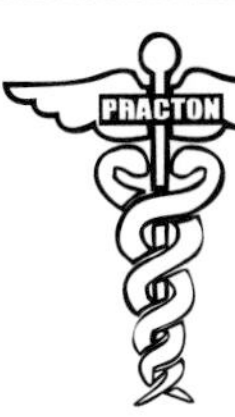

PRACTON MEDICAL GROUP, INC.

4567 BROAD AVENUE • WOODLAND HILLS, XY 12345-4700
OFFICE: (555) 486-9002 • FAX: (555) 488-7815

Fran Practon, M.D.
Gerald Practon, M.D.

Form 54

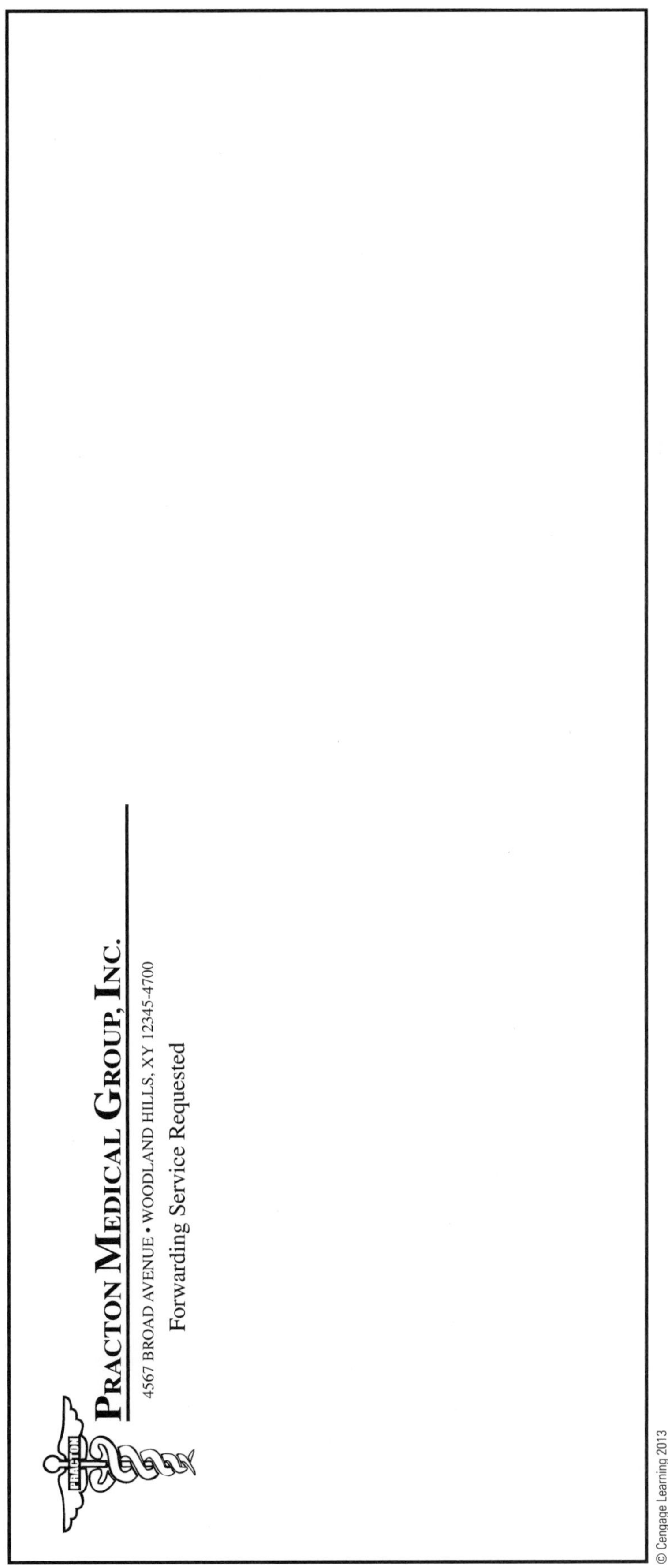
PRACTON
PRACTON MEDICAL GROUP, INC.
4567 BROAD AVENUE • WOODLAND HILLS, XY 12345-4700
Forwarding Service Requested
© Cengage Learning 2013

Form 55

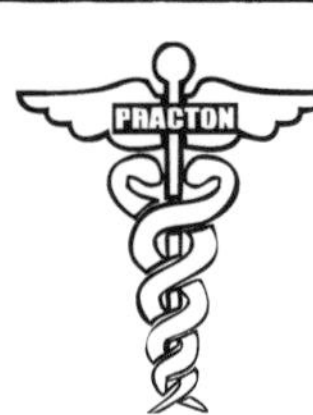

STATEMENT

PRACTON MEDICAL GROUP, INC.
4567 Broad Avenue
Woodland Hills, XY 12345-4700
Tel. 555-486-9002
Fax No. 555-488-7815

Phone No.(H)____________(W)____________ Birthdate____________
Insurance Co.________________________Policy No.____________

DATE	REFERENCE	DESCRIPTION	CHARGES	CREDITS		BALANCE
				PYMNTS.	ADJ.	
			BALANCE FORWARD →			

RB40BC-2-96

PLEASE PAY LAST AMOUNT IN BALANCE COLUMN ↑

THIS IS A COPY OF YOUR ACCOUNT AS IT APPEARS ON OUR RECORDS

Form 56

PRACTON MEDICAL GROUP, INC.

4567 BROAD AVENUE • WOODLAND HILLS, XY 12345-4700
OFFICE: (555) 486-9002 • FAX: (555) 488-7815

Fran Practon, M.D.
Gerald Practon, M.D.

AUTHORIZATION TO CHARGE CREDIT CARD

Patient Name ______________________________________

Cardholder Name ___________________________________

Credit Card Company________________________________

Card Number__________________ Expiration Date_________

I authorize __________________________ to charge my credit card $____________ on the ________ of each month until my balance of $________ is paid in full. I understand that if the charge is not accepted by my credit card company, I will immediately make the monthly payment to the practice.

I understand that I may cancel this authorization at any time, but by doing so I acknowledge that the balance owing will be due and payable in full.

______________________________ ______________

Signature Date

Form 57

FINANCIAL AGREEMENT

For PROFESSIONAL SERVICES rendered or to be rendered to :

Patient ______________________ Daytime Phone ______________

Parent if patient is a minor ______________________

1. Cash price for services .... $ ________
2. Cash down payment .... $ ________
3. Charges covered by insurance service plan................ $ ________
4. Unpaid balance of cash price .... $ ________
5. Amount financed (the amount of credit provided to you). .... $ ________
6. **FINANCE CHARGE** (the dollar amount the credit will cost you). ... $ ________
7. **ANNUAL PERCENTAGE RATE** (the cost of credit as a yearly rate) .... ________ %
8. Total of payments (5 + 6 above- The amount you will have paid when you have made all scheduled payments) .... $ ________
9. Total sales price (1 + 6 above-Sum of cash price, financing charge and any other amounts financed by the creditor, not part of the finance charge) .... $ ________

You have the right at anytime to pay the unpaid balance due under this agreement without penalty. You have the right at this time to receive an itemization of the amount financed.

☐ **I want an itemization** ☐ **I do not want an itemization**

Total of payments (# 8 above) is payable to Dr. ______________________ in __________ monthly installments of $ __________ each and __________ installments of $ ____________each. The first installment being payable on __________ 20 _____ and subsequent installments on the same day of each consecutive month until paid in full.

NOTICE TO PATIENT

Do not sign this agreement if it contains any blank spaces. You are entitled to an exact copy of any agreement you sign. You have the right at any time to pay the unpaid balance due under this agreement.

The patient (parent or guardian) agrees to be and is fully responsible for total payment of services performed in this office including any amounts not covered by any health insurance or prepayment program the responsible party may have. See your contract documents for any additional information about nonpayment, default, any required prepayment in full before the scheduled date and prepayment refunds and penalties.

Signature of patient or one parent if patient is a minor:

X ______________________________ Date: ______________

Doctor's Signature ______________________________

SCHEDULE OF PAYMENT

No.	Date Due	Amount of Installment	Date Paid	Amount Paid	Balance Owed
	Total Amount				
D.P.					
1					
2					
3					
4					
5					
6					
7					
8					
9					
10					
11					
12					
13					
14					
15					
16					
17					
18					
19					
20					
21					
22					
23					

Form 58

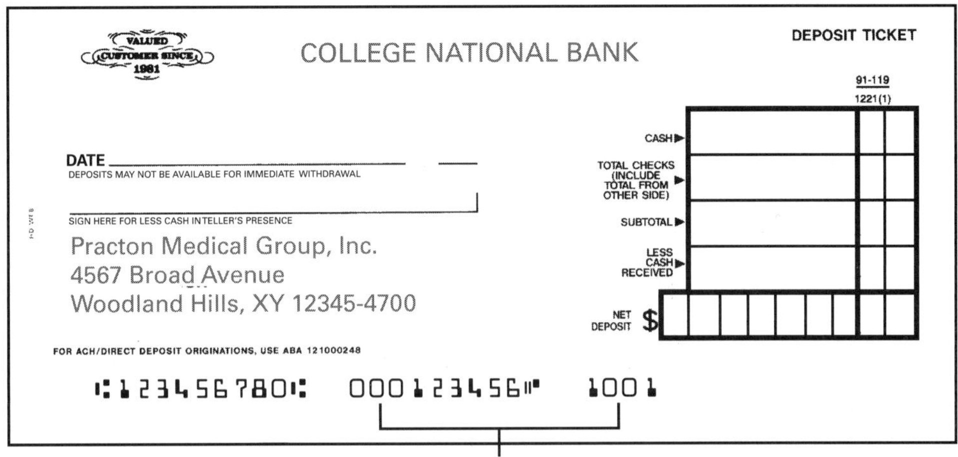
VALUED CUSTOMER SINCE 1981
COLLEGE NATIONAL BANK
DEPOSIT TICKET
91-119
1221(1)
DATE
DEPOSITS MAY NOT BE AVAILABLE FOR IMMEDIATE WITHDRAWAL
SIGN HERE FOR LESS CASH IN TELLER'S PRESENCE
Practon Medical Group, Inc.
4567 Broad Avenue
Woodland Hills, XY 12345-4700
CASH
TOTAL CHECKS (INCLUDE TOTAL FROM OTHER SIDE)
SUBTOTAL
LESS CASH RECEIVED
NET DEPOSIT $
FOR ACH/DIRECT DEPOSIT ORIGINATIONS, USE ABA 121000248
⑆123456780⑆ 000123456⑈ 1001

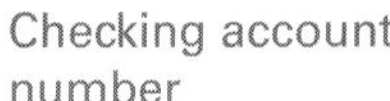
Checking account number

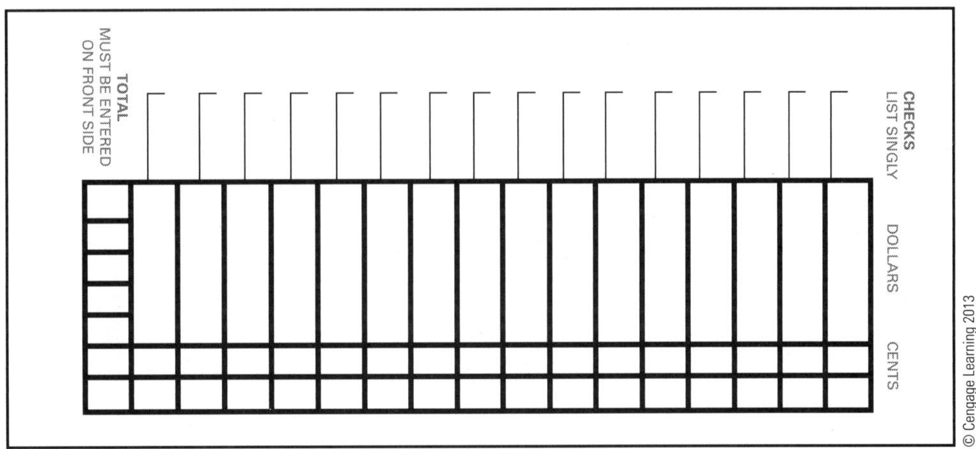
TOTAL MUST BE ENTERED ON FRONT SIDE
CHECKS LIST SINGLY
DOLLARS
CENTS

Form 59

Stationer's Corporation
340 West Main Street
Woodland Hills, XY 12345

STATEMENT

5-11-20XX

1 pkg pens	$10.00
1 box 3 x 5 cards	5.50
1 sm file box	8.00
subtotal	23.50
7% tax	1.65

TOTAL BALANCE DUE $25.15

Randolph Electrical Supply
458 State Street
Woodland Hills, XY 12345

STATEMENT

5-11-20XX

Small vacuum	$51.80
subtotal	51.80
7% tax	3.63

TOTAL BALANCE DUE $55.43

PRACTON MEDICAL GROUP, INC.
4567 Broad Avenue
Woodland Hills, XY 12345-4700

FOR INSTRUCTIONAL USE ONLY

DATE	ITEM	AMOUNT

485

3-2/310

PAY ______ **DOLLARS**

PAY TO THE ORDER OF	DATE	GROSS	DISC.

CHECK AMOUNT

$.

NOT VALID

THE FIRST NATIONAL BANK – Woodland Hills, XY 12345-4700
RB40BC-4-96

⑆1234567890⑆ 000123456⑈0485

PRACTON MEDICAL GROUP, INC.
4567 Broad Avenue
Woodland Hills, XY 12345-4700

FOR INSTRUCTIONAL USE ONLY

DATE	ITEM	AMOUNT

486

3-2/310

PAY ______ **DOLLARS**

PAY TO THE ORDER OF	DATE	GROSS	DISC.

CHECK AMOUNT

$.

NOT VALID

THE FIRST NATIONAL BANK – Woodland Hills, XY 12345-4700
RB40BC-4-96

⑆1234567890⑆ 000123456⑈0486

Form 60

BANK STATEMENT RECONCILIATION

FOUR EASY STEPS TO HELP YOU BALANCE YOUR CHECKBOOK

1. UPDATE YOUR CHECKBOOK
   - Compare and check off each transaction recorded in your check register with those listed on this statement. These include checks, direct deposits, direct debits, deposits, ATM transactions, etc.
   - Add interest and subtract service charges.

2. DETERMINE OUTSTANDING ITEMS
   - Use the charts below to list transactions shown in your check register but not included on this statement.
   - Include any from previous months.

OUTSTANDING CHECKS OR OTHER WITHDRAWALS					
CHECK NO.	AMOUNT		CHECK NO.	AMOUNT	
	$			$	
			TOTAL	$	

DEPOSITS NOT CREDITED		
DATE	AMOUNT	
	$	
TOTAL	$	

3. BALANCE YOUR ACCOUNT
   - Enter Ending Statement Balance shown on this statement. $ ______
   - Add deposits listed in your register and not shown on this statement. + ______
   - Subtract outstanding checks/withdrawals. - ______
   - **ADJUSTED TOTAL** (should agree with your checkbook balance) $ ______

4. IF THE BALANCE IN YOUR CHECKBOOK DOES NOT AGREE WITH THE ADJUSTED TOTAL, THEN
   - Check all addition and subtraction.
   - Make sure all outstanding checks, withdrawals, and deposits have been listed in the appropriate chart above.
   - Compare the amount of each check, withdrawal, and deposit in your checkbook with the amounts on this statement.
   - Review the figures on last month's statement.

Form 61

STATEMENT

PRACTON MEDICAL GROUP, INC.
4567 Broad Avenue
Woodland Hills, XY 12345-4700
Tel. 555-486-9002
Fax No. 555-488-7815

Phone No.(H)____________(W)________________ Birthdate________________
Insurance Co.________________________________Policy No.______________

DATE	REFERENCE	DESCRIPTION	CHARGES	CREDITS		BALANCE
				Pymnts	Adj	
	BALANCE FORWARD					

STATEMENT

PRACTON MEDICAL GROUP, INC.
4567 Broad Avenue
Woodland Hills, XY 12345-4700
Tel. 555-486-9002
Fax No. 555-488-7815

Phone No.(H)____________(W)________________ Birthdate________________
Insurance Co.________________________________Policy No.______________

DATE	REFERENCE	DESCRIPTION	CHARGES	CREDITS		BALANCE
				Pymnts	Adj	
	BALANCE FORWARD					

Form 62

STATEMENT

PRACTON MEDICAL GROUP, INC.
4567 Broad Avenue
Woodland Hills, XY 12345-4700
Tel. 555-486-9002
Fax No. 555-488-7815

Phone No.(H)____________(W)______________ Birthdate______________
Insurance Co.______________________________Policy No.____________

DATE	REFERENCE	DESCRIPTION	CHARGES	CREDITS		BALANCE
				Pymnts	Adj	
	BALANCE FORWARD					

STATEMENT

PRACTON MEDICAL GROUP, INC.
4567 Broad Avenue
Woodland Hills, XY 12345-4700
Tel. 555-486-9002
Fax No. 555-488-7815

Phone No.(H)____________(W)______________ Birthdate______________
Insurance Co.______________________________Policy No.____________

DATE	REFERENCE	DESCRIPTION	CHARGES	CREDITS		BALANCE
				Pymnts	Adj	
	BALANCE FORWARD					

Form 63

STATEMENT

PRACTON MEDICAL GROUP, INC.
4567 Broad Avenue
Woodland Hills, XY 12345-4700
Tel. 555-486-9002
Fax No. 555-488-7815

Phone No.(H)____________(W)______________ Birthdate_______________
Insurance Co.________________________________Policy No.______________

DATE	REFERENCE	DESCRIPTION	CHARGES	CREDITS		BALANCE
				Pymnts	Adj	
	BALANCE FORWARD					

STATEMENT

PRACTON MEDICAL GROUP, INC.
4567 Broad Avenue
Woodland Hills, XY 12345-4700
Tel. 555-486-9002
Fax No. 555-488-7815

Phone No.(H)____________(W)______________ Birthdate_______________
Insurance Co.________________________________Policy No.______________

DATE	REFERENCE	DESCRIPTION	CHARGES	CREDITS		BALANCE
				Pymnts	Adj	
	BALANCE FORWARD					

Form 64

STATEMENT

PRACTON MEDICAL GROUP, INC.
4567 Broad Avenue
Woodland Hills, XY 12345-4700
Tel. 555-486-9002
Fax No. 555-488-7815

Phone No.(H)____________(W)____________ Birthdate____________
Insurance Co.________________________Policy No.____________

DATE	REFERENCE	DESCRIPTION	CHARGES	CREDITS		BALANCE
				Pymnts	Adj	
	BALANCE FORWARD					

STATEMENT

PRACTON MEDICAL GROUP, INC.
4567 Broad Avenue
Woodland Hills, XY 12345-4700
Tel. 555-486-9002
Fax No. 555-488-7815

Phone No.(H)____________(W)____________ Birthdate____________
Insurance Co.________________________Policy No.____________

DATE	REFERENCE	DESCRIPTION	CHARGES	CREDITS		BALANCE
				Pymnts	Adj	
	BALANCE FORWARD					

Form 65

STATEMENT

PRACTON MEDICAL GROUP, INC.
4567 Broad Avenue
Woodland Hills, XY 12345-4700
Tel. 555-486-9002
Fax No. 555-488-7815

Phone No.(H)____________(W)______________ Birthdate______________
Insurance Co.______________________________Policy No.______________

DATE	REFERENCE	DESCRIPTION	CHARGES	CREDITS Pymnts	Adj	BALANCE
	BALANCE FORWARD					

STATEMENT

PRACTON MEDICAL GROUP, INC.
4567 Broad Avenue
Woodland Hills, XY 12345-4700
Tel. 555-486-9002
Fax No. 555-488-7815

Phone No.(H)____________(W)______________ Birthdate______________
Insurance Co.______________________________Policy No.______________

DATE	REFERENCE	DESCRIPTION	CHARGES	CREDITS Pymnts	Adj	BALANCE
	BALANCE FORWARD					

Form 66

STATEMENT

PRACTON MEDICAL GROUP, INC.
4567 Broad Avenue
Woodland Hills, XY 12345-4700
Tel. 555-486-9002
Fax No. 555-488-7815

Phone No.(H)____________(W)______________ Birthdate______________
Insurance Co.______________________________Policy No.______________

DATE	REFERENCE	DESCRIPTION	CHARGES	CREDITS		BALANCE
				Pymnts	Adj	
	BALANCE FORWARD					

STATEMENT

PRACTON MEDICAL GROUP, INC.
4567 Broad Avenue
Woodland Hills, XY 12345-4700
Tel. 555-486-9002
Fax No. 555-488-7815

Phone No.(H)____________(W)______________ Birthdate______________
Insurance Co.______________________________Policy No.______________

DATE	REFERENCE	DESCRIPTION	CHARGES	CREDITS		BALANCE
				Pymnts	Adj	
	BALANCE FORWARD					

Form 67

STATEMENT

PRACTON MEDICAL GROUP, INC.
4567 Broad Avenue
Woodland Hills, XY 12345-4700
Tel. 555-486-9002
Fax No. 555-488-7815

Phone No.(H)____________(W)______________ Birthdate______________
Insurance Co.____________________________Policy No.______________

DATE	REFERENCE	DESCRIPTION	CHARGES	CREDITS		BALANCE
				Pymnts	Adj	
	BALANCE FORWARD					

STATEMENT

PRACTON MEDICAL GROUP, INC.
4567 Broad Avenue
Woodland Hills, XY 12345-4700
Tel. 555-486-9002
Fax No. 555-488-7815

Phone No.(H)____________(W)______________ Birthdate______________
Insurance Co.____________________________Policy No.______________

DATE	REFERENCE	DESCRIPTION	CHARGES	CREDITS		BALANCE
				Pymnts	Adj	
	BALANCE FORWARD					

Form 68

STATEMENT

PRACTON MEDICAL GROUP, INC.
4567 Broad Avenue
Woodland Hills, XY 12345-4700
Tel. 555-486-9002
Fax No. 555-488-7815

Phone No.(H)____________(W)_______________ Birthdate_______________
Insurance Co.________________________________Policy No.______________

DATE	REFERENCE	DESCRIPTION	CHARGES	CREDITS Pymnts	CREDITS Adj	BALANCE
	BALANCE FORWARD					

STATEMENT

PRACTON MEDICAL GROUP, INC.
4567 Broad Avenue
Woodland Hills, XY 12345-4700
Tel. 555-486-9002
Fax No. 555-488-7815

Phone No.(H)____________(W)_______________ Birthdate_______________
Insurance Co.________________________________Policy No.______________

DATE	REFERENCE	DESCRIPTION	CHARGES	CREDITS Pymnts	CREDITS Adj	BALANCE
	BALANCE FORWARD					

Form 69

STATEMENT

PRACTON MEDICAL GROUP, INC.
4567 Broad Avenue
Woodland Hills, XY 12345-4700
Tel. 555-486-9002
Fax No. 555-488-7815

Phone No.(H)____________(W)_______________ Birthdate_______________
Insurance Co.______________________________Policy No.______________

DATE	REFERENCE	DESCRIPTION	CHARGES		CREDITS Pymnts		CREDITS Adj		BALANCE	
	BALANCE FORWARD									

STATEMENT

PRACTON MEDICAL GROUP, INC.
4567 Broad Avenue
Woodland Hills, XY 12345-4700
Tel. 555-486-9002
Fax No. 555-488-7815

Phone No.(H)____________(W)_______________ Birthdate_______________
Insurance Co.______________________________Policy No.______________

DATE	REFERENCE	DESCRIPTION	CHARGES		CREDITS Pymnts		CREDITS Adj		BALANCE	
	BALANCE FORWARD									

Form 70

STATEMENT

PRACTON MEDICAL GROUP, INC.
4567 Broad Avenue
Woodland Hills, XY 12345-4700
Tel. 555-486-9002
Fax No. 555-488-7815

Phone No.(H)____________(W)______________ Birthdate______________
Insurance Co.______________________________Policy No.______________

DATE	REFERENCE	DESCRIPTION	CHARGES	CREDITS Pymnts	CREDITS Adj	BALANCE
	BALANCE FORWARD					

STATEMENT

PRACTON MEDICAL GROUP, INC.
4567 Broad Avenue
Woodland Hills, XY 12345-4700
Tel. 555-486-9002
Fax No. 555-488-7815

Phone No.(H)____________(W)______________ Birthdate______________
Insurance Co.______________________________Policy No.______________

DATE	REFERENCE	DESCRIPTION	CHARGES	CREDITS Pymnts	CREDITS Adj	BALANCE
	BALANCE FORWARD					

Form 71

STATEMENT

PRACTON MEDICAL GROUP, INC.
4567 Broad Avenue
Woodland Hills, XY 12345-4700
Tel. 555-486-9002
Fax No. 555-488-7815

Phone No.(H)____________(W)______________ Birthdate____________
Insurance Co.____________________________Policy No.____________

DATE	REFERENCE	DESCRIPTION	CHARGES	CREDITS Pymnts	CREDITS Adj	BALANCE
	BALANCE FORWARD					

STATEMENT

PRACTON MEDICAL GROUP, INC.
4567 Broad Avenue
Woodland Hills, XY 12345-4700
Tel. 555-486-9002
Fax No. 555-488-7815

Phone No.(H)____________(W)______________ Birthdate____________
Insurance Co.____________________________Policy No.____________

DATE	REFERENCE	DESCRIPTION	CHARGES	CREDITS Pymnts	CREDITS Adj	BALANCE
	BALANCE FORWARD					

Form 72

STATEMENT

PRACTON MEDICAL GROUP, INC.
4567 Broad Avenue
Woodland Hills, XY 12345-4700
Tel. 555-486-9002
Fax No. 555-488-7815

Phone No.(H)____________(W)______________ Birthdate______________
Insurance Co.______________________________Policy No.______________

DATE	REFERENCE	DESCRIPTION	CHARGES	CREDITS		BALANCE
				Pymnts	Adj	
	BALANCE FORWARD					

STATEMENT

PRACTON MEDICAL GROUP, INC.
4567 Broad Avenue
Woodland Hills, XY 12345-4700
Tel. 555-486-9002
Fax No. 555-488-7815

Phone No.(H)____________(W)______________ Birthdate______________
Insurance Co.______________________________Policy No.______________

DATE	REFERENCE	DESCRIPTION	CHARGES	CREDITS		BALANCE
				Pymnts	Adj	
	BALANCE FORWARD					

Form 73

STATEMENT

PRACTON MEDICAL GROUP, INC.
4567 Broad Avenue
Woodland Hills, XY 12345-4700
Tel. 555-486-9002
Fax No. 555-488-7815

Phone No.(H)____________(W)_______________ Birthdate_______________
Insurance Co.________________________________Policy No.______________

DATE	REFERENCE	DESCRIPTION	CHARGES	CREDITS		BALANCE
				Pymnts	Adj	
	BALANCE FORWARD					

STATEMENT

PRACTON MEDICAL GROUP, INC.
4567 Broad Avenue
Woodland Hills, XY 12345-4700
Tel. 555-486-9002
Fax No. 555-488-7815

Phone No.(H)____________(W)_______________ Birthdate_______________
Insurance Co.________________________________Policy No.______________

DATE	REFERENCE	DESCRIPTION	CHARGES	CREDITS		BALANCE
				Pymnts	Adj	
	BALANCE FORWARD					

Form 74

STATEMENT

PRACTON MEDICAL GROUP, INC.
4567 Broad Avenue
Woodland Hills, XY 12345-4700
Tel. 555-486-9002
Fax No. 555-488-7815

Phone No.(H)____________(W)______________ Birthdate______________
Insurance Co.______________________________Policy No.______________

DATE	REFERENCE	DESCRIPTION	CHARGES	CREDITS		BALANCE
				Pymnts	Adj	
	BALANCE FORWARD					

STATEMENT

PRACTON MEDICAL GROUP, INC.
4567 Broad Avenue
Woodland Hills, XY 12345-4700
Tel. 555-486-9002
Fax No. 555-488-7815

Phone No.(H)____________(W)______________ Birthdate______________
Insurance Co.______________________________Policy No.______________

DATE	REFERENCE	DESCRIPTION	CHARGES	CREDITS		BALANCE
				Pymnts	Adj	
	BALANCE FORWARD					

Form 75

FAMILY HEALTH MAGAZINE
3490 Broadway Street
New York, NY 10010

0136

June 26, 20XX

16-66/1220

PAY TO THE ORDER OF Gerald Practon, M.D. $50.00

Fifty and NO/100 DOLLARS

VOID

BANK OF AMERICA NT&SA

⑆122000661⑆0136⑈ 10386⑈60402⑈

COLONY BOYS SCHOOL
659 Manchester Avenue
Woodland Hills, XY 12345

785

June 26, 20XX

16-36/208
1220

Pay to the Order of Fran Practon, M. D. $ 75.00

Seventy-five and no/100 Dollars

VOID

BARCLAYS BANK

memo lecture

⑆122000360⑆0785 208913379⑈

Adrienne Cane
6502 North J Street
Woodland Hills, XY 12345
Tel. 555/498-2110

0425

June 26, 20XX

16-4
1220

PAY TO THE ORDER OF Practon Medical Group, Inc. $50.00

Fifty and no/100 DOLLARS

VOID

SECURITY PACIFIC NATIONAL BANK

Adrienne Cane

⑆122000043⑆0425⑈ 229⑈048596⑈

Form 76

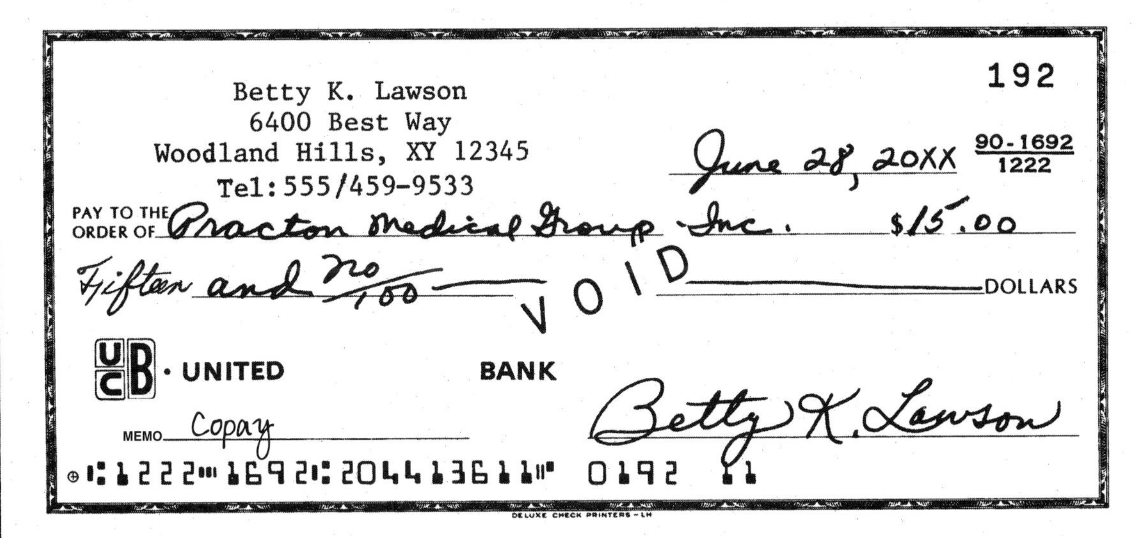

Betty K. Lawson
6400 Best Way
Woodland Hills, XY 12345
Tel:555/459-9533

192

June 28, 20XX 90-1692/1222

PAY TO THE ORDER OF Practon Medical Group Inc. $15.00

Fiften and no/100 DOLLARS

VOID

UCB · UNITED BANK

MEMO Copay

Betty K. Lawson

⑆1222⑈1692⑆2044136111⑈ 0192 11

DELUXE CHECK PRINTERS - LH

Jody F. Swinney
4300 Saunders Road
Woodland Hills, XY 12345
Tel: 555/908-6605

No. 150

June 28, 20XX 16-8/1220

Pay to the order of Practon Medical Group, Inc. $15.00

Fifteen and no/100 DOLLARS

VOID

CROCKER NATIONAL BANK

Memo

Jody F. Swinney

⑆122000085⑆0150 1400506010⑈0150

Form 77

DATE	REFERENCE	DESCRIPTION	CHARGES	CREDITS PYMNTS.	CREDITS ADJ.	BALANCE	PREVIOUS BALANCE	NAME

This is your RECEIPT for this amount
This is a STATEMENT of your account to date

Please present this slip to receptionist before leaving office.

PRACTON MEDICAL GROUP, INC.
4567 Broad Avenue
Woodland Hills, XY 12345-4700
Tel. 555-486-9002
Fax. No. 555-488-7815

Thank You!

ROA – Received on Account

OT – Other ______________________

NEXT APPOINTMENT ______________ 147

RB40BC-3-96

DATE	REFERENCE	DESCRIPTION	CHARGES	CREDITS PYMNTS.	CREDITS ADJ.	BALANCE	PREVIOUS BALANCE	NAME

This is your RECEIPT for this amount
This is a STATEMENT of your account to date

Please present this slip to receptionist before leaving office.

PRACTON MEDICAL GROUP, INC.
4567 Broad Avenue
Woodland Hills, XY 12345-4700
Tel. 555-486-9002
Fax. No. 555-488-7815

Thank You!

ROA – Received on Account

OT – Other ______________________

NEXT APPOINTMENT ______________ 148

RB40BC-3-96

DATE	REFERENCE	DESCRIPTION	CHARGES	CREDITS PYMNTS.	CREDITS ADJ.	BALANCE	PREVIOUS BALANCE	NAME

This is your RECEIPT for this amount
This is a STATEMENT of your account to date

Please present this slip to receptionist before leaving office.

PRACTON MEDICAL GROUP, INC.
4567 Broad Avenue
Woodland Hills, XY 12345-4700
Tel. 555-486-9002
Fax. No. 555-488-7815

Thank You!

ROA – Received on Account

OT – Other ______________________

NEXT APPOINTMENT ______________ 149

RB40BC-3-96

DATE	REFERENCE	DESCRIPTION	CHARGES	CREDITS PYMNTS.	CREDITS ADJ.	BALANCE	PREVIOUS BALANCE	NAME

This is your RECEIPT for this amount
This is a STATEMENT of your account to date

Please present this slip to receptionist before leaving office.

PRACTON MEDICAL GROUP, INC.
4567 Broad Avenue
Woodland Hills, XY 12345-4700
Tel. 555-486-9002
Fax. No. 555-488-7815

Thank You!

ROA – Received on Account

OT – Other ______________________

NEXT APPOINTMENT ______________ 150

RB40BC-3-96

Form 78

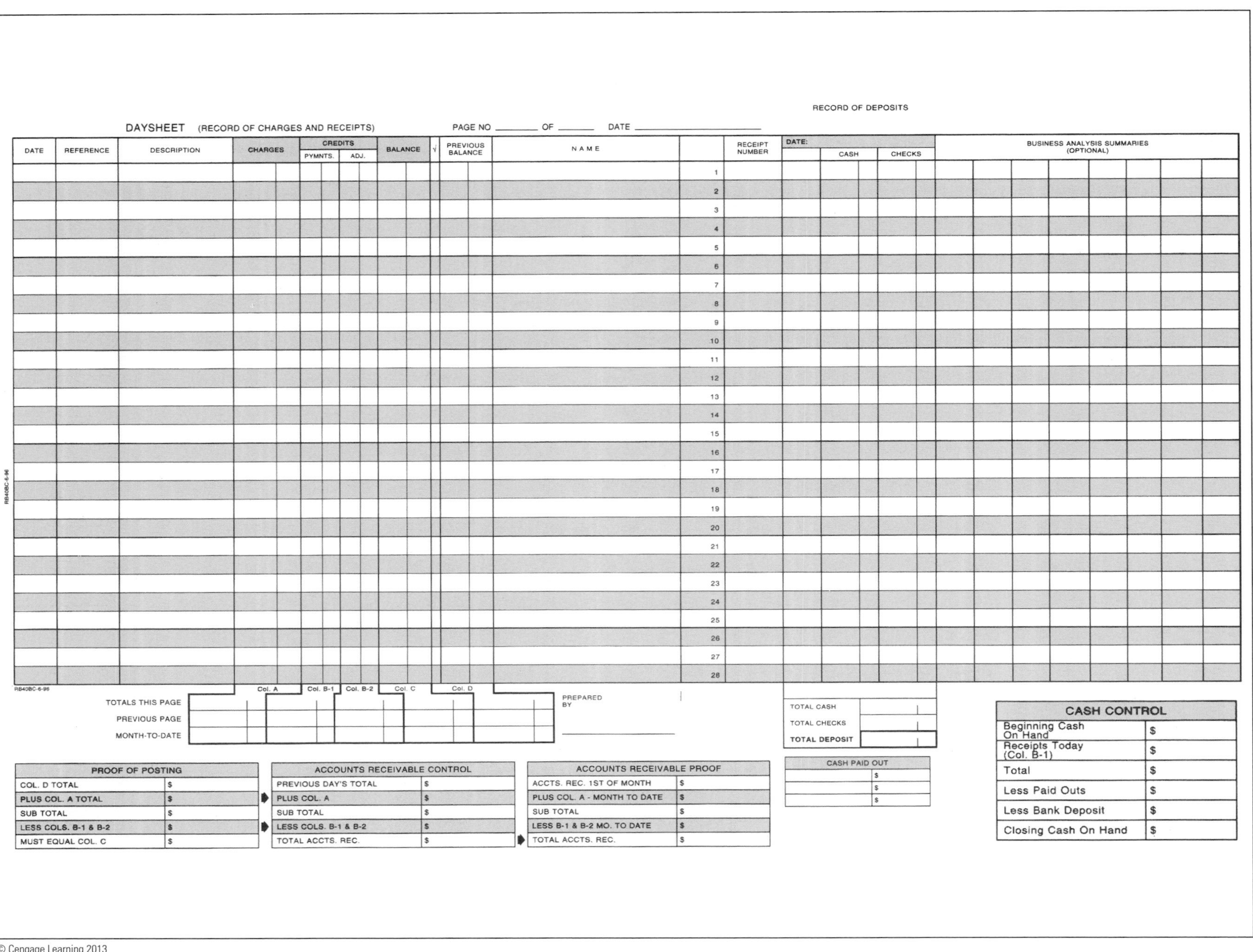

RECORD OF DEPOSITS

DAYSHEET (RECORD OF CHARGES AND RECEIPTS) PAGE NO ______ OF ______ DATE ______

DATE	REFERENCE	DESCRIPTION	CHARGES	CREDITS PYMNTS.	CREDITS ADJ.	BALANCE	√	PREVIOUS BALANCE	NAME		RECEIPT NUMBER	DATE:	CASH	CHECKS	BUSINESS ANALYSIS SUMMARIES (OPTIONAL)
										1					
										2					
										3					
										4					
										5					
										6					
										7					
										8					
										9					
										10					
										11					
										12					
										13					
										14					
										15					
										16					
										17					
										18					
										19					
										20					
										21					
										22					
										23					
										24					
										25					
										26					
										27					
										28					

RB40BC-6-96

	Col. A	Col. B-1	Col. B-2	Col. C	Col. D
TOTALS THIS PAGE					
PREVIOUS PAGE					
MONTH-TO-DATE					

PREPARED BY ______

TOTAL CASH	
TOTAL CHECKS	
TOTAL DEPOSIT	

CASH PAID OUT	
	$
	$
	$

PROOF OF POSTING	
COL. D TOTAL	$
PLUS COL. A TOTAL	$
SUB TOTAL	$
LESS COLS. B-1 & B-2	$
MUST EQUAL COL. C	$

ACCOUNTS RECEIVABLE CONTROL	
PREVIOUS DAY'S TOTAL	$
PLUS COL. A	$
SUB TOTAL	$
LESS COLS. B-1 & B-2	$
TOTAL ACCTS. REC.	$

ACCOUNTS RECEIVABLE PROOF	
ACCTS. REC. 1ST OF MONTH	$
PLUS COL. A - MONTH TO DATE	$
SUB TOTAL	$
LESS B-1 & B-2 MO. TO DATE	$
TOTAL ACCTS. REC.	$

CASH CONTROL	
Beginning Cash On Hand	$
Receipts Today (Col. B-1)	$
Total	$
Less Paid Outs	$
Less Bank Deposit	$
Closing Cash On Hand	$

Form 79

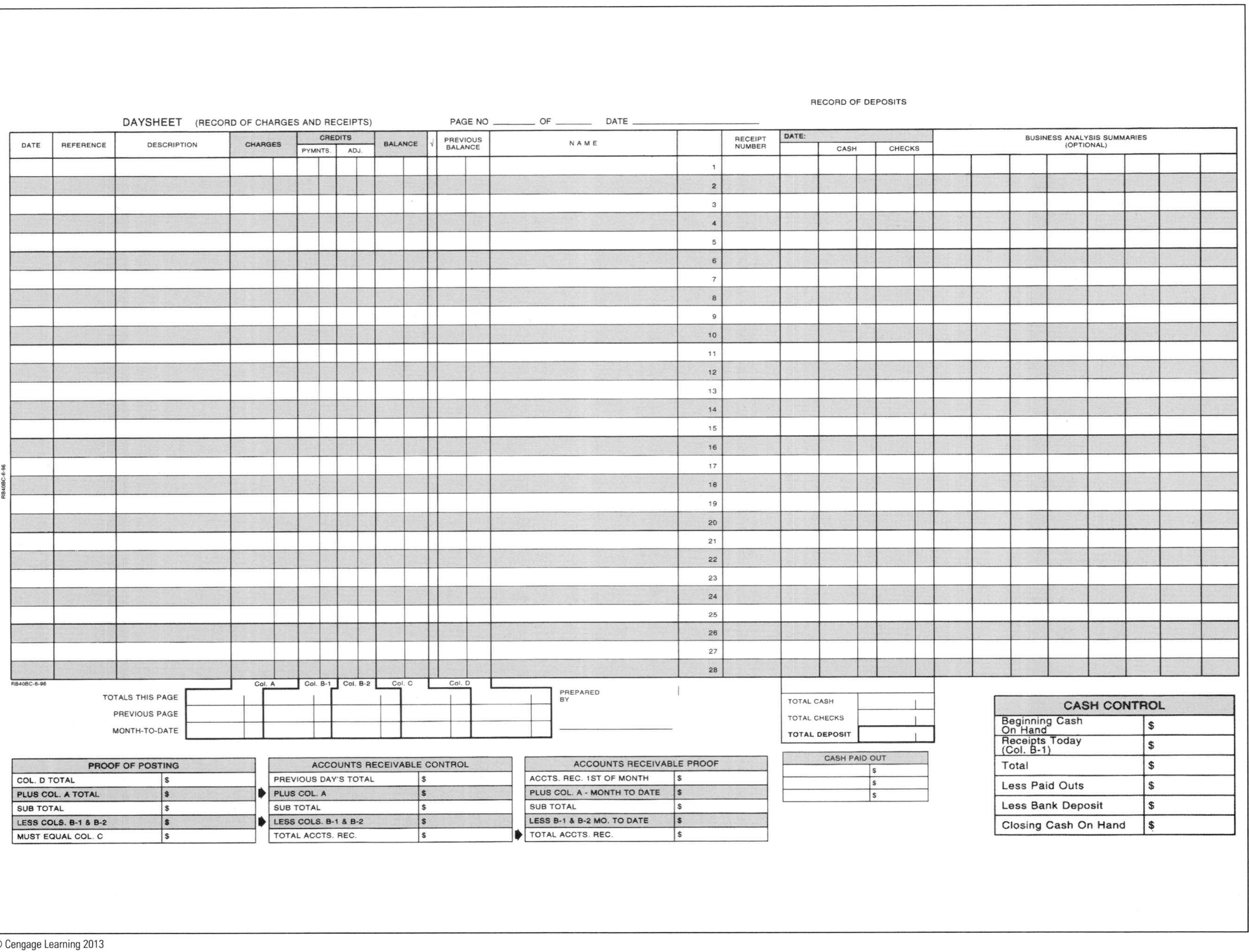

RECORD OF DEPOSITS

DAYSHEET (RECORD OF CHARGES AND RECEIPTS) PAGE NO ______ OF ______ DATE ____________

DATE	REFERENCE	DESCRIPTION	CHARGES	CREDITS PYMNTS.	CREDITS ADJ.	BALANCE	√	PREVIOUS BALANCE	NAME		RECEIPT NUMBER	DATE:	CASH	CHECKS	BUSINESS ANALYSIS SUMMARIES (OPTIONAL)
										1					
										2					
										3					
										4					
										5					
										6					
										7					
										8					
										9					
										10					
										11					
										12					
										13					
										14					
										15					
										16					
										17					
										18					
										19					
										20					
										21					
										22					
										23					
										24					
										25					
										26					
										27					
										28					

RB40BC-6-96

	Col. A	Col. B-1	Col. B-2	Col. C	Col. D
TOTALS THIS PAGE					
PREVIOUS PAGE					
MONTH-TO-DATE					

PREPARED BY ____________

TOTAL CASH	
TOTAL CHECKS	
TOTAL DEPOSIT	

PROOF OF POSTING	
COL. D TOTAL	$
PLUS COL. A TOTAL	$
SUB TOTAL	$
LESS COLS. B-1 & B-2	$
MUST EQUAL COL. C	$

ACCOUNTS RECEIVABLE CONTROL	
PREVIOUS DAY'S TOTAL	$
PLUS COL. A	$
SUB TOTAL	$
LESS COLS. B-1 & B-2	$
TOTAL ACCTS. REC.	$

ACCOUNTS RECEIVABLE PROOF	
ACCTS. REC. 1ST OF MONTH	$
PLUS COL. A - MONTH TO DATE	$
SUB TOTAL	$
LESS B-1 & B-2 MO. TO DATE	$
TOTAL ACCTS. REC.	$

CASH PAID OUT	
	$
	$
	$

CASH CONTROL	
Beginning Cash On Hand	$
Receipts Today (Col. B-1)	$
Total	$
Less Paid Outs	$
Less Bank Deposit	$
Closing Cash On Hand	$

Form 80

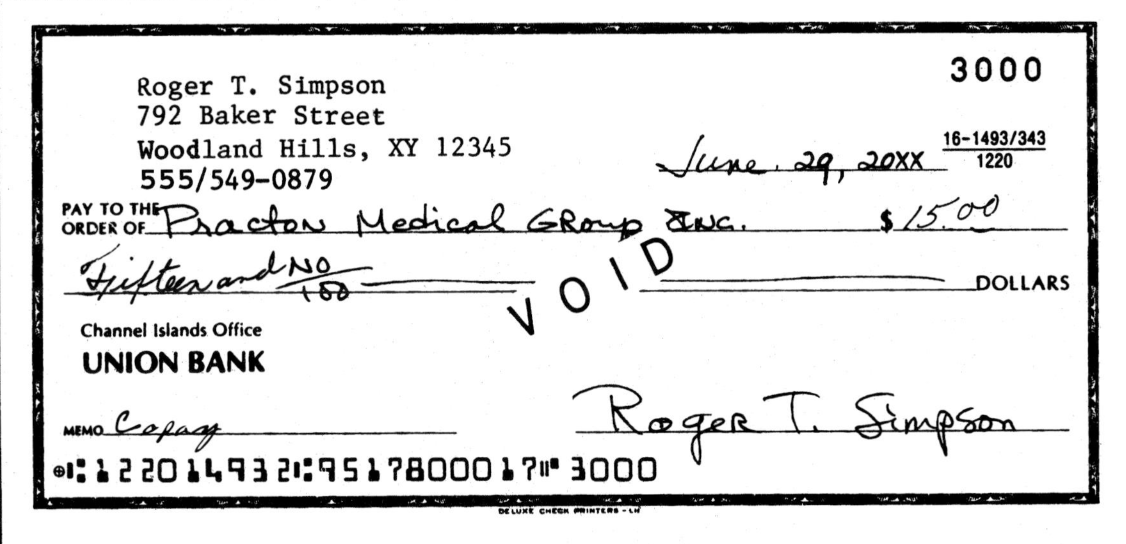

Roger T. Simpson
792 Baker Street
Woodland Hills, XY 12345
555/549-0879

3000

June 29, 20XX

16-1493/343
1220

PAY TO THE ORDER OF Practon Medical Group Inc. $ 15.00

Fifteen and NO/100 DOLLARS

VOID

Channel Islands Office
UNION BANK

MEMO Copay

Roger T. Simpson

⑆1220149321⑆9517800017⑈ 3000

DELUXE CHECK PRINTERS - LH

Bank of A. Levy

No 553

June 29, 20XX 90-372/1222

Pay to the Order of Practon Medical Group, Inc. $

Two and no/100 Dollars

VOID

Jack J. Johnson
5490 Olive Mill Road
Woodland Hills, XY 12345

Memo Copay

Signed Jack J. Johnson

⑆122203727⑆0553⑆2145⑈878⑈

Prudential Insurance Company
4680 Cowper Street
Woodland Hills, XY 12345

189

June 27,20XX

90-3219
1222

PAY TO THE ORDER OF Practon Medical Group, Inc.----- --------- $ 15.00

Fifteen and No/100-------------- ------------------- DOLLARS

VOID

OJAI VALLEY STATE BANK

HARLAND 8 TS-810

FOR completion life ins form

⑆122232196⑆0189⑈ 260⑈ 100742⑈

Form 81

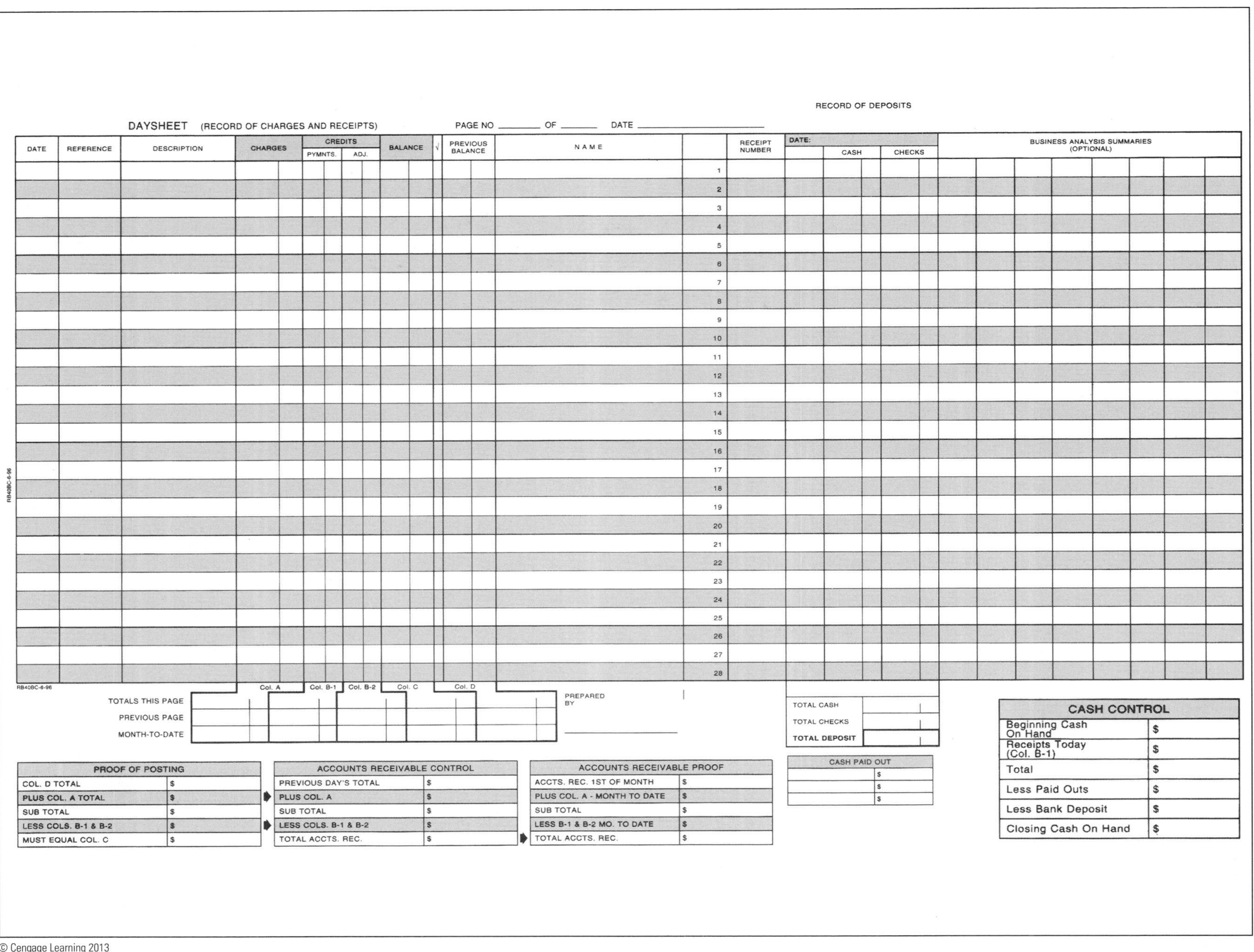

DAYSHEET (RECORD OF CHARGES AND RECEIPTS) PAGE NO ______ OF ______ DATE ______

RECORD OF DEPOSITS

DATE	REFERENCE	DESCRIPTION	CHARGES	CREDITS PYMNTS.	CREDITS ADJ.	BALANCE	√	PREVIOUS BALANCE	NAME		RECEIPT NUMBER	DATE: CASH	CHECKS	BUSINESS ANALYSIS SUMMARIES (OPTIONAL)
										1				
										2				
										3				
										4				
										5				
										6				
										7				
										8				
										9				
										10				
										11				
										12				
										13				
										14				
										15				
										16				
										17				
										18				
										19				
										20				
										21				
										22				
										23				
										24				
										25				
										26				
										27				
										28				

RB40BC-6-96

	Col. A	Col. B-1	Col. B-2	Col. C	Col. D
TOTALS THIS PAGE					
PREVIOUS PAGE					
MONTH-TO-DATE					

PREPARED BY ______

TOTAL CASH	
TOTAL CHECKS	
TOTAL DEPOSIT	

PROOF OF POSTING	
COL. D TOTAL	$
PLUS COL. A TOTAL	$
SUB TOTAL	$
LESS COLS. B-1 & B-2	$
MUST EQUAL COL. C	$

ACCOUNTS RECEIVABLE CONTROL	
PREVIOUS DAY'S TOTAL	$
PLUS COL. A	$
SUB TOTAL	$
LESS COLS. B-1 & B-2	$
TOTAL ACCTS. REC.	$

ACCOUNTS RECEIVABLE PROOF	
ACCTS. REC. 1ST OF MONTH	$
PLUS COL. A - MONTH TO DATE	$
SUB TOTAL	$
LESS B-1 & B-2 MO. TO DATE	$
TOTAL ACCTS. REC.	$

CASH PAID OUT	
	$
	$
	$

CASH CONTROL	
Beginning Cash On Hand	$
Receipts Today (Col. B-1)	$
Total	$
Less Paid Outs	$
Less Bank Deposit	$
Closing Cash On Hand	$

Form 82

Rachel T. O'Brien
5598 East 17 Street
Woodland Hills, XY 12345
555/566-2119

4800

16-21/204
1220

June 30, 20XX

pay to the order of Practon Medical Group, Inc. $ 10.00

Ten and NO/100 dollars

VOID

UNITED BANK

Rachel T. O'Brien

⑆122000218⑆ 2045028431⑈ 4800 11

Recycled and Recyclable

Joseph C. Smith
P.O. Box 4301
Woodland Hills, XY 12345
555/549-1124

217

June 30, 20XX

90-2055
1222

PAY TO THE ORDER OF Practon Medical Group, Inc. $ 75.00

Seventy Five and no/100 DOLLARS

VOID

SAMPLE VOID

SECURITY PACIFIC NATIONAL BANK

For PE + lab test

Joseph C. Smith

⑈000217⑈ ⑆1222⑉2055⑆437⑉123456⑈

Form 83

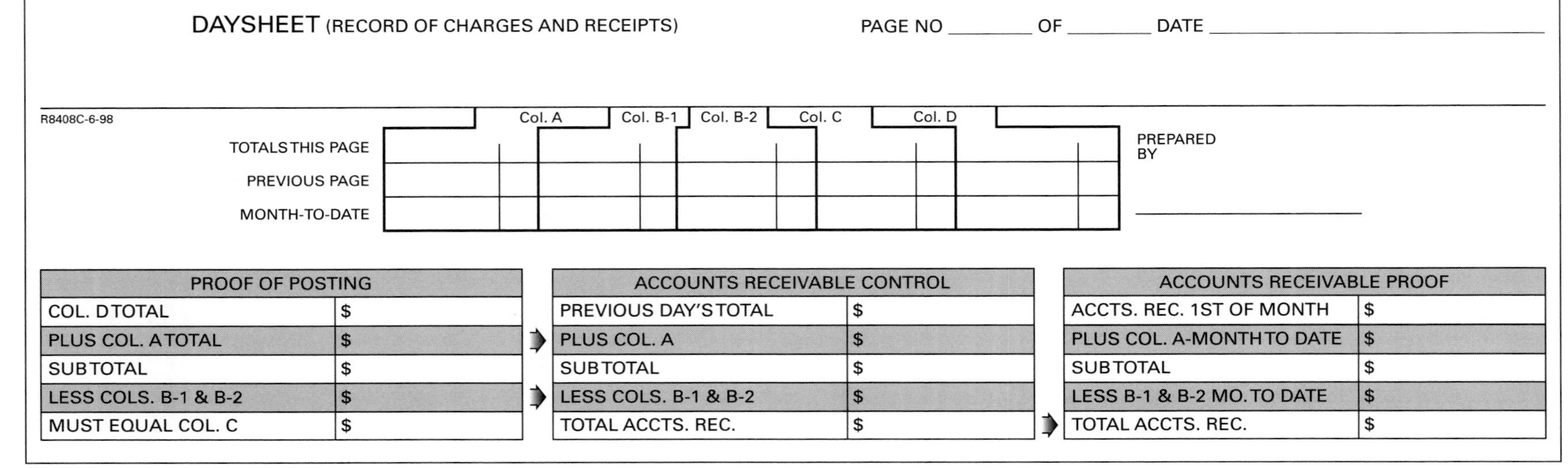

DAYSHEET (RECORD OF CHARGES AND RECEIPTS)

PAGE NO ________ OF ________ DATE ____________________

R8408C-6-98

	Col. A	Col. B-1	Col. B-2	Col. C	Col. D
TOTALS THIS PAGE					
PREVIOUS PAGE					
MONTH-TO-DATE					

PREPARED BY ____________________

PROOF OF POSTING	
COL. D TOTAL	$
PLUS COL. A TOTAL	$
SUBTOTAL	$
LESS COLS. B-1 & B-2	$
MUST EQUAL COL. C	$

ACCOUNTS RECEIVABLE CONTROL	
PREVIOUS DAY'S TOTAL	$
PLUS COL. A	$
SUBTOTAL	$
LESS COLS. B-1 & B-2	$
TOTAL ACCTS. REC.	$

ACCOUNTS RECEIVABLE PROOF	
ACCTS. REC. 1ST OF MONTH	$
PLUS COL. A-MONTH TO DATE	$
SUBTOTAL	$
LESS B-1 & B-2 MO. TO DATE	$
TOTAL ACCTS. REC.	$

Form 84

MANAGED CARE PLAN
TREATMENT AUTHORIZATION REQUEST

TO BE COMPLETED BY PRIMARY CARE PHYSICIAN OR OUTSIDE PROVIDER

Health Net	☐	Met Life	☐
Pacificare	☐	Travelers	☐
Secure Horizons	☐	Pru Care	☐

Patient Name_______________________________Date_______________________

M____ F____ Birthdate_______________ Home telephone number_________________

Address____

Primary Care Physician__________________________Member ID#________________

Referring Physician_____________________________Member ID#________________

Referred to__________________________ Address___________________________

_________________________________ Office telephone no.____________________

Diagnosis Code__________ Diagnosis____

Diagnosis Code__________ Diagnosis____

Treatment Plan____

Authorization requested for procedures/tests/visits:

Procedure Code__________ Description_______________________________________

Procedure Code__________ Description_______________________________________

Facility to be used__________________________Estimated length of stay____________

Office ☐ Outpatient ☐ Inpatient ☐ Other ☐

List of potential consultants (e.g., anesthetists, assistants, or medical/surgical):

____

Physician's signature____

TO BE COMPLETED BY PRIMARY CARE PHYSICIAN

PCP Recommendations____________________________________PCP Initials______

Eligibility checked_________________Effective date__________________________

TO BE COMPLETED BY UTILIZATION MANAGEMENT

Authorized__________________________ Not authorized_________________________

Deferred____________________________ Modified______________________________

Authorization Request #____

Comments____

Form 85

1500

HEALTH INSURANCE CLAIM FORM

APPROVED BY NATIONAL UNIFORM CLAIM COMMITTEE 08/05

PICA | PICA

CARRIER

1. MEDICARE (Medicare #) | MEDICAID (Medicaid #) | TRICARE CHAMPUS (Sponsor's SSN) | CHAMPVA (Member ID#) | GROUP HEALTH PLAN (SSN or ID) | FECA BLK LUNG (SSN) | OTHER (ID)

1a. INSURED'S I.D. NUMBER (For Program in Item 1)

2. PATIENT'S NAME (Last Name, First Name, Middle Initial)

3. PATIENT'S BIRTH DATE MM DD YY SEX M F

4. INSURED'S NAME (Last Name, First Name, Middle Initial)

5. PATIENT'S ADDRESS (No., Street)

6. PATIENT RELATIONSHIP TO INSURED Self Spouse Child Other

7. INSURED'S ADDRESS (No., Street)

CITY STATE

8. PATIENT STATUS Single Married Other

CITY STATE

ZIP CODE TELEPHONE (Include Area Code) ( )

Employed Full-Time Student Part-Time Student

ZIP CODE TELEPHONE (Include Area Code ( )

9. OTHER INSURED'S NAME (Last Name, First Name, Middle Initial)

10. IS PATIENT'S CONDITION RELATED TO:

11. INSURED'S POLICY GROUP OR FECA NUMBER

a. OTHER INSURED'S POLICY OR GROUP NUMBER

a. EMPLOYMENT? (Current or Previous) YES NO

a. INSURED'S DATE OF BIRTH MM DD YY SEX M F

b. OTHER INSURED'S DATE OF BIRTH MM DD YY SEX M F

b. AUTO ACCIDENT? YES NO PLACE (State)

b. EMPLOYER'S NAME OR SCHOOL NAME

c. EMPLOYER'S NAME OR SCHOOL NAME

c. OTHER ACCIDENT? YES NO

c. INSURANCE PLAN NAME OR PROGRAM NAME

d. INSURANCE PLAN NAME OR PROGRAM NAME

10d. RESERVED FOR LOCAL USE

d. IS THERE ANOTHER HEALTH BENEFIT PLAN? YES NO *If yes,* return to and complete item 9 a-d.

READ BACK OF FORM BEFORE COMPLETING & SIGNING THIS FORM.

12. PATIENT'S OR AUTHORIZED PERSON'S SIGNATURE I authorize the release of any medical or other information necessary to process this claim. I also request payment of government benefits either to myself or to the party who accepts assignment below.

SIGNED DATE

13. INSURED'S OR AUTHORIZED PERSON'S SIGNATURE I authorize payment of medical benefits to the undersigned physician or supplier for services described below.

SIGNED

PATIENT AND INSURED INFORMATION

14. DATE OF CURRENT: MM DD YY ILLNESS (First symptom) OR INJURY (Accident) OR PREGNANCY(LMP)

15. IF PATIENT HAS HAD SAME OR SIMILAR ILLNESS. GIVE FIRST DATE MM DD YY

16. DATES PATIENT UNABLE TO WORK IN CURRENT OCCUPATION FROM MM DD YY TO MM DD YY

17. NAME OF REFERRING PROVIDER OR OTHER SOURCE

17a. 17b. NPI

18. HOSPITALIZATION DATES RELATED TO CURRENT SERVICES FROM MM DD YY TO MM DD YY

19. RESERVED FOR LOCAL USE

20. OUTSIDE LAB? YES NO $ CHARGES

21. DIAGNOSIS OR NATURE OF ILLNESS OR INJURY (Relate Items 1, 2, 3 or 4 to Item 24E by Line)

1. ___ . ___ 3. ___ . ___

2. ___ . ___ 4. ___ . ___

22. MEDICAID RESUBMISSION CODE ORIGINAL REF. NO.

23. PRIOR AUTHORIZATION NUMBER

	24. A. DATE(S) OF SERVICE From MM DD YY To MM DD YY	B. PLACE OF SERVICE	C. EMG	D. PROCEDURES, SERVICES, OR SUPPLIES (Explain Unusual Circumstances) CPT/HCPCS MODIFIER	E. DIAGNOSIS POINTER	F. $ CHARGES	G. DAYS OR UNITS	H. EPSDT Family Plan	I. ID. QUAL.	J. RENDERING PROVIDER ID. #
1									NPI	
2									NPI	
3									NPI	
4									NPI	
5									NPI	
6									NPI	

25. FEDERAL TAX I.D. NUMBER SSN EIN

26. PATIENT'S ACCOUNT NO.

27. ACCEPT ASSIGNMENT? (For govt. claims, see back) YES NO

28. TOTAL CHARGE $

29. AMOUNT PAID $

30. BALANCE DUE $

31. SIGNATURE OF PHYSICIAN OR SUPPLIER INCLUDING DEGREES OR CREDENTIALS (I certify that the statements on the reverse apply to this bill and are made a part thereof.)

SIGNED DATE

32. SERVICE FACILITY LOCATION INFORMATION

a. NPI b.

33. BILLING PROVIDER INFO & PH # ( )

a. NPI b.

PHYSICIAN OR SUPPLIER INFORMATION

NUCC Instruction Manual available at: www.nucc.org

APPROVED OMB-0938-0999 FORM CMS-1500 (08-05)

Centers for Medicare and Medicaid Services.

Form 86

1500

HEALTH INSURANCE CLAIM FORM

APPROVED BY NATIONAL UNIFORM CLAIM COMMITTEE 08/05

PICA | PICA

CARRIER

1. MEDICARE (Medicare #) | MEDICAID (Medicaid #) | TRICARE CHAMPUS (Sponsor's SSN) | CHAMPVA (Member ID#) | GROUP HEALTH PLAN (SSN or ID) | FECA BLK LUNG (SSN) | OTHER (ID)

1a. INSURED'S I.D. NUMBER (For Program in Item 1)

2. PATIENT'S NAME (Last Name, First Name, Middle Initial)

3. PATIENT'S BIRTH DATE MM DD YY SEX M F

4. INSURED'S NAME (Last Name, First Name, Middle Initial)

5. PATIENT'S ADDRESS (No., Street)

6. PATIENT RELATIONSHIP TO INSURED Self Spouse Child Other

7. INSURED'S ADDRESS (No., Street)

CITY STATE

8. PATIENT STATUS Single Married Other

CITY STATE

ZIP CODE TELEPHONE (Include Area Code) ( )

Employed Full-Time Student Part-Time Student

ZIP CODE TELEPHONE (Include Area Code ( )

9. OTHER INSURED'S NAME (Last Name, First Name, Middle Initial)

10. IS PATIENT'S CONDITION RELATED TO:

11. INSURED'S POLICY GROUP OR FECA NUMBER

a. OTHER INSURED'S POLICY OR GROUP NUMBER

a. EMPLOYMENT? (Current or Previous) YES NO

a. INSURED'S DATE OF BIRTH MM DD YY SEX M F

b. OTHER INSURED'S DATE OF BIRTH MM DD YY SEX M F

b. AUTO ACCIDENT? YES NO PLACE (State)

b. EMPLOYER'S NAME OR SCHOOL NAME

c. EMPLOYER'S NAME OR SCHOOL NAME

c. OTHER ACCIDENT? YES NO

c. INSURANCE PLAN NAME OR PROGRAM NAME

d. INSURANCE PLAN NAME OR PROGRAM NAME

10d. RESERVED FOR LOCAL USE

d. IS THERE ANOTHER HEALTH BENEFIT PLAN? YES NO *If yes,* return to and complete item 9 a-d.

READ BACK OF FORM BEFORE COMPLETING & SIGNING THIS FORM.

12. PATIENT'S OR AUTHORIZED PERSON'S SIGNATURE I authorize the release of any medical or other information necessary to process this claim. I also request payment of government benefits either to myself or to the party who accepts assignment below.

SIGNED ______ DATE ______

13. INSURED'S OR AUTHORIZED PERSON'S SIGNATURE I authorize payment of medical benefits to the undersigned physician or supplier for services described below.

SIGNED ______

PATIENT AND INSURED INFORMATION

14. DATE OF CURRENT: MM DD YY ◀ ILLNESS (First symptom) OR INJURY (Accident) OR PREGNANCY(LMP)

15. IF PATIENT HAS HAD SAME OR SIMILAR ILLNESS. GIVE FIRST DATE MM DD YY

16. DATES PATIENT UNABLE TO WORK IN CURRENT OCCUPATION FROM MM DD YY TO MM DD YY

17. NAME OF REFERRING PROVIDER OR OTHER SOURCE

17a.

17b. NPI

18. HOSPITALIZATION DATES RELATED TO CURRENT SERVICES FROM MM DD YY TO MM DD YY

19. RESERVED FOR LOCAL USE

20. OUTSIDE LAB? YES NO $ CHARGES

21. DIAGNOSIS OR NATURE OF ILLNESS OR INJURY (Relate Items 1, 2, 3 or 4 to Item 24E by Line)

1. ___ . ___

2. ___ . ___

3. ___ . ___

4. ___ . ___

22. MEDICAID RESUBMISSION CODE ORIGINAL REF. NO.

23. PRIOR AUTHORIZATION NUMBER

24. A. DATE(S) OF SERVICE From MM DD YY To MM DD YY	B. PLACE OF SERVICE	C. EMG	D. PROCEDURES, SERVICES, OR SUPPLIES (Explain Unusual Circumstances) CPT/HCPCS MODIFIER	E. DIAGNOSIS POINTER	F. $ CHARGES	G. DAYS OR UNITS	H. EPSDT Family Plan	I. ID. QUAL.	J. RENDERING PROVIDER ID. #
1								NPI	
2								NPI	
3								NPI	
4								NPI	
5								NPI	
6								NPI	

25. FEDERAL TAX I.D. NUMBER SSN EIN

26. PATIENT'S ACCOUNT NO.

27. ACCEPT ASSIGNMENT? (For govt. claims, see back) YES NO

28. TOTAL CHARGE $

29. AMOUNT PAID $

30. BALANCE DUE $

31. SIGNATURE OF PHYSICIAN OR SUPPLIER INCLUDING DEGREES OR CREDENTIALS (I certify that the statements on the reverse apply to this bill and are made a part thereof.)

SIGNED DATE

32. SERVICE FACILITY LOCATION INFORMATION

a. NPI b.

33. BILLING PROVIDER INFO & PH # ( )

a. NPI b.

PHYSICIAN OR SUPPLIER INFORMATION

NUCC Instruction Manual available at: www.nucc.org

APPROVED OMB-0938-0999 FORM CMS-1500 (08-05)

Centers for Medicare and Medicaid Services.

Form 87

1500

HEALTH INSURANCE CLAIM FORM

APPROVED BY NATIONAL UNIFORM CLAIM COMMITTEE 08/05

PICA | PICA

CARRIER

1. MEDICARE (Medicare #) | MEDICAID (Medicaid #) | TRICARE CHAMPUS (Sponsor's SSN) | CHAMPVA (Member ID#) | GROUP HEALTH PLAN (SSN or ID) | FECA BLK LUNG (SSN) | OTHER (ID)

1a. INSURED'S I.D. NUMBER (For Program in Item 1)

2. PATIENT'S NAME (Last Name, First Name, Middle Initial)

3. PATIENT'S BIRTH DATE MM DD YY SEX M F

4. INSURED'S NAME (Last Name, First Name, Middle Initial)

5. PATIENT'S ADDRESS (No., Street)

6. PATIENT RELATIONSHIP TO INSURED Self Spouse Child Other

7. INSURED'S ADDRESS (No., Street)

CITY STATE

8. PATIENT STATUS Single Married Other

CITY STATE

ZIP CODE TELEPHONE (Include Area Code) ( )

Employed Full-Time Student Part-Time Student

ZIP CODE TELEPHONE (Include Area Code ( )

9. OTHER INSURED'S NAME (Last Name, First Name, Middle Initial)

10. IS PATIENT'S CONDITION RELATED TO:

11. INSURED'S POLICY GROUP OR FECA NUMBER

a. OTHER INSURED'S POLICY OR GROUP NUMBER

a. EMPLOYMENT? (Current or Previous) YES NO

a. INSURED'S DATE OF BIRTH MM DD YY SEX M F

b. OTHER INSURED'S DATE OF BIRTH MM DD YY SEX M F

b. AUTO ACCIDENT? YES NO PLACE (State)

b. EMPLOYER'S NAME OR SCHOOL NAME

c. EMPLOYER'S NAME OR SCHOOL NAME

c. OTHER ACCIDENT? YES NO

c. INSURANCE PLAN NAME OR PROGRAM NAME

d. INSURANCE PLAN NAME OR PROGRAM NAME

10d. RESERVED FOR LOCAL USE

d. IS THERE ANOTHER HEALTH BENEFIT PLAN? YES NO ***If yes,*** return to and complete item 9 a-d.

READ BACK OF FORM BEFORE COMPLETING & SIGNING THIS FORM.

12. PATIENT'S OR AUTHORIZED PERSON'S SIGNATURE I authorize the release of any medical or other information necessary to process this claim. I also request payment of government benefits either to myself or to the party who accepts assignment below.

SIGNED ______ DATE ______

13. INSURED'S OR AUTHORIZED PERSON'S SIGNATURE I authorize payment of medical benefits to the undersigned physician or supplier for services described below.

SIGNED ______

PATIENT AND INSURED INFORMATION

14. DATE OF CURRENT: MM DD YY ILLNESS (First symptom) OR INJURY (Accident) OR PREGNANCY(LMP)

15. IF PATIENT HAS HAD SAME OR SIMILAR ILLNESS. GIVE FIRST DATE MM DD YY

16. DATES PATIENT UNABLE TO WORK IN CURRENT OCCUPATION FROM MM DD YY TO MM DD YY

17. NAME OF REFERRING PROVIDER OR OTHER SOURCE

17a.

17b. NPI

18. HOSPITALIZATION DATES RELATED TO CURRENT SERVICES FROM MM DD YY TO MM DD YY

19. RESERVED FOR LOCAL USE

20. OUTSIDE LAB? YES NO $ CHARGES

21. DIAGNOSIS OR NATURE OF ILLNESS OR INJURY (Relate Items 1, 2, 3 or 4 to Item 24E by Line)

1. ___ . ___ 3. ___ . ___

2. ___ . ___ 4. ___ . ___

22. MEDICAID RESUBMISSION CODE ORIGINAL REF. NO.

23. PRIOR AUTHORIZATION NUMBER

24. A. DATE(S) OF SERVICE From MM DD YY To MM DD YY	B. PLACE OF SERVICE	C. EMG	D. PROCEDURES, SERVICES, OR SUPPLIES (Explain Unusual Circumstances) CPT/HCPCS MODIFIER	E. DIAGNOSIS POINTER	F. $ CHARGES	G. DAYS OR UNITS	H. EPSDT Family Plan	I. ID. QUAL.	J. RENDERING PROVIDER ID. #
1								NPI	
2								NPI	
3								NPI	
4								NPI	
5								NPI	
6								NPI	

25. FEDERAL TAX I.D. NUMBER SSN EIN

26. PATIENT'S ACCOUNT NO.

27. ACCEPT ASSIGNMENT? (For govt. claims, see back) YES NO

28. TOTAL CHARGE $

29. AMOUNT PAID $

30. BALANCE DUE $

31. SIGNATURE OF PHYSICIAN OR SUPPLIER INCLUDING DEGREES OR CREDENTIALS (I certify that the statements on the reverse apply to this bill and are made a part thereof.)

SIGNED DATE

32. SERVICE FACILITY LOCATION INFORMATION

a. NPI b.

33. BILLING PROVIDER INFO & PH # ( )

a. NPI b.

PHYSICIAN OR SUPPLIER INFORMATION

NUCC Instruction Manual available at: www.nucc.org

APPROVED OMB-0938-0999 FORM CMS-1500 (08-05)

Centers for Medicare and Medicaid Services.

Form 88

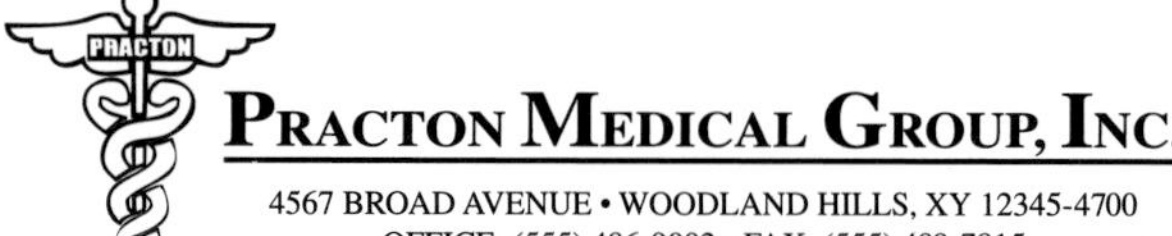

4567 BROAD AVENUE • WOODLAND HILLS, XY 12345-4700
OFFICE: (555) 486-9002 • FAX: (555) 488-7815

Fran Practon, M.D.
Gerald Practon, M.D.

PATIENT COMPLAINT DOCUMENT

Date of complaint ______________________ Account number __________

Patient name _________________________ Account balance __________

Complaint ____

____

____

____

Action taken to resolve complaint ________________________________

____

____

____

________________________________ ____________________
Employee signature Date

Form 89

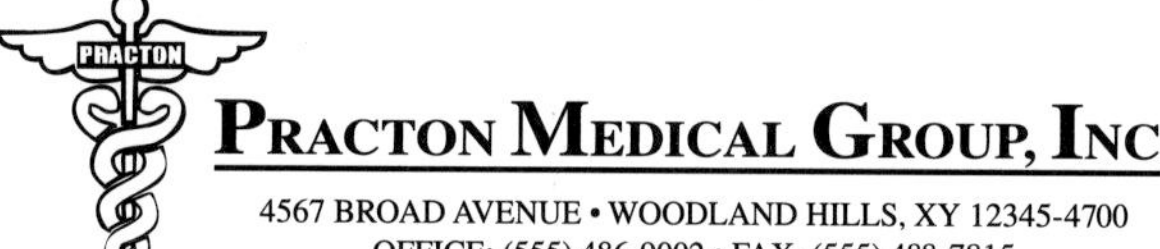

PRACTON MEDICAL GROUP, INC.

4567 BROAD AVENUE • WOODLAND HILLS, XY 12345-4700
OFFICE: (555) 486-9002 • FAX: (555) 488-7815

Fran Practon, M.D.
Gerald Practon, M.D.

PATIENT COMPLAINT DOCUMENT

Date of complaint ______________________ Account number __________

Patient name ______________________ Account balance __________

Complaint ____

____

____

____

Action taken to resolve complaint ______________________________

____

____

____

______________________________ ____________________
Employee signature Date

Form 90

Inventory Control Sheet/Maintenance Log

Name of Equipment	Manufacturer	Model No.	Warranty	Date Purchased	Purchase Price	Dates Serviced			

Form 91

medical arts press®

ORDER FORM

67000_B

SOURCE CODE	CUSTOMER NUMBER

1-A *BILL TO:* Party responsible for payment. If name and address are not correct, please make changes below. We cannot ship to a P.O. Box. If P.O. Box is shown, please fill in street address in "Ship To" area at right.

Name(s) ______
(include Dergee/Title)
______

Address ______
______

City/State/ZIP ______

Office Phone (____) ______ FAX Phone (____) ______

E-Mail Address: ______

For question...
Call ______
Phone (____) ______

To serve you bettter...
Practice Specialty ______
______ No. of Doctors ______

1-B *SHIP TO:* (Fill in only if different from "BILL TO".)
For delivery, We must have a street address.
We cannot ship to a P.O. Box.

Name(s) ______
______

Address ______
______
______

City ______

State/Zip ______

2 *PLEASE SEND ME:* Fill in only those areas that apply to you order.

Please Fill In As Applicable

QUANTITY	CATALOG NUMBER	DESCRIPTION	MESSAGE	INK COLOR(S)	TYPE STYLE	LAYOUT NO.	LOGO NO.	PRODUCT COLOR	SIZE	YEAR	START NO.	TOTAL AMOUNT

COUPON CODE(S) If you have any coupon or discount codes, please enter them here: ______ ______ ______ ______

MERCHANDISE TOTAL	
Handling Fee	FREE
Sales Tax: Medical Arts Press collects tax in all states that have a sales/use tax. Please add tax at applicable rate.	
*Rush Delivery	
TOTAL	

***For Rush Delivery specify:** ☐ **UPS Next Day** ☐ **UPS 2nd Day** Check the box at left if desired. You will be billed for rush shipping and handling charges.

☐ **RX BLANKS** (Complete the following information 85 it pertains to your state requirements)
DEA No. ______
License No. ______

☐ **MEDICAL INSURANCE CLAM FORMS** (Only complete the following if tou want it printed on your forms.)
Box 25: SSN No. ______ or Group No. ______
Box 33: PIN No. ______ or EIN No. ______

Courtesy of Medical Arts Press, PO Box 43200, Minneapolis, MN 55443-0200; Telephone (800) 328-2179; Web site: http//www.medicalartspress.com.

Form 92

ORDER FORM

photocopy this form for ordering convenience

24 HOUR FAX LINE: 800-555-1213

TOLL FREE DIRECT ORDER LINE

1-800-555-1212

Office Supply International
100 Main Street
Woodland Hills, XY

PLEASE FILL IN YOUR CUSTOMER NUMBER IF YOU HAVE PURCHASED FROM US BEFORE:

NAME ______
ADDRESS ______
CITY/STATE/ZIP ______
SPECIALTY ______
TELEPHONE ______
SHIP TO (IF DIFFERENT FROM ABOVE) ______

If you are a new customer, or have recently moved, help us expedite your order by providing us with your state registration number.
State License # ______
Expiration Date ______

PRODUCT PART NUMBER	PAGE #	PRODUCT DESCRIPTION	PKG SIZE	UNITS	QTY	EXTN

TOTAL OF MERCHANDISE	
STATE TAX (CA, IN, KY, OH, WA, WV)	
SHIPPING & HANDLING	
TOTAL	

IF YOU WISH TO PAY FOR YOUR ORDER BY CREDIT CARD, PLEASE COMPLETE THE FOLLOWING INFORMATION:

☐ VISA ☐ MASTERCARD ☐ DISCOVER ☐ PREFERRED CUSTOMER CARD

YOUR CARD # : ______

SIGNATURE ______ CARD EXP. DATE ______

THANK YOU FOR YOUR ORDER!

Form 93

medical arts press®

ORDER FORM

67000_B

SOURCE CODE	CUSTOMER NUMBER

1-A *BILL TO:* Party responsible for payment. If name and address are not correct, please make changes below. We cannot ship to a P.O. Box. If P.O. Box is shown, please fill in street address in "Ship To" area at right.

Name(s) ____________
(include Dergee/Title)
____

Address ____________
____

City/State/ZIP ____________

Office Phone (   ) ____________ FAX Phone (   ) ____________

E-Mail Address: ____________

For question...
Call ____________
Phone (   ) ____________

To serve you bettter...
Practice Specialty ____________
____________ No. of Doctors ______

1-B *SHIP TO:* (Fill in only if different from "BILL TO".)
For delivery, We must have a street address.
We cannot ship to a P.O. Box.

Name(s) ____________
____

Address ____________
____
____

City ____________

State/Zip ____________

2 *PLEASE SEND ME:* Fill in only those areas that apply to you order.

Please Fill In As Applicable

QUANTITY	CATALOG NUMBER	DESCRIPTION	MESSAGE	INK COLOR(S)	TYPE STYLE	LAYOUT NO.	LOGO NO.	PRODUCT COLOR	SIZE	YEAR	START NO.	TOTAL AMOUNT

COUPON CODE(S) If you have any coupon or discount codes, please enter them here:

MERCHANDISE TOTAL	
Handling Fee	FREE
Sales Tax: Medical Arts Press collects tax in all states that have a sales/use tax. Please add tax at applicable rate.	
*Rush Delivery	
TOTAL	

***For Rush Delivery specify:** ☐ **UPS Next Day** ☐ **UPS 2nd Day** Check the box at left if desired. You will be billed for rush shipping and handling charges.

☐ **RX BLANKS** (Complete the following information 85 it pertains to your state requirements)
DEA No. ____________
License No. ____________

☐ **MEDICAL INSURANCE CLAM FORMS** (Only complete the following if tou want it printed on your forms.)
Box 25: SSN No. ____________ or Group No. ____________
Box 33: PIN No. ____________ or EIN No. ____________

Courtesy of Medical Arts Press, PO Box 43200, Minneapolis, MN 55443-0200; Telephone (800) 328-2179; Web site: http//www.medicalartspress.com.

Form 94

medical arts press®

ORDER FORM

67000_B

1-A BILL TO: Party responsible for payment. If name and address are not correct, please make changes below. We cannot ship to a P.O. Box. If P.O. Box is shown, please fill in street address in "Ship To" area at right.

Name(s) (include Dergee/Title) ______

Address ______

City/State/ZIP ______

Office Phone ( ) ______ FAX Phone ( ) ______

E-Mail Address: ______

For question... Call ______ Phone ( ) ______

To serve you bettter... Practice Specialty ______ ______ No. of Doctors ______

SOURCE CODE	CUSTOMER NUMBER

1-B SHIP TO: (Fill in only if different from "BILL TO".) For delivery, We must have a street address. We cannot ship to a P.O. Box.

Name(s) ______

Address ______

City ______

State/Zip ______

2 PLEASE SEND ME: Fill in only those areas that apply to you order.

Please Fill In As Applicable

QUANTITY	CATALOG NUMBER	DESCRIPTION	MESSAGE	INK COLOR(S)	TYPE STYLE	LAYOUT NO.	LOGO NO.	PRODUCT COLOR	SIZE	YEAR	START NO.	TOTAL AMOUNT

COUPON CODE(S) If you have any coupon or discount codes, please enter them here:

***For Rush Delivery specify:** ☐ **UPS Next Day** ☐ **UPS 2nd Day** Check the box at left if desired. You will be billed for rush shipping and handling charges.

☐ **RX BLANKS** (Complete the following information 85 it pertains to your state requirements)

DEA No. ______

License No. ______

☐ **MEDICAL INSURANCE CLAM FORMS** (Only complete the following if tou want it printed on your forms.)

Box 25: SSN No. ______ or Group No. ______

Box 33: PIN No. ______ or EIN No. ______

MERCHANDISE TOTAL	
Handling Fee	FREE
Sales Tax: Medical Arts Press collects tax in all states that have a sales/use tax. Please add tax at applicable rate.	
*Rush Delivery	
TOTAL	

Courtesy of Medical Arts Press, PO Box 43200, Minneapolis, MN 55443-0200; Telephone (800) 328-2179; Web site: http//www.medicalartspress.com.

Form 95

TRAVEL EXPENSE REPORT

TRIP BEGINNING ______________________ TRIP ENDING ______________________

	SAT		SUN		MON		TUES		WED		THURS		FRI		SAT		
DATE																	**TOTALS**
LODGING																	
BREAKFAST																	
LUNCH																	
DINNER																	
LOCAL FARES																	
AUTO EXPENSES																	
PARKING FEES																	
PHONE/E-MAIL																	
ENTERTAINMENT																	
TIPS																	
TOLLS																	
OTHER/MISC.																	
TOTALS																	

Description of Business Purpose/Locations

____

____

____

Form 96

RECORD OF CHECKS DRAWN ON ____________________ CHECK REGISTER

MONTH OF ______________ ______PAGE NO.________

	Paid to	Date	Gross Amount		Discount			Amount of check		Check Number
								Balance Forward →		
1										
2										
3										
4										
5										
6										
7										
8										
9										
10										
11										
12										
13										
14										
15										
16										
17										
18										
19										
20										
21										
22										
23										
24										
25										
26										
27										
28										
29										
30										
			(A)		(B)			(C)		

PROOF FORMULAS:

DISBURSEMENTS – COL'S (B) + (C) = (A)

COL (A) TOTAL = TOTAL OF COLUMNS USED FOR EXPENSE DISTRIBUTION

Form 97

MONTH OF ______________ 20XX

Page 2

(MEMO) BANK BALANCE			(MEMO) BANK DEPOSIT		1 Medical Supplies	2 Office Upkeep	3 Salaries	4 Rent Upkeep	5 Utilities	6 Office Supplies	7 Taxes	8 Books Journals	9 Auto Upkeep	10 Landry Cleaning	11 Promo Entertainment
			Date	Amount											
		1													
		2													
		3													
		4													
		5													
		6													
		7													
		8													
		9													
		10													
		11													
		12													
		13													
		14													
		15													
		16													
		17													
		18													
		19													
		20													
		21													
		22													
		23													
		24													
		25													
		26													
		27													
		28													
		29													
		30													

Form 98

	EXPENSE DISTRIBUTION												Page 3
	(MEMO) BANK DEPOSIT		13	14	15	16	17	18	19	20	21	22	MISCELLANEOUS
			Business Travel	Collections	NSF Checks	Professional Meetings	Business Insurance	Contributions	Parking	Telephone	Life Insurance		Description / Amt
	Date	Amount											
1													
2													
3													
4													
5													
6													
7													
8													
9													
10													
11													
12													
13													
14													
15													
16													
17													
18													
19													
20													
21													
22													
23													
24													
25													
26													
27													
28													
29													
30													

Form 99

PRACTON MEDICAL GROUP, INC.
4567 Broad Avenue
Woodland Hills, XY 12345-4700

FOR INSTRUCTIONAL USE ONLY

DATE	ITEM	AMOUNT

479

3-2/310

PAY ______________________ DOLLARS

PAY TO THE ORDER OF	DATE	GROSS	DISC.

CHECK AMOUNT $.

NOT VALID

THE FIRST NATIONAL BANK – Woodland Hills, XY 12345-4700
RB40BC-4-96

⑈123450⑆ 000123456⑈ 0479

PRACTON MEDICAL GROUP, INC.
4567 Broad Avenue
Woodland Hills, XY 12345-4700

FOR INSTRUCTIONAL USE ONLY

DATE	ITEM	AMOUNT

480

3-2/310

PAY ______________________ DOLLARS

PAY TO THE ORDER OF	DATE	GROSS	DISC.

CHECK AMOUNT $.

NOT VALID

THE FIRST NATIONAL BANK – Woodland Hills, XY 12345-4700
RB40BC-4-96

⑈123450⑆ 000123456⑈ 0480

PRACTON MEDICAL GROUP, INC.
4567 Broad Avenue
Woodland Hills, XY 12345-4700

FOR INSTRUCTIONAL USE ONLY

DATE	ITEM	AMOUNT

481

3-2/310

PAY ______________________ DOLLARS

PAY TO THE ORDER OF	DATE	GROSS	DISC.

CHECK AMOUNT $.

NOT VALID

THE FIRST NATIONAL BANK – Woodland Hills, XY 12345-4700
RB40BC-4-96

⑈123450⑆ 000123456⑈ 0481

Form 100

PRACTON MEDICAL GROUP, INC.
4567 Broad Avenue
Woodland Hills, XY 12345-4700

FOR INSTRUCTIONAL USE ONLY

DATE	ITEM	AMOUNT	

482 3-2/310

PAY ______________________ **DOLLARS**

PAY TO THE ORDER OF	DATE	GROSS		DISC.	

CHECK AMOUNT $.

NOT VALID

THE FIRST NATIONAL BANK – Woodland Hills, XY 12345-4700
RB40BC-4-96

⑈123456780⑆ 000123456⑈ 0482

PRACTON MEDICAL GROUP, INC.
4567 Broad Avenue
Woodland Hills, XY 12345-4700

FOR INSTRUCTIONAL USE ONLY

DATE	ITEM	AMOUNT	

483 3-2/310

PAY ______________________ **DOLLARS**

PAY TO THE ORDER OF	DATE	GROSS		DISC.	

CHECK AMOUNT $.

NOT VALID

THE FIRST NATIONAL BANK – Woodland Hills, XY 12345-4700
RB40BC-4-96

⑈123456780⑆ 000123456⑈ 0483

PRACTON MEDICAL GROUP, INC.
4567 Broad Avenue
Woodland Hills, XY 12345-4700

FOR INSTRUCTIONAL USE ONLY

DATE	ITEM	AMOUNT	

484 3-2/310

PAY ______________________ **DOLLARS**

PAY TO THE ORDER OF	DATE	GROSS		DISC.	

CHECK AMOUNT $.

NOT VALID

THE FIRST NATIONAL BANK – Woodland Hills, XY 12345-4700
RB40BC-4-96

⑈123456780⑆ 000123456⑈ 0484

Form 101

PRACTON MEDICAL GROUP, INC.
4567 Broad Avenue
Woodland Hills, XY 12345-4700

FOR INSTRUCTIONAL USE ONLY

DATE	ITEM	AMOUNT

485

3-2/310

PAY ________________ DOLLARS

PAY TO THE ORDER OF	DATE	GROSS	DISC.

CHECK AMOUNT

$.

NOT VALID

THE FIRST NATIONAL BANK – Woodland Hills, XY 12345-4700
RB40BC-4-96

⑈123456780⑆ 000123456⑈ 0485

PRACTON MEDICAL GROUP, INC.
4567 Broad Avenue
Woodland Hills, XY 12345-4700

FOR INSTRUCTIONAL USE ONLY

DATE	ITEM	AMOUNT

486

3-2/310

PAY ________________ DOLLARS

PAY TO THE ORDER OF	DATE	GROSS	DISC.

CHECK AMOUNT

$.

NOT VALID

THE FIRST NATIONAL BANK – Woodland Hills, XY 12345-4700
RB40BC-4-96

⑈123456780⑆ 000123456⑈ 0486

PRACTON MEDICAL GROUP, INC.
4567 Broad Avenue
Woodland Hills, XY 12345-4700

FOR INSTRUCTIONAL USE ONLY

DATE	ITEM	AMOUNT

487

3-2/310

PAY ________________ DOLLARS

PAY TO THE ORDER OF	DATE	GROSS	DISC.

CHECK AMOUNT

$.

NOT VALID

THE FIRST NATIONAL BANK – Woodland Hills, XY 12345-4700
RB40BC-4-96

⑈123456780⑆ 000123456⑈ 0487

Form 102

PRACTON MEDICAL GROUP, INC.
4567 Broad Avenue
Woodland Hills, XY 12345-4700

FOR INSTRUCTIONAL USE ONLY

DATE	ITEM	AMOUNT

488 3-2/310

PAY ____________________ **DOLLARS**

PAY TO THE ORDER OF	DATE	GROSS	DISC.

CHECK AMOUNT $ [.]

NOT VALID

THE FIRST NATIONAL BANK – Woodland Hills, XY 12345-4700
RB40BC-4-96

⑈123456780⑆ 000123456⑈ 0488

PRACTON MEDICAL GROUP, INC.
4567 Broad Avenue
Woodland Hills, XY 12345-4700

FOR INSTRUCTIONAL USE ONLY

DATE	ITEM	AMOUNT

489 3-2/310

PAY ____________________ **DOLLARS**

PAY TO THE ORDER OF	DATE	GROSS	DISC.

CHECK AMOUNT $ [.]

NOT VALID

THE FIRST NATIONAL BANK – Woodland Hills, XY 12345-4700
RB40BC-4-96

⑈123456780⑆ 000123456⑈ 0489

PRACTON MEDICAL GROUP, INC.
4567 Broad Avenue
Woodland Hills, XY 12345-4700

FOR INSTRUCTIONAL USE ONLY

DATE	ITEM	AMOUNT

490 3-2/310

PAY ____________________ **DOLLARS**

PAY TO THE ORDER OF	DATE	GROSS	DISC.

CHECK AMOUNT $ [.]

NOT VALID

THE FIRST NATIONAL BANK – Woodland Hills, XY 12345-4700
RB40BC-4-96

⑈123456780⑆ 000123456⑈ 0490

Form 103

PRACTON MEDICAL GROUP, INC.
4567 Broad Avenue
Woodland Hills, XY 12345-4700

FOR INSTRUCTIONAL USE ONLY

DATE	ITEM	AMOUNT

491

3-2/310

PAY _______________ DOLLARS

PAY TO THE ORDER OF	DATE	GROSS	DISC.

CHECK AMOUNT $.

NOT VALID

THE FIRST NATIONAL BANK – Woodland Hills, XY 12345-4700
RB40BC-4-96

⑈123456780⑆ 000123456⑈ 0491

PRACTON MEDICAL GROUP, INC.
4567 Broad Avenue
Woodland Hills, XY 12345-4700

FOR INSTRUCTIONAL USE ONLY

DATE	ITEM	AMOUNT

492

3-2/310

PAY _______________ DOLLARS

PAY TO THE ORDER OF	DATE	GROSS	DISC.

CHECK AMOUNT $.

NOT VALID

THE FIRST NATIONAL BANK – Woodland Hills, XY 12345-4700
RB40BC-4-96

⑈123456780⑆ 000123456⑈ 0492

PRACTON MEDICAL GROUP, INC.
4567 Broad Avenue
Woodland Hills, XY 12345-4700

FOR INSTRUCTIONAL USE ONLY

DATE	ITEM	AMOUNT

493

3-2/310

PAY _______________ DOLLARS

PAY TO THE ORDER OF	DATE	GROSS	DISC.

CHECK AMOUNT $.

NOT VALID

THE FIRST NATIONAL BANK – Woodland Hills, XY 12345-4700
RB40BC-4-96

⑈123456780⑆ 000123456⑈ 0493

Form 104

PRACTON MEDICAL GROUP, INC.
4567 Broad Avenue
Woodland Hills, XY 12345-4700

FOR INSTRUCTIONAL USE ONLY

DATE	ITEM	AMOUNT	

494

3-2/310

PAY ______________________________ DOLLARS

PAY TO THE ORDER OF	DATE	GROSS		DISC.	

CHECK AMOUNT

$.

NOT VALID

THE FIRST NATIONAL BANK – Woodland Hills, XY 12345-4700
RB40BC-4-96

⑈123456780⑆ 000123456⑈ 0494

Form 105

PRACTON MEDICAL GROUP, INC.
4567 Broad Avenue
Woodland Hills, XY 12345-4700

FOR INSTRUCTIONAL USE ONLY

DATE	ITEM	AMOUNT	

495

3-2
310

PAY ______________________________ DOLLARS

PAY TO THE ORDER OF	DATE	GROSS		DISC.	

CHECK AMOUNT

$.

NOT VALID

THE FIRST NATIONAL BANK – Woodland Hills, XY 12345-4700
RB40BC-4-96

⑈123456780⑆ 000123456⑈ 0495

Form 106

PETTY CASH RECEIPT ENVELOPE

From ____________ **20XX To** ______________ **20XX** **Paid by Check No.** _________

Entered	Audited	Approved	Paid

Date	No.	Paid to:	Item	Account	Amount	

Office Fund Amount $ __________ **Receipts Paid** $ __________

Total Receipts and Cash $ __________ **Cash on Hand** $ __________

(Over or Short) $ __________ **TOTAL** $ __________

DISTRIBUTION OF PETTY CASH

									Totals

Form 107

BANK STATEMENT RECONCILIATION

FOUR EASY STEPS TO HELP YOU BALANCE YOUR CHECKBOOK

1. UPDATE YOUR CHECKBOOK
   - Compare and check off each transaction recorded in your check register with those listed on this statement. These include checks, direct deposits, direct debits, deposits, ATM transactions, etc.
   - Add interest and subtract service charges.

2. DETERMINE OUTSTANDING ITEMS
   - Use the charts below to list transactions shown in your check register but not included on this statement.
   - Include any from previous months.

OUTSTANDING CHECKS OR OTHER WITHDRAWALS				
CHECK NO.	AMOUNT		CHECK NO.	AMOUNT
	$			$
			TOTAL	$

DEPOSITS NOT CREDITED		
DATE	AMOUNT	
	$	
TOTAL	$	

3. BALANCE YOUR ACCOUNT
   - Enter Ending Statement Balance shown on this statement. $ ______
   - Add deposits listed in your register and not shown on this statement. + ______
   - Subtract outstanding checks/withdrawals. - ______
   - **ADJUSTED TOTAL** (should agree with your checkbook balance) $ ______

4. IF THE BALANCE IN YOUR CHECKBOOK DOES NOT AGREE WITH THE ADJUSTED TOTAL, THEN
   - Check all addition and subtraction.
   - Make sure all outstanding checks, withdrawals, and deposits have been listed in the appropriate chart above.
   - Compare the amount of each check, withdrawal, and deposit in your checkbook with the amounts on this statement.
   - Review the figures on last month's statement.

Form 108

PAYROLL REGISTER FOR PERIOD ENDING: ____________

EMPLOYEE NAME	EARNINGS						DEDUCTIONS								
	No. of Exempts	Hours Worked	Hourly Rate	Reg. Pay	Over-time	Gross Pay	FICA	Fed. Inc. Tax	State Inc. Tax	SDI	Medicare	Other	TOTAL DEDUC.	Check No.	NET PAY

Form 109

EMPLOYEE EARNING RECORD

Name____________________ Date of Hire____________________

Address____________________ Date of Birth____________________

____________________ Position____________________PT/FT

Telephone____________________ No. of Exemptions____________________S/M

Social Security Number____________ Rate of Pay____________________ hr/wk/mo

		EARNINGS			DEDUCTIONS								
Period Ended	Hours Worked	Reg. Pay	Over-time	Gross Pay	FICA	Fed. Inc. Tax	State Inc. Tax	SDI	Medicare	Other	TOTAL DEDUC.	NET PAY	Year to Date

Form 110

Form W-4 (2012)

Purpose. Complete Form W-4 so that your employer can withhold the correct federal income tax from your pay. Consider completing a new Form W-4 each year and when your personal or financial situation changes.

Exemption from withholding. If you are exempt, complete **only** lines 1, 2, 3, 4, and 7 and sign the form to validate it. Your exemption for 2011 expires February 16, 2012. See Pub. 505, Tax Withholding and Estimated Tax.

Note. If another person can claim you as a dependent on his or her tax return, you cannot claim exemption from withholding if your income exceeds $950 and includes more than $300 of unearned income (for example, interest and dividends).

Basic instructions. If you are not exempt, complete the **Personal Allowances Worksheet** below. The worksheets on page 2 further adjust your withholding allowances based on itemized deductions, certain credits, adjustments to income, or two-earners/multiple jobs situations.

Complete all worksheets that apply. However, you may claim fewer (or zero) allowances. For regular wages, withholding must be based on allowances you claimed and may not be a flat amount or percentage of wages.

Head of household. Generally, you may claim head of household filing status on your tax return only if you are unmarried and pay more than 50% of the costs of keeping up a home for yourself and your dependent(s) or other qualifying individuals. See Pub. 501, Exemptions, Standard Deduction, and Filing Information, for information.

Tax credits. You can take projected tax credits into account in figuring your allowable number of withholding allowances. Credits for child or dependent care expenses and the child tax credit may be claimed using the **Personal Allowances Worksheet** below. See Pub. 919, How Do I Adjust My Tax Withholding, for information on converting your other credits into withholding allowances.

Nonwage income. If you have a large amount of nonwage income, such as interest or dividends, consider making estimated tax payments using Form 1040-ES, Estimated Tax for Individuals. Otherwise, you may owe additional tax. If you have pension or annuity income, see Pub. 919 to find out if you shouldadjust your withholding on Form W-4 or W-4P.

Two earners or multiple jobs. If you have a working spouse or more than one job, figure the total number of allowances you are entitled to claim on all jobs using worksheets from only one Form W-4. Your withholding usually will be most accurate when all allowances are claimed on the Form W-4 for the highest paying job and zero allowances are claimed on the others. See Pub. 919 for details.

Nonresident alien. If you are a nonresident alien, see Notice 1392, Supplemental Form W-4 Instructions for Nonresident Aliens, before completing this form.

Check your withholding. After your Form W-4 takes effect, use Pub. 919 to see how the amount you are having withheld compares to your projected total tax for 2011. See Pub. 919, especially if your earnings exceed $130,000 (Single) or $180,000 (Married).

Personal Allowances Worksheet (Keep for your records.)

A Enter "1" for **yourself** if no one else can claim you as a dependent . . . . . A ______

B Enter "1" if:
- You are single and have only one job; or
- You are married, have only one job, and your spouse does not work; or
- Your wages from a second job or your spouse's wages (the total of both) are $1,500 or less.

. . . B ______

C Enter "1" for your **spouse.** But, you may choose to enter "-0-" if you are married and have either a working spouse or more than one job. (Entering "-0-" may help you avoid having too little tax withheld.) . . . . . C ______

D Enter number of **dependents** (other than your spouse or yourself) you will claim on your tax return . . . . . D ______

E Enter "1" if you will file as **head of household** on your tax return (see conditions under **Head of household** above) . . E ______

F Enter "1" if you have at least $1,900 of **child or dependent care expenses** for which you plan to claim a credit . . . F ______
(**Note.** Do **not** include child support payments. See Pub. 503, Child and Dependent Care Expenses, for details.)

G **Child Tax Credit** (including additional child tax credit). See Pub. 972, Child Tax Credit, for more information.
- If your total income will be less than $61,000 ($90,000 if married), enter "2" for each eligible child; then **less** "1" if you have three or more eligible children.
- If your total income will be between $61,000 and $84,000 ($90,000 and $119,000 if married), enter "1" for each eligible child plus "1" **additional** if you have six or more eligible Children . . . . . G ______

H Add lines A through G and enter total here. (**Note.** This may be different from the number of exemptions you claim on your tax return.) ▶ H ______

For accuracy, **complete all worksheets that apply.**
- If you plan to **itemize** or **claim adjustments to income** and want to reduce your withholding, see the **Deductions and Adjustments Worksheet** on page 2.
- If you have **more than one job** or are **married and you and your spouse both work** and the combined earnings from all jobs exceed $40,000 ($10,000 if married), see the **Two-Earners/Multiple Jobs Worksheet** on page 2 to avoid having too little tax withheld.
- If **neither** of the above situations applies, **stop here** and enter the number from line H on line 5 of Form W-4 below.

--------------- **Cut here and give Form W-4 to your employer. Keep the top part for your records.** ---------------

Form **W-4**
Department of the Treasury
Internal Revenue Service

Employee's Withholding Allowance Certificate

▶ **Whether you are entitled to claim a certain number of allowances or exemption from withholding is subject to review by the IRS. Your employer may be required to send a copy of this form to the IRS.**

OMB No. 1545-0074
2012

1 Type or print your first name and middle initial.	Last name	2 **Your social security number**
Home address (number and street or rural route)	3 ☐ Single ☐ Married ☐ Married, but withhold at higher Single rate. **Note.** If married, but legally separated, or spouse is a nonresident alien, check the "Single" box.	
City or town, state, and ZIP code	4 **If your last name differs from that shown on your social security card, check here. You must call 1-800-772-1213 for a replacement card.** ▶ ☐	

5 Total number of allowances you are claiming (from line **H** above **or** from the applicable worksheet on page 2) | 5 |
6 Additional amount, if any, you want withheld from each paycheck . . . . . | 6 | $
7 I claim exemption from withholding for 2011, and I certify that I meet **both** of the following conditions for exemption.
- Last year I had a right to a refund of **all** federal income tax withheld because I had **no** tax liability **and**
- This year I expect a refund of **all** federal income tax withheld because I expect to have **no** tax liability.

If you meet both conditions, write "Exempt" here . . . . . ▶ | 7 |

Under penalties of perjury, I declare that I have examined this certificate and to the best of my knowledge and belief, it is true, correct, and complete.

Employee's signature
(This form is not valid unless you sign it.) ▶ **Date** ▶

8 Employer's name and address (Employer: Complete lines 8 and 10 only if sending to the IRS.)	9 Office code (optional)	10 Employer identification number (EIN)

For Privacy Act and Paperwork Reduction Act Notice, see page 2. Cat. No. 10220Q Form **W-4** (2012)

Internal Revenue Service, www.irs.gov.

Form 111

EMPLOYEE BENEFITS

Benefit	**Employer Pays**	**Employee Pays**
Medical Insurance	$________________	$________________
Life Insurance	$________________	$________________
Accident Insurance	$________________	$________________
Disability Insurance	$________________	$________________
Worker's Compensation	$________________	$________________
Holiday # _____	$________________	$________________
Vacation # _____	$________________	$________________
Sick Leave # _____	$________________	$________________
Personal Leave	$________________	$________________
Education	$________________	$________________
Incentive Bonus	$________________	$________________
Retirement	$________________	$________________
Uniforms	$________________	$________________
Other	$________________	$________________
Total benefits	$________________	$________________

Hourly wage or salary of employee $________________

Gross wage for 20_____ $________________

Total employment package $________________

Employee Name:________________________________ Date:________

Form 112

EMPLOYMENT APPLICATION FORM

Directions: Answer all questions using black ink (print).

PERSONAL INFORMATION

(LAST NAME)	(FIRST NAME)	(MI)	
ADDRESS – STREET	CITY	STATE	ZIP

PHONE NUMBER: SOCIAL SECURITY NUMBER:

POSITION DESIRED:

EXPECTED SALARY OR HOURLY WAGE:

EDUCATION

NAME OF SCHOOL	ADDRESS	DATE(S)	DEGREE/CERTIFICATE
HIGH SCHOOL			
VOCATIONAL/TECHNICAL			
COLLEGE			
OTHER			

WORK EXPERIENCE – Give present position (or last position held) first.

JOB TITLE	EMPLOYER	ADDRESS	DATES

DUTIES PERFORMED:

JOB TITLE	EMPLOYER	ADDRESS	DATES

DUTIES PERFORMED:

JOB TITLE	EMPLOYER	ADDRESS	DATES

DUTIES PERFORMED:

REFERENCES – List three persons (other than relatives) who have known you for at least 2 years.

NAME/TITLE	ADDRESS	TELEPHONE NUMBER

APPLICANT'S SIGNATURE ______________________________ DATE______________

Form 113

PREEMPLOYMENT WORKSHEET

Employment objective: ____

Driver's license number: ____

Date of birth: ____________ U.S. citizen? Yes ____ No __

Physical disabilities that need to be taken into consideration for job modifications: _____

____

Volunteer activities: ____

Memberships in professional organizations: ___________________________

____

Personal interests: ____

____

SKILLS: ____________________________

Typing/Keying rate: _____WPM ____________________________

Other: ____________________________ ____________________________

____________________________ ____________________________

____________________________ ____________________________

____________________________ ____________________________

____________________________ ____________________________

____________________________ ____________________________

____________________________ ____________________________

____________________________ ____________________________

____________________________ ____________________________

____________________________ ____________________________

____________________________ ____________________________

Form 114

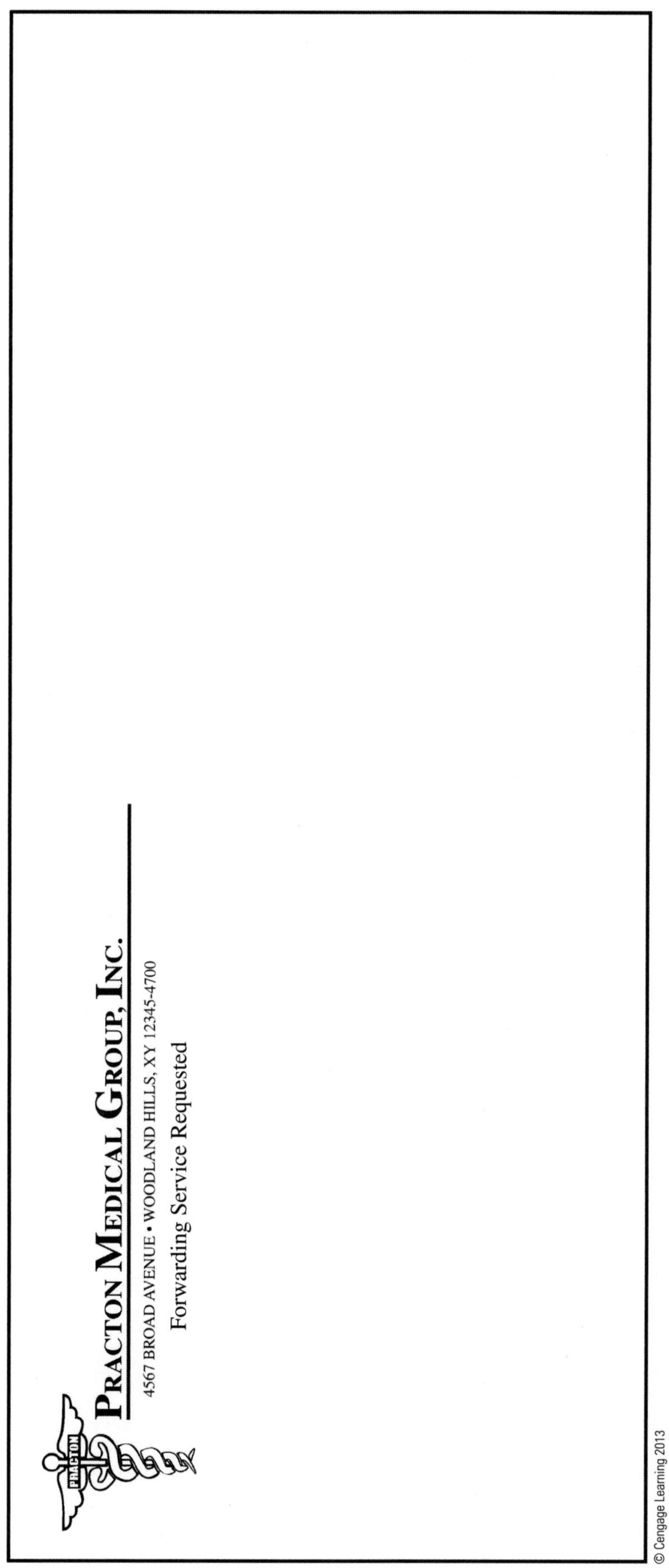

PRACTON MEDICAL GROUP, INC.
4567 BROAD AVENUE • WOODLAND HILLS, XY 12345-4700
Forwarding Service Requested

Form 115

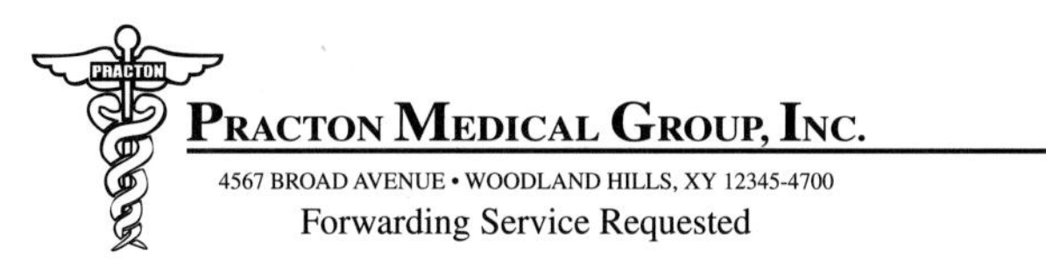
PRACTON
PRACTON MEDICAL GROUP, INC.
4567 BROAD AVENUE • WOODLAND HILLS, XY 12345-4700
Forwarding Service Requested

Form 116

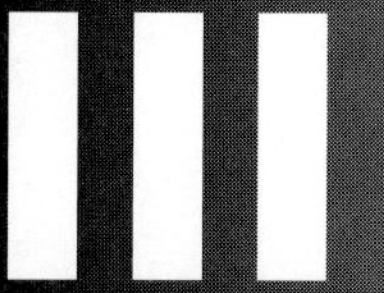

PART III

Appendix for Practon Medical Group, Inc.

- Introduction
- Medical Practice Reference Material
- Office Policies
- Payment Policies and Health Insurance Protocol
- Fee Schedule
- *CPT* Modifiers
- *HCPCS Level II* Codes

INTRODUCTION

To gain practical experience and put theory to work, assume that you have been hired to work as an administrative medical assistant for a husband-and-wife team; Dr. Fran T. Practon is a family practitioner (FP) and Dr. Gerald M. Practon is a general practitioner (GP). Their practice is called Practon Medical Group, Inc., and they are on the staff of College Hospital. You will be presented with realistic scenarios and will perform tasks in the *Workbook* Job Skills as if you were employed in their office. Use this reference material for data required in the assignments.

MEDICAL PRACTICE REFERENCE MATERIAL

Practon Medical Group, Inc.
4567 Broad Avenue
Woodland Hills, XY 12345-4700
Telephone Number: (555) 486-9002
Fax Number: (555) 488-7815
Group National Provider Identification Number (NPI): 36640210XX
Group Tax Identification Number (EIN): 20-8765432
Medicare Durable Medical Equipment (DME) Supplier Number: 33420985XX

Fran T. Practon, MD
State License Number: C 1503X
National Provider Identification (NPI) Number: 65499947XX
Federal Tax Identification Number (EIN): 73-40313XX

Gerald M. Practon, MD
State License Number: C 1402X
National Provider Identification (NPI) Number: 46278897XX
Federal Tax Identification Number (EIN): 78-51342XX

College Hospital
4500 Broad Avenue
Woodland Hills, XY 12345-4700
Telephone Number: (555) 487-6789
Fax Number: (555) 487-6790
Hospital National Provider Identification Number: 54378601XX

OFFICE POLICIES

The office policies set by Drs. Fran and Gerald Practon appear on the next several pages. Refer to them for daily routines, office appointment scheduling, telephone procedures, and filling practices as you complete the *Workbook* Job Skills. Account information is also included to help determine fees and office policies regarding charges.

Daily Routine

Both physicians prefer that the medical assistant call the answering service for messages right after the office is opened and office machines are turned on. Incoming mail should be opened and sorted when it arrives. Correspondence is to be mailed the same day it is dictated. Chart notes are to be placed in each patient's medical record as soon as possible after the dictation is received, typically within 72 hours.

Office Hours

Office hours are 9:00 a.m. to 5:00 p.m. Monday through Friday. The lunch hour is from 12:00 noon to 1:00 p.m. Both physicians leave the office at 3:00 p.m. on Wednesdays and reserve one morning each week for surgery and additional hospital responsibilities; Gerald reserves Tuesday mornings and Fran reserves Thursday mornings. Each physician covers the office while the other is at the hospital. No elective appointments are scheduled between 11:30 a.m. and noon or between 4:30 p.m. and 5:00 p.m. to allow time for callbacks, work-ins, emergencies, and dictation. An asterisk (*) distinguishes Fran's patients from Gerald's when physician verification is necessary. *Record office hours information on a 3" by 5" card for easy reference.*

Appointments

Both physicians work by appointment. New patients receiving a complete physical examination or consultation are scheduled for one hour. Routine follow-up appointments for established patients are scheduled for half an hour. Brief office visits for services such as suture removals, cast checks, dressing changes, injections, and blood pressure checks are scheduled for 15-minute appointments. Appointments should be scheduled at the earliest time available and consecutively when possible. Check with the physician regarding time frames for office procedures and hospital surgeries. House calls are discouraged but, if necessary, are made after 5:00 p.m.

Patients should be specific in outlining the nature of their medical problem so appropriate time is allowed. If multiple problems exist and are made known by the patient, additional time will be allotted. There is no charge if appointments are cancelled 24 hours in advance; uncancelled appointments are billed at one-half the usual fee. *Record appointment information on the back of the office hours 3" by 5" card for easy reference.* Refer to Table IV-3 in Part IV of the *Workbook* for appointment terms and their abbreviations.

Telephone Calls

The medical assistant answers most inquiries so the physicians need not leave patients during examinations to answer the telephone. When a medical emergency arises or a telephone call is received from another physician, it may be necessary to knock on the door of the treatment room and advise the physician of the urgency of the telephone call or ask the physician if he or she wishes to take the call. When the assistant is unable to give a complete answer to a question asked via telephone, the physician is consulted and typically reviews the medical record and either calls back the same day or has a member of the staff make the call-back. Routine calls that the physicians personally return are made after 11:30 a.m., during the lunch hour, or after 4:30 p.m. Generally, there is no charge for telephone calls.

Filing

The "Patient Information" (registration) form is stapled to the left inside area of the file folder. Correspondence in reference to a patient is filled under the patient's name. Folders are filed alphabetically according to rules established by the Association of Records Managers and Administrators (ARMA), and material is filled chronologically within each section of the file folder. Sections include (starting from the front of the chart):

Progress notes
Consultations
Operative reports
Laboratory test reports
Radiology reports

In lieu of file folder dividers, sections may be indicated with a colored sheet of paper, titled according to the section. The history and physical report as well as the discharge summary are filed along with the operative report for the patient's hospital encounter.

History and physical reports for new patients or yearly examinations and progress notes for established patients are filed under "Progress Notes" in the right portion of the file folder in chronological order. Ledger cards are kept alphabetically in a special file container; however, in our mock situation, place them in front of the patient's file folder behind the "Patient Information" form.

PAYMENT POLICIES AND HEALTH INSURANCE PROTOCOL

After a patient is seen, the fee is determined by referring to the *CPT** code listing and the correct column in the fee schedule. The fee is posted to the patient's ledger card and entered on the daily journal (daysheet). All monies received by mail are posted in the same manner on the day they arrive. The first statement is given to the patient at the time of service or sent shortly thereafter. Successive statements are sent every 30 days according to a schedule set by the first date of service.

Uninsured patients are expected to pay at the time of service. Professional discounts are not typically allowed; however, uninsured or cash patients who pay the entire bill in cash at the time of service are allowed a 20% discount. If either physician treats an uninsured physician, a professional discount or no charge is considered. Financial hardship cases are reviewed case by case.

Patients who have health insurance coverage are expected to pay copayments prior to services being rendered. Insured patients are responsible for the total amount of the bill at the time services are rendered and will receive regular statements after the date of service; however, their insurance company is billed by Practon Medical Group, Inc., and patients can wait until the insurance company pays their portion before paying the coinsurance amount. If the insurance payment is delayed, the patient is responsible for paying the bill and contacting the insurance company to help resolve the problem.

When coding insurance claims, use codes from the Standard Code Set, which has been developed by the Centers for Medicare and Medicaid Services (CMS). Codes in this standard that apply to billing outpatient medical claims include:

- *International Classification of Diseases, 10th Revision, Clinical Modification (ICD-10-CM)*—diagnostic codes
- *Current Procedural Terminology (CPT)**—also referred to as *HCPCS Level I* codes for procedures and services
- *Healthcare Common Procedure Coding System (HCPCS)—HCPCS Level II* codes

When coding diagnoses using *ICD-10-CM*, refer to the following example, which illustrates how to locate a code by the main term found in the diagnostic statement.

Note: To identify the main term, ask, "What is wrong with the patient?" The additional term may state where the problem is (anatomic site), identify the *time frame* in which the patient is experiencing the problem (e.g., acute, subacute, chronic), or further define the *type* of problem (e.g., *alcoholic* liver disease).

Example of Main Terms

Diagnostic Statement	Main Term	ICD-10-CM Codes	ICD-9-CM Codes	Additional Term
muscle atrophy	atrophy	M62.50	728.2	muscle—where
chronic bronchitis	bronchitis	J42	491.9	chronic—time frame
allergic conjunctivitis (chronic)	conjunctivitis	H10.45	372.14	allergic—type
recurrent depression	depression	F33.9	296.30	recurrent—time frame
nasal (bone) fracture	fracture	S02.2xxA	802.0	nasal—where

For information regarding filing health insurance claim forms, refer to Chapter 16 and the CMS-1500 Field-by-Field Instructions in Appendix A of the *textbook*. Both physicians bill using their group tax identification number (see Field 25) and their group national provider identification number (see Field 33), not independently.

FEE SCHEDULE

Figure III-1 is the fee schedule for Practon Medical Group, Inc. Fees are listed numerically according to *CPT** code number as found in the codebook. Section titles of the codebook and subsection titles of the Surgery section are included for easy reference. All fees listed are examples only. Fees can vary according to the region of the United States (West, Midwest, South, and East), the type of community (urban, suburban, or rural), the type of practice (solo, group, and so forth), and the specialty of the practitioner, as well as the practice overhead, expense, and a number of other factors.

The seven columns in the fee schedule are as follows:

- **Column 1 (*CPT* Code Number)** lists selected code numbers from 2012 *Current Procedural Terminology.**
- **Column 2 (*CPT* Code Description)** contains abbreviated descriptions of procedures and services.
- **Column 3 (*Mock Fee)*** shows the physician's standard fees. These are used to bill private patients as well as those on Medicaid, TRICARE, and workers' compensation.
- **Column 4 (Medicare—Participating)** lists the allowed amounts Medicare approves for a physician with a contract. Medicare pays 80% of this fee, the patient pays 20%, and the difference between the allowed amount and the charged amount is written off the books as a courtesy adjustment.
- **Column 5 (Medicare—Nonparticipating)** shows the allowed amounts Medicare approves for noncontracted physicians. Medicare pays 80% of this fee, and 20% is collected from the patient (see comments under Limiting Charge).
- **Column 6 (Limiting Charge)** lists the highest amounts that a nonparticipating physician is allowed to bill for the service rendered. In addition to the 20% collected from the nonparticipating physician's allowed amount, the noncontracted physician can also collect the difference between the nonparticipating fee (charged amount) and the limiting charge from the patient.
- **Column 7 (Follow-Up Days)** lists the number of global follow-up days included in a surgical package.

Drs. Gerald and Fran Practon are both contracted with Medicare and use the participating fee unless otherwise stated.

FIGURE III-1 Fee schedule for Practon Medical Group, Inc., for reference when doing the *Workbook* Job Skills.

FRAN T. PRACTON, M.D.
Family Practice

GERALD M. PRACTON, M.D.
General Practice

Practon Medical Group, Inc.
4567 Broad Avenue
Woodland Hills, XY 12345-4700

FEE SCHEDULE

CPT Code No. and Description		Mock Fees	Medicare		
			Participating	Nonparticipating	Limiting Charge
EVALUATION AND MANAGEMENT*					
OFFICE	**New Patient**				
99201	Level I	33.25	30.43	28.91	33.25
99202	Level II	51.91	47.52	45.14	51.91
99203	Level III	70.92	64.92	61.67	70.92
99204	Level IV	106.11	97.13	92.27	106.11
99205	Level V	132.28	121.08	115.03	132.38
Established Patient					
99211	Level I	16.07	14.70	13.97	16.07
99212	Level II	28.55	26.14	24.83	28.55
99213	Level III	40.20	36.80	34.96	40.20
99214	Level IV	61.51	56.31	53.49	61.51
99215	Level V	96.97	88.76	84.32	96.97
HOSPITAL Observation Services (new or est pt)					
99217	Discharge	66.88	61.22	58.16	66.88
99218	D/C hx/exam SF/LC DM	74.22	67.91	64.54	74.22
99219	C hx/exam MC DM	117.75	107.78	102.39	117.75
99220	C hx/exam HC DM	147.48	134.99	128.24	147.48
Initial Hospital Care (new or est pt)					
99221	30 min	73.00	66.82	63.48	73.00
99222	50 min	120.80	110.57	105.04	120.80
99223	70 min	152.98	140.03	133.03	152.98
Subsequent Hospital Care					
99231	15 min	37.74	34.55	32.82	37.74
99232	25 min	55.56	50.85	48.31	55.56
99233	35 min	76.97	70.45	66.93	76.97
99238	Discharge (30 min or less)	65.26	59.74	56.75	65.26
99239	more than 30 min				
CONSULTATIONS office (new or est pt)					
99241	Level I	51.93	47.54	45.16	51.93
99242	Level II	80.24	73.44	69.77	80.24
99243	Level III	103.51	94.75	90.01	103.51
99244	Level IV	145.05	132.77	126.13	145.05
99245	Level V	195.48	178.93	169.98	195.48
Inpatient (new/est pt)					
99251	Level I	53.29	48.78	46.34	53.29
99252	Level II	80.56	73.74	70.05	80.56
99253	Level III	106.10	97.12	92.26	106.10

*See Table 17-2 and Table 17-3 in Chapter 17 of the *textbook* for more description on E/M codes 99201 through 99255.

FIGURE III-1 Fee schedule (*continued*)

CPT Code No. and Description		Mock Fees	Medicare		
			Participating	Nonparticipating	Limiting Charge
99254	Level IV	145.26	132.96	126.31	145.26
99255	Level V	196.55	179.91	170.91	196.55
EMERGENCY DEPARTMENT (new/est pt)					
99281	PF hx/exam SF DM	24.32	22.26	21.15	24.32
99282	EPF hx/exam LC DM	37.02	33.88	32.19	37.02
99283	EPF hx/exam MC DM	66.23	60.62	57.59	66.23
99284	D hx/exam MC DM	100.71	92.18	87.57	100.71
99285	C hx/exam HC DM	158.86	145.41	138.14	158.86
CRITICAL CARE SERVICES					
99291	First 30–74 min	208.91	191.22	181.66	208.91
+99292*	Each addl 30 min	102.02	92.46	87.84	102.02
NURSING FACILITY (initial new/est pt)					
99304	D/C hx/exam SF/LC DM	64.11	58.68	55.75	64.11
99305	C hx/exam MC DM	90.55	82.88	78.74	90.55
99306	C hx/exam HC DM	136.76	125.18	118.92	136.76
Subsequent (new/est pt)					
99307	PF hx/exam SF DM	37.95	34.74	33.00	37.95
99308	EPF hx/exam LC DM	55.11	50.44	47.92	55.11
99309	D hx/exam MC DM	69.61	63.72	60.53	69.61
99310	C hx/exam HC DM	83.12	77.11	74.88	83.12
DOMICILIARY, REST HOME, CUSTODIAL CARE New patient					
99324	PF hx/exam SF DM	46.10	42.20	40.09	46.10
99325	EPF hx/exam LC DM	65.02	59.52	56.54	65.02
99326	D hx/exam MC DM	86.18	78.88	74.94	86.18
99327	C hx/exam MC DM	105.77	113.54	109.40	105.77
99328	C hx/exam HC DM	123.98	131.06	127.62	123.98
Established patient					
99334	PF hx/exam SF DM	37.31	34.15	32.44	37.31
99335	EPF hx/exam LC DM	49.22	45.05	42.80	49.22
99336	D hx/exam MC DM	60.61	55.47	52.70	60.61
99337	C hx/exam MC/HC DM	72.03	77.65	74.12	72.03
HOME SERVICES New patient					
99341	PF hx/exam SF DM	70.32	64.37	61.15	70.32
99342	EPF hx/exam LC DM	91.85	84.07	79.87	91.85
99343	D hx/exam MC DM	120.24	110.06	104.56	120.24
99344	C hx/exam MC DM	131.04	122.16	116.98	131.04
99345	C hx/exam HC DM	148.67	132.59	124.88	148.67
Established patient					
99347	PF hx/exam SF DM	54.83	50.19	47.68	54.83
99348	EPF hx/exam LC DM	70.06	64.13	60.92	70.06
99349	D hx/exam MC DM	88.33	80.85	76.81	88.33
99350	C hx/exam M//HC DM	101.36	94.54	88.21	101.36
PROLONGED SERVICES WITH CONTACT Outpatient					
+99354	First hour	96.67	88.76	84.32	96.97
+99355	Each addl 30 min	96.97	88.76	84.32	96.97

(*continues*)

*The symbol + indicates an add-on code in *CPT* 2012.

FIGURE III-1 Fee schedule (*continued*)

CPT Code No. and Description		Mock Fees	Medicare*		
			Participating	Nonparticipating	Limiting Charge
Inpatient					
+99356	First hour	96.42	88.25	83.84	96.42
+99357	Each addl 30 min	96.42	88.25	83.84	96.42
PROLONGED SERVICES WITHOUT DIRECT CONTACT					
99358	First hour	90.00			
+99359	Each addl 30 min	90.00			
PHYSICIAN STANDBY SERVICE					
99360	Each 30 min	95.00			
CASE MANAGEMENT SERVICES					
Team Conferences					
99366	Face-to-face; health care prof 30 min	102.00			
99367	Non-face-to-face; health care prof 30 min	93.00			
99368	Non-physician prof	85.00			
CARE PLAN OVERSIGHT SERVICES					
99374	Home health pt 15–29 min	93.40	85.49	81.22	93.40
99375	greater than 30 min	118.00			
PREVENTIVE MEDICINE New Patient					
99381	Infant under age 1 year	50.00			
99382	1–4 years	50.00			
99383	5–11 years	45.00			
99384	12–17 years	45.00			
99385	18–39 years	50.00			
99386	40–64 years	50.00			
99387	65 years and over	55.00			
Established Patient					
99391	Infant under age 1 year	35.00			
99392	1–4 years	35.00			
99393	5–11 years	30.00			
99394	12–17 years	30.00			
99395	18–39 years	35.00			
99396	40–64 years	35.00			
99397	65 years and over	40.00			
COUNSELING (new/est pt)					
Individual—Preventive					
99401	15 min	35.00			
99402	30 min	50.00			
99403	45 min	65.00			
99404	60 min	80.00			
Group—Preventive					
99411	30 min	30.00			
99412	60 min	50.00			

*Some services and procedures may not be considered a benefit under the Medicare program, and when listed on a claim form, no reimbursement may be received. However, it is important to include these codes when billing because Medicare policies may change without an individual knowing of a new benefit. For this reason, some of the services shown in this mock fee schedule do not have any amounts listed under the three Medicare columns.

FIGURE III-1 Fee schedule (*continued*)

CPT Code No. and Description		Mock Fees	Medicare*		
			Participating	Nonparticipating	Limiting Charge
Other Preventive Medicine Services					
99420	Health hazard appraisal	50.00			
99429	Unlisted preventive med serv	variable			
NON-FACE-TO-FACE-PHYSICIAN SERVICES					
Telephone Calls					
99441	Simple/brief (5–10 min)	30.00			
99442	Intermediate (11–20 min)	40.00			
99443	Complex (21–30 min)	60.00			
NEWBORN CARE (Evaluation)					
99460	Hosp or birthing center care	102.15	93.50	88.83	102.15
99461	other than hosp or birth room	110.16	100.83	95.79	110.16
99462	Subsequent hospital care	54.02	49.44	46.97	54.02
99463	History & exam; discharge same day	240.55	220.18	209.17	240.55
99464	Newborn stabilization	248.97	239.22	231.23	248.97
99465	Newborn resuscitation	255.98	234.30	222.59	255.98
NEONATAL AND PEDIATRIC INTENSIVE CARE					
99468	Initial (28 days or younger)	933.89	887.20	1,020.28	933.89
99469	Subsequent (28 days or younger)	410.80	390.26	448.80	410.80
99471	Initial (29 days–24 mo)	784.38	745.16	856.93	784.38
99472	Subsequent (29 days–24 mo)	399.77	379.78	436.75	399.77
99475	Initial (2–5 yrs)	565.70	537.42	618.03	565.70
99476	Subsequent (2–5 yrs)	343.00	325.85	374.73	343.00
ANESTHESIOLOGY					
Anesthesiology fees are presented here for *CPT* codes. However, each case would require unit values indicating time, e.g., every 15 minutes would be worth $55. Some anesthetists may list a surgical code with a modifier indicating anesthesiologist for carriers that do not acknowledge anesthesia codes.					
QUALIFYING CIRCUMSTANCES					
+99100	Anes for pt under 1 yr/over 70	55.00			
+99116	Anes complicated by use of total hypothermia	275.00			
+99135	Anes complicated by use of hypotension	275.00			
+99140	Anes complicated by emer cond	110.00			
PHYSICAL STATUS MODIFIER CODES					
P-1	Normal healthy patient	variable			
P-2	Patient with mild systemic disease	variable			
P-3	Patient with severe systemic disease	55.00			
P-4	Patient with severe systemic disease (constant threat to life)	110.00			
P-5	Moribund pt not expected to survive for 24 hr without operation	165.00			
P-6	Declared brain-dead pt organs being removed for donor	variable			

(*continues*)

*Some services and procedures may not be considered a benefit under the Medicare program, and when listed on a claim form, no reimbursement may be received. However, it is important to include these codes when billing because Medicare policies may change without an individual knowing of a new benefit. For this reason, some of the services shown in this mock fee schedule do not have any amounts listed under the three Medicare columns.

FIGURE III-1 Fee schedule (*continued*)

CPT Code No. and Description	Mock Fees	Medicare* Participating	Medicare* Nonparticipating	Medicare* Limiting Charge
HEAD				
00160 Anes for proc nose & accessory sinuses: NOS	275.00			
00172 Anes repair cleft palate	165.00			
THORAX				
00400 Anes for proc integumentary system extremities, ant trunk, and perineum	165.00			
00402 Anes breast reconstruction	275.00			
00546 Anes pulmonary resection with thoracoplasty	275.00			
SPINE & SPINAL CORD				
00600 Anes cervical spine and cord	550.00			
LOWER ABDOMEN				
00800 Anes for proc lower ant abdominal wall	165.00			
00840 Anes intraperitoneal proc lower abdomen: NOS	330.00			
00842 amniocentesis	220.00			
PERINEUM				
00914 Anes TURP	275.00			
00942 Anes colporrhaphy, colpotomy, vaginectomy	220.00			
UPPER LEG				
01210 Anes open proc hip joint: NOS	330.00			
01214 total hip replacement	440.00			
UPPER ARM AND ELBOW				
01740 Anes open/arthroscopic proc elbow; NOS	220.00			
01758 exc cyst/tumor humerus	275.00			
RADIOLOGIC PROCEDURES				
01922 Anes noninvasive imaging/rad. therapy	385.00			

*Some services and procedures may not be considered a benefit under the Medicare program, and when listed on a claim form, no reimbursement may be received. However, it is important to include these codes when billing because Medicare policies may change without an individual knowing of a new benefit. For this reason, some of the services shown in this mock fee schedule do not have any amounts listed under the three Medicare columns.

FIGURE III-1 Fee schedule (*continued*)

CPT Code No. and Description		Mock Fees	Medicare Participating	Medicare Non-participating	Medicare Limiting Charge	Follow-Up Days*
INTEGUMENTARY SYSTEM						
10060	I & D furuncle, cyst, paronychia; single	75.92	69.49	66.02	75.92	10
11100	Biopsy of skin, SC tissue &/or mucous membrane; 1 lesion	65.43	59.89	56.90	65.43	0
11200	Removal skin tags; up to 15	55.68	50.97	48.42	55.68	10
11401	Exc benign lesion, 0.6–1.0 cm; trunk, arms, legs	95.62	87.53	83.15	96.62	10
11402	1.1–2.0 cm	121.52	111.23	105.67	121.52	10
11403	2.1–3.0 cm	151.82	138.97	132.02	151.82	10
11420	Exc benign lesion, 0.5 cm or less; scalp, neck, hands, feet, genitalia	75.44	69.05	65.60	75.44	10
11422	1.1–2.0 cm	131.35	120.23	114.22	131.35	10
11441	Exc benign lesion face, ears, eyelids, nose, lips, or mucous membrane; 0.6–1.0 cm dia or less	119.08	109.00	103.55	119.08	10
11602	Exc malignant lesion, trunk, arms, or legs; 1.1–2.0 cm dia	195.06	178.55	169.62	195.06	10
11720	Debridement of nails; 1–5	32.58	29.82	28.33	32.58	0
11721	6 or more	32.58	29.82	28.33	32.58	0
11730	Avulsion nail plate, partial or complete, simple repair; single	76.91	70.40	66.88	76.91	0
11750	Exc nail or nail matrix, partial or complete; permanent	193.45	177.07	168.22	193.45	10
12001	Simple repair (scalp, neck, axillae, ext genitalia, trunk, or extremities incl hands & feet); 2.5 cm or less	91.17	83.45	79.82	91.17	10
12011	Simple repair (face, ears, eyelids, nose, lips, or mucous membranes); 2.5 cm or less	101.44	92.85	88.21	101.44	10
12013	2.6–5.0 cm	123.98	113.48	107.81	123.98	10
12032	Repair, scalp axillae, trunk (intermediate) 2.6–7.5 cm	169.73	155.36	147.59	169.73	10
12034	7.6–12.5 cm	214.20	196.06	186.26	214.20	10

(*continues*)

Global Period

Various services are associated with an operative procedure when they are considered integral parts of that procedure. The global period refers to the time frame during which all services integral to the surgical procedure are covered by a single payment.

- 0 Services provided the day of the procedure are included in the fee schedule amount.
- 10 Services provided the day of and during the 10-day period following the surgical procedure are included in the fee schedule amount.
- 90 Services provided the day before, the day of, and during the 90-day period following the surgical procedure are included in the fee schedule amount.
- INC Services are included in the global period of another related service.
- N/A Not applicable

*Timeframes for the surgical follow-up days may vary according to insurance carrier and are listed as examples only.

FIGURE III-1 Fee schedule (*continued*)

CPT Code No. and Description		Mock Fees	Medicare			
			Participating	Non-participating	Limiting Charge	Follow-Up Days*
INTEGUMENTARY SYSTEM (*continued*)						
12051	Repair, intermediate, layer closure of wounds (face, ears, eyelids, nose, lips, or mucous membranes); 2.5 cm or less	167.60	153.41	145.74	167.60	10
17000	Destruction benign or premalignant lesion, first	37.38	34.58	32.85	37.38	10
+17003	2–14 lesions, each	19.41	17.77	16.88	19.41	NA
17110	Destruction benign lesions, other than skin tags (laser, electro-, cryo-, chemosurgery, curettement); up to 14 lesions	77.05	70.53	67.00	77.05	10
17111	15 or more lesions	88.92	81.39	77.32	88.92	10
19020	Mastotomy, drainage/ exploration; deep	237.36	217.26	206.40	237.36	90
19100	Biopsy, breast, needle core	96.17	88.03	83.63	96.17	0
19101	open, incisional	281.51	257.67	244.79	281.51	10
MUSCULOSKELETAL SYSTEM						
20610	Arthrocentesis, aspiration, or injection; major joint (shoulder, hip, knee) or bursa	52.33	47.89	45.50	52.33	0
21330	Nasal fracture, open treatment complicated	599.46	548.71	521.27	599.46	90
24066	Biopsy, deep, soft tissue, upper arm, elbow	383.34	350.88	333.34	383.34	90
27455	Osteotomy, proximal tibia	1248.03	1142.36	1085.24	1248.03	90
27500	Treatment closed femoral shaft fracture without manipulation	554.90	507.92	482.52	554.90	90
27530	Treatment closed tibial fracture, proximal, without manipulation	344.24	315.90	299.34	344.24	90
27750	Treatment closed tibial shaft fracture without manipulation	400.94	366.99	348.64	400.94	90
27752	with manipulation	531.63	486.62	462.29	531.63	90
29345	Appl long leg cast (thigh to toes)	123.23	112.80	107.16	123.23	0
29355	walker or ambulatory type	133.75	122.42	116.30	133.75	0
29425	Appl short leg walking cast	102.10	93.45	88.78	102.10	0
RESPIRATORY SYSTEM						
30110	Excision, simple nasal polyp	145.21	132.92	126.27	145.21	10
30520	Septoplasty	660.88	604.93	574.68	660.88	90
30903	Control nasal hemorrhage; anterior; complex	118.17	108.17	102.76	118.17	0
30905	Control nasal hemorrhage, posterior with posterior nasal packs; initial	190.57	174.43	165.71	190.57	0
30906	subsequent	173.01	158.36	150.44	173.01	0
31625	Bronchoscopy with biopsy	312.87	286.38	272.06	312.87	0
32310	Pleurectomy, parietal	1234.79	1130.24	1073.73	1234.79	90
32440	Pneumonectomy, total	1972.10	1805.13	1714.87	1972.10	90

*Time frames for the surgical follow-up days may vary according to insurance carrier and are listed as examples only.

FIGURE III-1 Fee schedule (*continued*)

CPT Code No. and Description		Mock Fees	Medicare Participating	Medicare Non-participating	Medicare Limiting Charge	Medicare Follow-Up Days*
CARDIOVASCULAR SYSTEM						
33020	Pericardiotomy	1289.25	1180.09	1121.09	1289.25	90
33206	Insertion of pacemaker; atrial	728.42	666.75	633.41	728.42	90
33208	AV	751.57	687.89	653.50	751.57	90
35301	Thromboendarterectomy with or without patch graft; carotid, vertebral, subclavian by neck incision	1585.02	1450.82	1378.28	1585.02	90
36005	Intravenous injection for contrast venography; extremity	59.18	54.17	51.46	59.18	0
36245	Catheter placement (selective) arterial system, ea first order	68.54	62.74	59.60	68.54	NA
36415	Routine venipuncture for collection of specimen(s)	10.00	—	—	—	XXX
38101	Splenectomy, partial	994.44	910.24	864.73	994.44	90
38510	Biopsy, open excision, deep cervical lymph node(s)	327.42	299.69	284.71	327.42	10
MEDIASTINUM/DIAPHRAGM/DIGESTIVE SYSTEM						
42820	T & A under age 12 years	341.63	312.71	297.07	341.63	90
42821	over age 12 years	410.73	375.96	357.16	410.73	90
43234	Upper GI endoscopy, simple primary exam	201.86	184.77	175.53	201.86	0
43235	Upper GI endoscopy incl esophagus, stomach, duodenum, or jejunum; diagnostic	238.92	218.69	207.76	238.92	0
43334	Repair hiatal hernia1	436.50	1314.87	1249.13	1436.50	90
43456	Dilation esophagus	254.52	232.97	221.32	254.52	0
43820	Gastrojejunostomy	971.86	889.58	845.10	971.86	90
44150	Colectomy, total, abdominal	1757.81	1608.98	1528.53	1757.81	90
44320	Colostomy or skin cecostomy	966.25	884.44	840.22	966.25	90
44950	Appendectomy	568.36	520.24	494.23	568.36	90
45308	Proctosigmoidoscopy with removal of single tumor/polyp	135.34	123.88	117.69	135.34	0
45315	multiple tumors/polyps	185.12	169.44	160.97	185.12	0
45330	Sigmoidoscopy, diagnostic, with/ without collection of specimen (by brushing or washing)	95.92	87.80	83.41	95.92	0
45380	Colonoscopy with biopsy	382.35	349.98	332.48	382.35	0
46255	Hemorrhoidectomy int & ext, single	503.57	460.94	437.89	503.57	90
46258	with fistulectomy	636.02	582.17	553.06	636.02	90
46600	Anoscopy; diagnostic	32.86	30.07	28.57	32.86	0
46614	with control of bleeding	182.10	166.68	158.35	182.10	0
46700	Anoplasty for stricture, adult	657.39	601.73	571.64	657.39	90
47600	Cholecystectomy	937.74	858.35	815.43	937.74	90
49505	Inguinal hernia repair, age 5 or over	551.07	504.41	479.19	551.07	90
49520	Repair, inguinal hernia, any age; recurrent	671.89	615.00	584.25	671.89	90

(*continues*)

*Time frames for the surgical follow-up days may vary according to insurance carrier and are listed as examples only.

FIGURE III-1 Fee schedule (*continued*)

			Medicare			
CPT Code No. and Description		Mock Fees	Participating	Non-participating	Limiting Charge	Follow-Up Days*
URINARY SYSTEM						
50080	Nephrostolithotomy, percutaneous	1323.93	1211.83	1151.24	1323.93	90
50780	Ureteroneocystostomy	1561.23	1429.84	1357.59	1561.23	90
51900	Closure of vesicovaginal fistula, abdominal approach	1196.32	1095.48	1040.71	1196.82	90
52000	Cystourethroscopy	167.05	152.90	145.26	167.05	0
52601	Transurethral electrosurgical resection of prostate	888.87	813.61	772.93	888.87	90
53040	Drainage of deep periurethral abscess	520.11	476.07	452.27	520.11	90
53230	Excision, female diverticulum (urethral)	859.69	786.91	747.56	859.69	90
53240	Marsupialization of urethral diverticulum, M or F	520.11	476.07	452.27	520.11	90
53620	Dilation, urethra, male	100.73	92.20	87.59	100.73	0
53660	Dilation, urethra, female	48.32	44.23	42.02	48.32	0
MALE/FEMALE GENITAL SYSTEM						
54150	Circumcision—clamp type	111.78	102.32	97.20	111.78	10
54520	Orchiectomy, simple	523.92	479.56	455.58	523.92	90
55700	Biopsy of prostate, needle or punch	156.22	142.99	135.84	156.22	0
55801	Prostatectomy, perineal subtotal	1466.56	1342.39	1275.27	1466.56	90
57265	Colporrhaphy AP with enterocele repair	902.24	825.85	784.56	902.24	90
57452	Colposcopy	84.18	77.05	73.20	84.18	0
57511	Cryocauterization of cervix	195.83	179.25	170.29	195.83	10
57520	Circumferential (cone) of cervix with or without D & C, cold knife or laser	387.08	354.30	336.59	387.08	90
58100	Endometrial biopsy	71.88	65.79	62.50	71.88	0
58120	D & C diagnostic and/or therapeutic (nonOB)	272.83	249.73	237.24	272.83	10
58150	TAH w/without salpingo-oophorectomy	1167.72	1068.85	1015.41	1167.72	90
58200	TAH, including partial vaginec-tomy, w/lymph node sampling	1707.24	1562.69	1484.56	1707.24	90
58210	with bilateral radical pelvic lymphadenectomy	2160.78	1977.83	1878.94	2160.78	90
58300	Insertion of intrauterine device	100.00	—	—	—	NA
58340	Hysterosalpingography with inj proc	73.06	66.87	63.53	73.06	0
58720	Salpingo-oophorectomy, complete or partial, unilateral or bilateral	732.40	670.39	636.87	732.40	90

*Time frames for the surgical follow-up days may vary according to insurance carrier and are listed as examples only.

FIGURE III-1 Fee schedule (*continued*)

CPT Code No. and Description		Mock Fees	Medicare			Follow-Up Days*
			Participating	Non-participating	Limiting Charge	
MATERNITY CARE AND DELIVERY						
59120	Surgical treatment of ectopic pregnancy; salpingectomy and/or oophorectomy	789.26	722.43	686.31	789.26	90
59121	without salpingectomy and/or oophorectomy	638.84	584.75	555.51	638.84	90
59130	abdominal pregnancy	699.12	639.93	607.93	699.12	90
59135	total hysterectomy, interstitial, uterine pregnancy	1154.16	1056.44	1003.62	1154.16	90
59136	partial uterine resection, interstitial uterine pregnancy	772.69	707.26	671.90	772.69	90
59140	cervical, with evacuation	489.68	448.22	425.81	489.68	90
59160	Curettage; postpartum	293.46	268.61	255.18	293.46	10
59400	OB care—routine with vag dlvy, inc antepartum/postpartum care	1864.30	1706.45	1621.13	1864.30	NA
59510	C-section, inc antepartum and postpartum care	2102.33	1924.33	1828.11	2102.33	NA
59515	C-section, inc postpartum care only	1469.80	1345.36	1278.09	1469.80	NA
59812	Treatment of incompl abortion, any trimester; completed surgically	357.39	327.13	310.77	357.39	90
NERVOUS SYSTEM						
61314	Craniotomy infratentorial	2548.09	2332.35	2215.73	2548.09	90
62270	Spinal puncture, lumbar; diagnostic	77.52	70.96	67.41	77.52	0
EYE AND OCULAR ADNEXA						
65091	Excision of eye, without implant	708.22	648.25	615.84	708.22	90
65205	Removal of foreign body, ext eye	56.02	51.27	48.71	56.02	0
65222	corneal, with slit lamp	73.81	67.56	64.18	73.81	0
69420	Myringotomy	97.76	89.48	85.01	97.76	10
RADIOLOGY, NUCLEAR MEDICINE, AND DIAGNOSTIC ULTRASOUND						
70120	X-ray mastoids, 1–2 views p/side	38.96	35.66	33.88	38.96	
70130	3 views p/side	56.07	51.33	48.76	56.07	
71010	X-ray chest, 1 view	31.95	29.24	27.78	31.95	
71020	2 views	40.97	37.50	35.63	40.97	
71030	compl, 4 views	54.02	49.44	46.97	54.02	
71060	Bronchography, bilateral	143.75	131.58	125.00	143.75	
72100	X-ray spine, lumbosacral, 2–3 views	43.23	39.57	37.59	43.23	
72114	complete, incl bending views, minimum 6	74.97	68.62	65.19	74.97	
73100	X-ray wrist, 2 views	31.61	28.94	27.49	31.61	

(*continues*)

*Time frames for the surgical follow-up days may vary according to insurance carrier and are listed as examples only.

FIGURE III-1 Fee schedule (*continued*)

CPT Code No. and Description		Mock Fees	Medicare		
			Participating	Non-participating	Limiting Charge
RADIOLOGY, NUCLEAR MEDICINE, AND DIAGNOSTIC ULTRASOUND (*continued*)					
73500	X-ray hip, 1 view	31.56	28.88	27.44	31.56
73540	X-ray pelvis & hips, infant or child, 2 views	37.94	34.73	32.99	37.94
73590	X-ray tibia & fibula, 2 views	33.35	30.53	29.00	33.35
73620	Radiologic exam, foot; 2 views	31.61	28.94	27.49	31.61
73650	X-ray calcaneus, 2 views	30.71	28.11	26.70	30.71
74241	Radiologic exam, upper gastro-intestinal tract, with/without delayed films with KUB	108.93	99.71	94.72	108.93
74245	with small bowel	161.70	148.01	140.61	161.70
74270	Barium enema	118.47	108.44	103.02	118.47
74290	Oral cholecystography	52.59	48.14	45.73	52.59
74400	Urography (pyelography), intravenous, with or without KUB	104.78	95.90	91.11	104.78
74410	Urography, infusion	116.76	106.87	101.53	116.76
74420	Urography, retrograde	138.89	127.13	120.77	138.89
75982	Percutaneous placement of drainage catheter	359.08	328.67	312.24	359.08
76805	Ultrasound, pregnant uterus, real time; after first trimester	154.18	141.13	134.07	154.18
+76810	each additional gestation	306.54	280.59	266.56	306.54
76946	Ultrasonic guidance for amniocentesis	91.22	83.49	79.32	91.22
77055	Mammography, unilateral	62.57	57.27	54.51	62.57
77056	bilateral	82.83	75.82	72.03	82.83
77300	Radiation dosimetry	97.58	89.32	84.85	97.58
77315	Teletherapy isodose plan, complex	213.59	195.51	185.73	213.59
78104	Bone marrow imaging, whole body	230.56	211.04	200.49	230.56
78215	Liver and spleen imaging	160.44	146.85	139.51	160.44
78800	Tumor localization, limited area	191.53	175.32	166.55	191.53
PATHOLOGY AND LABORATORY*					
Laboratory tests done as groups or combination "profiles" performed on multichannel equipment should be billed using the appropriate code number (80047 through 80076). Following is a list of the panels.					
80047	Basic metabolic panel (Calcium, ionized)	75.00			
80048	Basic metabolic panel (Calcium, total	75.00			
80050	General health panel	50.00			
80051	Electrolyte panel	50.00			
80053	Comprehensive metabolic panel	200.00			
80055	Obstetric panel	75.00			

*Mock fees for laboratory tests presented in this schedule may not be representative of fees in your region due to the variety of capitation and managed care contracts as well as discount policies made by laboratories. At the time of this edition, Medicare guidelines may or may not pay for automatic multichannel tests where a large number of tests are performed per panel. Some cases require documentation and a related diagnostic code for each test performed. Providers must have the CLIA Level of licensure to bill for tests, and test results must be documented.

FIGURE III-1 Fee schedule (*continued*)

CPT Code No. and Description		Mock Fees	Medicare		
			Participating	Non-participating	Limiting Charge
80061	Lipid panel	50.00			
80069	Renal function panel	150.00			
80074	Acute hepatitis panel	50.00			
80076	Hepatic function panel	75.00			
81000	Urinalysis (dip stick), non-automated, with microscopy	8.00	7.44	5.98	8.84
81001	automated, with microscopy	8.00	7.44	5.98	8.84
81002	non-automated, without microscopy	8.00	7.44	5.98	8.84
81015	Urinalysis, microscopy only	8.00	7.44	5.98	8.84
81025	Urine pregnancy test	10.00			
82565	Creatinine; blood	10.00	9.80	8.88	12.03
82951	Glucose tol test, 3 spec	40.00	41.00	36.80	45.16
+82952	each add spec beyond 3	30.00	28.60	25.97	32.16
83020	Hemoglobin, electrophoresis	25.00	20.00	19.94	23.93
83700	Lipoprotein, blood; electrophoretic separation	25.00	20.00	19.94	23.93
84478	Triglycerides, blood	20.00	19.20	15.99	21.87
84480	Triiodothyronine (T-3)	20.00	19.20	15.99	21.87
84520	Urea nitrogen; quantitative	25.00	20.99	19.94	23.93
84550	Uric acid; blood	20.00	19.20	15.99	21.87
84702	Gonadotropin, chorionic; quantitative	20.00	19.20	15.99	21.87
84703	qualitative	20.00	19.20	15.99	21.87
85018	Blood count, hemoglobin	20.00	19.20	15.99	21.87
85025	Complete blood count (CBC, Hgb, RBC, WBC, and platelet count), automated, differential WBC count	25.00	20.00	19.94	23.93
85032	manual count (each)	25.00	20.00	19.94	23.93
85097	Bone marrow, smear interpretation	73.52	67.29	63.93	73.52
85345	Coagulation time; Lee & White	20.00	19.20	15.99	21.87
86038	Antinuclear antibodies (ANA)	25.00	20.00	19.94	23.93
87081	Culture, screening; pathogenic organisms	25.00	20.00	19.94	23.93
87181	Sensitivity studies, antibiotic; per agent	20.00	19.20	15.99	21.87
87184	disk method, per plate (12 disks or less)	20.00	19.20	15.99	21.87
87210	Smear, primary source, wet mount with simple stain, for infectious agents	35.00	48.35	45.93	55.12
88150	Papanicolaou cytopath, manual screen (vag or cerv); phys supervision	35.00	48.35	45.93	55.12
88302	Surgical pathology (level II), gross & micro exam (skin, fingers, nerve, testis)	24.14	22.09	20.99	24.14
88305	Surgical pathology (level IV); bone marrow, interpret	77.69	71.12	67.56	77.69

(*continues*)

FIGURE III-1 Fee schedule (*continued*)

CPT Code No. and Description		Mock Fees	Medicare*		
			Participating	Non-participating	Limiting Charge
MEDICINE SECTION					
Immunization Administration and Products for Vaccines/Toxoids					
90471	Immunization admin. (inj.); one (single or combination)	2.50			
90473	Immunization admin. intranasal/oral; one (single or combination)	2.50			
90701	Diphtheria, tetanus, pertussis	34.00			
90703	Tetanus toxoid	28.00			
90712	Poliovirus vaccine, oral	28.00			
Psychiatry					
90804	Ind psychotherapy 20–30 min	73.70	67.46	64.09	73.30
90805	with E/M service	82.88	75.86	72.07	82.88
90806	Ind psychotherapy 45–50 min	110.23	100.89	95.98	110.23
90853	Group therapy	29.22	26.75	25.41	29.22
Hemodialysis					
90935	Hemodialysis with physician eval	117.23	107.31	101.94	117.23
90937	Hemodialysis with repeat eval	206.24	188.78	179.34	206.24
Gastroenterology					
91010	Esophageal motility with interpretation & report	69.82	63.91	60.71	69.82
91030	Esophagus, acid perfusion test	87.41	80.01	16.01	87.41
Ophthalmologic Services					
92004	Comprehensive eye exam; NP	90.86	83.17	79.01	90.86
92100	Tonometry (serial)	47.31	43.31	41.14	47.31
92230	Fluorescein angioscopy	55.49	50.79	48.25	55.49
92275	Electroretinography	81.17	74.29	70.58	81.17
92531	Spontaneous nystagmus	26.00			
Audiologic Function Tests					
92557	Comprehensive audiometry	54.33	49.73	47.24	54.33
92596	Ear protector measurements	26.81	24.54	23.31	26.81
Cardiography					
93000	Electrocardiogram (ECG)	34.26	31.36	29.79	34.26
93015	Treadmill ECG	140.71	128.80	122.36	140.71
93040	Rhythm ECG; 1–3 leads	18.47	16.90	16.06	18.47
Pulmonary					
94010	Spirometry	38.57	35.31	33.54	38.57
94060	Spirometry before and after bronchodilator	71.67	65.60	62.32	71.67
94150	Vital capacity, total	13.82	12.65	12.02	13.82
Allergy and Clinical Immunology					
95024	Intradermal tests	6.58	6.02	5.72	6.58
95044	Patch tests	8.83	8.08	7.68	8.83

*Some services and procedures may not be considered a benefit under the Medicare program, and when listed on a claim form, no reimbursement may be received. However, it is important to include these codes when billing because Medicare policies may change without an individual knowing of a new benefit. For this reason, some of the services shown in this mock fee schedule do not have any amounts listed under the three Medicare columns.

FIGURE III-1 Fee schedule (*continued*)

CPT Code No. and Description		Mock Fees	Medicare*		
			Participating	Non-participating	Limiting Charge
95115	Treatment for allergy, single inj	17.20	15.75	14.96	17.20
95117	two or more inj	22.17	20.29	19.28	22.17
95165	Prof service for super of preparation and antigens for allergen immunotherapy, single or multiple antigens, multiple-dose vials	3.63	3.33	3.16	3.63
Neurology & Neuromuscular Procedures					
95812	Electroencephalogram, 41–60 min	129.32	118.37	112.45	129.32
95819	awake and asleep	126.81	116.07	110.27	126.81
95860	Electromyography, needle, 1 extremity	88.83	81.31	77.24	88.83
95864	4 extremities	239.99	219.67	208.69	239.99
96102	Psychological testing (per hour)	80.95	74.10	70.39	80.95
Therapeutic Prophylactic and Diagnostic Injections					
96372	Therapeutic, prophylactic, or diagnostic inj; IM or SC	4.77	4.37	4.15	4.77
96374	IV push	21.33	19.53	18.55	21.33
Physical Medicine					
97024	Diathermy modality	14.27	13.06	12.41	14.27
97036	Hubbard tank, each 15 min	24.77	22.67	21.54	24.77
97110	Physical therapy, one or more areas; 15 min	23.89	21.86	20.77	23.89
97140	Manual therapy, one or more areas; 15 min	16.93	15.49	14.72	16.93
Special Services and Reports					
99000	Handling of specimen (transfer from Dr.'s office to lab)	5.00			
99050	Services requested after office hours in addition to basic service	25.00			
99056	Services normally provided in office requested by pt in location other than office	20.00			
99058	Office services provided on an emergency basis	65.00			
99070	Supplies and materials over and above those usually required (itemize drugs/materials)	25.00			
99080	Special reports: Insurance forms	10.00			
	Review of data to clarify pt's status	20.00			
	WC reports	50.00			
	WC extensive review report	250.00			

*Some services and procedures may not be considered a benefit under the Medicare program, and when listed on a claim form, no reimbursement may be received. However, it is important to include these codes when billing because Medicare policies may change without an individual knowing of a new benefit. For this reason, some of the services shown in this mock fee schedule do not have any amounts listed under the three Medicare columns.

CPT MODIFIERS*

−22	Increased procedural services (attach report to claim)
−23	Unusual anesthesia (pt requires general anesthetic instead of none or local anesthesia)
−24	Unrelated evaluation and management service by the same physician during a postoperative period
−25	Significant, separate identifiable evaluation and management service by the same physician on the day of a procedure
−26	Professional component (physician interpretation only, not technical component)
−32	Mandated services (e.g., consult requested by a third party payor)
−47	Anesthesia by surgeon
−50	Bilateral procedure
−51	Multiple procedures performed on the same day or at the same session
−52	Reduced services
−53	Discontinued procedure
−54	Surgical care only
−55	Postoperative management only
−56	Preoperative management only
−57	Decision for surgery (use with E/M service performed just prior to surg)
−58	Staged or related procedure or service by the same physician during the postoperative period
−59	Distinct procedural service
−62	Two surgeons (usually with different skills)
−63	Procedure performed on infants less than 4 kg
−66	Surgical team
−76	Repeat procedure by the same physician
−77	Repeat procedure by another physician
−78	Unplanned return to the operating room for a related procedure during the postoperative period
−79	Unrelated procedure or service by the same physician during the postoperative period
−80	Assistant surgeon
−81	Minimum assistant surgeon
−82	Assistant surgeon (when qualified resident surgeon not available)
−90	Reference (outside) laboratory procedures performed by a lab other than the treating physician
−91	Repeat clinical diagnostic laboratory test
−99	Multiple modifiers (use of two or more modifiers for a service)

HCPCS Level II CODES**

These codes have been selected from many *HCPCS* codes as examples. The fees stated are only examples.

		FEES
A0422	Ambulance service, oxygen supplies, life sustaining situation	$600.00
A4206	Syringe with needle; 1 cc	10.00
A5051	Ostomy pouch; one piece with barrier attached	15.00
A6410	Eye pad, sterile	15.00
A9150	Nonprescription drugs	10.00
B4034	Enteral feeding supply kit; syringe fed, per day	25.00
E0100	Cane; any material, adjustable or fixed	60.00
E0114	Crutches; underarm, other than wood	100.00
G0008	Administration, influenza virus vaccine	10.00
H0001	Alcohol and/or drug assessment	75.00
J0120	Injection, tetracycline, up to 250 mg	25.00
J0171	Injection, adrenalin, 0.1 mg	25.00
J0558	Injection, penicillin G, 100,000 units	25.00
J1460	Injection, gamma globulin, intramuscular, 1 cc	20.00
L0180	Cervical, multiple post collar	50.00
L3209	Surgical boot, child	50.00
M0075	Cellular therapy	70.00
P3001	Papanicolaou smear screening (up to 3), interpretation by physician	25.00

*For a full description of *CPT* modifiers with examples, see *textbook* Table 17-4.
**2012 *HCPCS Level II* codes used.

PART IV

Abbreviation Tables

TABLE IV-1
Address Abbreviations

Alley	ALY	East	E	Park	PK	Street	ST
Annex	ANX	Estates	ESTS	Parkway	PKWY	Suite	STE
Apartment	APT	Expressway	EXPY	Place	PL	Summit	SMT
Arcade	ARC	Extension	EXT	Plaza	PLZ	Terrace	TER
Association	ASSN	Freeway	FWY	Point	PT	Track	TRAK
Avenue	AVE	Grove	GRV	Port	PRT	Trail	TRL
Bayou	BYU	Harbor	HBR	Prairie	PR	Tunnel	TUNL
Beach	BCH	Heights	HTS	President	PRES	Turnpike	TPKE
Bend	BND	Hill	HL	Ranch	RNCH	Union	UN
Bluff	BLF	Hospital	HOSP	Rapids	RPDS	Valley	VLY
Bottom	BTM	Institute	INST	Ridge	RDG	Viaduct	VIA
Boulevard	BLVD	Isle	ISLE	River	RIV	Vice President	VP
Branch	BR	Island	IS	Road	RD	View	VW
Bridge	BRG	Junction	JCT	Room	RM	Village	VLG
Brook	BRK	Lake	LK	Route	RT	Ville	VL
Burg	BG	Lakes	LKS	Row	ROW	Vista	VIS
Bypass	BYP	Lane	LN	Run	RUN	Walk	WALK
Camp	CP	Mall	MALL	Rural	R	Way	WAY
Canyon	CYN	Manager	MGR	Secretary	SECY	Wells	WLS
Cape	CPE	Manor	MNR	Shoal	SHL	West	W
Causeway	CSWY	Mount	MT	Shore	SH		
Center	CTR	Mountain	MTN	South	S		
Circle	CIR	North	N	Southeast	SE		
Cliffs	CLFS	Northeast	NE	Southwest	SW		
Club	CLB	Northwest	NW	Spring	SPG		
Court	CT	Orchard	ORCH	Square	SQ		
Drive	DR	Palms	PLMS	Station	STA		

TABLE IV-2
Appointment and Patient Care Abbreviations

Abbreviation	Meaning
A	allergy; abortion
AB	antibiotic
abd, abdom	abdominal, abdomen
abt	about
Acc, acc	accommodation
acid	accident
adm	admit; admission; admitted
adv	advice
aet.	at the age of
$AgNO_3$	silver nitrate
AIDS	acquired immune deficiency syndrome
alb	albumin
ALL	allergy
a.m., AM	before noon
AMA	American Medical Association
an ck	annual check
an PX	annual physical examination
ant	anterior
ante	before
A & P	auscultation and percussion
AP	anterior posterior; anteroposterior; antepartum care
AP & L	anteroposterior and lateral
approx	approximate
apt	apartment
ASA	acetylsalicylic acid (Aspirin)
asap, ASAP	as soon as possible
ASCVD	arteriosclerotic cardiovascular disease
ASHD	arteriosclerotic heart disease
asst	assistant
auto	automobile
Ba	barium
BI	biopsy
BM	bowel movement
BMR	basal metabolic rate
BP, B/P	blood pressure
BP ck, BP ✓	blood pressure check
breast ck	breast check
Brev	Brevital (drug)
BS	blood sugar
BUN	blood urea nitrogen
Bx, BX	biopsy
C	cervical; centigrade; Celsius
C & S	culture and sensitivity
Ca, CA	cancer, carcinoma
canc, cncl	cancel, canceled
cast ck	cast check
Cauc	Caucasian
CBC	complete blood count
CC	chief complaint
CDC	calculated date of confinement
chem.	chemistry
CHF	congestive heart failure
chr	chronic
ck, ✓	check
CI	color index
cm	centimeter
CNS	central nervous system
CO, C/O	complains of
CO_2, CO2	carbon dioxide
comp	comprehensive
compl	complete
Con, CON, Cons, consult	consultation
Cont.	continue
COPD	chronic obstructive pulmonary disease
CPE, CPX	complete physical examination
C section, C/S	cesarean section
CT	computerized tomography
CV	cardiovascular
CVA	costovertebral angle; cardiovascular accident; cerebrovascular accident
CXR	chest x-ray
Cysto, cysto	cystoscopy
D & C	dilatation and curettage
dc	discontinue
DC	discharge, dressing change
del	delivery
Dg, dg, Dx, dx	diagnosis
diag.	diagnosis, diagnostic
diam.	diameter
diff.	differential
dilat	dilate
disch.	discharged
DNA	does not apply
DNKA	did not keep appointment
DNS	did not show
DOB	date of birth
dr, drsg	dressing
DSHA	does she have appointment
DTaP*	diphtheria, tetanus, and pertussis (vaccine)
Dx, Dg, dx	diagnosis
E	emergency
ECG	electrocardiogram; electrocardiograph
ED	emergency department
EDC	estimated date of confinement; due date for baby
EEG	electroencephalogram; electroencephalograph
EENT	eye, ear, nose, and throat
EKG	electrocardiogram; electrocardiograph
EMG	electromyogram, electromyelogram
epith.	epithelial
ER	emergency room
ESR	erythrocyte sedimentation rate
est.	established; estimated

(continues)

TABLE IV-2
Appointment and Patient Care Abbreviations (*continued*)

Abbreviation	Meaning	Abbreviation	Meaning
etiol.	etiology	inj., INJ	injection
EU	etiology unknown	int, INT	internal
Ex, exam.	examination	intermed	intermediate
exc.	excision	interpret	interpretation
ext	external	IPPB	intermittent positive pressure breathing
F	Fahrenheit; French (catheter)	IQ	intelligence quotient
FH	family history	IUD	intrauterine device
FHS	fetal heart sounds	IV, I.V.	intravenous
flu syn	influenza syndrome	IVP	intravenous pyelogram
fluor	fluoroscopy	JVD	jugulovenous distention
ft	foot; feet	K35	Kollmann (dilator)
FU, F/U	follow-up (visit)	KUB	kidneys, ureters, bladder
FUO	fever of unknown/undetermined origin	L	left; laboratory; living children; liter
FX, Fx	fracture	lab, LAB	laboratory
G	gravida (number of pregnancies)	lac	laceration
g, gm	gram	L&A, l/a	light and accommodation
GA	gastric analysis	L&W	living and well
GB	gallbladder	lat, LAT	lateral
GC	gonorrhea	LBP	low back pain
GGE	generalized glandular enlargement	lb(s)	pound(s)
GI	gastrointestinal	LLL	left lower lobe
GTT	glucose tolerance test	LLQ	left lower quadrant
GU	genitourinary	LMP	last menstrual period
Gyn, GYN	gynecology	lt., LT	left
H	hospital call	ltd.	limited
HA	headache	LUQ	left upper quadrant
HBP	high blood pressure	M	medication; married
HC	house call; hospital call; hospital consultation	MA	mental age
HCD	house call, day	med., MED	medicine
HCl	hydrochloric acid	mg	milligram(s)
HCN	house call, night	MH	marital history
hct	hematocrit	ml	milliliter(s)
HCVD	hypertensive cardiovascular disease	mm	millimeter(s)
HEENT	head, eyes, ears, nose, and throat	MM	mucous membrane
Hgb, Hb	hemoglobin	MMR	measles, mumps, rubella (vaccine)
hist	history	mo	month(s)
H_2O, H2O	water	MRI	magnetic resonance imaging
hosp	hospital	N	negative
H&P	history and physical	NA, N/A	not applicable
HPI	history of present illness	NaCl	sodium chloride
hr, hrs	hour, hours	NAD	no appreciable disease
HS	hospital surgery	neg.	negative
Ht, ht	height	New OB	new obstetric patient
HV	hospital visit	NFA	no future appointment
HX	history	NP, N/P, (N)	new patient
HX PX	history and physical examination	NPN	nonprotein nitrogen
I	injection	N/S, NS	no-show
I&D	incision and drainage	NTRA	no telephone requests for antibiotics
IC	initial consultation	N&V	nausea and vomiting
i.e.	that is	NYD	not yet diagnosed
IM	intramuscular	O_2, O2	oxygen
imp., IMP	impression	OB	obstetrical patient, obstetrics; prenatal care
inc	include		
inf, INF	infection, infected	OC	office call
inflam., INFL	inflammation	occ	occasional
init	initial	ofc	office

(*continues*)

TABLE IV-2
Appointment and Patient Care Abbreviations (*continued*)

OH	occupational history	ret, retn	return
OP, op.	operation, operative, outpatient	rev	review
OPD	outpatient department	Rh-	Rhesus negative (blood)
OR	operating room	RHD	rheumatic heart disease
orig.	original	RLQ	right lower quadrant
OT	occupational therapy	RO, R/O	rule out
OTC	over the counter	ROS	review of systems
OV	office visit	rt., R	right
P	pulse; preterm parity or deliveries before term	RT	respiratory therapy
		RTC	return to clinic
PA	posterior anterior, posteroanterior	RTO	return to office
P&A	percussion and auscultation	RUQ	right upper quadrant
PAP, Pap	Papanicolaou (test/smear)	RV	return visit
Para I	woman having borne one child (Para II, two children, and so on)	Rx, RX, R	prescription; any medication or treatment ordered
PBI	protein-bound iodine	S	surgery
PC	present complaint; pregnancy confirmation	SD	state disability
		SE	special examination
PD	permanent disability	sed rate	sedimentation rate
PE	physical examination	sep.	separated
perf.	performed	SH	social history
PERRLA, PERLA	pupils equal, round, react to light and to accommodation	SIG, sigmoido	sigmoidoscopy
		SLR	straight leg raising
pH	hydrogen ion concentration	slt	slight
PH	past history	Smr, sm.	smear
Ph ex	physical examination	S, M, W, D	single, married, widowed, divorced
phys.	physical	SOB	shortness of breath
PI	present illness	sp gr	specific gravity
PID	pelvic inflammatory disease	SubQ*	subcutaneous
p.m., PM	after noon	SR	suture removal; sedimentation rate
PMH	past medical history	STAT, stat.	immediately
PND	postnasal drip	STD	sexually transmitted disease
PO	postoperative check, phone order	strab	strabismus
P Op, Post-op	postoperative check	surg.	surgery
pos.	positive	Sx.	symptoms
post.	posterior	T	temperature; term parity or deliveries at term
postop	postoperative		
PP	postpartum care	T&A	tonsillectomy and adenoidectomy
Pre-op, preop	preoperative (office visit)	Tb, tbc, TB	tuberculosis
prep	prepare, prepared	TD	temporary disability
PRN, p.r.n.	as necessary	temp.	temperature
procto	proctoscopic (rectal) examination	TIA	transient ischemic attack
prog	prognosis	TMs	tympanic membranes
P&S	permanent and stationary	TPR	temperature, pulse, respiration
PSP	phenolsulfonphthalein	Tr.	treatment
Pt, pt	patient	TTD	total temporary disability
PT	physical therapy	TURB	transurethral resection of bladder
PTR	patient to return	TURP	transurethral resection of prostate
PX	physical examination	TX, Tx	treatment
R	right; residence call; report	U	unit
RBC, rbc	red blood cell	UA, U/A	urinalysis
Re:, re:	regarding	UCHD	usual childhood diseases
rec	recommend	UCR	usual, customary, and reasonable
re ch	recheck	UGI	upper gastrointestinal
re-exam, reex	reexamination	UPJ	ureteropelvic junction or joint
REF, ref	referral	UR, ur	urine
reg.	regular	URI	upper respiratory infection

(*continues*)

TABLE IV-2
Appointment and Patient Care Abbreviations (*continued*)

UTI	urinary tract infection	wk	week; work
vac	vaccine	wks	weeks
VD	venereal disease	WM, W/M	white male
VDRL	Venereal Disease Research Laboratory (test for syphilis)	WNL	within normal limits
		WR	Wassermann reaction (syphilis test)
W	work; white	WT, Wt, wt	weight
WBC, wbc	white blood cell or count; well baby care	x, X	x-ray(s); multiplied by
WF	white female	XR	x-ray(s)
WI, W/I	walk-in, work-in	yr	year
Symbols			
*	birth	−, ō	negative
c̄, /c, w/	with	±	negative or positive; indefinite
p̄	after	Ⓛ	left
s̄, /s, w/o	without	ⓜ	murmur
c̄c, −c̄/c	with correction (eyeglasses)	Ⓡ	right
		♂	male
s̄c, s̄/c	without correction (eyeglasses)	♀	female
+	positive	μ	micron

*Abbreviation approved by the Joint Commission as the preferred abbreviation.

TABLE IV-3
Appointment Terms and Their Abbreviations

Medical Term	Abbreviation	Medical Term	Abbreviation
abdominal	abd, abdom	immediately	stat
accident	accid	infection	inf
annual check	an ck	influenza syndrome	flu syn
annual physical examination	an PX/PE	injection	inj, INJ
antepartum care	AP	intrauterine device	IUD
blood pressure check	BP	laboratory follow-up	Lab FU, Lab F/U
breast check	breast ck	laceration	lac
cancel, canceled	canc	low back pain	LBP
cast check	cast ck	measles, mumps, rubella vac.	MMR
check	ck	new patient	(N), N/P, NP
chest x-ray	CXR, PA chest, AP chest	new obstetric patient	New OB
complete blood count	CBC	no future appointment	NFA
complete physical examination	CPX, CPE	no-show	N/S, NS
consultation	consult, cons, con	obstetric patient	OB
cystoscopy	cysto	office visit	OV
diagnosis	Dx, dx, dg, diag.	Papanicolaou smear	Pap
did not keep appointment	DNKA	physical examination	PE, PX, Ph ex, phys
did not show	DNS	postoperative check	PO, Post-op
dressing	dr, drsg	postpartum care	PP
dressing change	DC	pregnancy confirmation	PC
electrocardiogram	EKG, ECG	prenatal care	OB
electromyogram, electromyelogram	EMG	preoperative office visit	Pre-op, preop
		proctoscopic examination	procto
emergency	E	referral	REF, ref
emergency room	ER	return to clinic	RTC
follow-up visit	FU	return to office	RTO
fracture	FX, Fx	return visit	RV, ret, retn
glucose tolerance test	GTT	sigmoidoscopy	SIG, sigmoido
gynecological check	Gyn ck, GYN	suture removal	SR
headache	HA	walk-in, work-in	WI, W/I
house call	HC	weight	WT

TABLE IV-4
Bookkeeping Abbreviations and Definitions

AC or acct	account	EC, ER	error corrected	pt	patient
A/C	account current	Ex MO	express money order	PVT CK	private check
adj	adjustment			recd, recv'd	received
A/P	accounts payable	FLW/UP	follow-up	ref	refund
A/R	accounts receivable	fwd	forward	req	request
B/B	bank balance	IB	itemized bill	ROA	received on account
Bal fwd, B/F	balance forward	I/f	in full	snt	sent
BD	bad debt	ins, INS	insurance	T	telephoned
BSY	busy	inv	invoice	TB	trial balance
c/a, CS	cash on account	J/A	joint account	UCR	usual, customary, and reasonable
cc	credit card	LTTR	letter		
ck	check	MO	money order	w/o	write off
COINS	coinsurance	mo	month	$	money/cash
Cr	credit	msg	message	—	charge already made
CXL	cancel	NC, N/C	no charge	0	no balance due (zero balance)
DB	debit	NF	no funds		
DED	deductible	NSF	not sufficient funds	✓	posted
def	charge deferred	PD	paid	<$56.78>	credit symbols
disc, discnt	discount	pmt	payment		

TABLE IV-5
Collection Abbreviations

B	bankrupt	N1, N2	note one, note two (sent)	S	she or wife
BLG	belligerent	NA	no answer	SEP	separated
EO	end of month	NF/A	no forwarding address	SK	skip or skipped
EOW	end of week	NI	not in	SOS	same old story
FN	final notice	NLE	no longer employed	STO	she telephoned office
H	he or husband	NR	no record	T	telephoned
HHCO	have husband call office	NSF	not sufficient funds (check)	TB	telephoned business
HTO	he telephoned office	NSN	no such number	TR	telephoned residence
L1, L2	letter one, letter two (sent)	OOT	out of town	U/Emp	unemployed
LB	line busy	OOW	out of work	UTC	unable to contact
LD	long distance	Ph/Dsc	phone disconnected	Vfd/E	verified employment
LMCO	left message, call office	POW	payment on way	Vfd/I	verified insurance
LMVM	left message voice mail	PP	promise to pay		

TABLE IV-6
Physician Specialist and Health Care Professional Abbreviations

Physician Specialist	Abbreviation	Health Care Professional	Abbreviation
Doctor of Chiropractic	DC	Certified Coding Specialist; certified by the American Health Information Management Association	CCS
Doctor of Dental Surgery	DDS	Certified First Assistant (surgical)	CFA
Doctor of Dental Science	DDSc	Certified Laboratory Assistant; certified by the Registry of American Society of Clinical Pathologists	CLA (ASCP)
Doctor of Emergency Medicine	DEM	Certified Medical Transcriptionist	CMT
Doctor of Hygiene	DHy	Certified Nurse Midwife	CNM
Doctor of Medical Dentistry	DMD	Certified Professional Coder; certified by AAPC (formerly the American Academy of Professional Coders)	CPC
Doctor of Medicine	MD	Certified Registered Nurse Anesthetist	CRNA
Doctor of Optometry	OD	Certified Surgical Technician (2nd surgical asst.)	CST
Doctor of Ophthalmology	OphD	Emergency Medical Technician	EMT
Doctor of Osteopathy	DO	Health Information Management	HIM
Doctor of Pharmacy	Pharm D	Inhalation Therapist	IT
Doctor of Podiatry	DPM	Laboratory Technician Assistant	LTA
Doctor of Public Health	DPH	Licensed Practical Nurse	LPN
Doctor of Tropical Medicine	DTM	Licensed Vocational Nurse	LVN
Doctor of Veterinary Medicine	DVM	Master of Public Health	MPH
Doctor of Veterinary Surgery	DVS	Medical Technologist	MT (ASCP)
Fellow of the American Academy of Pediatrics	FAAP	Physician's Assistant—Certified	PA–C
Fellow of the American College of Obstetricians and Gynecologists	FACOG	Public Health Nurse	PHN
Fellow of the American College of Surgery	FACS	Registered Dietitian	RD
Senior Fellow	SF	Registered Nurse	RN
		Registered Nurse First Assistant (surgical)	RNFA
		Registered Nurse Practitioner	RNP
		Registered Occupational Therapist	ROT
		Registered Physical Therapist	RPT
		Registered Respiratory Therapist	RRT
		Registered Technologist (Radiology)	RT (R)
		Registered Technologist (Therapy)	RT (T)
		Visiting Nurse	VN

TABLE IV-7
Prescription Abbreviations* and Symbols

Abbreviation	Meaning
$\bar{a}$	before
$\overline{aa}$	of each
a.c.	before meals
ad lib.	as much as needed
a.m. or AM	morning
ante	before
aq.	aqueous/water
b.i.d.	two times a day
caps	capsule
$\bar{c}$	with
$\overline{cc}$	with meals
comp. or comp	compound
d	day
DC or D/C	discontinue
dos.	doses
DS	double strength
DSD	double starting dose
elix.	elixir
emul.	emulsion
et	and
ext.	extract
garg.	gargle
gm or g	gram
gr	grain
gt.	drop
gtt.	drops
h.	hour
h.s.	before bedtime (hour of sleep)
ID	intradermal
IM	intramuscular
inj.	injection; to be injected
IV or I.V.	intravenous
kg	kilogram
liq	liquid
M or m.	mix
mcg	microgram
mg or mgm	milligram (used instead of "cc" for cubic centimeter)
ml	milliliter
N.E. or ne	negative
noct.	night
NPO or n.p.o.	nothing by mouth
O_2	oxygen
o.d.	once a day
o.h.	every hour
oint	ointment

Abbreviation	Meaning
o.m.	every morning
o.n.	every night
OTC	over-the-counter (drugs)
oz	ounce
$\bar{p}$	after
p.c.	after meals
p.o.	by mouth (per os)
p.r.	per rectum
p.r.n. or PRN	whenever necessary
q.	every
q.a.m.	every morning
q.h.	every hour
q.h.s.	every night
q.i.d.	four times a day (not at night)
q.n.	every night
q.p.m.	every night
q.2 h.	every two hours
q.3 h.	every three hours
q.4 h.	every four hours
rep, REP	let it be repeated; Latin *repeto*
Rx	take (recipe), prescription
$\bar{s}$	without
SC or subq	subcutaneous
sat.	saturated
Sig.	write on label; give directions on prescription
SL	sublingual
sol.	solution
SR	sustained release
ss	one-half
stat or STAT	immediately
syr.	syrup
tab.	tablet
t.i.d.	three times a day
top	topically
Tr. or tinct.	tincture
tsp	teaspoon
vag.	vagina
X or x	times (X10d/times ten days)
i, ii, iii, iv; viii, etc.	1, 2, 3, 4; 8, etc.
5", 10", 15"	5, 10, 15 minutes, etc.
5°, 10°, 15°, or 5', 10', 15', etc.	5 hours, 10 hours, 15 hours, etc.
ʒ or dr.	dram (drachm)
℥ or oz.	ounce

*Many of these abbreviations are derived from Latin; they are usually typed in lowercase and with periods. Periods are especially important if without periods an abbreviation would spell a word; for example, b.i.d. without periods is bid.

TABLE IV-8
Two-Letter Abbreviations for the United States and Territories and Canadian Provinces

United States and Territories					
Alabama	AL	Kansas	KS	No. Mariana Islands	MP
Alaska	AK	Kentucky	KY	Ohio	OH
American Samoa	AS	Louisiana	LA	Oklahoma	OK
Arizona	AZ	Maine	ME	Oregon	OR
Arkansas	AR	Marshall Islands	MH	Palau	PW
California	CA	Maryland	MD	Pennsylvania	PA
Colorado	CO	Massachusetts	MA	Puerto Rico	PR
Connecticut	CT	Michigan	MI	Rhode Island	RI
Delaware	DE	Minnesota	MN	South Carolina	SC
District of Columbia	DC	Mississippi	MS	South Dakota	SD
Federated States of Micronesia	FM	Missouri	MO	Tennessee	TN
		Montana	MT	Texas	TX
Florida	FL	Nebraska	NE	Utah	UT
Georgia	GA	Nevada	NV	Vermont	VT
Guam	GU	New Hampshire	NH	Virginia	VA
Hawaii	HI	New Jersey	NJ	Virgin Islands, U.S.	VI
Idaho	ID	New Mexico	NM	Washington	WA
Illinois	IL	New York	NY	West Virginia	WV
Indiana	IN	North Carolina	NC	Wisconsin	WI
Iowa	IA	North Dakota	ND	Wyoming	WY
Canadian Provinces					
Alberta	AB	Northwest Territories	NT	Quebec	QC
British Columbia	BC	Nova Scotia	NS	Saskatchewan	SK
Manitoba	MB	Nunavut	NU	Yukon Territory	YT
New Brunswick	NB	Ontario	ON		
Newfoundland and Labrador	NL	Prince Edward Island	PE		

PART V

Medical Office Simulation Software (MOSS) 2.0

ABOUT MEDICAL OFFICE SIMULATION SOFTWARE (MOSS) 2.0

Medical Office Simulation Software (MOSS) 2.0 is generic practice management software, realistic in its look and functionality, which helps users prepare to work with any commercial software used in medical offices today. With a friendly, highly graphical interface, MOSS allows users to learn the fundamentals of medical office software packages in an educational environment.

The MOSS Computer Competency activities in Chapters 5, 7, 11, 15, and 16 in this *Workbook* are designed to be used with MOSS (single-user version).

MOSS INFORMATION, TRAINING, AND SUPPORT

Our MOSS Information, Training, and Support site (www.cengage.com/community/moss) includes many helpful resources:

- Tutorials that instruct on the various functionalities of MOSS
- User documentation
- FAQs
- And more!

For technical support related to MOSS, please contact Cengage Technical Support, Monday through Friday, from 8:30 a.m. to 6:30 p.m. eastern standard time:

- Phone: 1-800-648-7450
- Web: www.cengage.com/support

INSTALLATION AND SETUP INSTRUCTIONS

Following are installation instructions used to install the MOSS 2.0 program:

1. Close all open programs and documents.
2. Place the Medical Office Simulation Software 2.0 CD into your CD-ROM drive.
3. Medical Office Simulation Software 2.0 should begin setup automatically. Follow the on-screen prompts to install MOSS and Microsoft Access Runtime:
   - Click *Next*.
   - Click *I Accept* the terms of the license agreement.
   - Click *Next*.
   - Click the button next to *TYPICAL* as the setup type.
   - Click *Install*.
4. If MOSS does not begin setup automatically, follow these instructions:
   - Double-click on *My Computer*.
   - Double-click the *Control Panel* icon.
   - Double-click *Add/Remove Programs*.
   - Click the *Install* button, and follow the prompts as indicated in step 3.
5. When you finish installing MOSS, it will be accessible through the *Start* menu: **Start > Programs > MOSS v2.0**

GETTING STARTED WITH MOSS 2.0

Logon Instructions

1. When MOSS is launched, it brings up a logon window.
2. The default user name and password are already loaded for you. (The default user name and password is "Student1".)
3. Click *OK*. (See Figure V-1.)

FIGURE V-1 Logging in to MOSS.

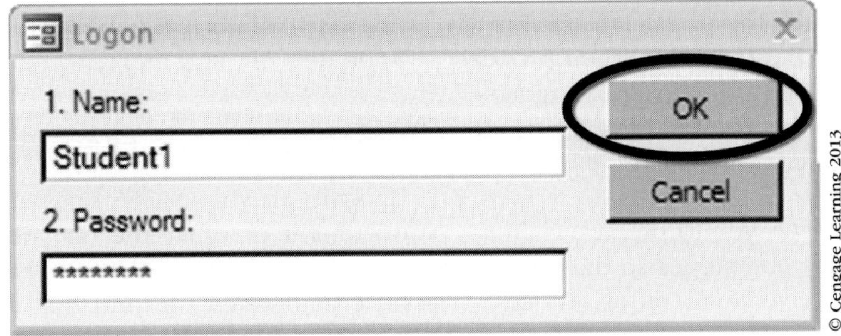

4. You are now at the *Main Menu* screen of MOSS.

Navigating within the Program

The *Main Menu* screen (Figure V-2) orients you to the general functions of most practice management software programs and includes buttons that provide access to specific areas. Clicking on a specific button will allow you to work in that area of the program. Alternatively, there is an icon bar along the top left to quickly access the areas of the software, or the user may choose to navigate the software by using the pull-down menus below the software title bar.

FIGURE V-2 The *Main Menu* screen.

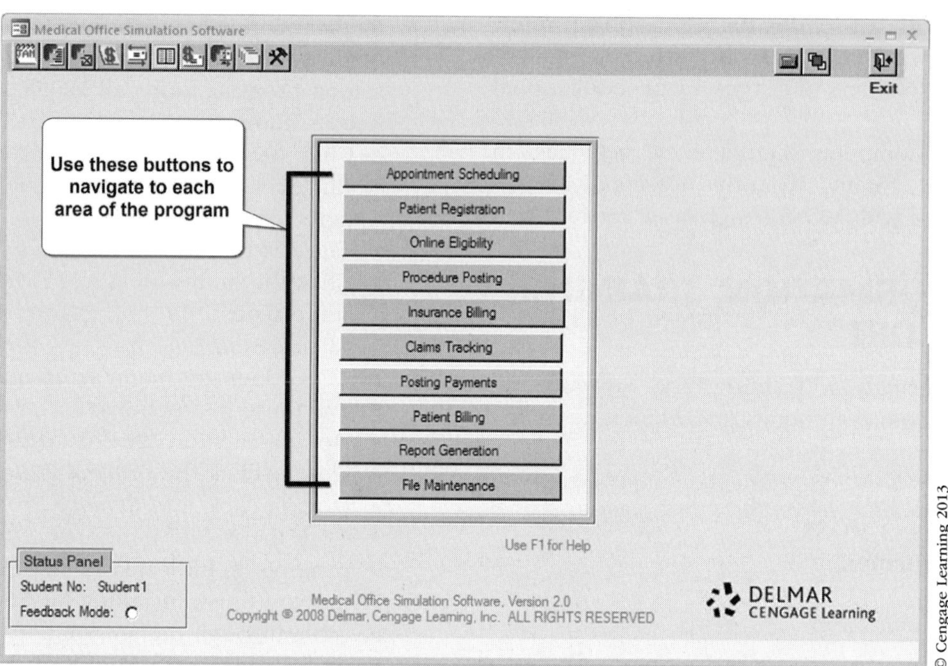

- **Patient Registration** allows you to input information about each patient in the medical practice, including demographic, HIPAA, and insurance information. From the *Main Menu* screen, click on the *Patient Registration* button to search for a patient, or to add a new patient, using the command buttons along the bottom of the patient selection dialog box.
- **Appointment Scheduling** allows you to make appointments and also cancel, reschedule, and search for appointments. MOSS allows for block scheduling, as well as several print features including appointment cards and daily schedules.
- **Procedure Posting** allows you to select services and procedures the physician has performed and apply patient fees. When procedures are input into the procedure posting system, the software assigns the fee to be charged according to the fee schedule for the patient's insurance type.
- **Insurance Billing** allows you to prepare claims to be sent to insurance companies so that the medical office can receive payment for services provided. You can generate and print a paper claim or simulate sending the claim electronically.
- **Claims Tracking** simulates receiving an electronic explanation of benefits (EOB) or remittance advice (RA) from an insurance carrier.
- **Posting Payments** allows you to input payments received by the practice from patients or insurance companies, as well as enter adjustments to the account.
- **Patient Billing** allows you to generate a billing statement to be sent directly to the patient to collect any outstanding balances.
- **File Maintenance** is a utility area of the program that contains common information used by various systems within the software. In this area, you can create and restore backup files, change your password, turn *Feedback Mode* and *Balloon Help* on and off, and more.

Creating Backup Files

Backing up your MOSS database is just like saving a document or other file on your computer. Creating a backup file allows you to save all the work you have completed up until that point. You may create a backup file of the work you have completed in the program at any time.

Backup files are very useful; for example, if you realize you have made a mistake and cannot correct it, you could restore a previous backup file and start the exercise over again. (Directions for restoring backup files are in the next section.)

We recommend creating a backup file after each chapter requiring MOSS.

Follow these steps to create a backup file:

1. Click on *File Maintenance*, and then click the button next to **2. Backup Database.**
2. Click *Yes* at the prompt.
3. Now, select a location to save your backup file. We recommend that you save the database on a flash drive (in most computers, this is your E:/ or F:/ computer drive). When saving your file, you may also choose to rename the file. You may rename the file anything you choose; **however, you must keep the file extension (.mde) in the file name. (See Figure V-3.)**

FIGURE V-3 Naming your backup file—keep the file extension (.mde) in the file name.

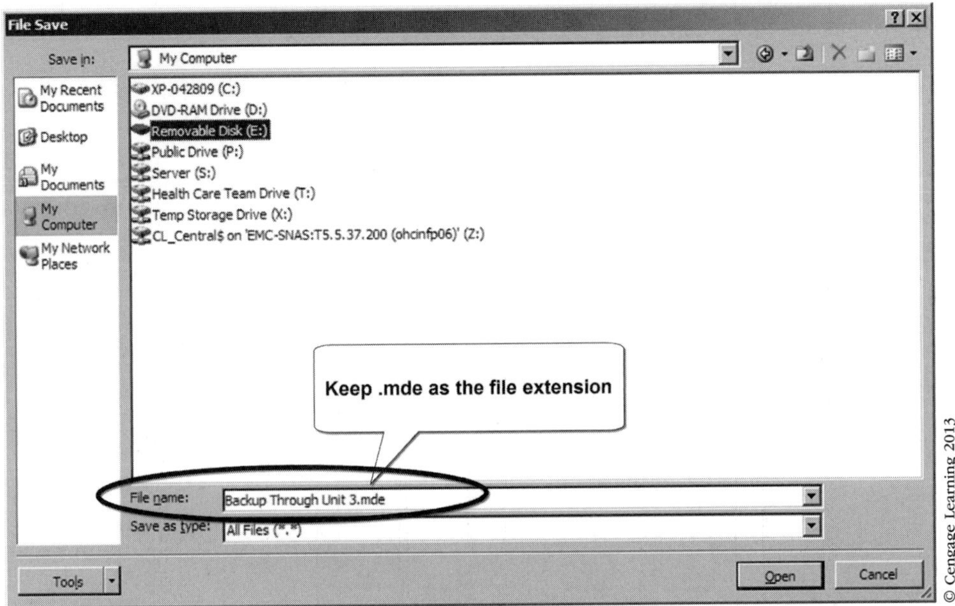

4. Click *Save* when you are finished. You will receive a prompt telling you that your file was completed successfully. Click *OK.*

Restoring Backup Files

The restore function allows you to return to a previous point in the program. For instance, if you realize you have made a mistake and cannot correct it, you could restore a previous backup file and start the exercise over again. You may restore a backup file of previous work you have saved in the program at any time. Please note that restoring a backup file is permanent; all entries you have entered after creating that backup file will no longer appear in the program.

Follow these steps to restore a backup file:

1. Click on *File Maintenance*, and then click the button next to **3. Restore Database**. Note that restoring a backup file is an irreversible process.
2. Click *Yes* at the prompt.
3. Click *Restore MOSS from Database* at the next prompt.
4. Click *Yes* at the following prompt. (Remember that restoring a backup file is an irreversible process.)
5. Find the backup file that you have created, click once to highlight it, and then click *OK.*
6. Click *Yes* at the following prompt.
7. Click the button *Return to MOSS.*
8. You have successfully restored your backup database. You will need to log in to the new database to start working.